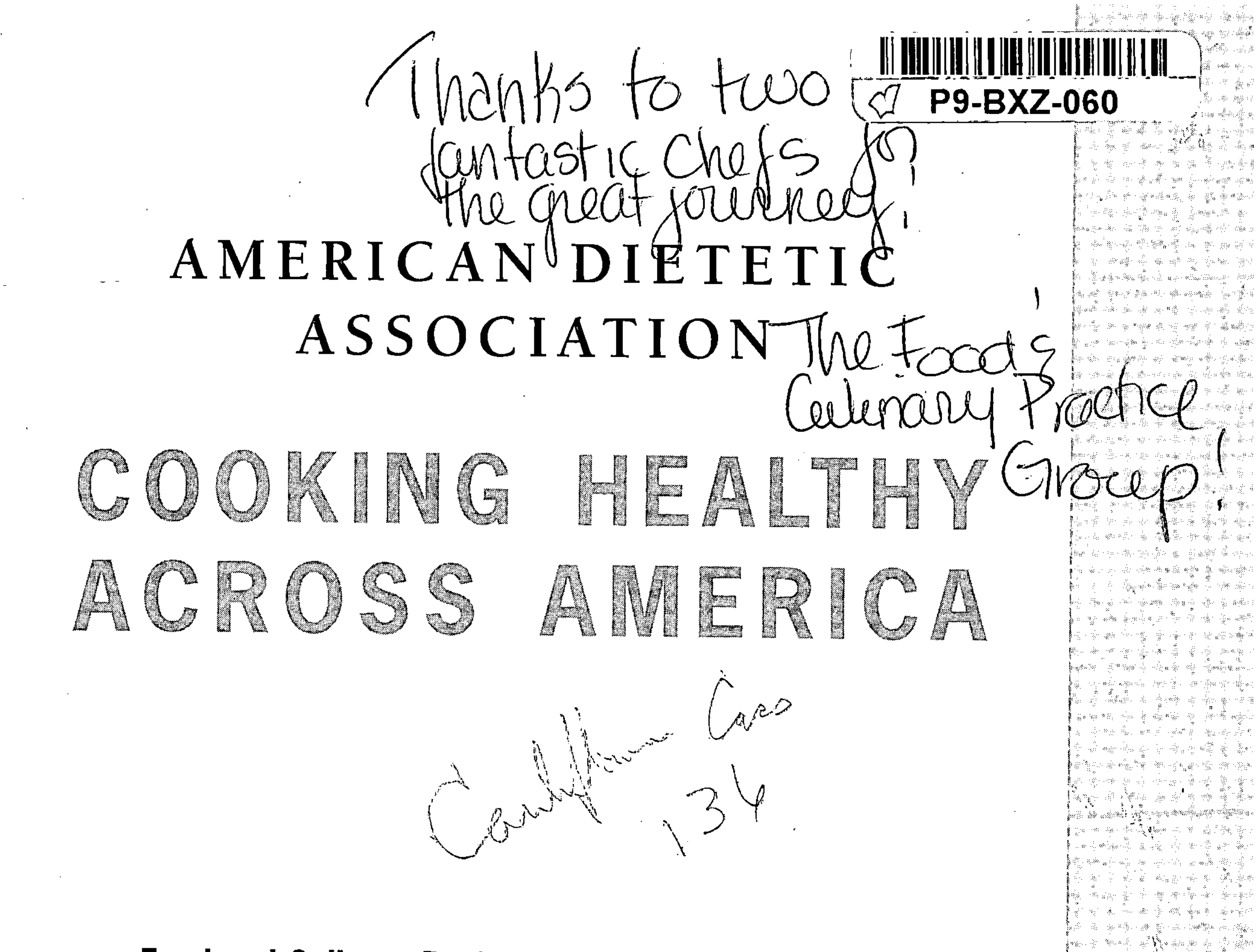

AMERICAN DIETETIC ASSOCIATION

COOKING HEALTHY ACROSS AMERICA

Food and Culinary Professionals, a Dietetic Practice Group of American Dietetic Association

Kristine Napier, M.P.H., R.D., editor

John Wiley & Sons, Inc.

This book is printed on acid-free paper. ♾

Published by John Wiley & Sons, Inc., Hoboken, New Jersey
Published simultaneously in Canada

Design and production by Navta Associates, Inc.

For general information about our other products and services, please contact our Customer Care Department within the United States at (800) 762-2974, outside the United States at (317) 572-3993 or fax (317) 572-4002.

Wiley also publishes its books in a variety of electronic formats. Some content that appears in print may not be available in electronic books. For more information about Wiley products, visit our web site at www.wiley.com.

Library of Congress Cataloging-in-Publication Data:

American Dietetic Association cooking healthy across America / American Dietetic Association, Food and Culinary Professionals ; Kristine Napier, editor.
p. cm.
Includes bibliographical references and index.
ISBN 0-471-68682-4 (cloth : alk. paper)
ISBN 0-47147430-4 (pbk.: alk. paper)
1. Cookery, American. 2. Nutrition. I. Napier, Kristine M. II. American Dietetic Association. Food and Culinary Professionals.
TX715.A51265 2004
641.5973—dc22
2004014934

Printed in the United States of America

10 9 8 7 6 5 4 3 2

Contents

Contents

Preface

Savor the flavors! The *American Dietetic Association Cooking Healthy across America* cookbook takes you on a culinary journey across our nation, from the kitchens of more than 1,500 culinary-focused registered dietitians. Created with a blend of food and nutrition expertise, this cookbook from the Food & Culinary Professionals (FCP) Dietetic Practice Group of the American Dietetic Association (ADA) brings together healthful eating and great taste as it celebrates American regional cuisine.

From our kitchens to yours, we've shared what FCP members do well: helping you prepare healthful food that's gourmet-delicious, too, with recipes that are easy to prepare for your busy lifestyle. You'll find stories from our own kitchens, our favorite family and regional recipes, our culinary secrets, and our healthy food prep tips and insights. We invite you and your family and friends to take a flavor adventure with us, enjoy regional and healthful food from the region where you live, and try new foods and recipes from the bounty of a far-off corner of our vast country.

The Food & Culinary Professionals bring culinary perspectives to the American Dietetic Association, the largest organization of food and nutrition professionals in the world. Within the ADA, the FCP dietetic practice group is committed to developing food expertise within the field of dietetics. By bringing food and nutrition together, our goal for the public is to help consumers make food choices that improve the quality both of their lives and their health.

In creating this remarkable cookbook, the Food & Culinary Professionals recognize and celebrate the capable editorship of FCP member Kristine

Napier, M.S., R.D., who gave graciously, generously, and expertly in support of member culinary talents and efforts and their nutrition expertise. We're grateful for the ADA publications staff for supporting FCP's commitment to reaching consumers with this health-focused cookbook, and to our ADA editors: Laura Brown, Kristen Short, and Diana Faulhaber. We are also pleased with John Wiley & Sons' enthusiasm for our book under the editorship of Tom Miller. Most important, we recognize the hundreds of FCP members who volunteered countless hours, wonderful recipes, and expert culinary and nutrition insights to make *American Dietetic Association Healthy Cooking across America* a unique cookbook for American consumers.

We invite you to set the table for good nutrition—and to join us in savoring the pleasures of the American table.

Roberta L. Duyff, M.S., R.D., F.A.D.A., C.F.C.S.
FCP Past Chair
Cookbook Chair

Edith Hogan, M.S., R.D.
FCP Chair

Acknowledgments

The Food and Culinary Professional Dietetic Practice Group of the American Dietetic Association acknowledges its many members and friends who gave their flavorful recipes and culinary nutrition contributions along with their time and resources in the visioning, recipe testing, recipe analysis, and review of *American Dietetic Association Cooking Healthy across America.* With their commitment we celebrate the pleasures of the table as we enjoy the bounty of healthful, regional cuisine.

Many thanks to the board members of the Food and Culinary Professionals Dietetic Practice Group who have given their leadership insights and expertise to *American Dietetic Association Cooking Healthy across America.*

Maria C. Alamo, M.P.H., R.D., L.D.
Esther Allen-White, M.S., R.D., L.D.
Barbara J. Alvarez, M.P.H., R.D., L.D.N.
Aarti Arora, M.P.H., R.D.
Linda Arpino, C.D.N., M.A., R.D.
Elizabeth Arvidson, R.D.
Bonnie Athas, R.D.
Pamela Aughe, R.D.
Judy Barbe, M.S., R.D.
Nancy Becker, M.S., R.D., L.D.
Paula Benedict, M.P.H., R.D.
Janice Newell Bissex, M.S., R.D.
Christina Blais, D.Pt., M.Sc.
Vivian Bradford, R.D.
Susan Braverman, M.S., R.D., C.D.N., F.A.D.A.
Elsa Ramirez Brisson, M.P.H., R.D.
Kitty Broihier, M.S., R.D.
Maureen Callahan, M.S., R.D.
Kathleen Carozza, M.A., R.D.
Monica L. Ceille, R.D., C.D.
Dorothy Chen-Maynard, Ph.D., R.D.
Marie Chrabaszewski, R.D.
Tami J. Cline, M.S., R.D., F.A.D.A., S.F.N.S.
Anita Crook, R.D., C.D.
Suzanne Render Curtis, Ph.D., R.D.
Mary Jo Cutler, M.S., R.D., L.D.
Sanna James Delmonico, M.S., R.D.
Rebecca Dowling, R.D.
Suzanne T. Duggan, R.D.
Roberta Larson Duyff, M.S., R.D., F.A.D.A., C.F.C.S.
Peggy Eastmond, R.D.
Beth Ebmeier, M.S., R.D., L.M.N.T.
Golda Ewalt, R.D., L.D.
Linda Ferber, M.S., R.D.

Madhu Gadia, M.S., R.D., C.D.E.
Ingrid Gangestad, R.D., L.D.
Maureen Garner, M.S., R.D., L.D.
Barbara Gollman, R.D.
Rita Storey Grandgenett, M.S., R.D.
Maggie Green, R.D., L.D., C.C.
Stephanie Green, R.D.
Stacy Haumea, R.D.
Jane M. Hemminger, R.D., L.D.
Alice Henneman, M.S., R.D.
Ann A. Hertzler, Ph.D., R.D., L.D.N.
Mary Abbott Hess, L.H.D., M.S., R.D., F.A.D.A.
Annette Hinton, C.E.C., R.D., L.D.
Ellen Hird, M.B.A., R.D.
Catherine Hoffmann, M.S., R.D.
Linda R. Hofmeister, M.M., R.D., L.D., F.A.D.A., C.H.E.
Edee Howard Hogan, R.D., L.D.
Jeannie Houchins, R.D.
Marsha Hudnall, M.S., R.D., C.D.
Karen Jacobsen, R.D.
Candace S. Johnson, R.D.
Lynnette Jones, M.S., M.B.A., R.D.
Regan Miller Jones, R.D., L.D.
Marilyn Baker Jouini, M.S., R.D., A.R.M.
Naomi Kakiuchi, R.D., C.D.
Sandy Kapoor, Ph.D., R.D., F.A.D.A.
Beverlee Kell, R.D.
Angela M. Kirke, R.D., L.D.
Pamela Kittler, M.S.
Susan C. Kosma, M.S., R.D., L.D.N.
Frances Largeman, R.D.
Judy Lee-Norris, M.P.H., R.D.
LaDonna Levik, R.D.
Julie Ann Lickteig, M.S., R.D., F.A.D.A.
Marjorie K. Livingston, M.S., R.D.
Carolyn K. Manning, M.A., R.D.
Caroline Margolis, R.D.
Martha Marino, M.A., R.D., C.D.
Linda Marmer, M.S., R.D., L.D.
Lori Martinez-Hassett, R.D.
Jim McGowan, R.D.
Carol Mergen, M.S., R.D.
Joanne B. Milkereit, M.H.S.A., R.D., C.D.E.
Lori A. Miller, R.D., L.D.
Libby Mills, M.S., R.D., L.D.
Angela M. Miraglio, M.S., R.D., F.A.D.A.
Laura L. Molseed, M.S., R.D., L.D.N.
Mary Etta Moorachian, Ph.D., R.D., C.C.P., C.F.C.S.
Cindy Moore, M.S., R.D., L.D., F.A.D.A.
Linda W. Moore, R.D., L.D.N.
Marlene M. Most, Ph.D., R.D., L.D.N., F.A.D.A.
Kristine Napier, M.P.H., R.D.
Jackie Newgent, R.D., C.D.N.
Alma Nocchi, R.D.
Jill Nussinow, M.S., R.D.
Melissa Stevens Ohlson, M.S., R.D., L.D.
Susan Kell Peletta, R.D.
Lisa C. Peterson, M.S., R.D., C.D.N.
Margaret Pfeiffer, M.S., R.D., C.D.
Michelle Plummer, M.S., R.D., C.D.
Lisa Poggas, M.S., R.D.
Catherine Powers, M.S., R.D.
Barbara J. Pyper, M.S., R.D., C.D., F.H.C.F.A., F.C.S.I.
Ruth Rauscher, R.D., M.A., L.M.N.T.
Alita E. Rethmeyer, Ed.D., R.D.
Dona Richwine, M.S., R.D.
Corrina Riemann, R.D.
Dr. Anne Rogan, R.D., C.D.N.
Deanna Rose, R.D., L.D.N.
Barrie Rosencrans, M.S., R.D., L.D.
Marie Fasano Ruggles, M.S., R.D.
Raeanne Sarazen, R.D.
Marjorie Sawicki, M.S., R.D., L.D.
Martine Scannavino, M.S., R.D., L.D.N.
Kathleen Schader, M.B.A., M.S., R.D., L.D.
Janice D. Schultz, M.S., R.D.
Geraldine C. Seinberg, B.S., R.D.
Lana Shepek, R.D., L.D.
Linda Simon, R.D.
Rebecca Sparks, R.D.
Ruth Stemler, M.S., R.D., L.D.
Julienne T. Stewart, M.S., R.D., L.D.N.
Hanna Strowman, M.M., R.D., L.D.N.
Lauren Swann, M.S., R.D., L.D.N.
Taiga Sudakin, R.D., L.D.
Mona R. Sutnick, Ed.D., R.D.
Patricia L. Bucci Szeliga, R.D., C.D.N., C.D.E.
Jessica Terry, R.D.
Laura Faler Thomas, M.Ed., R.D., L.D.
Robin Thomas, M.S., R.D., L.N.
Josephine Totten, R.D.
Lisa Turner, R.D.
Alamelu Vairavan, friend of the FCP
Brenda Bracewell Valera, R.D.
Maria Vargas, M.S., R.D.
Donna L. Weihofen, R.D., M.S.
Liz Weiss, M.S., R.D.
Diane A. Welland, M.S., R.D.
Diane Werner, R.D.
Page Westover, R.D.
Diane Wiggins, friend of the FCP
Paula Williams, R.D., C.E.C.
Deb Winders, M.S., R.D.
Beth P. Witherspoon, M.P.H., R.D.
Marion S. Wollmeringer, M.S., R.D., L.D.N.

Introduction

Kristine Napier, M.P.H., R.D.

Part of the fun of traveling to another city or state is tasting the food from that neck of the woods. A trip to Baltimore is hardly complete without sampling a crabcake. In Chicago, it's deep-dish pizza; in Philadelphia, cheesesteak; and in Memphis, slow-cooked barbecue. Indeed, the United States is a land of delectable eating, with differences often deliciously coming together on one block in our nation's big cities. Cultural diversity simmers with culinary traditions, creating an explosion of flavors still waiting to be discovered.

No wonder it's just not possible to wrap the definition of American cuisine into a neat package. Its culinary parts aren't even containable in a tower of kitchen bundles. The horn of plenty provides a great visual for the diversity in American cuisine, but there's culinary multiplicity at many levels: the ingredients, the spices, and the cooking methods.

Although American food is quite diverse, you'll find recurrent themes from the Atlantic to the Pacific and everywhere in between. Long before Europeans set foot on American soil, Native American people had learned to use the bounty of the land. They taught the settlers to plant the three sisters of Native American cuisine: corn, beans, and squash.

The ancient Native American practice of planting corn, beans, and squash together was passed down from their Latin American ancestors. Today's agricultural experts say it was a stroke of agricultural genius. It is a nutritionally sound strategy because of the complementing nutrients in these foods. Around rows of corn, tribes planted pole beans and squash. The bean sister, they knew from ancient rituals, would twine about and use the corn maiden for support. The squash sister would send vines along the rows between the corn plants, choking out weeds, shading the earth, and holding in moisture.

This "companion planting," say agricultural experts, has even more complex advantages. Bean roots have bacterial colonies on them that capture nitrogen gas from the air. In turn, they release nitrogen into the soil. While all plants need nitrogen, corn is an especially nitrogen-needy plant. Indian legends abound about the three sisters who should always be planted, eaten, and celebrated together.

While tribes throughout Central, South, and North America planted the three sisters, both beans and squash, and, of course, corn, are thought to have tropical beginnings. Many tribes call the combined three foods sustainers of life, and they continue to play a vital role in defining American cuisine. While they were cooked, baked, simmered, or stewed in distinctly differently ways in each corner of the country, the triad retains its starring role in recipes across the continent. Southerners frequently cook up plenty of grits, cornbread, and hoppin' John. New Englanders bake plenty of baked beans and succotash. Tortillas and pinto beans are a natural pair in the Southwest. Pumpkin pie, of course, is an American favorite on Thanksgiving and all year.

Food across the nation reflects our cultural and ethnic diversity. For centuries, the demand for practicality has played a significant role in the foods that have been served over campfires and on American tables. It's the story of family traditions intertwined with wealth or poverty, land, religion, and economics.

The food of our nation over time is also the story of life itself. It is an intricately woven tale of learning new food customs from the native people, and also of importing familiar foodways from homelands far away. Overall, it is the steps of discovering how to sustain life in times of feast and famine.

As nutrition professionals, we are fascinated by the lessons we've learned from the people and their foods that have touched this great land. Some of the foodways point to nutrition strategies that can sustain us in good health, such as the three sisters.

The Chinese, for example, teach us to extract from every ingredient multiple layers of pleasurable qualities. Their plate is an exquisite palette of colors and textures; indeed, one already feels satisfied by simply looking at the food. Chinese cuisine, ubiquitous on restaurant row from the South to the Northwest, boasts two other nutrition secrets: using many different types of vegetables is an excellent way to reap a wider variety of nutrients. Today, we encourage everyone to focus on choosing a rainbow array of fruits and vegetables to have a better chance of getting all the essential nutrients. The cultural choice of eating with chopsticks has another nutrition secret: eating slowly is a simple yet important way to eat appropriate amounts of food. Even if you don't use chopsticks, try eating more slowly so that you can taste every delicious bite you eat and so that you give your body a chance to realize you have eaten.

Tribes native to the Caribbean barbecued food in ground pits because it was their only option for cooking. Grilling food is an excellent way to reduce dietary fat and calories.

African food culture is not only soul-satisfying, but also rich in nutrition quality. Using little bits of many different ingredients out of necessity, their diets were more nutritionally sound than the plantation owners who ate significant quantities of just a few foods.

Celebrate your heritage and explore American regionalism with our recipes. Enjoy excellent versions of foods that have become all-American, as well as foods that fuse together regions, cultures, and ethnicities. Some are old-fashioned; all have contemporary appeal.

In this book we take you on a journey through culinary time and place, starting with the New England colonies. Savor the delicious details of food history and regional foodways. The stories are sure to make you hungry to try new recipes. In each regional chapter, you'll find recipes for all meal occasions—including dessert. Indeed, we believe that food is a celebration of life. Enjoying delicious food every single day is key to feeding the human body. More than nutrients, we need variety and exquisite taste—we need to tickle every taste bud every day. Doing so is one key strategy to enjoying appropriate portions, which is quintessential to achieving and maintaining a healthy body weight.

We've included our best cooking secrets with each recipe to help you try new recipes and to diversify your own diet. In the back of the book, you'll find everything you need to know about buying, storing, and cooking meat. Ever wonder how to choose a ripe mango or pineapple? Do you need help in storing vegetables for longer keeping? You'll find such details in the last chapters.

PART 1

Cooking Healthy Every Day

1

NEW ENGLAND

Simple, Sturdy Foods

Kitty Broihier, M.S., R.D., and Kristine Napier, M.P.H., R.D.

The simple, sturdy foods of New England reflect both the English origins of our country and the harsh conditions faced by the early colonists. They also speak of tradition, of comfort food, and of one-pot meals. Many traditional recipes that remain Northeastern favorites (indeed, national ones) give us a peek back in time to the days when food was used essentially for simple sustenance. Other enduring recipes attributed to New England cooking originated with northeastern Native American tribes.

Before the Pilgrims

The Wampanoag Nation enjoyed an abundance of food from northeastern forests, fields, streams, and the generous Atlantic Ocean. Indigenous foods included blueberries, cranberries, currants, grapes, persimmons, and strawberries. The three sisters—corn, beans, and squash—had traveled to northeastern lands, and were important ingredients for their sustenance. Game, including the wild turkey, was abundant. The cold, long winters yielded maple syrup, an ingredient which was not available in many other parts of the country. "Forest sugar," as the Indians called it, was the only flavoring they added to foods. They added it to everything from popcorn to meat and boiled fish.

According to lore, maple syrup was discovered when a Native American woman was cooking a pot of moose stew. Too busy to go to the nearby stream for water to add to the stew, she filled her pail with "water" dripping from a nearby tree. When she tasted the finished stew, she found that the meat was in a deliciously sweet and thick syrup instead of gravy. They called the maple trees *sheesheegummawis*, which means "sap flows fast."

Traditional New England Food with Native American Beginnings

The clambake is thought to originate with the Narragansett and Penobscot tribes, who steamed their clams in beach pits lined with hot rocks and seaweed. After layering clams, crabs, lobster, and corn with seaweed, they covered the pit and allowed the foods to steam for hours.

Succotash, probably the first one-pot meal, was the Narraganset word for "fragments." Native Americans taught colonists up and down the eastern seaboard how to make it by cooking corn and beans together to make an easy, filling meal. In the New England colonies, it was sweetened with maple syrup; in the southern colonies, bear fat flavored the succotash. Sunflower seeds, pine nuts, or other available nuts were used to round out the dish.

Even Boston baked beans probably originated with northeastern Native American tribes who simmered dried beans with maple syrup for days. Today's recipes for baked beans are associated with the city of Boston (still called Bean Town), where colonial Puritan women baked beans on Saturday to avoid cooking on the Sabbath. They served the beans for Saturday dinner and as leftovers for Sunday breakfast and lunch. Boston brown bread, too, was a recipe adapted from local Native Americans, who prepared corn bread by steaming. With time, the colonists made brown bread with a mixture of flours.

New England Colonists Arrive

The Pilgrims had a very lean beginning in America after arriving off Cape Cod in 1620. The growing season was short and the soil peppered with rocks. They were not hunters or fishers.

The Pilgrims and Thanksgiving

By the fall of 1621, their first crops were ready for harvest. At harvest time, the Plymouth colonists invited guests from the Wampanoag Nation for a fall harvest celebration. Their feast (often called the first Thanksgiving) lasted three days. The menu included many foods we know today, including turkey, squash, and corn. It also included codfish and bass, fish that were plentiful in the nearby Atlantic.

According to Plimouth Plantation historians, the first true Thanksgiving didn't come until two years later. The 1621 autumn harvest celebration was not a religious thanksgiving day in the eyes of the Pilgrims. Rather, it was a secular celebration that included games, which would have been unthinkable as part of a religious Thanksgiving. The actual first declared Thanksgiving occurred in 1623, after a providential rain shower saved the colony's crops.

The first cookbook in America, published in 1796, was filled with recipes for foods native to this land. It also included many recipes dating to colonial Thanksgiving, including pumpkin pie and stuffed turkey. The turkey stuffing recipe hasn't changed much from this more than 200-year-old recipe, which called for bread, butter, salt pork, eggs, sweet marjoram, summer savory, parsley, sage, and salt (Mom's Stuffing, page 31).

CHEWING GUM AND THE PILGRIMS

Chewing gum probably started with northeastern Native Americans, who chewed resin from black spruce trees to ease hunger pangs. Pilgrims learned this hunger-easing technique from their neighbors. The first commercial chewing gum manufacturing plant, built in Maine in about 1850, followed the Indian practice and flavored the gum with spruce resin.

TURKEY TRIVIA

Turkeys are native to the Americas. The origin of the turkey's name, though, is uncertain. Some believe the name comes from one way the turkey "speaks"—its soft "turk, turk, turk." Others think the colonists confused the bird with one they had seen in Europe, the guinea cock, which was imported into Europe from Africa through Turkey. Indeed, the English colonists called it the "turkie-bird." Still others maintain that the head of the bird resembles a Turkish fez.

Benjamin Franklin wanted the turkey to be the national symbol of the United States. When the bald eagle was chosen instead, he said: "I wish the Bald Eagle had not been chosen as the representative of our country: he is a Bird of bad moral character: like those among Men who live by Sharping and Robbing, he is generally poor and very often lousy. The Turkey is a much more respectable Bird, and withal a true original native of North America."

The Colonists Develop "American" Food Ways

During their first century in America, the colonists kept many of their British food ways. Their breakfast mush, or pudding, was characteristic of their morning meals back in England. Wheat did not grow well, though, so they were forced to bake with corn instead. During their first, lean days in America, the colonists made Hasty Pudding—originally made in Britain with flour and other ingredients—using just water and cornmeal. They whisked together the meager, plain ingredients with a birch twig whisk. Often, the raw pudding was wrapped in a loose, floured sack and boiled for several hours. So why were these puddings called hasty if they took so long to cook? Other puddings of the day took up to ten hours to cook. As the pudding steamed in the water, it swelled and filled the sack. Sometimes, puddings were also served with other meals, or as the entire meal when food was sparse. When available, meat became the dominating food in meals, despite the ready availability of fruits and edible greens.

When the New England colonists learned from the Native Americans how to tap maple trees for syrup, they added it to their Hasty Pudding. In later years, when food became more abundant, they added milk, molasses, and eggs.

Breakfast also became more diverse. The colonists started adding cold meat, bread, milk, and fruit pies. Apple pies were their favorite. In winter, they made stacks of pies and froze them in sheds. Each morning, they warmed a frozen pie by the fireplace for breakfast.

Apples were not native to America; the Pilgrims brought the seeds with them. Apple pie, in fact, is a British invention (All-American Apple Pie, page 54). Soon, though, it became a universal American favorite. The poor of New England called it "house pie."

From their Native American neighbors, the British settlers learned how to cultivate and use corn, squash, beans, and cranberries. They made chowders with the vegetables, as their neighbors had; the beans were turned into baking beans and other bean dishes in the Native American way. The colonists took their main meal—what we call dinner or supper—in early afternoon when their labor-intensive chores were finished and they were famished.

Despite the diversity, though, food and cooking in colonial New England remained survivalist in nature, reflecting frontier life that demanded practicality.

Sweets and Whimsical Cookies

Adding sugar to seasonal fruit was a simple way for the colonists to enjoy dessert. The colonists, like their Native American friends, enjoyed many wild fruits. They described the wild strawberries as four times larger than the ones they ate in England. Fruits were stewed with sugar and thickened with a grain (today, we would use cornstarch) to make Flummery, a dessert enjoyed in Britain (Wild Blueberry Sauce, page 62).

New England colonial cooks became known for creating fabulous cookies quickly in a no-nonsense fashion. They are also remembered for the whimsical names they gave to their cookie creations. Jolly Boys, Tangle Breeches, Kinkawoodles, and Snickerdoodles were just some cookies with New England colonial beginnings whose names are just pure fun (Soft Snickerdoodles, page 60). (We do note that while most food historians believe that Snickerdoodles have New England roots, some think the cookies originated in the middle colonies with the Pennsylvania Dutch.)

Approaching the Twentieth Century

Mary J. Lincoln founded the Boston Cooking School in 1879, at least partly in an effort to bring a certain standard of cooking into American homes. Soon, a home economics movement began, and Lincoln's cookbooks became core books in the ensuing curricula. Home economists wanted to improve nutrition and kitchen hygiene in American homes, hoping to apply scientific principles just under development. This home economics movement dovetailed with nutrition science, which was dawning on the science frontier. The first vitamin was discovered just as the nineteenth century turned into the twentieth.

Wicked Good Foods in Maine

From Maine-style chowder to whoppie pies, some "wicked good" foods hail from Maine. Ayuh. (That's the Maine way of saying "Uh-huh," "Yep," or "Yes, I agree." Frequently, this statement seems to just appear at the end of peoples' sentences for no apparent reason other than to perhaps indicate that they've finished saying what they wanted to say on that subject.) Let's take a look at two of the absolute best and simplest in the New England tradition: lobster and Maine wild blueberries.

Lobster

Visit Maine without enjoying at least one lobster dinner and you just haven't visited Maine. Lobster is practically synonymous with the state of Maine, and most people who visit look forward to getting lobster a little cheaper (and a little fresher) than they could in their home state.

While some tourists pay to go on lobster boat tours where they can see a day's catch up close, many others don't bother to view live lobsters. Frankly, lobsters aren't that attractive. If you've only seen them cooked, you might be surprised to know that when they're alive, they are an ugly greenish brown color. They don't turn bright orangey red until they're cooked, when the other shell pigments that mask the orange color are destroyed. For some, the fact that lobsters are not particularly attractive at all makes it easier to plunge them into boiling water. For others, seeing them alive makes the cooked product quite inedible later. If you're one of those people, stay out of the kitchen when a lobster is present.

A Brief Maine Lobster History

While lobster is now looked upon by many as a delicacy, it was not always so. Local Native Americans only ate lobster when they couldn't catch any fish, preferring instead to use lobster as fishing bait or as crop fertilizer. The early settlers weren't too fond of lobster, either, considering it to be fit only for the poor. In fact, generally, only indentured servants and prisoners were fed lobster. It's said that during the American Revolution, British prisoners of war threatened to revolt if they had to eat any more lobster. According to information from the Gulf of Maine Aquarium (GMA), servants in Massachusetts even specified in their contracts that they would not be forced to eat lobster more than three times per week.

By the nineteenth century the opinion about lobster had changed, and the demand from New York and Boston increased. Gathering lobster by hand was abandoned as trap fishing came into existence in Maine around 1850, according to the GMA. Today, Maine is the largest lobster-trapping state in the nation.

Enjoying Lobster, the Maine Way

Getting superfresh lobsters and cooking them at home is wonderful, but so is going to a lobster pound when you don't feel like cooking. Lobster pounds (the name comes from the word *impound*, as lobsters need to be kept alive while awaiting shipping or delivery) were set up around the turn of the twentieth century so that tourists could buy lobsters, watch them being cooked in large, wood-fired cooking pots, and enjoy them on the spot. The lobster pound protocol requires a good deal of assertiveness, especially if you arrive at the lunch or dinner hour. Be prepared to shout your order over the din of other people placing an order and clanging lobster pots. Order by the weight of the live lobster, or choose the exact spiney creature you want from the tank. Your lobster (and accompaniments such as mussels and corn on the cob) are tied into a string bag and then plunged into boiling water.

Tourists love lobster pounds (as do many native Mainers), and it's no wonder. There's something about the simplicity, the freshness of the lobster, and the ease of eating outside that add up to a very primal, satisfying experience. Eating at a lobster pound is something that every visitor to Maine should experience.

There's much more that can be done with lobster than just boiling it. Mainers are historically a frugal bunch, and since lobster was abundant and many people made their living catching lobsters, there are myriad traditional recipes for using lobster. Many have very simple ingredients, such as lobster stew (a milk-based, thin, chowder-type soup) and lobster rolls (a simple lobster salad served on a grilled hot dog bun with lettuce). Fancier, more complicated "company's coming" recipes also evolved, including such favorites as lobster bisque, baked stuffed lobster, and lobster pie. These days, for fun, there's even an establishment in Bar Harbor, Maine, that features lobster ice cream among its offerings.

The classic Maine lobster bake is a real experience in humble cooking. Mainers don't really cook like this, of course, as it's impractical, but for show (and at occasions such as weddings or conventions) nothing beats the spectacle of a lobster bake. The most traditional method includes digging a big pit on the beach and baking or steaming lobsters, clams, mussels, and corn on the cob over a layer of hot rocks. Seaweed is placed between layers of seafood and corn to provide moisture. Because it's such a time-intensive procedure, not to mention physically demanding, most people hire caterers to do lobster bakes in Maine. Although lobster bakes are not always done the traditional way (on the beach, with the pit, and so on), the results are still delicious. After all, it's hard to go wrong with fresh lobster.

Wild Blueberries

If you've never tasted a wild blueberry, you're in for a melt-in-your-mouth surprise when you do. These tiny berries, one of only four fruits native to North America, are especially flavorful, despite their diminutive size. Unlike cultivated "high bush" blueberries that most people know, wild blueberries seem to explode with flavor. With so much flavor, a few berries go a long way—a small handful is perfectly fine. This is a good thing, because unless you have your own blueberry patch, wild blueberries can be pricey and rather hard to come by, even in Maine. Just a sprinkle over a bowl of cereal or cup of yogurt is all you need to get a true taste of Maine (Wild Blueberry Sauce, page 62).

A Little History on the Little Berry

For Native Americans, wild blueberries were a staple food, and much revered. When early settlers arrived, the Native Americans taught them how to burn the blueberry fields (a method of pruning the plants) to encourage berry growth, as well as how to use the blueberries for medicinal purposes. Today, although the blueberry fields are still occasionally burned to control certain insects and diseases, most blueberry fields are pruned by mechanical mowing. Harvesting the berries is no easy task—it's usually done by hand using a special blueberry rake. Mechanical harvesters are now sometimes used, but less than 10 percent of the fields in Maine employ this technique, according to the University of Maine Cooperative Extension.

While they're still referred to as "wild," the berries are, to a large extent, cultivated as well. If they weren't, there wouldn't be any blueberry farmers, per se; they'd just be blueberry gatherers. These days, the name seems to refer more to the native species, the most abundant of which is *Vaccinium angustifolium*, or the "low sweet blueberry."

Maine grows wild blueberries on 60,000 acres, making it the largest producer of wild blueberries in the world. There are seven companies that operate blueberry processing plants in Maine, and one fresh-pack cooperative. Given the extremely fragile and perishable nature of wild blueberries, they have to be processed for shipping long distances. During the Civil War, the blueberries were canned and then shipped to the Union troops. Today freezing has replaced canning as the preservation method of choice. Ninety-nine percent of Maine's wild blueberry crop is frozen (although some of these berries are canned later), and less than 1 percent of the crop is sold fresh.

The Berry Popular Wild Blueberry

Wild blueberries are generally used in the same culinary ways that high bush blueberries are: in baking, jams, and pies. Since most of the Maine blueberry crop is processed, you'll find the berries in plenty of other packaged foods, such as blueberry muffin mixes, canned pie fillings, and preserves. They're considered a premium berry, and often appear in some fashion on high-end restaurants' dessert menus in big cities during the late summer. In Maine, some companies make candy out of them, use them in baked goods, dry them, or make syrup from them. Now that blueberries are getting lots of press as "the number one antioxidant fruit," they seem to be popping up everywhere and in all sorts of food products. Keep an eye out for them on your supermarket shelf in one form or another (canned, frozen, or as an ingredient in something else). If you live in Maine, you're lucky enough to freeze large amounts of blueberries during their fleeting season and use them in cooking and baking all year—enjoying a taste of summer in the dead of winter.

Other Maine Foods of Note

This wouldn't be a decent snapshot of the Maine culinary scene without mentioning a few other items that native Mainers enjoy, including:

- Italians. Midwesterners might call this sandwich of sliced meat and vegetables on a submarine bun a "hoagie"; in other parts of the country, it might be called a grinder or sub sandwich. I have yet to eat an Italian, but I have chuckled over seeing signs in convenience stores along the highway boasting: "We've Got Loaded Italians!" No one can say Mainiacs don't have a sense of humor.
- Whoppie pies. This is a dessert featuring two soft, cookie-shaped chocolate cakes with a marshmallow and cream filling. They're large in size—some are almost hamburger-size—and, therefore, good for sharing at the end of a meal.
- Needhams. These are a Maine version of the Mounds bar. You can find them at candy stores or even at the grocery store sold in a rather large, plain box (not at the checkout candy rack).
- Red hot dogs. The Jordan Meat Company makes these hot dogs, which are bright red and stay that way even after cooking, thanks to the inclusion of red dye. They don't taste like regular hot dogs; they taste more like a bland kind of sausage, just a little spicy and with a rather thick casing. Unless you grew up eating these hot dogs, you may not count them among your favorite foods.

PINEAPPLES IN COLONIAL NEW ENGLAND?

Pineapples often appear in colonial woodcarvings or paintings, which is odd, given that pineapples did not grow in New England. American sailors returning from the tropics carried them home and placed them on doorsteps to signal their safe return. In this way, pineapples became associated with hospitality.

All-American Muesli

Lisa C. Peterson, M.S., R.D., C.D.N.

Serves: 4
Hands-on time: 5 minutes
Standing time: overnight (minimum of 8 hours)

Muesli, originated at the end of the nineteenth century by the Swiss nutritionist Dr. Bircher-Benner, is now a nutrient- and fiber-rich breakfast food across the United States. Muesli can contain any raw or toasted cereals, dried fruits, nuts, bran, wheat germ, sugar, yogurt, milk, and/or fruit juice. This recipe is the version we enjoy most in our Connecticut home. Commercial versions are often called granola.

- ¾ cup rolled oats (not instant)
- ¼ cup toasted wheat germ
- ¼ cup milled or ground flaxseed
- 1 cup vanilla (or any flavor) nonfat yogurt
- 3 tablespoons honey
- ¼ cup lemon juice
- 1 apple (peel on), grated or chopped finely
- 1 cup fresh or dried berries
- 2 tablespoons chopped walnuts (or other nuts)

Combine the oats, wheat germ, flaxseed, and 2 cups water in a medium-size bowl. Stir well. Cover and refrigerate overnight.

Stir in the yogurt, honey, lemon juice, and apple. Divide among 4 bowls. Top each with the berries and nuts.

NUTRITION PER SERVING	
Serving size	¾ cups
Calories	300 kcal
Fat	7 g
Saturated fat	0.5 g
Cholesterol	0 mg
Sodium	45 mg
Carbohydrates	52 g
Dietary fiber	6 g
Protein	11 g

Pumpkin Cranberry Muffins

Janice Newell Bissex, M.S., R.D.

The New England colonists would have loved these muffins. And so will you, at breakfast and for dessert. Double the batch and freeze some.

Serves: 12 or 18
Hands-on time: 15 minutes
Cooking time: 25 minutes

- 1 cup all-purpose flour
- 1 cup whole wheat flour
- 1 cup sugar
- 1 cup very finely chopped walnuts or pecans
- 2 teaspoons baking powder
- 1 teaspoon ground cinnamon
- ½ teaspoon baking soda
- ½ teaspoon salt
- 4 eggs, beaten lightly
- 1 15-ounce can 100% pure pumpkin
- ½ cup canola oil
- ¼ cup low-fat milk
- 1 cup dried cranberries

Preheat the oven to 350°F. Coat 12 large or 18 medium-size muffin cups with vegetable oil spray. Whisk together the flour, whole wheat flour, sugar, walnuts or pecans, baking powder, cinnamon, baking soda, and salt in a large bowl. In a separate bowl, combine the eggs, pumpkin, canola oil, and milk. Add to the dry mixture along with the dried cranberries and stir to combine. Spoon the batter into the prepared muffin cups.

Bake for about 25 minutes (large) or 20 minutes (medium-size) or until a wooden toothpick inserted in the center comes out clean.

NUTRITION PER SERVING	
Serving size	1 large muffin
Calories	360 kcal
Fat	19 g
Saturated fat	2 g
Cholesterol	70 mg
Sodium	240 mg
Carbohydrates	45 g
Dietary fiber	4 g
Protein	6 g

NUTRITION PER SERVING	
Serving size	1 medium-size muffin
Calories	240 kcal
Fat	12 g
Saturated fat	1.5 g
Cholesterol	45 mg
Sodium	160 mg
Carbohydrates	30 g
Dietary fiber	3 g
Protein	4 g

Chocolate Banana Peanut Butter Smoothie

Catherine Hoffmann, M.S., R.D.

Serves: 1

Hands-on time: 5 minutes

If you love chocolate–peanut butter cups, this smoothie will become a healthy staple in your home. I send it out from my home state of Maine across the United States to every chocolate lover I know!

1 cup fat-free chocolate milk or low-fat chocolate soy milk
1 ripe banana
1 tablespoon peanut butter
4 to 6 ice cubes

Combine all the ingredients in a blender or a food processor; blend until smooth.

NUTRITION PER SERVING	
Serving size	1 smoothie
Calories	330 kcal
Fat	13 g
Saturated fat	2.5 g
Cholesterol	0 mg
Sodium	180 mg
Carbohydrates	44 g
Dietary fiber	4 g
Protein	15 g

Pumpkin Cheesecake Smoothie

Catherine Hoffmann, M.S., R.D.

The vanilla yogurt makes this smoothie taste like pumpkin cheesecake. You'll think it should be in a pie shell. The flavor is reminiscent of fall in Maine.

Serves: 2
Hands-on time: 5 minutes

- 1 cup canned pumpkin
- 1 cup low-fat vanilla yogurt
- 1 cup fat-free milk
- ½ teaspoon ground cinnamon
- ¼ teaspoon vanilla extract
- 2 teaspoons sugar
- sprinkle of nutmeg

Combine all the ingredients except the nutmeg in a blender or a food processor. Blend until smooth. Pour into a glass and garnish with a sprinkle of nutmeg.

VARIATION

For a nuttier taste and another burst of nutrition, add ¼ cup toasted wheat germ to the blender. (Calories increase to 270 per serving and fiber bumps up 1 gram.)

NUTRITION PER SERVING	
Serving size	1½ cups
Calories	210 kcal
Fat	1 g
Saturated fat	0 g
Cholesterol	5 mg
Sodium	150 mg
Carbohydrates	41 g
Dietary fiber	4 g
Protein	12 g

Apricot Peach Smoothie

Catherine Hoffmann, M.S., R.D.

Serves: 1
Hands-on time: 5 minutes

Canned apricots make this a snap to prepare wherever you are in the States, but you can substitute fresh if you like (as I do much of the year in Maine).

1 cup low-fat peach yogurt
6 canned apricot halves
½ cup nonfat milk
4 to 6 ice cubes
½ teaspoon vanilla extract (optional)

Combine all the ingredients in a blender or a food processor. Blend until smooth.

NUTRITION PER SERVING	
Serving size	1 smoothie
Calories	220 kcal
Fat	0.5 g
Saturated fat	0 g
Cholesterol	5 mg
Sodium	180 mg
Carbohydrates	42 g
Dietary fiber	3 g
Protein	14 g

Koenigsberger Klops (German Meatballs)

Marion S. Wollmeringer, M.S., R.D., L.D.N.

There are several towns called Koenigsberg in Germany. The largest, near Berlin, is probably the origin of this old family favorite, which we still cook in our Boston home. Many of the millions of people of German heritage who settled in Boston in large waves as the nineteenth century turned to the twentieth also continue to make this delicacy.

Serves: 12
Hands-on time: 20 minutes
Cooking time: 20 minutes

MEATBALLS
2 slices white bread, torn into small pieces
2 cups warm water
1¼ pounds lean ground beef or turkey
1 medium onion, chopped (about ¾ cup)
¼ cup liquid egg substitute
½ teaspoon salt
½ teaspoon garlic powder
½ teaspoon dry mustard
¼ teaspoon black pepper
¼ teaspoon dried marjoram leaves
vegetable oil cooking spray

SAUCE
4 cups cold water
⅓ cup flour
4 reduced-sodium beef or chicken bouillon cubes (1 bouillon cube = 1 teaspoon bouillon granules)
⅓ cup Dijon mustard or 1 tablespoon dry mustard
⅓ cup capers (optional)
2 teaspoons lemon juice

Meatballs

Preheat oven to 400°F. Soak the bread in warm water for 10 minutes. Squeeze out excess water. Mix the bread with the beef, onion, egg substitute, and seasonings. Shape the mixture into 24 bite-size balls. Place the meatballs in a 15½-by-10½-by-1-inch baking pan. Bake 20 minutes or until a thermometer inserted into the meatballs registers 165°F. Discard the fat.

COOK'S TIP

For convenience, unbaked meatballs can be added to the prepared sauce and simmered for 20 minutes or until done. However, using this alternate method will increase the amount of fat in the sauce.

NUTRITION NUGGET

Reduced-sodium beef (or chicken) bouillon cubes (or granules) cut the sodium by about one-third. While 1 cube of regular bouillon has about 1,000 mg, 1 cube of reduced-sodium has about 666 mg.

NUTRITION PER SERVING	
Serving size	2 meatballs plus 2 teaspoons sauce
Calories	130 kcal
Fat	5 g
Saturated fat	2 g
Cholesterol	16 mg
Sodium	440 mg
Carbohydrates	8 g
Dietary fiber	1 g
Protein	12 g

Koenigsberger Klops *(continued)*

Sauce

Mix the flour and water in a medium saucepan. Add the bouillon cubes. Bring to a boil; reduce heat and cook, stirring constantly, for 5 minutes or until the sauce is slightly thickened. Add the mustard, capers, and lemon juice. Add the baked meatballs to the sauce and simmer 5 minutes to blend flavors.

Cod, Potato, and Horseradish Cakes

Kristine Napier, M.P.H., R.D.

Cod was a staple for the New England colonists and remains nearly that today. The mild flavor of cod is accented with horseradish and pickle relish to create these easy appetizers. Make the cakes twice as big and enjoy them for dinner.

Serves: 12
Hands-on time: 30 minutes
Cooking time: 45 minutes

- 1 pound red potatoes (peel on), scrubbed and cubed
- 6 cloves garlic, peeled and chopped
- 1 pound cod
- ⅓ cup water
- 2 tablespoons lemon juice
- ⅓ cup nonfat milk
- 1 tablespoon butter
- 3 tablespoons reduced-fat cream cheese
- 1 teaspoon salt
- black pepper to taste
- 1 tablespoon sweet pickle relish
- 1 tablespoon horseradish (or to taste)
- 3 tablespoons canola oil

Combine the potatoes and garlic in a medium-size saucepan; cover with water. Cover and bring to a boil. Reduce heat and simmer until the potatoes are fork tender, about 30 minutes.

Meanwhile, combine the cod, water, and lemon juice in a medium-size nonstick skillet. Cover and simmer until the cod flakes easily with a fork, about 7 to 15 minutes.

Drain the potatoes and garlic and return to the saucepan. Add the milk, butter, and cream cheese; warm over low heat 5 minutes. Remove from heat. Mash the potatoes by hand or with a mixer.

Mince the cod; add to the mashed potatoes, along with salt, pepper, pickle relish, and horseradish. Heat 1 tablespoon oil in batches in a large nonstick skillet over medium-high to high heat. Drop the cod-potato mixture by heaping tablespoons into very hot oil. Cook each side 2 to 3 minutes, or just until browned. Repeat in batches until all of the mixture is cooked.

FOOD TRIVIA
Scrod is young cod and haddock. Cod grow up to 100 pounds in both the Pacific and North Atlantic Oceans and are available year round.

COOK'S TIP
Cod can be baked, poached, braised, broiled, and fried.

FOOD TRIVIA
Missionaries traveling from New England to Hawaii packed salt cod for their long trip.

NUTRITION PER SERVING

Serving size	2 cakes
Calories	140 kcal
Fat	5 g
Saturated fat	1.5 g
Cholesterol	25 mg
Sodium	260 mg
Carbohydrates	12 g
Dietary fiber	1 g
Protein	10 g

Vineyard Stuffed Quahogs (or Clams)

Mary Jo Cutler, M.S., R.D., L.D.

Serves: 6
Hands-on time: 45 minutes
Cooking time: 25 minutes (includes steaming clams and baking stuffed clams)

I generally make this recipe using quahogs or clams that I have dug in a salt-water pond on Martha's Vineyard. Quahogs (also called chowders) and cherrystone and littleneck clams are all in the same family and differ by size. Quahogs are more than three inches long, cherrystones are two and a half to three inches, and littlenecks are one to two and a half inches (it is illegal to take anything smaller than one inch). Because they are so sweet and tender, I usually just steam the littlenecks and the smaller cherrystones, and serve the tougher quahogs and large cherrystones stuffed. The fresh corn is my nod to the Native Americans who first introduced us to quahogs and clams, though they probably did not make a stuffed version.

12 quahogs or large cherrystone clams (freshly harvested or purchased at a fish market)
1 cup dry white wine, optional
1 tablespoon olive oil
1 shallot, chopped
1 clove garlic, minced
1 tablespoon chopped roasted red pepper (from a jar)
½ cup plain bread crumbs, preferably fresh
¼ cup corn, preferably from a freshly steamed ear of corn
salt and pepper to taste
seafood cocktail sauce, optional

Steaming the Clams

Carefully rinse the quahogs or clams in several changes of water to remove sand and grit. If the quahogs are fresh out of the mud, they should be soaked in a large bowl sprinkled with cornmeal, which helps to draw out the sand. The soaking should be followed by several rinsings.

Place about 2 inches of water in a large pot. Add wine, if desired. Bring to a boil and gently add one layer of clams. Remove the clams from the liquid as they open. This will take from 3 to 10 minutes, depending on the clam size. Reserve the clam broth.

Remove the clams from their shells when they are cool enough to handle. When removing the clam meat, also remove the muscle, which connects the clam to the shell. It may be necessary to use a knife to remove the muscle. Reserve the shells for later use.

NUTRITION PER SERVING

Serving size	2 stuffed clams
Calories	140 kcal
Fat	3.5 g
Saturated fat	0 g
Cholesterol	15 mg
Sodium	270 mg
Carbohydrates	14 g
Dietary fiber	0 g
Protein	7 g

Clam Stuffing

Roughly chop the clam meat in a food processor.

Heat the olive oil in a large skillet; add the chopped shallot and garlic; sauté for about 5 minutes. Add the chopped red pepper and continue to sauté for 1 minute. Add the corn and the bread crumbs and sauté 1 more minute. Remove the pan from the heat.

Add the chopped clams and stir. If the mixture is dry, add clam broth until sufficiently moist. Add salt and pepper to taste.

Stuffing the Clams

Preheat oven to 375°F.

Separate the halves of the clamshells, reserving the best 12 half shells. Discard the remaining half shells. Rinse the shells so they are free of sand. Place about 2 tablespoons of stuffing in each half shell. Bake for approximately 15 minutes or until lightly browned.

Serve hot with optional seafood cocktail sauce as a condiment.

Turkey-Sage Wontons

Kristine Napier, M.P.H., R.D.

Serves: 12
Hands-on time: 20 minutes
Cooking time: 10 minutes

Think of Thanksgiving and you can't help but think of that first one in New England. The wonderful aroma of a baking turkey soon comes to mind. If you don't have leftover turkey, purchase smoked turkey breast meat to make this appetizer. If you haven't worked with wonton wrappers, don't be intimidated—they're very kind to first-time chefs.

- vegetable oil cooking spray
- 2 carrots, peeled and shredded
- 5 green onions, chopped finely
- 2 tablespoons minced fresh sage leaves
- 1 rib celery, chopped finely
- 8 ounces (1 cup) cooked turkey, chopped finely
- ½ teaspoon salt
- black pepper to taste
- 24 wonton wrappers (3 inch by 3 inch)
- 1 tablespoon butter, melted

Preheat oven to 400°F. Coat 24 mini-muffin cups with vegetable oil spray. Combine the carrots, onions, sage, celery, turkey, salt, and pepper in a medium-size bowl; mix well. Place one wonton wrapper into each muffin cup; press into the middle. Fill the muffin cups evenly with the mixture. Fold each corner of the wonton wrapper into the center of the cup. Flip the filled wonton over. Brush the wontons with the melted butter.

Bake 10 minutes, or until golden brown. Remove from the pan. Serve hot, bottom side up.

SHOPPING TIP
When buying fresh sage, look for leaves free of black spots, wilting, curling, or wet spots.

COOK'S TIP
Store fresh sage up to 4 days in the refrigerator wrapped in a wet paper towel and tucked into a tightly sealed plastic bag.

NUTRITION PER SERVING

Serving size	2 wontons
Calories	80 kcal
Fat	2 g
Saturated fat	1 g
Cholesterol	10 mg
Sodium	210 mg
Carbohydrates	11 g
Dietary fiber	1 g
Protein	5 g

Omi's German Cucumber Salad

Marion S. Wollmeringer, M.S., R.D., L.D.N.

It's easy to prepare our family's prized German recipes in Massachusetts, especially during the summer when cucumbers are so plentiful in gardens.

Serves: 4
Hands-on time: 10 minutes
Refrigeration time: 30 minutes

1 to 2 medium cucumbers, peeled and thinly sliced (about 2½ cups)
1 cup water
¼ cup white distilled vinegar
2½ tablespoons finely chopped onion (½ medium)
1 tablespoon sugar
1 teaspoon salt
1 teaspoon dried dill weed, or 2 tablespoons chopped fresh dill
⅛ teaspoon freshly ground pepper

Place the cucumbers in a medium-size bowl. Mix the water, vinegar, onion, sugar, salt, dill, and pepper in a small bowl. Pour over the cucumbers. Refrigerate 30 minutes.

COOK'S TIP

Omi, my grandmother, sprinkled 1 teaspoon of salt over the cucumbers and let them stand for 30 minutes to draw out liquid. She then rinsed, drained, and followed the rest of the recipe. You'll get a more intense cucumber flavor with this method.

NUTRITION PER SERVING	
Serving size	¾ cup
Calories	25 kcal
Fat	0 g
Saturated fat	0 g
Cholesterol	0 mg
Sodium	590 mg
Carbohydrates	6 g
Dietary fiber	Less than 1 g
Protein	1 g

Creamy Ranch-Style Dressing

Kathleen Schader, M.B.A., M.S., R.D., L.D.

Serves: 16
Hands-on time: 5 minutes

Nothing showcases fresh tossed greens more than a homemade dressing. This one is so easy to whisk together, and you're likely to have all the ingredients on hand, even in the midst of a long New Hampshire winter.

- ½ cup reduced-fat mayonnaise
- 1 cup fat-free buttermilk
- 1 cup nonfat plain yogurt
- 1½ teaspoons onion powder
- ½ teaspoon garlic powder
- 1 tablespoon chopped parsley

Mix all the ingredients in a medium-size bowl, and blend well with a whisk.

SUBSTITUTIONS

Use 1 small onion, minced, in place of the onion powder; 1 or 2 cloves of garlic, minced, can replace the garlic powder.

SERVING SUGGESTION

Use as a dip for fresh veggies.

COOK'S TIP

Refrigerate leftovers in a tightly sealed container and enjoy them for up to 1 week.

NUTRITION PER SERVING	
Serving size	2 tablespoons
Calories	30 kcal
Fat	0.5 g
Saturated fat	0 g
Cholesterol	0 mg
Sodium	100 mg
Carbohydrates	4 g
Dietary fiber	0 g
Protein	1 g

German Classic Red Cabbage

Marion S. Wollmeringer, M.S., R.D., L.D.N.

Simmer together red cabbage and apples and you've got the makings of traditional Bavarian Red Cabbage—or German Classic Red Cabbage, as others know it. In both my Boston home and the one I left behind in Germany, I know many versions, including this quick one.

Serves: 4
Hands-on time: 5 minutes
Cooking time: 35 minutes

vegetable oil cooking spray
1 16-ounce jar sweet-and-sour red cabbage
1 medium yellow onion, chopped
1 tart apple (such as Granny Smith), peel on, chopped

Coat a medium-size saucepan with the cooking spray. Add the cabbage, onion, and apple. Bring to a boil; reduce heat, and cover. Simmer gently 35 minutes or until the mixture is tender, stirring occasionally. Serve warm.

COOK'S TIP

Instead of cooking on the stove, place the cabbage, the onion, and the apple in a 2-quart casserole dish and microwave on high for 20 to 25 minutes, stirring every 5 minutes.

NUTRITION PER SERVING	
Serving size	½ cup
Calories	200 kcal
Fat	0 g
Saturated fat	0 g
Cholesterol	0 mg
Sodium	20 mg
Carbohydrates	51 g
Dietary fiber	2 g
Protein	1 g

Double Apricot Glazed Winter Vegetables

Lisa Turner, R.D.

Serves: 6
Hands-on time: 10 minutes
Cooking time: 15 minutes

Eating a variety of vegetables can be difficult during long winters in the north. Let a variety of root vegetables come to the rescue. Here is a savory combination of carrots, rutabagas, and turnips to warm your soul on cold, winter nights, flavored delicately with a touch of apricot. These vegetables are great served as leftovers all week.

3 carrots, scrubbed with skin on
1 small rutabaga, peeled
1 turnip, peeled
2 tablespoons water

GLAZE
2 tablespoons apricot all-fruit preserves
½ cup water
½ cup chopped dried apricots

Slice the carrots thinly. Slice the rutabaga and the turnip; cut slices into thin sticks. Combine the vegetables in a microwave-safe bowl with 2 tablespoons water. Cover and cook on high for 10 to 15 minutes, stirring every 5 minutes until the vegetables are tender. Or steam the vegetables on the stovetop 20 to 25 minutes until fork tender.

To Glaze
Combine the apricot preserves, ½ cup water, and the dried apricots in a heavy small saucepan. Bring to a boil; boil gently, stirring, until the mixture has thickened.

Drain the vegetables and place in a serving dish; pour glaze evenly over the top and toss.

VARIATION

Substitute orange marmalade for the apricot and omit the dried apricots. Sprinkle ¼ cup chopped fresh parsley before serving.

NUTRITION PER SERVING	
Serving size	¾ cup
Calories	0 kcal
Fat	0 g
Saturated fat	0 g
Cholesterol	0 mg
Sodium	35 mg
Carbohydrates	20 g
Dietary fiber	3 g
Protein	1 g

Mom's Stuffing

Suzanne Duggan, R.D.

Plain and simple comfort food at its best, accented with fresh mushrooms. This recipe is reminiscent of the stuffing made by the Pilgrims for their feast in America.

Serves: 12
Hands-on time: 30 minutes
Cooking time: 30 to 45 minutes (depending on pan)

- vegetable oil cooking spray
- 1 loaf white bread, sliced
- 1 pound mushrooms, sliced
- 1 large onion, chopped
- 4 stalks celery, diced
- 1 14-ounce can reduced-sodium chicken broth
- 1½ cups liquid egg substitute
- 1 tablespoon dried dill
- 1½ teaspoons salt
- 1 teaspoon black pepper

Lay the bread out on clean towels or baking sheets overnight to dry.

Preheat oven to 325°F. Spray a 2-quart casserole dish with the nonstick cooking spray.

Cube the bread. Combine all the ingredients in a large bowl; mix well. Spoon evenly into the casserole dish.

Bake for 30 to 45 minutes, or until lightly golden.

NUTRITION PER SERVING	
Serving size	1 cup
Calories	150 kcal
Fat	3 g
Saturated fat	0.5 g
Cholesterol	0 mg
Sodium	580 mg
Carbohydrates	23 g
Dietary fiber	2 g
Protein	9 g

Vermont Celebration Beans

Lisa C. Peterson, M.S., R.D., C.D.N.

Serves: 8
Hands-on time: 10 minutes
Cooking time: 1 hour
Baking time: 3 hours

Summer picnics in Vermont demand baked beans, and my mom rose to the occasion with this family-favorite recipe. While she baked them in classic heavy, brown-glazed pottery, any baking vessel that can be tightly covered works. Reduced-fat kielbasa replaces the recipe's original salt pork to remove some of the fat—but none of the flavor!

- 1 pound (2 cups) dry navy beans
- 1 teaspoon salt
- ⅓ cup brown sugar
- ¼ cup dark molasses
- 1 tablespoon apple cider vinegar
- 1 medium-size onion, minced
- ¾ teaspoon dry mustard
- 2 8-ounce cans tomato sauce
- ½ pound reduced-fat kielbasa, sliced thinly

Rinse and sort the beans, discarding shriveled beans. In a 3-quart saucepan, combine the beans with enough water to cover by 1 inch. Bring to a boil; cover and simmer for 1 hour. Reserve 2½ cups bean liquid, then drain the rest.

Preheat oven to 300°F. Combine the beans, reserved liquid, salt, brown sugar, molasses, vinegar, onion, mustard, and tomato sauce in a 2-quart oven-safe dish or bean pot. Arrange the kielbasa over top. Cover tightly with a lid or foil.

Bake 2½ hours, stirring occasionally. Remove the cover; continue baking 30 minutes more. Serve hot.

SHOPPING TIP

If you can find them, try substituting soldier or great northern beans for the navy beans.

SERVING SUGGESTION

Like the salt pork in the original recipe, the kielbasa is used primarily for its flavor, but it also makes this a one-pot meal.

SUBSTITUTIONS

Reduce the sodium in this recipe by using no-salt-added tomato sauce. Or substitute three 14- or 15-ounce cans great northern beans for the dry. Rinse and drain, combine with the remaining ingredients (do not add the water), stir, and bake uncovered for 1 hour.

NUTRITION PER SERVING

Serving size	¾ cup
Calories	360 kcal
Fat	9 g
Saturated fat	3 g
Cholesterol	20 mg
Sodium	960 mg
Carbohydrates	56 g
Dietary fiber	15 g
Protein	18 g

Black Lantern's Curried Butternut Squash Soup

Deb Winders, M.S., R.D.

What better way to warm up a cool fall and an even colder winter in New Hampshire than with a thick butternut squash soup? The Indian curry paste adds another layer of warmth.

Serves: 8
Hands-on time: 15 minutes
Cooking time: 30 minutes

- 3 tablespoons unsalted butter
- 1 to 2 large onions, chopped
- 1 to 2 tablespoons hot Indian curry paste
- 6 cups vegetable broth
- 4 pounds butternut squash, peeled and cut into 2-inch pieces
- 1 12-ounce can lite coconut milk
- ½ cup reduced-fat sour cream
- cilantro sprigs for garnish

Melt the butter in a large Dutch oven or kettle. Sauté the onion in the butter until softened. Add the hot curry paste and stir until well blended. Add the vegetable broth and squash; bring to a boil. Reduce heat to low and simmer until the squash is very tender, 20 to 25 minutes.

Remove from heat. Purée the squash in a blender or with an immersion stick blender until very smooth. Return the soup to the kettle and add the lite coconut milk. Heat the soup to 165°F. Ladle into bowls and garnish with a dollop of sour cream and cilantro.

SHOPPING TIP
My favorite brand of hot curry paste is Patak's.

COOK'S TIP
Different varieties of winter squash, such as acorn, butternut, and pumpkin can often be substituted for one another in recipes, although the seasonings used to bring out their flavors may vary.

NUTRITION NUGGET
Adding vegetable-based soups to your diet is an easy and delicious way to boost your intake of vegetables.

NUTRITION PER SERVING	
Serving size	1½ cups
Calories	190 kcal
Fat	7 g
Saturated fat	4 g
Cholesterol	15 mg
Sodium	790 mg
Carbohydrates	33 g
Dietary fiber	8 g
Protein	5 g

Butternut Squash Bisque

Kathleen Schader, M.B.A., M.S., R.D., L.D.

Serves: 4
Hands-on time: 20 minutes
Cooking time: 25 to 30 minutes

This is a delicious fall soup enjoyed by New Englanders after the harvest and through the winters. It's a favorite comfort food in our New Hampshire home.

2 tablespoons canola oil
2 medium-size onions, chopped coarsely
1 rib celery, sliced
2 cloves garlic, minced
1 to 2 tablespoons minced fresh ginger
¼ to ½ teaspoon black pepper
3 to 3½ pounds butternut squash, peeled, seeded, and chopped into 1-inch pieces
2 14½-ounce cans reduced-sodium chicken or vegetable broth
½ cup skim milk (optional)
¼ cup roasted pumpkin seeds for garnish

Heat the oil in a heavy saucepan; add the onions, celery, garlic, ginger, and pepper; cook over medium heat for 5 minutes, or until the vegetables are softened. Stir frequently; do not brown. Add the squash and broth, cover, and bring to a boil; reduce heat and simmer for 20 to 25 minutes or until the squash is tender.

Purée the soup in batches in a blender; return to the pot. Or, purée in a pot using a hand blender.

Garnish with pumpkin seeds before serving.

Toasted Pumpkin Seeds

Combine 1 cup green (not roasted) pumpkin seeds and 1 teaspoon canola oil in a 9- or 10-inch heavy skillet; toss. Cook and stir over medium heat about 6 to 8 minutes or until the seeds are puffed and golden. Add ¼ teaspoon salt; toss. Cooled seeds can be stored in the refrigerator in a tightly sealed container for up to 3 months.

SERVING SUGGESTION

In addition to or in place of toasted pumpkin seeds, garnish the soup with chives or ground ginger.

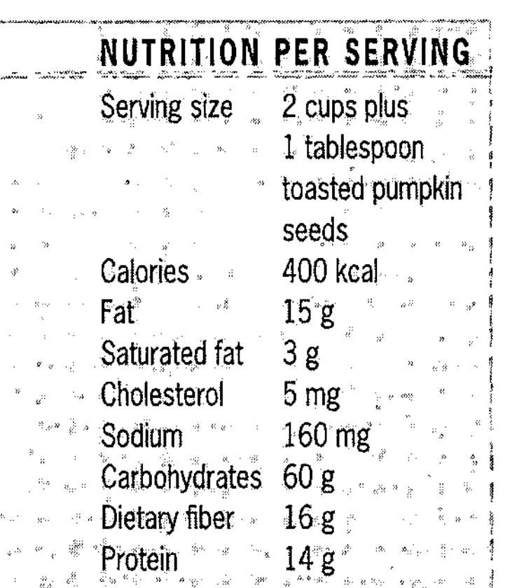

NUTRITION PER SERVING	
Serving size	2 cups plus 1 tablespoon toasted pumpkin seeds
Calories	400 kcal
Fat	15 g
Saturated fat	3 g
Cholesterol	5 mg
Sodium	160 mg
Carbohydrates	60 g
Dietary fiber	16 g
Protein	14 g

No-Nonsense New England Clam Chowder

Janice Newell Bissex, M.S., R.D., and Liz Weiss, M.S., R.D.

For a quick clam chowder brimming with flavor and good nutrition without the usual cup of cream, try this simple, no-fuss chowder. With just a few pantry staples like canned minced clams, creamed corn, and shell-shaped pasta, this hearty and healthy soup can be on the table in a flash—whether you live in New England, California, or anywhere in between.

Serves: 4
Hands-on time: 10 minutes
Cooking time: 20 minutes

- 4 ounces uncooked medium-size pasta shells (about 1½ cups)
- 2 cups 1% low-fat milk
- ¼ cup all-purpose flour
- 1 teaspoon onion powder
- ⅛ teaspoon dried thyme
- 2 6½-ounce cans minced clams
- 1 15-ounce can cream-style corn
- 1 tablespoon dry sherry or wine

Cook the pasta according to package directions. Drain and set aside.

In a medium-size saucepan, combine the milk, flour, onion powder, and thyme; whisk until well blended. Stir in the clams and the corn, and turn heat to high. Bring the mixture to a simmer, stirring constantly. Reduce the heat to medium low and continue to simmer and stir until the soup thickens slightly, about 2 minutes. Stir in the cooked pasta and sherry. Heat through and serve piping hot.

SUBSTITUTIONS

Substitute 1 small onion, minced, for the onion powder. You can also substitute an equal quantity of cooking sherry or dry white wine for the dry sherry. Alternatively, use 1 to 2 teaspoons of Worcestershire sauce.

NUTRITION PER SERVING	
Serving size	1 cup
Calories	390 kcal
Fat	4 g
Saturated fat	1 g
Cholesterol	65 mg
Sodium	170 mg
Carbohydrates	56 g
Dietary fiber	2 g
Protein	34 g

Creamy Asparagus Soup

Kathleen Schader, M.B.A., M.S., R.D., L.D.

Serves: 4
Hands-on time: 15 minutes
Cooking time: 20 minutes

Fresh spring asparagus soup is a delicious starter for any meal, especially in New Hampshire where the first spears celebrate the end of the snow (to be sure, though, it's good all year). This creamy soup has all of the flavor of a cream soup—no one will be able to tell there is such a small amount of fat in it.

1 tablespoon butter
1 medium-size onion, coarsely chopped
1 rib celery, sliced
¼ to ½ teaspoon pepper
1 pound fresh asparagus, washed, woody stems removed, cut into 1-inch pieces
2 14½-ounce cans reduced-sodium chicken broth
2 to 3 tablespoons minced fresh dill (or 2 to 3 teaspoons dried dill)
3 tablespoons all-purpose flour
½ cup nonfat milk
freshly ground black pepper, optional

Melt the butter in a large saucepan. Add the onion and celery and cook over medium heat until soft, not browned, about 5 minutes. Add the pepper, asparagus, and chicken broth. Cover and bring the mixture to a boil. Reduce heat and simmer uncovered about 8 to 10 minutes or until the asparagus is tender.

Purée in batches in a blender, or purée in saucepan with a hand blender. Return the soup to the saucepan. Stir in the dill.

Mix the flour and skim milk in a small bowl until smooth. Whisk into the soup, and heat (do not boil) until thickened. Add additional pepper, if desired.

SERVING SUGGESTIONS

Add 1 tablespoon of low-fat plain yogurt to each bowl of soup; swirl just before serving. Sprinkle 1 teaspoon of minced fresh dill on each serving.

NUTRITION PER SERVING

Serving size	1½ cups
Calories	130 kcal
Fat	5 g
Saturated fat	2.5 g
Cholesterol	10 mg
Sodium	150 mg
Carbohydrates	17 g
Dietary fiber	4 g
Protein	8 g

Hearty Maine Fish Chowder

Kitty Broihier, M.S., R.D.

During the fall and winter months I serve this chowder as the main course to nearly all my guests, whether they're "from away" or native Mainers. It has a classic taste, a traditional thinner, milky Maine chowder consistency (though it does use flour as a thickener, which is not the traditional Maine method), and a lot less of the fat that makes some cream-based chowders so overwhelming.

Serves: 8
Hands-on time: 20 minutes
Cooking time: 40 minutes

- vegetable oil cooking spray
- 5 slices (about 5 ounces) Canadian bacon, chopped
- 4 tablespoons butter
- 1¼ cups chopped onions
- 1 cup chopped celery
- 1½ teaspoons dried thyme leaves, optional (or 1½ tablespoons fresh thyme)
- 3 tablespoons flour
- 4 cups fish stock (prepared from fish bouillon cubes or fish soup base)
- 2 cups diced potatoes, scrubbed, unpeeled
- 2½ pounds mixed white fish (such as cod, haddock, or wolf fish) cut into 1½-inch pieces (okay to use frozen)
- 1½ cups fat-free half-and-half (or more, depending on desired consistency)
- ½ teaspoon salt
- pinch black pepper
- 2 tablespoons chopped chives or green onion tops, optional garnish

Spray the bottom of a medium-size stockpot with the cooking spray. Add the Canadian bacon and cook over medium heat until lightly browned and slightly crisp, stirring constantly. Stir in the butter, onions, celery, and thyme. Cook 5 minutes, or until the onions are soft and translucent. Using a wire whisk, whisk in flour and continue stirring and cooking a minute or two, until the flour is well incorporated and all of the vegetables are coated.

Pour in the fish stock, a little at a time, while continuing to whisk constantly. (The mixture will be very thick at first and gradually get thinner.) Continue until all fish stock has been incorporated. Reduce heat, add the potatoes, and simmer 10 to 15 minutes, or until potatoes are tender, stirring and scraping the bottom of the pot occasionally.

Add the fish pieces and cook another 5 to 10 minutes or until all fish pieces are cooked through. Stir in the fat-free half-and-half, adding more if the chowder seems too thick. Add salt and pepper. Taste and adjust the seasonings, if necessary. Heat through, but do not boil. Ladle into bowls and garnish with the chopped chives or green onions, if desired.

SHOPPING TIPS

This recipe works wonderfully with fish that's been frozen, so stock up when your favorite white fish is on sale. Also, fish pieces that are not nice enough to serve as an entrée (such as thinner tail ends or trimmed pieces) are perfect for chowder.

SERVING SUGGESTIONS

In Maine, we serve chowder with Nabisco Crown Pilot Crackers, a thick, hard white cracker that's usually only available in New England. Saltine crackers, oyster crackers, or a nice, crusty bread is fine, too. Complete the meal with a green salad and a fruit-based dessert for a filling, healthful dinner.

NUTRITION PER SERVING	
Serving size	1¼ cups
Calories	400 kcal
Fat	21 g
Saturated fat	8 g
Cholesterol	135 mg
Sodium	690 mg
Carbohydrates	14 g
Dietary fiber	2 g
Protein	36 g

Yankee Gumbo

Lisa C. Peterson, M.S., R.D., C.D.N.

Serves: 10 generously
Hands-on time: 30 minutes
Cooking time: 1 hour, 15 minutes

This dish is a winner at our annual Kentucky Derby party. We use locally smoked pork loin or chicken breasts instead of traditional fresh oysters to give this dish a Yankee spin. Perfect for entertaining, it can be prepared to near completion the day before—just add the crab and shrimp 30 minutes before serving.

¼ cup canola oil
⅔ cup all-purpose flour
2 medium-size onions, diced
1 celery rib, diced
1 medium-size green bell pepper, diced
2 garlic cloves, peeled and minced
½ teaspoon ground white pepper
¼ teaspoon garlic powder
¼ teaspoon ground black pepper
¼ teaspoon sweet paprika
½ teaspoon dried thyme
½ teaspoon dried oregano
7 14-ounce cans reduced-sodium chicken broth
1 8-ounce can tomato sauce
½ pound andouille or other spicy smoked sausage, sliced
1 15-ounce can chopped tomatoes, with juice
½ pound smoked chicken breasts (remove skin) or pork loin, diced
2 cups fresh or frozen okra, sliced
¾ pound fresh or frozen crab meat
1 pound peeled, deveined shrimp (medium or large)
salt, hot pepper sauce, and cayenne pepper to taste
1½ cups hot cooked white rice

In a large kettle or Dutch oven, heat the oil over medium heat. Blend in the flour, stirring constantly with a wire whisk. Cook and stir for 8 to 10 minutes until medium brown.

Add the onions, celery, and green pepper and stir over medium heat 5 minutes. Add the garlic, white pepper, garlic powder, black pepper, paprika, thyme, and oregano; stir 3 minutes. Stir in the broth and tomato sauce; whisk until smooth. Reduce heat and simmer 45 minutes. Separately, in a saucepan combine the sausage with enough water to cover. Simmer 5 minutes. Drain and reserve.

Add the chopped tomatoes, chicken or pork, okra, and reserved sausage; heat through. Note that the gumbo may be made to this point and refrigerated overnight. Reheat and continue instructions about 30 minutes before serving. Gently stir in the crab and shrimp; simmer 10 to 15 minutes or until the shrimp is pink and firm. Season to taste. Serve hot in individual bowls with 2 tablespoons rice spooned into the center.

SUBSTITUTION

If you are allergic to shellfish, substitute 2 pounds of cod or other white fish for the crab and shrimp.

NUTRITION PER SERVING	
Serving size	1½ cups
Calories	390 kcal
Fat	17 g
Saturated fat	4.5 g
Cholesterol	130 mg
Sodium	1080 mg
Carbohydrates	26 g
Dietary fiber	3 g
Protein	33 g

Savory Roasted Salmon and Green Beans

Marsha Hudnall, M.S., R.D., C.D.

This delightfully gentle but distinctive Asian-inspired salmon recipe was created in Vermont. The leftovers are great cold, or heated and served with rice.

Serves: 4
Hands-on time: 5 minutes
Cooking time: 20 minutes

1½ pounds salmon fillet
1 pound fresh green beans, trimmed
1 tablespoon grated fresh ginger
3 cloves garlic, minced
¼ cup reduced-sodium soy sauce

Place the salmon fillet skin side down in an oven-safe 9-by-13-inch glass baking dish. Arrange the green beans around the salmon. Combine the ginger, garlic, and soy sauce in a small bowl; mix well. Pour over the salmon and beans. Cover tightly and marinate at least 2 hours and up to 8 hours in the refrigerator.

Preheat the oven to 400°F. Baste the salmon and beans with the sauce. Roast uncovered 15 to 20 minutes or until the salmon flakes easily with a fork.

SUBSTITUTION

If fresh green beans are out of season, use the French-cut frozen green beans instead. Marinate thawed beans with salmon, but do not add them to the pan when salmon is placed in the oven. Instead, add them after cooking the salmon 5 to 8 minutes.

COOK'S TIP

The quantities of grated fresh ginger, minced garlic, and soy sauce may be varied to your taste.

NUTRITION PER SERVING

Serving size	4 ounces roasted salmon plus ¾ cup cooked beans
Calories	290 kcal
Fat	11 g
Saturated fat	1.5 g
Cholesterol	95 mg
Sodium	610 mg
Carbohydrates	9 g
Dietary fiber	4 g
Protein	36 g

Connecticut Coast Shrimp Salad Pitas

Lisa C. Peterson, M.S., R.D., C.D.N.

Serves: 8
Hands-on time: 10 minutes
Cooking time: 5 minutes
Chill time: 2 hours

We love shrimp on the Connecticut coast, where it's easy to get. If you live inland (or you just want a shortcut), use fully cooked or frozen and thawed shrimp.

2 pounds large, raw shrimp (not peeled)
1 cup reduced-fat sour cream, or crème fraiche
¾ cup low-fat mayonnaise
1 tablespoon ketchup
⅓ cup chopped fresh dill
4 green onions, chopped
pepper to taste
4 pita rounds, halved
1 large red onion, sliced very thinly
8 large lettuce leaves, preferably Boston lettuce

Bring a large pot of water to a boil; add the shrimp all at once. Bring the water back to a boil; simmer the shrimp 2 minutes. Drain the shrimp; immerse in cold water. When cool, peel and devein the shrimp. Halve lengthwise; reserve.

Combine the sour cream, mayonnaise, ketchup, dill, green onions, and pepper; mix well. Add the shrimp. Chill at least 2 hours.

To assemble the sandwiches, fill each pita half with onion slices, lettuce, and about ⅔ cup shrimp salad. Serve immediately.

VARIATIONS

Make this with crab, lobster, or an artificial seafood. Sprinkle in red pepper sauce to spice it up.

NUTRITION PER SERVING	
Serving size	½ stuffed pita
Calories	230 kcal
Fat	2.5 g
Saturated fat	0 g
Cholesterol	170 mg
Sodium	460 mg
Carbohydrates	25 g
Dietary fiber	3 g
Protein	27 g

Turkey Pot Pie

Mary Jo Cutler, M.S., R.D., L.D.

I developed this recipe as a way to use leftover Thanksgiving turkey in our New England home. I usually make it on the Saturday after Thanksgiving and serve it for a casual supper meal with friends. Since we cook our Thanksgiving turkey on a Weber grill with wood chips, the turkey and the gravy have a wonderful smoked flavor that enhances the taste of the pie. Instead of often-used carrots, I use sweet potatoes to add a more interesting flavor.

Serves: 8
Hands-on time: 1 hour
Cooking time: 1 hour

2 9-inch purchased pie crusts

FILLING
3 cups turkey meat, light and dark (smoked if possible), chopped
2 sweet potatoes, peeled and chopped
3 medium-size red potatoes, cubed (not peeled)
1 10-ounce package frozen baby peas, thawed
1 teaspoon dry tarragon (or 1 tablespoon chopped fresh)
1 teaspoon dry parsley (or 1 tablespoon chopped fresh)
½ teaspoon black pepper
other herbs and spices as desired

SAUCE
3 tablespoons cornstarch
3 cups cold nonfat milk
2 tablespoons butter
pepper to taste
1 cup reduced-sodium chicken broth

Preheat oven to 375°F. Place one crust in a deep-dish pie plate. Line with waxed paper and fill with dry beans or weights. Bake for 15 minutes. Remove from the oven to a cooling rack. Remove beans and wax paper. Meanwhile, boil the potatoes for 5 to 10 minutes until tender, but not falling apart.

Line the pie crust with the turkey. Add the potatoes and peas. Combine the tarragon, parsley, black pepper, and other herbs and spices as desired. Sprinkle over vegetables in the pie plate.

NUTRITION PER SERVING	
Serving size	⅛ pie wedge
Calories	260 kcal
Fat	7 g
Saturated fat	3 g
Cholesterol	50 mg
Sodium	180 mg
Carbohydrates	26 g
Dietary fiber	4 g
Protein	23 g

Turkey Pot Pie
(continued)

Combine the cornstarch and milk in a medium pan, stirring until smooth. Add the butter and pepper. Bring to a boil, stirring constantly; reduce heat, lightly boil 1 minute. Add the gravy or broth; stir and cook until thickened. Pour the sauce over the meat and vegetables in the pie plate. Cover the pie with top crust; crimp edges. Make six ½-inch slits in the crust to allow steam to escape. Bake at 375°F for about 1 hour, until contents are bubbling through the slits in the crust.

New England Blue Ribbon Meatloaf

Lisa C. Peterson, M.S., R.D., C.D.N.

This is perhaps my mom's greatest culinary achievement. In my Connecticut home, I've tried other meatloaf recipes, just to be rebellious, but I keep coming back to this one. Like any great meatloaf, this one is scrumptious both warm and cold late at night.

Serves: 6
Hands-on time: 10 minutes
Cooking time: 80 minutes

- vegetable oil cooking spray
- 1 pound extra-lean ground beef
- 1 cup dry seasoned bread crumbs
- 1 large egg, lightly beaten
- 1 medium-size onion, minced
- 1 8-ounce can tomato sauce, divided
- 2 tablespoons white wine vinegar
- 2 tablespoons Dijon or yellow mustard
- 2 tablespoons brown sugar
- 3 tablespoons chopped parsley, optional

Preheat oven to 375°F. Coat a 9-by-4-inch loaf pan with the cooking spray.

Combine the beef, bread crumbs, egg, onion, and ½ cup tomato sauce; mix well but don't beat the mixture. Form into a loaf with a ridge down the center. Place into a loaf pan.

In a small bowl, combine the remaining ½ cup tomato sauce, vinegar, mustard, and brown sugar; whisk until smooth. Pour over the meat. Cover the pan tightly with foil. Bake 40 minutes. Remove the foil; continue baking 30 to 40 more minutes, or until the meat thermometer reaches 160°F. Serve hot, garnished with the chopped parsley.

VARIATION

Try using different types of flavored canned tomato sauce, like roasted garlic or bell pepper and onion.

NUTRITION PER SERVING	
Serving size	⅙ of loaf
Calories	260 kcal
Fat	9 g
Saturated fat	3 g
Cholesterol	65 mg
Sodium	950 mg
Carbohydrates	24 g
Dietary fiber	2 g
Protein	21 g

Shoreline Shepherd's Pie

Lisa C. Peterson, M.S., R.D., C.D.N.

Serves: 8
Hands-on time: 20 minutes
Cooking time: 40 minutes

I've been working for the southeastern Connecticut shoreline soup kitchens for years. The menus are balanced for nutrition and variety, and I am often asked to contribute shepherd's pie as a one-pot meal that meets these high standards for nutrition. This English pub classic is satisfying and easy-to-make, and the recipe can be easily doubled and tripled. If you have a smaller family, enjoy two to three meals from this batch—and an easy week of cooking and cleanup.

MASHED POTATOES

1½ pounds (about 2 to 3 large) russet or Idaho potatoes, peeled and diced
vegetable oil cooking spray
¼ cup nonfat milk
2 tablespoons butter
4 ounces (½ cup) nonfat cream cheese
½ teaspoon salt
⅛ to ¼ teaspoon white pepper

FILLING

1 pound extra-lean ground beef
1 medium-size onion, chopped
2 carrots, peeled and diced
2 stalks celery, diced
1 teaspoon dried thyme (or 1 tablespoon fresh thyme)
½ teaspoon black pepper
⅛ teaspoon grated nutmeg
3 tablespoons all-purpose flour
1 14-ounce can reduced-sodium beef broth

2 cups frozen, canned, or fresh corn kernels

Boil the potatoes in salted water until fork tender.

Brown the beef with the onion, carrots, celery, thyme, pepper, and nutmeg in a large nonstick skillet over medium high heat, breaking up the meat as you do, about 10 to 12 minutes. Stir in the flour. Pour in the broth and simmer, stirring, until slightly thickened, about 3 to 5 minutes. Remove from heat.

Preheat oven to 375°F. Spray a 2-quart casserole with vegetable oil spray.

VARIATION

Try using other lean ground meats for all or some of the beef in the recipe. A traditional English variation calls for ground lamb, but veal, buffalo, or emu can be used, too.

NUTRITION PER SERVING

Serving size	1½ cups
Calories	250 kcal
Fat	6 g
Saturated fat	3 g
Cholesterol	40 mg
Sodium	330 mg
Carbohydrates	33 g
Dietary fiber	4 g
Protein	18 g

Drain the potatoes and return to the pan. Add the milk, butter, cream cheese, salt, and pepper. Heat over low heat briefly until butter melts. (See tip regarding hot liquids for mashing potatoes.) Mash by hand or with an electric mixer.

Transfer the meat mixture to a prepared casserole dish. Spread the corn evenly over the meat. Spoon the potato mixture evenly over the corn. Bake for 30 to 40 minutes, or until the top is lightly browned and the casserole is bubbling around the edges of the potatoes.

COOK'S TIP

Heating milk, butter, and cream cheese before mashing potatoes makes your finished potatoes creamier and smoother.

New England Steak Milanese

Lisa C. Peterson, M.S., R.D., C.D.N.

Serves: 6 generously
Hands-on time: 15 minutes
Cooking time: 10 minutes

My kids love steak and anything with tomato sauce. This Italian-inspired dish that I make in my Connecticut home is easy to fix and great for reheating later, such as when you're helping out a friend with a home-cooked dinner or contributing to a potluck meal, a New England tradition that began with the colonists.

- ½ cup seasoned dry bread crumbs
- 2 tablespoons grated Parmesan cheese
- 2 eggs
- 6 4-ounce cube steaks
- pepper to taste
- 2 tablespoons canola oil
- 2 cups hot prepared marinara sauce

In a shallow bowl, combine the bread crumbs and the cheese; set aside. In another shallow bowl, beat the eggs with 1 tablespoon water.

Lightly season the steaks with pepper (may not be necessary depending on your tastes and how seasoned your bread crumbs are). Heat the oil in a large nonstick pan.

Dip the steaks into the eggs and then into the bread crumb mixture, dredging through the crumbs well. Fry in hot oil over medium heat about 4 minutes on each side or until cooked through. Serve hot with ½ cup marinara sauce poured over each steak.

SHOPPING TIP
There are many kinds of sauce you can use—marinara, spaghetti, or pasta sauce. Just choose your favorite kind and flavor—or make your own!

FOOD TRIVIA
Milanese (mee-lah-NAY-zay) means "in the style of Milan."

NUTRITION PER SERVING

Serving size	1 piece steak plus ⅓ cup sauce
Calories	470 kcal
Fat	34 g
Saturated fat	12 g
Cholesterol	150 mg
Sodium	730 mg
Carbohydrates	16 g
Dietary fiber	2 g
Protein	24 g

Calzones

Marion S. Wollmeringer, M.S., R.D., L.D.N.

While some people think calzones originated in New Haven, Connecticut, some food historians say these half-moon-shaped, stuffed pizzas originated in Naples, Italy. Calzone is the Italian word for "pocket sandwich." Here are two wonderful calzone variations, but calzones can be filled with any combinations of meat, cheese, and vegetables. This baked version is exceptionally delicious and low in fat.

Serves: 6
Hands-on time: 1 hour
Cooking time: 15 to 20 minutes

DOUGH

3 cups stirred all-purpose flour
1½ teaspoons active dry yeast
½ teaspoon salt
1 cup warm water (130°F.)
1 tablespoon plus 1 teaspoon olive oil
vegetable oil cooking spray

Sift the flour, yeast, and salt together into a large mixer bowl. Slowly add the warm water and 1 tablespoon olive oil. Mix on low speed or stir with a large mixing spoon until the dough pulls away from the sides of the bowl, about 2 to 3 minutes. Knead the dough on a lightly floured surface until smooth and elastic, about 3 to 4 minutes. Cover with a cloth and let rise 20 to 30 minutes. While dough rises, prepare filling of choice (recipes follow).

Preheat oven to 450°F.

Divide the dough into 6 individual balls. On a very lightly floured surface, roll each ball into a 6- to 7-inch circle.

Place each dough circle on a square of parchment paper. Divide the filling equally between the 6 circles of dough; place on the lower half of each circle. Fold the top half of the dough over the filling. Seal the dough by pinching a narrow seam or pressing with the tines of a fork. To make sure the filling is distributed throughout the dough, press the top of the filled sealed dough very gently. A tight seal is needed or the filling will leak out. Check the back of the dough edge for a tight seal. Place each calzone and parchment on a cookie sheet. A jelly roll or pizza pan with a small lip can be used to catch leaks.

Repeat with the remaining dough balls.

Bake for about 18 to 20 minutes or until the dough is lightly browned and slightly puffed. Remove from the baking sheet to a cooling rack. Brush the tops with olive oil. Serve hot or warm.

PREPARATION TIPS

Stirring the flour before measuring will ensure the proper consistency of the dough.

HOW MUCH WATER FOR THE DOUGH?

The amount of water needed depends on the humidity of your kitchen and on the dryness of the flour. The dough should be only slightly sticky. Add 1 or 2 tablespoons flour if the dough is too sticky.

COOK'S TIP

A pizza stone may be used; follow the instructions specific to your stone. This dough may be used to make pizzas.

Calzones *(continued)*

NUTRITION PER SERVING

Serving size	1 calzone
Calories	370 kcal
Fat	13 g
Saturated fat	7 g
Cholesterol	40 mg
Sodium	450 mg
Carbohydrates	46 g
Dietary fiber	2 g
Protein	17 g

SUBSTITUTION

Frozen spinach may be used instead of fresh. Thaw 1 package or ½ bag (7½ ounces) frozen chopped spinach in the microwave 3 minutes on high. Let cool; squeeze out excess liquid, yielding about 1 cup spinach.

PREPARATION TIP

If the filling is prepared ahead, cover tightly and refrigerate no more than 1 to 2 hours. Too long in the refrigerator causes the filling to get too watery. The salt in the cheese pulls water out of the fresh spinach.

NUTRITION PER SERVING

Serving size	1 calzone
Calories	330 kcal
Fat	8 g
Saturated fat	2.5 g
Cholesterol	10 mg
Sodium	360 mg
Carbohydrates	49 g
Dietary fiber	4 g
Protein	14 g

Cheesy Florentine Filling

1 medium-size garlic clove, peeled
2½ cups chopped fresh spinach
1 cup part skim ricotta cheese
1¼ cup (5 ounces) shredded fontina (or fontinella) cheese

Place the garlic clove and spinach in a food processor bowl fitted with a metal blade. Pulse 10 to 12 times, or until the spinach is finely chopped.

Combine the ricotta and fontina cheeses in a 3-quart mixing bowl. Add the garlic and the spinach mixture. Stir well.

Use a slightly heaping ⅓ cup of cheese mixture for each calzone.

Mushroom and Mozzarella Cheese Filling

1 tablespoon olive oil
2 medium-size onions, chopped (about 2 cups)
1 medium-size garlic clove, peeled and minced
3 cups thin sliced button mushrooms (about 8 ounces)
⅛ teaspoon salt
⅛ teaspoon fresh ground pepper
1 cup (4 ounces) shredded mozzarella cheese, divided

Heat the olive oil in a 10-inch skillet. Sauté the onions and garlic until the onions are transparent, about 4 to 5 minutes. Remove to a dish and set aside.

In the same pan, sauté the mushrooms until they ooze their juices, about 6 to 7 minutes. Combine with onion mixture; add the salt and pepper. Mix well. If the filling is prepared ahead, cover tightly and refrigerate 8 hours or overnight.

Use ⅓ cup of filling for each calzone. Sprinkle with 3 tablespoons mozzarella cheese before closing.

Grilled Chicken with Roasted Red Pepper Pasta Sauce

Lisa C. Peterson, M.S., R.D., C.D.N.

Serves: 6
Hands-on time: 10 minutes

1½ pounds boneless, skinless chicken breast, grilled or roasted and then chilled
2 cloves garlic, peeled
½ medium-size onion, cut into 2 pieces
1 12-ounce jar roasted red peppers (in brine), drained
½ cup low-fat mayonnaise
2 tablespoons reduced-fat sour cream
hot pepper sauce to taste
1 tablespoon Dijon mustard
2 tablespoons fresh herbs (choose from parsley, chives, basil, oregano, tarragon, etc.)

Place the garlic cloves and onion in a food processor bowl; pulse until finely minced. Add the remaining ingredients; process until smooth, scraping down the sides of the bowl occasionally. Cover and refrigerate 1 hour or overnight. Slice the chicken; place the strips on a serving platter and drizzle the sauce over the top.

SHOPPING TIP
Choose herbs based on the entrée that the finished sauce will accompany. For example, if parsley and rosemary are in the entrée, match the flavors with your sauce. Avoid mixing too many herb flavors.

NUTRITION PER SERVING	
Serving size	3 to 4 chicken strips plus ⅓ cup sauce
Calories	250 kcal
Fat	10 g
Saturated fat	2.5 g
Cholesterol	86 mg
Sodium	280 mg
Carbohydrates	7 g
Dietary fiber	2 g
Protein	30 g

Pleasing Pumpkin Ice Cream Pie

Alice Henneman, M.S., R.D.

Serves: 8
Hands-on time: 20 minutes
Freezing time: About 4 hours or until firm

The New England colonists heartily embraced the pumpkin, a multi-purpose fruit that became a traditional Thanksgiving food. They used it as a side-dish, soup, dessert, and even made beer of it. This pie can be prepared in advance.

1 quart (4 cups) vanilla ice cream or frozen yogurt, softened
1 15- to 16-ounce can pure pumpkin
¼ cup sugar
1½ to 2 teaspoons pumpkin pie spice
1 9- or 10-inch reduced-fat graham cracker pie crust
fat-free whipped topping, optional

Soften the ice cream or frozen yogurt by storing in the refrigerator for 25 to 30 minutes, or at room for temperature for 10 to 15 minutes.

Mix the pumpkin, sugar, and spice; stir in the softened ice cream and mix well. Pour into the pie crust and freeze, uncovered, until firm, about 4 hours.

COOK'S TIPS

The lower the fat content of ice cream and frozen yogurt, the faster it may melt. Avoid repeatedly softening and refreezing ice cream and frozen yogurt as this makes the texture icy. For longer storage, seal with freezer-quality foil or a plastic freezer bag with the air sealed out. Or pack the pumpkin/ice cream mixture into a tightly sealed container. It will keep for up to two weeks.

NUTRITION NUGGET

To omit the calories and fat of the crust, pour ¾ cup of the pumpkin mixture into 8 custard cups, cover, and freeze.

NUTRITION PER SERVING

Serving size	⅛ of pie with vanilla ice cream
Calories	320 kcal
Fat	15 g
Saturated fat	6 g
Cholesterol	30 mg
Sodium	230 mg
Carbohydrates	46 g
Dietary fiber	2 g
Protein	4 g

NUTRITION PER SERVING

Serving size	⅛ of pie with low-fat frozen yogurt
Calories	290 kcal
Fat	9 g
Saturated fat	2.5 g
Cholesterol	5 mg
Sodium	230 mg
Carbohydrates	48 g
Dietary fiber	2 g
Protein	6 g

Cover with plastic wrap until ready to serve. For longer storage, seal tightly with heavy duty aluminum foil. Remove from the freezer 15 minutes before serving. Top with whipped topping, if desired.

SUBSTITUTIONS

If you don't have pumpkin pie spice, for each teaspoon of pumpkin pie spice, you can substitute the following: ½ teaspoon ground cinnamon, ¼ teaspoon ground ginger, ⅛ teaspoon ground nutmeg, and ⅛ teaspoon ground cloves. If you're missing some of these spices, it might be simplest just to buy pumpkin pie spice. Additional uses of pumpkin pie spice are as a flavoring for sweet potatoes, acorn squash, and French toast. Or, add it to baked products such as banana bread, zucchini bread, and carrot cake; use about a ½ teaspoon per cup of batter.

NUTRITION NUGGET

Pumpkin is a good source of beta-carotene, a nutrient that may help reduce the risk of developing certain types of cancer, and offers possible protection against heart disease. Don't limit serving this dessert to just holidays!

Broiled Strawberries with Balsamic Vanilla Sauce

Kathleen Schaderr, M.B.A., M.S., R.D., L.D.

Serves: 4
Hands-on time: 10 minutes
Cooking time: 35 minutes

This tangy blend of flavors is perfect on just-picked berries. You can enjoy this recipe year round as a luscious low-calorie dessert. The New England colonists (who lived in my backyard) said that strawberries in America were four times larger than the ones they ate in England.

- ½ cup balsamic vinegar
- 1 4-inch vanilla bean or 2 teaspoons vanilla extract
- 4 prunes (cherry flavor works well), diced
- 1 tablespoon brown sugar
- butter-flavored cooking spray
- 1 quart strawberries, washed, hulled, stem sides cut off (to help them sit securely in pan)
- 8 ounces low-fat vanilla yogurt, or 2 cups low-fat frozen yogurt, optional

Combine the vinegar, vanilla, prunes, and brown sugar in a small saucepan. Bring to a boil, reduce heat, and cook until reduced in volume by half, about 30 minutes. If using a real vanilla bean, remove from sauce. The sauce can be stored in the refrigerator for up to 1 week.

Preheat broiler. Spray an oven-safe pan with the cooking spray, and arrange the whole berries stem side down in pan. The berries should be touching. Pour the sauce over the berries, and broil, 3 to 4 inches from heat, for 3 to 5 minutes.

Serve plain or with ¼ cup low-fat vanilla yogurt or ½ cup low-fat frozen yogurt.

NUTRITION PER SERVING

Serving size	1 cup broiled strawberries plus 2 tablespoons sauce
Calories	100 kcal
Fat	0.5 g
Saturated fat	0 g
Cholesterol	0 mg
Sodium	10 mg
Carbohydrates	23 g
Dietary fiber	4 g
Protein	1 g

Cinnamon Raisin Apple Indian Pudding

Kristine Napier, M.P.H., R.D.

Serve this version of a New England colonial favorite for breakfast or dessert.

Serves: 9
Hands-on time: 15 minutes
Baking time: 1 hour

- vegetable oil cooking spray
- 1 quart (4 cups) nonfat milk
- ⅔ cup yellow cornmeal
- ¼ cup packed brown sugar
- 1 teaspoon ground cinnamon
- 1 teaspoon salt
- 2 eggs, lightly beaten
- ½ cup packed raisins
- 4 apples (peel on), cored and chopped

Preheat oven to 350°F. Spray a 9-inch square baking dish with the cooking spray.

In a heavy saucepan, heat the milk to boiling. Whisk in the cornmeal. Cook and stir until thick, about 3 minutes.

Remove from heat. Stir in the brown sugar, cinnamon, and salt. Stir in the eggs, raisins, and apples. Pour into a prepared pan and bake for 60 minutes.

SUBSTITUTION

The colonists used molasses (instead of brown sugar). Substitute an equal amount of molasses to make it this way.

VARIATION

Omit the apples (prepare recipe as directed).

NUTRITION PER SERVING	
Serving size	1 cup
Calories	200 kcal
Fat	1 g
Saturated fat	Less than 0.5 g
Cholesterol	29 mg
Sodium	270 mg
Carbohydrates	43 g
Dietary fiber	3.5 g
Protein	6 g

All-American Apple Pie

Naomi Kakiuchi, R.D., C.D.

Serves: 10
Hands-on time: 30 minutes
Baking time: 40 to 50 minutes

In every corner of the United States, people have a special place in their hearts for apple pie, which originated in the Northeast. Although there are many variations, nothing beats a traditional apple filling cuddled in a flaky pastry. Served warm or cool, with ice cream or cheese, it's a true American comfort food.

- 2 unbaked 8-inch or 9-inch pie shells (recipe follows for Mom's Best Pie Crust)
- 5 cups peeled, cored, and sliced apples (about 2 pounds)
- 3 tablespoons fresh lemon juice
- ¾ cup sugar
- 2 heaping tablespoons flour
- 1 teaspoon cinnamon
- ¼ teaspoon nutmeg
- ⅛ teaspoon salt
- 2 teaspoons butter

Preheat oven to 400°F. Prepare the pie crust.

Sprinkle the apples with lemon juice.

In a large bowl, stir together the sugar, flour, cinnamon, nutmeg, and salt. Add the apples and toss lightly. Spoon into a pastry-lined pie plate. Dot with butter. Cover with the top crust and crimp the edges together. Cut slits in the top crust to allow steam to escape.

Bake until the crust is browned and the filling bubbles through the slits, about 40 to 50 minutes.

NUTRITION PER SERVING	
Serving size	⅒ of pie
Calories	260 kcal
Fat	11 g
Saturated fat	3 g
Cholesterol	15 mg
Sodium	150 mg
Carbohydrates	39 g
Dietary fiber	2 g
Protein	3 g

Mom's Best Pie Crust

Makes 2 two-crust 8-inch or 9-inch pies

- 1 egg
- 4 tablespoons cold water
- 1 tablespoon vinegar
- 3 cups all-purpose flour
- ½ teaspoon salt
- 1 cup shortening

Beat the egg, cold water, and vinegar; set aside.

Stir together the flour and the salt. Using two knives or a pastry blender, cut in the shortening until the mixture resembles coarse crumbs. Add the egg mixture, stirring with a fork to form a ball.

Divide the dough into 2 equal parts. Cut each piece of dough in half and shape the halves into rounds. Roll each round to ⅛-inch thickness on a floured surface to fit an 8-inch or 9-inch pie pan. (If you are making only one pie, freeze half in a tightly sealed plastic bag.)

Dessert Calzones

Marion S. Wollmeringer, M.S., R.D., L.D.N.

Serves: 16
Hands-on time: 1 hour
Baking time: 15 to 20 minutes

Yes, the same dough used to make main dish calzones can be used to make a great dessert. Freeze some before baking for an easy, impressive dessert later.

Dessert Calzone Dough

3 cups stirred all-purpose flour (about 12 ounces)
1½ teaspoons active dry yeast
½ teaspoon salt
1 cup warm water (130°F.)
1 tablespoon olive oil
vegetable oil cooking spray
about 1 teaspoon olive oil or melted butter, optional
filling (recipe follows)

Sift together the flour, yeast, and salt into a large mixer bowl. Slowly add the warm water and olive oil. Mix on low speed, or stir with a large mixing spoon, until the dough pulls away from the sides of the bowl, about 2 to 3 minutes. Knead the dough on a lightly floured surface until smooth and elastic, about 3 to 4 minutes. Cover with a cloth and let rise 20 to 30 minutes. Prepare filling while dough rises.

Preheat oven to 450°F.

Divide the dough into 8 individual balls. On a very lightly floured surface, roll each ball into a 5-inch to 6-inch circle. Place each dough circle on a square of parchment paper. Divide the filling equally between the dough circles, placing it on the lower half of each circle. Fold the top half of the dough over the filling. Seal the dough by pinching a narrow seam or pressing with the tines of a fork. To make sure the filling is distributed throughout the dough, press the top of the filled sealed dough very gently. A tight seal is needed or the filling will leak out. Check the back of the dough edge for a tight seal. Place the calzone and parchment paper on a cookie sheet sprayed with the vegetable oil cooking spray. A jelly roll or pizza pan with a small lip can be used to catch leaks.

Repeat with the remaining dough balls. (If freezing some for later, do so at this point.)

PREPARATION TIP

Stirring the flour before measuring or weighing it will ensure the proper consistency of the dough.

HOW MUCH WATER FOR THE DOUGH?

The amount of water needed depends on the humidity of your kitchen and on the dryness of the flour. The dough should be only slightly sticky. Add 1 or 2 tablespoons flour if the dough is too sticky.

NUTRITION PER SERVING

Serving size	½ calzone
Calories	185 kcal
Fat	5 g
Saturated fat	3 g
Cholesterol	15 mg
Sodium	165 mg
Carbohydrates	29 g
Dietary fiber	1 g
Protein	6 g

Bake for about 15 to 20 minutes, or until the dough is lightly browned and slightly puffed. Remove from the baking sheet to a cooling rack.

Brush the tops with melted butter, if desired.

Serve hot or warm.

Dessert Calzone Filling

2½ cups (10 ounces) chopped dried apricots, peaches, pears, cranberries, cherries, or a combination

8 ounces Brie cheese, cut into 1-ounce pieces

Use a scant ⅓ cup dried fruit (1¼ ounces) and 1 ounce Brie cheese for each calzone.

COOK'S TIP

To prepare frozen calzones, place the still frozen calzone on a baking sheet coated with vegetable oil cooking spray. Place in a cold oven; turn the oven to 350°F. Bake for 25 to 30 minutes, or until golden brown.

COOK'S TIP

Use a baking stone. A pizza stone may be used; follow the instructions specific to your stone.

SUBSTITUTIONS

Whipped light cream cheese or low-fat ricotta cheese may be used instead of the Brie. Spread 2 heaping tablespoons (1 ounce) on half of each circle before adding the fruit filling.

VARIATION

This dough may be used to make pizzas.

Roza's Plum Pie (Zwetschgen Kucken)

Marion S. Wollmeringer, M.S., R.D., L.D.N.

Serves: 10
Hands-on time: 30 to 45 minutes
Baking time: 40 to 45 minutes

My mother was not a baker, but once a year she made a plum pie for my father's birthday. I think it must have been her mother's recipe. When I was old enough, I took over this task and have baked this pie every fall in my Boston kitchen when Italian prune plums are in season. My mother-in-law, who came from the Rhine, did not use the streusel; she slit the tops of the plums so they made attractive peaks and sprinkled the pie with confectioners' sugar when it came out of the oven.

1 cup all-purpose flour
¼ cup sugar
½ teaspoon baking powder
pinch of salt
¼ cup plus 1 tablespoon cold unsalted butter, cut into cubes
1 large egg
2 pounds Italian prune plums (about 28)
almond streusel (recipe follows), optional
confectioners' sugar, optional
whipping cream, beaten, optional

Blend the flour, sugar, baking powder, and salt in a food processor, pulsing 4 or 5 times. Add the butter and pulse 6 to 8 times, until rolled oat-size pieces form. Add the egg and pulse for about 1 minute, until the egg is well distributed and a dough forms.

Turn the dough out on a cold work surface. Knead about 1 minute or until smooth and doughy. Do not overwork, as it will become soft and sticky. Roll out the dough on a well-floured surface to form an 11-inch circle. Transfer to a 9-inch glass pie pan. Fold the edges over to form a rim; crimp the edges. Hold the pan up to the light to see that the dough is evenly distributed.

Preheat oven to 375°F.

Wash the plums; cut in half and remove pits. Place the plums upright in concentric circles on top of the crust. Add the remaining halves to fill in gaps. If using almond streusel, crumble it evenly over fruit. If the pie is made without streusel, slit the tops of the plums so attractive peaks form as the pie bakes. Bake for 40 minutes or until the crust is lightly

COOK'S TIP
If the dough becomes warm and sticky, wrap in plastic, flatten, and refrigerate 15 to 30 minutes.

NUTRITION PER SERVING

Serving size	1/10 of pie without streusel
Calories	170 kcal
Fat	7 g
Saturated fat	4 g
Cholesterol	35 mg
Sodium	45 mg
Carbohydrates	26 g
Dietary fiber	2 g
Protein	3 g

NUTRITION PER SERVING

Serving size	1/10 of pie with streusel
Calories	370 kcal
Fat	16 g
Saturated fat	9 g
Cholesterol	60 mg
Sodium	50 mg
Carbohydrates	53 g
Dietary fiber	2 g
Protein	4 g

browned. (Look at the bottom.) If not using streusel, sprinkle the pie with confectioners' sugar when it comes out of the oven.

Allow the pie to cool. Serve it with whipped cream, if desired.

Make the dough by hand: Sift together the flour, baking powder, and salt. Form sifted ingredients into a wreath on a working surface. Place the sugar in the middle of the wreath. Stir the egg into the sugar until well mixed. Distribute butter cubes over the flour. Quickly work the flour and butter into the sugar-egg mixture. Press with the heel of your hand to blend the butter into the flour mixture. This process is somewhat like kneading dough. (You could do this with a fork; fingers can be too warm.) Wrap in plastic wrap and chill at least 1 hour.

Almond Streusel

½ cup unsalted butter
1⅓ cups all-purpose flour
¾ cup sugar
1 teaspoon almond extract

Melt the butter over medium heat; allow to cool 5 minutes.

Combine the flour and sugar in a small bowl; mix in the butter and almond extract.

SUBSTITUTIONS

Up to 1 tablespoon plus 2 teaspoons of unsalted corn oil margarine can be substituted for an equal quantity of butter (do not use low-fat margarine). 2½ pounds tart apples (such as Macintosh) can be used in place of plums. Peel, core and slice thinly; toss with lemon juice and then follow remaining instructions.

SHOPPING TIP

Italian prune plums are usually available in late August or early September. Summer plums can be used if Italian prune plums are not available. If the pie is made with summer plums, do not crowd the pie pan because plums may weep and cause boilover.

Soft Snickerdoodles

Kristine Napier, M.P.H., R.D.

Serves: 60
Hands-on time: 30 minutes
Chill time: 1 hour
Baking time: 6 to 8 minutes

While the history of the snickerdoodle is as mixed up as the sound of the name, most food historians agree that snickerdoodles are a New England "confection" made with flour, nuts, and dried fruits (especially currants). Somehow, over the years, the nuts and fruits seem to have disappeared. I've put them back for history's sake, and the result is magnificent!

- 2 tablespoons plus 1⅓ cups sugar, divided
- 1 tablespoon ground cinnamon, divided
- 1 cup butter, softened (2 sticks)
- ¾ cup liquid egg substitute
- 2 teaspoons vanilla extract
- 2 cups all-purpose flour
- ¾ cup whole-wheat flour
- 1 teaspoon baking soda
- ½ teaspoon salt
- 2 teaspoons cream of tartar
- 1 cup chopped peanuts
- 1 cup currants
- 1 cup sweetened dried cranberries
- vegetable oil cooking spray

In a shallow bowl, combine 2 tablespoons sugar and 1 teaspoon cinnamon; set aside.

Cream the butter and 1⅓ cups sugar by hand or with an electric mixer; add the egg substitute and vanilla extract.

In a separate bowl, sift together the flours, baking soda, salt, cream of tartar, and 2 teaspoons cinnamon. Add the sifted ingredients to the creamed mixture; stir or beat until well blended. Stir in the peanuts, currants, and cranberries.

Shape generous teaspoons of dough into 1-inch balls and roll in the cinnamon-sugar mixture. Place in a large bowl; refrigerate for one hour.

Preheat oven to 400°F. Lightly coat 2 cookie sheets with the cooking spray. Place the cinnamon-sugar coated balls 2 inches apart on the prepared cookie sheets. Bake the snickerdoodles for 6 to 8 minutes or until lightly browned. Remove to wire racks to cool.

COOK'S TIP

Chilling the dough before baking makes cookies softer after baking. Baking on the shorter side (6 minutes) also helps produce a softer cookie.

NUTRITION PER SERVING

Serving size	1 cookie
Calories	100 kcal
Fat	4.5 g
Saturated fat	2 g
Cholesterol	10 mg
Sodium	45 mg
Carbohydrates	13 g
Dietary fiber	Less than 1 g
Protein	2 g

Hulda's Geburtstag's Kuchen (Pound Cake)

Marion S. Wollmeringer, M.S., R.D., L.D.N.

My dad remembers his German grandmother, Pauline, making this cake. She would sit with the bowl between her knees, stirring and stirring, as his mom, Hulda, learned to do. Now, in my Boston home, I make this family treasure with my Kitchen Aid mixer.

Serves: 20
Hands-on time: 10 to 15 minutes
Baking time: 1 hour for Bundt pan; 50 to 55 minutes for 2 4½-by-8½-inch loaf pans

- 2 cups plus 2 tablespoons sifted all-purpose flour
- 2 teaspoons baking powder
- 1 cup (2 sticks) plus 2 tablespoons unsalted butter, softened
- 1¼ cups sugar
- 6 large eggs
- 1½ to 2 teaspoons lemon or orange rind (1 large)
- 1 teaspoon vanilla extract

Preheat oven to 375°F. Butter a Bundt pan.

Sift the flour and the baking powder into a small bowl; set aside.

Add the butter to a medium-size mixing bowl; using an electric mixer, beat on medium speed until smooth and fluffy. Beat in the sugar, then the eggs, and then the lemon rind and vanilla. Gradually beat in the combined flour and baking powder on low speed. Continue mixing on medium speed until the batter is smooth.

Pour the batter into a prepared Bundt pan. Bake 1 hour or until the cake is golden and a toothpick inserted into the center comes out clean. Remove immediately from the pan and let cool on a rack.

VARIATIONS

Two 8½-by-4½-inch loaf pans can be used in place of the Bundt pan. Decrease baking time to 55 minutes. Add some fruit: one apple, sliced or ½ cup raisins may be stirred into the batter after the combined flour and baking powder have been mixed in.

COOK'S TIP

As the cake bakes, uncooked batter rises and causes a split in the center. This must be baked through.

NUTRITION PER SERVING	
Serving size	1/20 of cake
Calories	210 kcal
Fat	12 g
Saturated fat	7 g
Cholesterol	90 mg
Sodium	20 mg
Carbohydrates	23 g
Dietary fiber	0 g
Protein	3 g

Wild Blueberry Sauce

Kitty Broihier, M.S., R.D.

Serves: 8
Hands-on time: 5 minutes
Cooking time: about 15 minutes

Although you can still find them growing wild in many places, wild blueberries are also a cultivated crop here in Maine. At my house, we buy a couple flats of them every summer. After we've eaten our fill, made jam, and canned some blueberry syrup, I freeze the rest (unwashed) to use in place of regular blueberries throughout the year. This blueberry sauce is great on pancakes or as a dessert sauce over sorbet, fruit, or angel food cake. It's not overly sweet and it takes just a few minutes to prepare.

- ½ cup sugar
- 2 tablespoons cornstarch
- ½ cup cold water
- 2 cups fresh or thawed wild blueberries, washed
- 1 teaspoon lemon zest
- 1 tablespoon fresh lemon juice
- ½ teaspoon cinnamon
- dash nutmeg, optional

Whisk together the sugar, cornstarch, and water in a medium-size saucepan. Stir in the berries. Turn heat to medium high and bring the mixture to a boil, stirring occasionally. Reduce heat to medium and continue to cook, stirring occasionally, until the sauce thickens.

Remove the sauce from heat and stir in the lemon zest, lemon juice, cinnamon, and nutmeg. Serve warm or cooled.

SHOPPING TIP

Fresh wild blueberries are usually only available in New England because they're highly perishable and don't travel well. However, commercially frozen or canned wild blueberries are widely available in the supermarket.

FOOD TRIVIA

The New England colonists often stewed berries and sugar (or maple syrup) to make desserts such as Flummery. This recipe is reminiscent of Flummery, except that Flummery usually had more thickening added so that it could be molded.

NUTRITION PER SERVING

Serving size	¼ cup
Calories	80 kcal
Fat	0 g
Saturated fat	0 g
Cholesterol	0 mg
Sodium	0 mg
Carbohydrates	19 g
Dietary fiber	Less than 1 g
Protein	0 g

2

MID-ATLANTIC STATES

Maryland Crab Feasts to Philly Cheesesteaks

Laura L. Molseed, M.S., R.D., L.D.N.; Frances Largeman, R.D.;
Ellen Garippa; and Kristine Napier, M.P.H., R.D.

The Mid-Atlantic States—once the middle colonies—claim several culinary firsts, including:

- The American café and pastry shop (New York City's Delmonico's Steak House)
- Amusement park foods, such as those found at New York's Coney Island

These states were first inhabited by a group of English immigrants led by Captain John Smith. "Heaven and earth never agreed better to frame a place for man's habitation," said Captain Smith about Chesapeake Bay, where he and his fellow Englishman first settled. Watered well by the Potomac and nearly fifty other rivers, the fertile land was perfect for the settlers to build rice, cotton, and tobacco plantations. They also grew a rainbow range of fruit trees, whose fruit further diversified the cuisine and nutritional profile.

The fruits of Chesapeake Bay and the surrounding Atlantic flavor much of the food in the Mid-Atlantic states. They're complemented by distinctive

The New York Cook Book (Marie Martinelo, 1892) is one of a number of volumes in the Rare Book and Special Collections Division of the Library of Congress that have been consulted by, among others, film art directors trying to create an authentic period feel of the cuisine in their productions. Cuisine, like fashion, changes with time.

ethnic foods that serve as a reflection of many people who populated the land. Other food traditions reflect the creativity and ingenuity of hard-working immigrants. Although north of the Mason-Dixon line, the African influence on food was profound. Let's take a look at some of the culinary traditions they established, as well as the twists and turns of bowls, spoons, and kettles over time to today.

Maryland: From Seafood and Biscuits to Legendary Cakes

Savor Maryland's first cookbooks and you'll discover that state's rich culinary history in its "receipts," as recipes were once called. Three centuries of recipes reveal recurrent themes and ingredients: seafood, corn, and biscuits. Be adventurous and simmer some of the more unusual recipes, such as Muskrat Soup or Brunswick Stew (made with chicken, squirrel, and lima beans).

BEAT THOSE BISCUITS

Biscuits accompanied most meals in nineteenth-century Maryland. The recipe is simple, but the instructions require a good bit of elbow grease. The process calls for beating the biscuit dough with a mallet, a rolling pin, the flat of an axe, or some other heavy object. Some cooks also ran the dough through a beaten biscuit machine, which looks very much like an old-fashioned clothes wringer. The consistency of beaten biscuits is not light and fluffy, but rather hard and crisp. The dough must be beaten for about thirty minutes—just enough time to vent any serious frustrations (and burn off some calories)! Our breakfast strawberry shortcake recipe includes old-fashioned biscuits, but doesn't require this much beating.

My Lady, My Lord

Lady Baltimore Cake is the stuff of legends. This moist, three-layered white cake with a succulent filling of raisins, nuts, and figs, and occasionally other fruit, is covered with fluffy white frosting. The novelist Owen Wister first mentioned the cake in his 1906 novel, *Lady Baltimore*. Legend has it that a young woman gave Wister such a cake, which he later described in his novel. Other folklore says the cake originated with the first Lord Baltimore's wife, who served it at afternoon tea.

Regardless of its origins, the various recipes for this delicious white cake always include raisins, figs, vanilla, and chopped walnuts or pecans. Some recipes call for adding cognac to the frosting. John Shields, in *The Chesapeake Bay Cookbook,* says that Tupperware salespersons who traditionally served Lady Baltimore Cake at home sales events once swore by the "cognac trick" to help increase sales.

What would a lady be without her lord? The story goes that Lord Baltimore, the first governor of Maryland, was appalled at all the egg yolks that went to waste making Lady Baltimore's cake. Along with his trusty head cook, he concocted a rich cake made with egg yolks. He certainly outdid his wife with his frosting, which included almonds, walnuts, vanilla, candied cherries, and also macaroon crumbs and sweet sherry.

Serious About Seafood

Crabs and Old Bay Seasoning go hand-in-hand, or claw-in-claw, as it may be. Ubiquitous in Mid-Atlantic seafood cookery, Old Bay's motto is "Entice with Spice"—and that it does. The recipe for this spice medley is under wraps, but it includes salt, pepper, mustard, pimiento, cloves, bay leaves, mace, cardamom, ginger, and paprika. Marylanders use this wondrous concoction on—and in—everything from crabs to Bloody Marys and, in between, potato chips.

The port town of Baltimore was originally planned to help farmers ship their wares outside the area; the city remains one of the country's most important ports. Baltimore has plentiful friendly locals, known as Baltimoreans, and—part of the year—delicious-to-eat crabs.

Crab Feasts

Ask any Baltimorean what their favorite summer weekend family pastime is, and the answer is often the crab feast. You'll find crab feasts in backyards or crab houses—the latter also called "crab hackeries." Crab hackeries are fun, casual establishments, lined with tables covered in newsprint or brown paper. These roll-up-your-sleeves, good-time celebrations start with boiling a huge pot of water, indoors or out, and then steaming live blue crabs. The crab's Latin name is *Calinectes sapidus,* which means "savory beautiful swimmer." You'll hear complaining about "whacking them into bits" to harvest the sweet flesh, but no one *truly* minds. The reward is just too delicious. In *The Chesapeake Bay Cookbook,* Shield writes: "The crab feast is a Chesapeake social ritual. It is performed for the pleasure and bonding of family and friends."

Blue crabs are in season from May through October. The males are called "jimmies" and the females are "sooks" during the hard-shell stage. When the old shell has been shed and the new one is just forming, the crabs are referred to as soft-shell crabs and are considered quite a delicacy.

Preparing for an old-fashioned crab feast couldn't be easier. You need only fresh, live crabs, a huge vessel in which to steam them, Old Bay Seasoning, newspapers for placemats, and mallets or hammers for cracking the shells. Beer or ginger beer is considered the essential best accompaniment for this wonderfully simple supper.

Crab Cakes

A visit to Maryland or Washington, D.C., wouldn't be complete without sampling crab cakes—an amalgam of fresh crabmeat, bread crumbs, and seasoning.

One *must* use fresh crabmeat, say Marylanders, or a crab cake just isn't a crab cake. However, for those of you in Wisconsin, Nebraska, or Arizona, don't despair; we tested the two recipes in this book (pages 77 and 89), with canned and frozen crabmeat, and we can attest that they are still very good.

Lump crabmeat is the integral ingredient in any self-respecting crab cake. Lump refers to lean, big pieces of crab with absolutely no shell or cartilage. Other key ingredients include mayonnaise, Old Bay Seasoning, and Worcestershire sauce or hot sauce. Tartar sauce, made with more mayonnaise, pickles, and onion is the traditional accompaniment for crab cakes. The cakes are often served with another Chesapeake favorite, coleslaw.

New Jersey: Wolf's Peaches and Submarine Sandwiches

Travel over New Jersey's country roads and you'll see for yourself why freshness is first in New Jersey kitchens. The state is the third largest producer of green peppers. Tomatoes, too, are an important crop. But that's not the most important story of the tomato and New Jersey. The history of the tomato is far more delicious.

Tomatoes: Alias Wolf's Peaches?

The tomato was once feared as a deadly poison because it is a member of the nightshade family of plants. This is why tomatoes were called "Wolf's Peaches." The state of New York banned their consumption in 1820 because officials were convinced that eating tomatoes would cause sudden death.

The image of the tomato changed one day in the 1830s on the steps of the Salem, New Jersey, courthouse. Colonel Robert Gibbon Johnson announced that he would eat an entire basket of Wolf's Peaches. With thousands of onlookers and a marching band playing a somber tune, Colonel Johnson said: "The time will come when this luscious, scarlet apple . . . will form the foundation of a great garden industry, and will be . . . eaten, and enjoyed as an edible food . . . and to help speed that enlightened day, to prove that it will not strike you dead—I am going to eat one right now!" Try our Garden Fresh Tomato Basil Pasta (page 292) or Garlic-Basil-Balsamic Marinated Sliced Tomatoes on a Bed of Cucumbers (page 80).

Submarine Sandwiches

No one can say for sure what came first: the Submarine, the Hoagie, the Grinder, the Dagwood, the Hero, or the Po' Boy sandwich. We have a hunch it may be the Submarine, one version of a king-sized sandwich filled with meats, vegetables, and other trimmings.

Most food historians think the original concept for these sandwiches came from the Italians who immigrated to New York in the late 1800s. No doubt many families claim they were the first to use the name "Submarine Sandwich," but the best story goes to the family of Dominic Conti, who

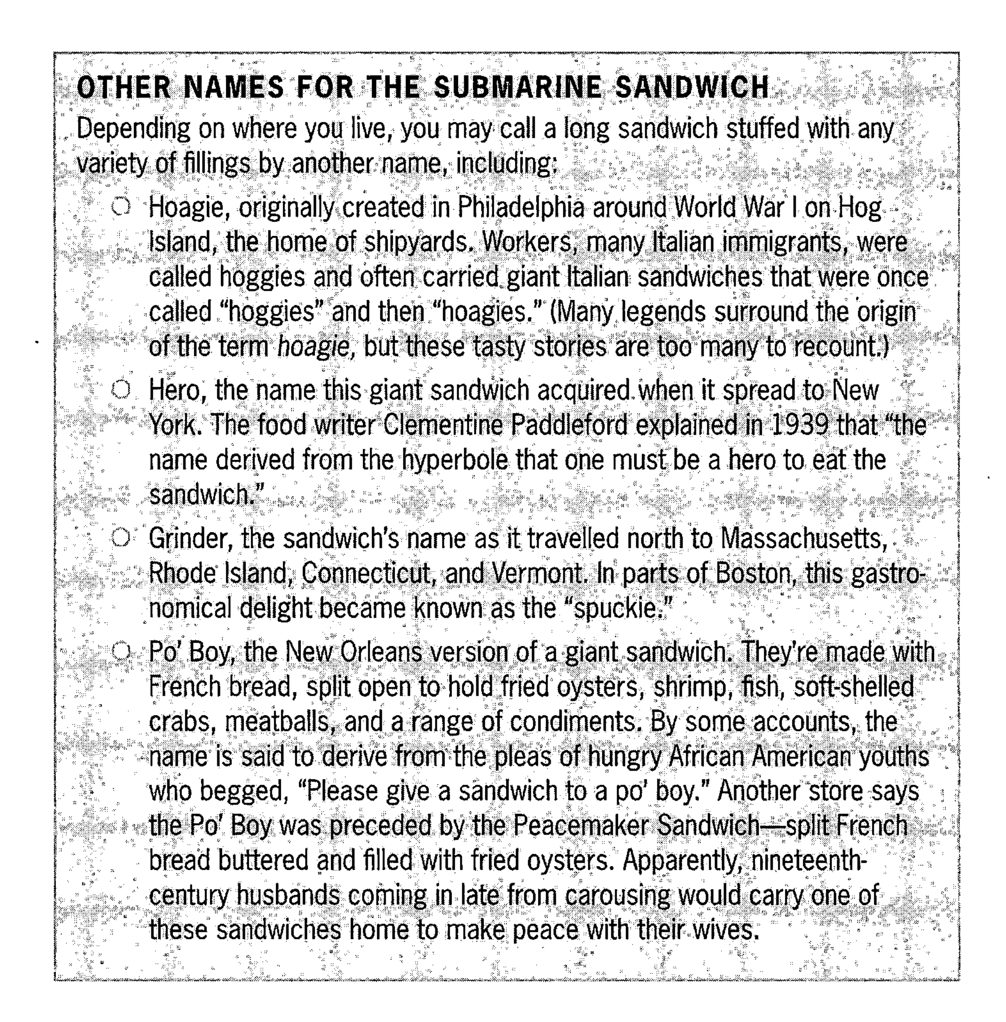

OTHER NAMES FOR THE SUBMARINE SANDWICH

Depending on where you live, you may call a long sandwich stuffed with any variety of fillings by another name, including:

- Hoagie, originally created in Philadelphia around World War I on Hog Island, the home of shipyards. Workers, many Italian immigrants, were called hoggies and often carried giant Italian sandwiches that were once called "hoggies" and then "hoagies." (Many legends surround the origin of the term *hoagie,* but these tasty stories are too many to recount.)
- Hero, the name this giant sandwich acquired when it spread to New York. The food writer Clementine Paddleford explained in 1939 that "the name derived from the hyperbole that one must be a hero to eat the sandwich."
- Grinder, the sandwich's name as it travelled north to Massachusetts, Rhode Island, Connecticut, and Vermont. In parts of Boston, this gastronomical delight became known as the "spuckie."
- Po' Boy, the New Orleans version of a giant sandwich. They're made with French bread, split open to hold fried oysters, shrimp, fish, soft-shelled crabs, meatballs, and a range of condiments. By some accounts, the name is said to derive from the pleas of hungry African American youths who begged, "Please give a sandwich to a po' boy." Another store says the Po' Boy was preceded by the Peacemaker Sandwich—split French bread buttered and filled with fried oysters. Apparently, nineteenth-century husbands coming in late from carousing would carry one of these sandwiches home to make peace with their wives.

traveled to the United States in 1895 from Montella, Italy. He opened Dominic Conti's Grocery Store on Mill Street in Paterson, New Jersey. There, he sold many traditional Italian sandwiches built on long crusty rolls and filled with cold cuts, lettuce, tomatoes, peppers, onions, oil, vinegar, and Italian spices. There was always a layer of cheese next to each slice of bread, so the bread wouldn't get soggy. When Mr. Conti went to see the *Holland I* in 1927 (the first experimental 14-foot submarine), he said, "It looks like the sandwich I sell at my store." Thus, the sandwich was—apparently—dubbed the submarine.

Pennsylvania: Philly Cheesesteaks, Pierogies, Italian Wedding Soup, and More

Travel from eastern to western Pennsylvania, and you'll discover fabulously interesting ethnic pockets of recipes. From the Philly Cheesesteak (Philly Cheesesteak Potato Packets, page 94) and Philly Soft Pretzels (Philly Soft Pretzel Bread Pudding with Chocolate, page 100) to Polish sausage, the highlights are many. Let's sample a few.

Pennsylvania is a treasure trove for food cultures and traditions. A true melting pot, the Pittsburgh area retains many of its ethnic areas and traditions. While most of the Old World languages and clothing have disappeared, many of the foods and accompanying customs survive today. Pockets of ethnic areas and neighborhoods are known not only for their culture, but also for traditional foods, restaurants, and food purveyors, where you can find almost any specialty product that you desire.

Many Cultures

Germans first inhabited Pennsylvania in the 1700s. They were farmers and ship builders and practiced Mennonite, Jewish, or Lutheran faiths. They led thrifty and sober lifestyles. Their traditional staple foods were fairly bland, but heavy, featuring sausage, eggs, ham, and pork. Vegetables they grew and harvested were generally sold rather than cooked to lighten up their family meals.

As the eighteenth century turned into the nineteenth, Germans were followed to Western Pennsylvania by the Scots and the Irish. Then the steel and tin mills and coal mines brought a culinary revolution. Russian, Hungarian, Polish, Ukrainian, and Slovakian men immigrated to the area to work in the steel mills and coal mines so they could send money to their families in the Old World. Their lifestyle defined the culinary flavors. The men lived in boarding houses and worked long hours. Inexpensive, fat-laden, and calorie-dense foods made up the typical menus for the men—economical food that kept them going for long hours. The men often cooked together and prepared large portions. They would pack their meals in tin cans to take to the mill for lunch the next day. The tin cans were ideal containers, as the lunches could be warmed in the can, over the fire in the mills.

Kielbasa, sauerkraut (page 96), halusky (noodle dumplings), mushroom and bean soups, pierogies, goulash, "pigs in a blanket," cabbage rolls, and a variety of other cabbage dishes were typical foods. (See Unstuffed Cabbage Casserole, page 97 and Bavarian Red Cabbage, page 82.) Many of these are still staples for western Pennsylvania families. Kielbasa will always be found at local tailgate parties, and mushroom soup is served in many households on New Year's Eve for good luck. Pierogies—which are pasta pockets filled with mashed potatoes alone, mashed potatoes with onions and cheese, sweet potatoes, sauerkraut, or a sweet filling—are boiled or sautéed with butter and onions and are found on many family dinner tables. In the fall, a few of the remaining Polish churches have pierogie sales. The ladies of the church prepare pierogies in the traditional way and residents throughout the area place their orders weeks in advance. Drive-through pierogie restaurants can be found in Pittsburgh, and trendy restaurants now serve pierogie pizza. Mashed potatoes, cheese, and onions baked on pizza dough is a fabulous treat!

Northern Italians also arrived in the 1800s to work in the mills. Their countrymen from the Italian south followed and were the ethnic group that brought most of the lasting culinary traditions to the area. These workers supported the rapidly expanding area with their carpentry skills and businesses, including specialty food shops and restaurants. Italian restaurants and food stores are still in abundance in the area.

Celebrations and Holidays

Celebrations and holidays have provided some of the most enduring food traditions. Best known by all western Pennsylvanians are Italian Wedding Soup (page 85), cookie tables, and Christmas Eve fish dinners. Wedding soup is standard fare at most weddings in western Pennsylvania. The soup is served to provide the happy couple with stamina for the wedding night. Wedding soup originally had nothing to do with the wedding celebration. In the Old Country, it was just a bad translation that led to this lasting tradition. *Minestra maritata* means only "married soup." When something is *maritata*, it "works well together." For the soup, this simply means that the vegetables and meat in a clear broth are a wonderful combination. Regardless, you will find wedding soup as the first course at many Pittsburgh wedding receptions as well as on menus in both Italian and non-Italian restaurants and cafeterias throughout the area.

Another custom found at most area weddings and other family celebrations is the cookie table. Although not specific to any culture or ethnicity, cookie tables have been a part of most family celebrations for generations. The history of the beginning of the cookie table is unclear. Many feel that it evolved from a variety of European traditions. At weddings in Germany, Poland, and many Slovakian countries, a sweet or pastry was given to the couple as a gift, to the guests as a thank-you, or to the villagers as a sign of good luck for the couple. In Italy, candy-coated almonds were given to the guests during the reception. Cookies may have become a part of the wedding celebration in this country, as so many of the immigrants were poor.

Another theory is that the cookie table is a symbol of the merging of two families. The families of the bride and groom, aunts and cousins included, provide a mix of their favorite cookies that are blended together on the table. Today, families still cook for weeks on end before the big occasion, or for those with little time, many area bakeries now provide a variety of delectable treats. Often the cookies disappear long before the wedding cake has been cut. There are not any standard cookies for a cookie table, but you can be fairly certain to find Italian love knots, nut rolls, ladylocks, thumbprint cookies, pizzelles—and, of course, chocolate chip cookies, which were named Pennsylvania's official cookie in 2003 (Must-Have Chocolate Chip Cookies, page 101).

The Christmas and New Year's holidays also have many culinary customs that are observed throughout Pennsylvania. Christmas Eve for those of Polish and Italian heritage is the biggest feast of the year. Polish families believed that Christmas Eve was a magical evening. It was the one night of the year that animals could speak and the water in the family or town well turned to wine at midnight. Christmas Eve dinners were a big event, also surrounded with much superstition. The meal must include an odd number of courses, typically seven, nine, or eleven. There must not be an odd number of people at the table, and most dishes are based on fish. One of the most common fish dishes served is baccala, made with dried, salted cod. For Italians, primarily those of southern Italian heritage, the "seven fish dinner" is a common practice. The significance of seven fish has many tales and possible meanings. They include a celebration of the seven days for the creation, the seven catholic sacraments, Mary and Joseph's seven-day journey to Bethlehem, the seven sins of the world, the seven hills of Rome, or the seven wonders of the world. Whatever the origin, the dinner is one of the biggest of the year for most families. The fish served varies according to the family, but common dishes include smelt, calamari (both fried and boiled), shrimp, baccala, eel, and linguine with clam sauce. Other pasta dishes (Saffron Seafood Pasta, page 91) are served and dinner is finished with the Italian dessert bread, panettone.

New Year's Eve and New Year's Day have numerous traditions and superstitions of their own. Mushroom and bean soups are served by many cultures on New Year's Eve for good luck in the new year. Pork and sauerkraut (German Sauerkraut, page 96) are traditional items brought by German and Polish settlers. Eating pork on New Year's Day is supposed to "root out your fortune," while eating chicken on New Year's Day is said to "bury your fortune." Cabbage is a symbol of prosperity and good luck, and sauerkraut and "pigs in a blanket" are a common part of the dinner spread. Italian families celebrate with lasagna (White Lasagna with Creamed Mushrooms, page 296), veal, pepperoni, and rum cake.

The ethnic centers in Pennsylvania provide a range of ideas and lend creativity to the cuisine of the area. While traditional foods remain a significant part of the diet and family gatherings, restaurants and chefs have begun to capitalize on the flavors and styles of traditional cuisine and are creating trendy new foods in their eating establishments. Yes, some of our ancestors are likely turning over in their graves as one ethnic culinary tradition fuses with another, but that is a characteristic of American cuisine.

Melon Smoothie

Rebecca Sparks, R.D.

Serves: 2
Hands-on time: 5 minutes

When melon is plentiful, as it is in July and August in New Jersey, freeze extra so that you can enjoy this refreshing smoothie for breakfast, dessert, or a snack in the winter.

½ cantaloupe, cut up and frozen
1 cup fat-free vanilla yogurt
1 cup vanilla soy milk, or 1 cup nonfat milk
½ cup orange juice
½ teaspoon cinnamon

Place all ingredients in a blender and process until smooth. Serve immediately.

VARIATION

To bump up the fiber, add 2 to 4 tablespoons milled or ground flaxseed before blending. (2 tablespoons adds about 1 gram fiber per serving.)

NUTRITION PER SERVING	
Serving size	1¼ cups
Calories	210 kcal
Fat	0.5 g
Saturated fat	0 g
Cholesterol	5 mg
Sodium	160 mg
Carbohydrates	40 g
Dietary fiber	Less than 1 g
Protein	11 g

Parmesan Tomato Asparagus Frittata

Kristine Napier, M.P.H., R.D.

Created in honor of the state of New Jersey, where tomatoes were boldly introduced into American culture, this one-step omelet combines three wonderful ingredients to produce a burst of gentle yet definitive flavor.

Serves: 4
Hands-on time: 10 minutes
Cooking time: 20 minutes

- vegetable oil cooking spray
- 2 medium-size tomatoes, thinly sliced
- ½ pound very thin fresh asparagus spear tips (3 inches in length, including tip)
- ½ cup Parmesan cheese, shredded (divided use)
- 4 large eggs, gently beaten
- ¼ teaspoon salt

Spray a large nonstick skillet with the vegetable oil spray; place over medium-low heat. Place half of the tomato slices on the bottom of the pan, overlapping. Top with half of the asparagus. Repeat. Sprinkle with half of the Parmesan cheese. Pour the egg over the top; sprinkle with salt. Cover and cook over low heat 20 minutes.

Slide the omelet onto a large serving platter. Sprinkle with the remaining Parmesan cheese.

COOK'S TIP
Use the leftover asparagus to make Creamy Asparagus Soup (page 36).

NUTRITION NUGGET
Reduce cholesterol, fat, and calories by substituting 1 cup liquid egg substitute for the four eggs.

NUTRITION PER SERVING

Serving size	¼ omelet
Calories	140 kcal
Fat	8 g
Saturated fat	3.5 g
Cholesterol	220 mg
Sodium	380 mg
Carbohydrates	5 g
Dietary fiber	1 g
Protein	11 g

Strawberry Shortcake

Kristine Napier, M.P.H., R.D.

Serves: 6
Hands-on time: 15 minutes
Baking time: 12 to 15 minutes

A great combination of all-time favorite Maryland beaten biscuits and early-summer-plentiful strawberries, this recipe is as great for a dessert as it is for breakfast.

- ½ cup all-purpose flour
- ⅓ cup whole wheat flour
- 3 tablespoons divided, plus 2 teaspoons sugar
- 2 teaspoons baking powder
- ½ teaspoon baking soda
- ½ teaspoon salt
- 2 tablespoons extra-virgin olive oil
- ½ cup nonfat milk
- 6 cups fresh strawberries
- 2 cups nonfat vanilla yogurt (choose one with 90 calories per 6 ounce)

Preheat oven to 450°F. Combine the flours, 3 tablespoons sugar (reserve 2 teaspoons for biscuit tops), baking powder, baking soda, and salt in a medium-size bowl. Add the oil and milk; beat with a spoon 30 to 40 strokes.

Drop 6 heaping tablespoons of batter onto an ungreased baking sheet. Bake 12 to 14 minutes, or until lightly golden brown. (After baking, remove from the pan to cool for 5 minutes.)

Meanwhile, slice the strawberries and place in a large bowl. Mix 1 cup sliced strawberries with 2 tablespoons sugar in a small bowl; mash with a fork. Alternatively, purée in a food processor. Pour mashed or puréed strawberries over the sliced berries; stir to mix. Set aside.

To serve, break each biscuit in half; place in a bowl. Top with ¾ cup strawberries and ⅓ cup yogurt.

VARIATION

Try nonfat lemon yogurt for a tangier version.

COOK'S TIP

Freeze completely cooled biscuits in a tightly sealing bag or container up to 1 month.

NUTRITION PER SERVING	
Serving size	1 biscuit, ¾ cup strawberries, ⅓ cup yogurt
Calories	260 kcal
Fat	5 g
Saturated fat	0.5 g
Cholesterol	5 mg
Sodium	360 mg
Carbohydrates	49 g
Dietary fiber	4 g
Protein	7 g

Lamb-Stuffed Grape Leaves

Jackie Newgent, R.D., C.D.N.

They might look like "green cigars" to those not familiar with them, but they're delicacies to those who know them. Luckily, stuffed grape leaves are becoming mainstream—even in Middle America. The leaves are available packed in brine. They can be picked fresh off grapevines, too. This dish always brings back fond family memories of picking leaves off grapevines throughout northeast Ohio—whether behind my house or off less-traveled roads. The best part, besides eating this delightful finger food, is having the whole family pitch in stuffing and rolling the leaves. I still make them in my New York City home, where ethnic recipes like this Lebanese one fuse together to form a colorful cuisine.

Serves: 8
Hands-on time: 45 minutes
Cooking time: 1 hour, 15 minutes

1½ pounds ground lamb
3 onions, finely chopped
1 cup uncooked basmati rice
1 teaspoon sea salt
1 teaspoon freshly ground black pepper, or to taste
1 teaspoon ground cinnamon
½ teaspoon ground allspice
¼ cup minced fresh dill
¼ cup minced fresh mint
3 tablespoons finely chopped toasted pine nuts, optional
3 tablespoons finely chopped or puréed currants, optional
1 1-pound jar grape leaves
juice of 1 large lemon
1 tablespoon butter, melted

Combine the lamb, onions, rice, salt, pepper, cinnamon, allspice, dill, mint, and, if using, pine nuts and currants. Stir in ¼ cup water and mix well.

Drain the brine from the jar of grape leaves. Rinse the leaves well. Lay out on paper towels and pat dry. Place a heaping tablespoon of meat and rice mixture in the center of a leaf's dull side. Roll the leaf tightly, folding the edges over and rolling toward the point of the leaf.

SUBSTITUTION

Use 3 tablespoons bottled lemon juice if you do not have a fresh lemon.

NUTRITION PER SERVING	
Serving size	7 to 8 stuffed leaves
Calories	400 kcal
Fat	20 g
Saturated fat	8 g
Cholesterol	85 mg
Sodium	580 mg
Carbohydrates	30 g
Dietary fiber	1 g
Protein	26 g

Lamb-Stuffed Grape Leaves *(continued)*

Cover the bottom of a Dutch oven or a large saucepan with torn leaves. Arrange the rolls in layers on top of the torn leaves. Pour water over the rolls until just covered. Drizzle with lemon juice and melted butter. Cover with a heavy plate to keep the rolls from opening during cooking. Cover the saucepan and cook over low heat for 1 hour and 15 minutes. Remove from heat and keep covered until time to serve. Serve warm.

Corn Bread–Crusted Crab Cakes

Frances Largeman, R.D.

Slightly southern, definitely Chesapeake, these corn bread–encrusted crab cakes are a delightful variation of the traditional version. Make a batch of corn bread from a mix the day before to make the crumbs, or try the Moist Corn Bread recipe on page 168. Lump crabmeat from the animal's back fin is preferred over shredded meat from the rest of the crab, but frozen or canned are okay, too, such as fresh-pack pasteurized claw meat.

Serves: 12 as an appetizer or 6 as a main course
Hands-on time: 15 minutes
Cooking time: 15 minutes

4 3-by-3-inch pieces corn bread, dried overnight
1 pound fresh lump crabmeat, shell removed
⅓ cup chopped flat-leaf parsley
3 scallions, chopped
1 medium-size red bell pepper, minced
2 tablespoons freshly squeezed lemon juice
1 tablespoon nonfat milk
2 teaspoons hot sauce
¼ teaspoon salt
¼ teaspoon pepper
2 egg whites, lightly beaten
2 tablespoons reduced-fat mayonnaise
3 tablespoons canola oil
lemon wedges and parsley sprigs for garnish

SAUCE
2 tablespoons reduced-fat mayonnaise
1 to 2 teaspoons Old Bay seasoning

Place the dried corn bread in a food processor; process until crumbed. Set aside.

Combine 1½ cups crumbs, the crab, parsley, scallions, red pepper, lemon juice, milk, hot sauce, salt, pepper, egg whites, and mayonnaise. Mix well and set aside. (May be covered and refrigerated for up to a day.)

Place the remaining corn bread crumbs in a flat pan.

Divide the crabmeat mixture into 12 portions and shape into patties. Squeeze gently to remove excess moisture. Roll the patties in the corn bread crumbs.

Heat 1½ tablespoons oil in a large nonstick skillet over medium-high heat. Add 6 patties and cook for 4 minutes, or until golden brown. Turn patties and cook for another 4 minutes. Transfer to a plate. Add the remaining oil to the skillet, and cook the rest of the patties.

Combine the mayonnaise and Old Bay seasoning to create a sauce.

SHOPPING TIP
Crab cakes can be made with frozen or canned crabmeat.

NUTRITION PER SERVING

Serving size	2 crab cakes
Calories	280 kcal
Fat	11 g
Saturated fat	1.5 g
Cholesterol	95 mg
Sodium	1,530 mg
Carbohydrates	20 g
Dietary fiber	2 g
Protein	22 g

Philly Steak Quesadillas

Laura Faler Thomas, M.Ed., R.D., L.D.

Serves: 12 as an appetizer or 4 as a main course
Hands-on time: 15 minutes
Cooking time: 10 minutes

Enjoy the classic taste of the Philly cheesesteak in the form of a quesadilla—fusion cuisine at its best!

- vegetable oil cooking spray
- 1 green bell pepper, thinly sliced
- 1 yellow bell pepper, thinly sliced
- 1 red bell pepper, thinly sliced
- 1 medium-size onion, thinly sliced
- 1 cup shredded part-skim Mozzarella cheese (4 ounces)
- 6 10-inch flour tortillas
- 4 ounces thinly sliced deli roast beef

Coat a large nonstick skillet with the cooking spray, and cook the peppers and onion 5 minutes or until crisp-tender. Remove from the pan; keep warm. Do not wash the pan.

Sprinkle 2 tablespoons cheese over each of 3 tortillas. Top each evenly with roast beef. Sprinkle the remaining cheese evenly over the top of the roast beef. Top each with another tortilla.

Cook each quesadilla in the skillet over medium-high heat, 1 minute per side, or until the cheese is melted. Cut each into 4 wedges; serve with the cooked vegetables.

NUTRITION PER SERVING

Serving size	3 wedges, main course
Calories	500 kcal
Fat	14 g
Saturated fat	5 g
Cholesterol	30 mg
Sodium	960 mg
Carbohydrates	70 g
Dietary fiber	6 g
Protein	24 g

NUTRITION PER SERVING

Serving size	1 wedge, appetizer
Calories	170 kcal
Fat	4.5 g
Saturated fat	2 g
Cholesterol	10 mg
Sodium	320 mg
Carbohydrates	23 g
Dietary fiber	2 g
Protein	8 g

Tangy Vegetable Dip

Robin Thomas, M.S., R.D., L.N.

This great dip will make vegetables disappear. We also love it as a seafood cocktail sauce in our Maryland home. Versatile indeed, it's also an excellent accompaniment to roast beef.

Serves: 6
Hands-on time: 5 minutes
Chill time: overnight

- 1 cup reduced-fat sour cream, or low-fat plain yogurt
- ½ cup bottled chili sauce
- 1½ teaspoons Worcestershire sauce
- 1½ teaspoons prepared horseradish

Whisk together all ingredients; chill.

VARIATION
Omit the Worcestershire sauce or horseradish, and adjust the remaining ingredients to taste.

COOK'S TIP
Store leftovers up to a week or 10 days, covered tightly, in the refrigerator.

NUTRITION PER SERVING	
Serving size	¼ cup
Calories	60 kcal
Fat	1 g
Saturated fat	0.5 g
Cholesterol	5 mg
Sodium	680 mg
Carbohydrates	10 g
Dietary fiber	0 g
Protein	2 g

Garlic-Basil-Balsamic Marinated Sliced Tomatoes on a Bed of Cucumbers

Kristine Napier, M.P.H., R.D.

Serves: 6.
Hands-on time: 15 minutes
Marinating time: 1 hour

Slightly trendy, but definitely garden fresh, this recipe is at home in New Jersey, where tomato farming is so important to the economy, and anywhere else.

- 4 cloves garlic, minced
- ½ cup minced fresh basil, divided
- 2 tablespoons extra-virgin olive oil
- ¼ cup balsamic vinegar
- 1 tablespoon sugar
- 4 ripe unpeeled tomatoes, sliced thinly
- 2 garden fresh or 1 English unpeeled cucumber, scrubbed, dried, and chopped coarsely
- freshly ground black pepper to taste

Combine the garlic, ¼ cup basil, oil, vinegar, and sugar in a shallow glass dish. Add the tomato slices. Spoon the mixture over the tomatoes evenly. Marinate at room temperature 1 hour, stirring once and turning the tomatoes.

Make a bed of chopped cucumbers and the remaining ¼ cup basil. Spoon the sliced tomatoes evenly over the top. Sprinkle with freshly ground black pepper.

Serve the remaining marinade as an optional topping.

NUTRITION PER SERVING	
Serving size	1 cup
Calories	90 kcal
Fat	1 g
Saturated fat	0.5 g
Cholesterol	0 mg
Sodium	10 mg
Carbohydrates	11 g
Dietary fiber	2 g
Protein	2 g

Roasted Spring Asparagus

Frances Largeman, R.D.

Asparagus doesn't last long in the Mid-Atlantic region, only the months of May and June. Although you can grill, steam, or broil asparagus, I especially love it roasted. This tasty and simple dish goes well with chicken, lamb, or fish.

Serves: 8
Hands-on time: 10 minutes
Cooking time: 20 minutes

1 pound thin asparagus spears
1 tablespoon extra-virgin olive oil
½ teaspoon salt
¼ to 1 teaspoon freshly ground pepper, or to taste
2 teaspoons truffle oil, optional

Preheat oven to 425°F.

Clean and trim the asparagus. Peel the ends if the spears are thick.

Drizzle a roasting pan with the olive oil and lay the asparagus evenly in the pan. Turn to coat with the oil. Season with salt and pepper.

Roast the asparagus for approximately 20 minutes, or until the stalks are tender yet crisp. Remove from the pan and transfer to a serving dish. Drizzle with the truffle oil, if using. Serve warm or at room temperature.

FOOD TRIVIA

Asparagus is a member of the lily family.

COOK'S TIP

Truffle oil is olive oil that has been infused with the flavor of black truffles; it imparts a rich, earthy flavor to cooked foods.

SHOPPING TIPS

Whether you bring home stalks from the farmer's market or from your local grocery, make sure the spears are firm and fresh looking and the tips are tightly closed. Asparagus should be eaten within a few days for the best flavor. The best way to store asparagus in the refrigerator is to cut off an inch from the stalk and stand the spears upright in an inch or two of water, covered with a plastic bag.

NUTRITION NUGGET

Asparagus is a great source of folate, iron, and potassium. This vegetable is also high in vitamins A and C.

FOOD TRIVIA

In addition to the common green color, asparagus also comes in purple and white varieties. The purple asparagus turns green when cooked. The prized white variety is cultivated by covering the stalks with mounds of earth to prevent the development of chlorophyll, which creates the green hue.

NUTRITION PER SERVING	
Serving size	About 6 spears
Calories	30 kcal
Fat	2 g
Saturated fat	0 g
Cholesterol	0 mg
Sodium	150 mg
Carbohydrates	3 g
Dietary fiber	1 g
Protein	1 g

Bavarian Red Cabbage

Susan Braverman, M.S., R.D., C.D.N., F.A.D.A.

Serves: 6
Hands-on time: 15 minutes
Cooking time: 40 minutes

In New York, we know German dishes well from my Pennsylvania neighbors. Such recipes are a staple due to the immigrants who brought their rich German heritage.

- 2 tablespoons canola oil
- small head of red cabbage (about 3 pounds), shredded
- 2 tart green apples, chopped
- 2 bay leaves
- ½ teaspoon ground cloves
- ½ teaspoon ground ginger
- ½ teaspoon salt
- 1 tablespoon sugar
- 3 tablespoons lemon juice

Heat the oil in a large, heavy soup kettle. Add the cabbage and brown about 4 to 6 minutes, stirring occasionally.

Add the apples, bay leaves, cloves, ginger, salt, sugar, and 1½ cups water. Bring to a boil; reduce heat, cover, and simmer 30 minutes.

Remove and discard the bay leaves. Stir in the lemon juice.

NUTRITION PER SERVING	
Serving size	2 cups
Calories	130 kcal
Fat	5 g
Saturated fat	0 g
Cholesterol	0 mg
Sodium	220 mg
Carbohydrates	23 g
Dietary fiber	6 g
Protein	3 g

Maryland Oyster Stew

Edee Howard Hogan, R.D., L.D.

Make this delicious stew with fresh Maryland oysters or canned ones. Just be sure to try this incredibly easy version of a classic. You'll find it's great for Sunday supper with oyster crackers, a nice salad, and warm fruit cobbler for dessert.

Serves: 8
Hands-on time: 10 minutes
Cooking time: 15 minutes

¼ cup flour
1 cup plus 5 cups nonfat milk
½ cup butter
1 quart shucked oysters with liquid
1 teaspoon salt
¼ teaspoon pepper
½ teaspoon paprika, or to taste
1 tablespoon chopped parsley
oyster crackers

Stir the flour into 1 cup milk until smooth; set aside.

Melt the butter in a 3-quart double boiler or a heavy saucepan. Add the oysters with their own liquid and bring just to the boiling point, but *do not boil*. Slowly stir in the milk and the flour mixture (stir first), the remaining 5 cups milk, and the salt, pepper, and paprika. Heat until the edges of the oysters curl. Stir in the parsley.

Serve immediately with oyster crackers.

SUBSTITUTION

Substitute three 6½-ounce cans oysters for the fresh.

NUTRITION PER SERVING	
Serving size	1½ cups
Calories	290 kcal
Fat	18 g
Saturated fat	10 g
Cholesterol	115 mg
Sodium	520 mg
Carbohydrates	17 g
Dietary fiber	0 g
Protein	15 g

Bethany Beach Summer Green Soup

Edee Howard Hogan, R.D., L.D.

Serves: 8
Hands-on time: 20 minutes
Cooking time: 25 to 35 minutes

This soup is standard fare at our Bethany Beach, Maryland, home. The combination of zucchini, which is always plentiful at the shore in the summer, and peas creates a rich buttery soup. When our grandchildren come to visit, they get the job of shelling the peas—but they don't mind because they love the soup!

- 3 tablespoons extra-virgin olive oil
- 2 medium-size onions, chopped
- 3 cloves garlic, chopped
- 4 medium-size zucchini, unpeeled, sliced
- 1½ teaspoons salt
- ½ teaspoon pepper
- 1 tablespoon dried thyme
- 4 cups homemade chicken stock, or 2 14-ounce cans reduced-sodium chicken broth
- 1 10-ounce package frozen petite peas, or 2 cups fresh peas (about 2 pounds in the pod)
- 1 tablespoon lemon juice
- ½ cup reduced-fat sour cream, optional garnish
- sprigs of fresh dill and/or thyme for garnish

In a heavy soup kettle, combine the oil, onions, and garlic over medium-low heat. Sauté 4 to 5 minutes, or until translucent. Add the zucchini, salt, pepper, thyme, and chicken stock. Cover and simmer 10 minutes. Add the peas; cover and simmer 5 to 7 minutes more, or until the vegetables are tender.

Remove from heat; stir in the lemon juice. Mash the vegetables with a potato masher for a chunky soup, blend in a food processor for a smoother soup, or use a blender for very smooth soup. If using a blender, cool the soup first and do not fill the blender container more than half full, as hot liquids expand.

Serve the soup with a dollop of sour cream in the middle; swirl in a pretty design for a festive look. Garnish with fresh herb sprigs if desired.

COOK'S TIP
Soup can be stored, tightly covered, for up to 4 days in the refrigerator.

NUTRITION PER SERVING	
Serving size	1 cup
Calories	150 kcal
Fat	8 g
Saturated fat	2.5 g
Cholesterol	10 mg
Sodium	500 mg
Carbohydrates	14 g
Dietary fiber	3 g
Protein	6 g

Italian Wedding Soup

Laura L. Molseed, M.S., R.D., L.D.N.

A classic Italian soup made of chicken broth, small meatballs, greens, and pastina. This soup is traditionally served as the first course at many wedding celebrations in western Pennsylvania. It is said to give the bride and groom stamina for the evening!

Serves: 6
Hands-on time: 40 minutes
Cooking time: 30 minutes

- 1 tablespoon olive oil
- 1 medium-size onion, chopped
- 1 clove garlic, minced
- 6 cups chicken stock or low-sodium chicken broth
- 1 carrot, cut into 1-inch long julienne
- 1 tablespoon chopped fresh oregano or 1 teaspoon dried
- 1½ cups shredded escarole, spinach, or arugula
- 20 to 30 1-inch meatballs (recipe follows)
- 1 cup cubed cooked chicken (6 ounces uncooked)
- ½ cup uncooked pastina (any quick-cooking small pasta such as *acini di pepe*)
- 1 teaspoon salt
- ¼ teaspoon pepper, or to taste
- ¾ cup grated Parmesan cheese

Heat the oil in an 8-quart stockpot over medium heat. Add the onion and the garlic. Sauté until translucent. Add the chicken stock, carrot, and oregano. Cook over medium heat for 5 minutes or until the broth is hot. Add the escarole, meatballs, chicken, pastina, salt, and pepper. Cook until the pastina is cooked and the meatballs and chicken are heated through, about 10 minutes.

Serve in a soup bowl topped with 2 tablespoons Parmesan cheese.

COOK'S TIP
You can make the meatballs ahead and freeze in batches for this soup. Meatballs not used for the soup can be frozen and used later.

NUTRITION PER SERVING	
Serving size	2 cups plus about 5 or 6 meatballs
Calories	311 kcal
Fat	12 g
Saturated fat	6.5 g
Cholesterol	85 mg
Sodium	870 mg
Carbohydrates	14 g
Dietary fiber	1 g
Protein	35 g

Italian Wedding Soup *(continued)*

Meatballs

1 pound extra-lean ground beef
½ pound ground veal
½ cup bread crumbs
1 tablespoon fresh flat-leaf parsley, finely chopped
1 tablespoon fresh oregano, finely chopped
½ teaspoon garlic powder

Preheat oven to 350°F.

Mix the beef, veal, bread crumbs, parsley, oregano, and garlic powder thoroughly. Shape into 1-inch meatballs. Place the meatballs on a rimmed baking sheet. Bake for 10 minutes or until a thermometer inserted into the meatballs registers 160°F, turning once during baking.

Remove the meatballs from the baking sheet. Place on a paper towel to drain. Makes about 70 meatballs.

Native American Roasted Corn Soup

Lori A. Miller, R.D., L.D.

This soup is based on a traditional recipe from the Native Americans living in the Mohawk valley of New York. An all-day task, the soup was originally made with salt pork and dried white corn (similar to hominy) that had to be cooked in ashes to remove the tough outer covering of the kernels.

Serves: 6
Hands-on time: 30 minutes
Cooking time: 45 minutes

- 1 teaspoon melted butter
- 5 cobs fresh corn
- ½ teaspoon canola oil
- ½ pound pork, cut into cubes
- 6 cups water
- 1 15-ounce can dark kidney beans, undrained
- ½ teaspoon salt
- ⅛ teaspoon ground black pepper

Preheat broiler. Brush the melted butter onto the corn. Broil 6 inches from the broiler for 10 minutes. Turn the corn over; broil 10 minutes longer. Cool. Cut the kernels from the cob and set aside.

Heat the canola oil in a large heavy saucepan. Sear the pork cubes on all sides, stirring constantly for 10 minutes. Add the water, roasted corn, kidney beans, salt, and pepper. Bring to a boil, reduce heat to low, and simmer for 45 minutes longer.

FOOD TRIVIA
The Navaho Indians use canned hominy and add plenty of chilies and onions to give this a southwestern zip.

SUBSTITUTION
Canned hominy is a quick substitution for the 5 cups of corn.

FOOD TRIVIA
Traditionally, many tribes base their cooking on very basic Native American flavors.

COOK'S TIP
Roasting the corn and searing the meat are natural cooking techniques that create more intense flavors.

NUTRITION PER SERVING	
Serving size	1½ cups
Calories	200 kcal
Fat	5 g
Saturated fat	1.5 g
Cholesterol	25 mg
Sodium	380 mg
Carbohydrates	28 g
Dietary fiber	6 g
Protein	14 g

Lox and Salmon Chowder

Mona R. Sutnick, Ed.D., R.D.

Serves: 4
Hands-on time: 15 minutes
Cooking time: 40 minutes

From the mid-Atlantic seaboard, this delightfully gentle but boldly rich soup is sure to become a favorite of anyone who loves lox.

- 1 tablespoon extra-virgin olive oil
- 1 medium-size onion, chopped
- 2 large potatoes, scrubbed and diced (about 1 pound)
- 2 ribs celery, chopped
- 2 carrots, trimmed and sliced thinly
- 2 14-ounce cans reduced-sodium vegetable broth, or 1½ cups fish stock
- ¼ pound (4 ounces) lox, chopped
- ½ pound (8 ounces) salmon filet, skin removed, cut into bite-size chunks
- ⅓ cup all-purpose flour
- 1 cup nonfat milk
- ¼ teaspoon black pepper
- 2 tablespoons chopped fresh dill

Heat the oil in a medium-heavy kettle over medium-low heat; sauté the onion until translucent, about 5 minutes. Add the potatoes, celery, carrots, and broth. Bring to a boil; cover, reduce heat, and simmer for 20 minutes.

Add the lox and the salmon to the pot and simmer, uncovered, 10 minutes, or until the vegetables are tender and the salmon fillet flakes with a fork.

Blend the flour into the milk until smooth; stir into the chowder. Cook, stirring, until the mixture thickens, about 5 minutes. Stir in the pepper and the dill.

SUBSTITUTION
Looking for more calcium? Substitute 1 cup fat-free evaporated milk for the flour and milk mixture.

NUTRITION PER SERVING	
Serving size	1½ cups
Calories	420 kcal
Fat	10 g
Saturated fat	2.5 g
Cholesterol	45 mg
Sodium	780 mg
Carbohydrates	54 g
Dietary fiber	5 g
Protein	28 g

Maryland Crab Cakes

Edee Howard Hogan, R.D., L.D.

A visit to Chesapeake Bay wouldn't be complete without crab cakes. Now you can make them at home, no matter where you live. Substitute canned or frozen crabmeat for the fresh—just don't tell Marylanders.

Serves: 6
Hands-on time: 35 minutes
Cooking time: 8 to 10 minutes
Chill time: 4 or more hours

- 1 pound Maryland lump or backfin crabmeat, or frozen or canned
- 1 egg, beaten
- 3 tablespoons reduced-fat mayonnaise
- 1 tablespoon finely chopped parsley
- 2 teaspoons Worcestershire sauce
- 1 teaspoon dry English mustard
- 1 teaspoon salt
- ¼ teaspoon white pepper
- 1 teaspoon Old Bay seafood seasoning
- ½ cup plain bread crumbs
- 1 tablespoon butter
- 1 tablespoon canola oil
- parsley sprigs
- lemon wedges

Remove the cartilage from the crabmeat carefully to avoid breaking up the pieces.

Combine the egg, mayonnaise, parsley, Worcestershire sauce, mustard, salt, pepper, and seafood seasoning. Fold the crabmeat gently into the mixture. Form into 6 cakes. Spread the bread crumbs on wax paper. Coat both sides of the crab cakes until they are well covered. Refrigerate for at least 4 hours.

Heat the butter and oil in a skillet. Cook the crab cakes until browned, about 5 minutes on each side. Garnish with a parsley sprig and a lemon wedge.

SERVING SUGGESTION
Make 18 small cakes to serve as appetizers.

COOK'S TIP
Spice it up by increasing the amount of Old Bay seasoning to satisfy your taste buds.

NUTRITION PER SERVING	
Serving size	1 crab cake
Calories	130 kcal
Fat	2.5 g
Saturated fat	0.5 g
Cholesterol	105 mg
Sodium	900 mg
Carbohydrates	9 g
Dietary fiber	0 g
Protein	18 g

Anna's Salmon Cakes

Robin Thomas, M.S., R.D., L.N.

Serves: 2
Hands-on time: 10 minutes
Cooking time: 10 minutes

Crab cakes are famous here in Maryland, but not always practical or affordable. This quick and easy recipe uses ingredients that can be kept on hand for preparation on busy days. Anna was my mother-in-law who prepared simple but delicious meals. This is one of the recipes she typed up for me when I married her son.

1 7½-ounce can salmon, drained, skin removed
¼ cup plain, dry bread crumbs
½ cup finely chopped red onion
2 tablespoons chopped fresh dill, or 1 teaspoon dried
1 egg, lightly beaten
1 tablespoon reduced-fat mayonnaise
2 teaspoons horseradish
vegetable oil cooking spray

Mix all the ingredients except the cooking spray in a medium-size bowl.

Form into 4 equal-size patties.

Coat a medium nonstick pan with the cooking spray; heat over medium-high heat.

Cook the salmon cakes on both sides until golden brown.

SUBSTITUTION
Chili sauce may be used instead of horseradish.

NUTRITION NUGGET
This is an easy and inexpensive way to reel in omega-3s, fish fat with anti-inflammatory properties that may also help fight heart disease.

NUTRITION PER SERVING

Serving size	2 patties
Calories	280 kcal
Fat	11 g
Saturated fat	2.5 g
Cholesterol	155 mg
Sodium	300 mg
Carbohydrates	16 g
Dietary fiber	1 g
Protein	27 g

Saffron Seafood Pasta

Lori Martinez-Hassett, R.D.

Chesapeake Bay seafood fused with Italian pasta and Middle Eastern saffron creates a delightfully distinct—but easy to prepare—dish. If you haven't cooked with saffron, this is a perfect recipe to start with. It lends not only a distinct flavor, but also a beautiful golden hue.

Serves: 6
Hands-on time: 35 minutes
Cooking time: 25 minutes

- 2 tablespoons olive oil
- 1 large onion, chopped
- 4 cloves garlic, minced
- 1 14½-ounce can diced tomatoes
- 1 12-ounce can tomato paste
- ½ teaspoon saffron threads
- ¼ cup chopped basil
- ¼ cup chopped flat-leaf parsley
- 1 teaspoon salt
- ½ teaspoon freshly ground pepper
- 1 cup fish stock (purchased or use recipe on page 459 in the California-Hawaii chapter)
- 1½ pounds mixed shellfish and finfish (shrimp, scallops, bass, cod, etc.)
- 6 cups cooked pasta
- fresh basil or parsley for garnish

Heat the oil over medium heat in a 4- or 5-quart pan. Sauté the onion and garlic until the onion is soft.

Stir together the tomatoes, tomato paste, saffron threads, basil, parsley, salt, and pepper. Add to the pan and simmer 15 to 20 minutes over medium heat. Gradually add the fish stock, ¼ cup at a time. Note that the sauce should be slightly thin in consistency.

Add the seafood and continue cooking, about 3 to 5 minutes. The fish and scallops will be opaque. Do not overcook.

Serve over the pasta; garnish with fresh chopped basil or parsley.

SHOPPING TIPS
Try frozen shellfish and fillets to cut down on costs. Purchase saffron threads for best flavor; crush just before using.

FOOD TRIVIA
Saffron comes from the purple crocus plant.

NUTRITION PER SERVING

Serving size	1½ cups sauce, 1 cup cooked pasta
Calories	430 kcal
Fat	7 g
Saturated fat	1 g
Cholesterol	90 mg
Sodium	850 mg
Carbohydrates	60 g
Dietary fiber	8 g
Protein	31 g

Delmarva Chicken

Edee Howard Hogan, R.D., L.D.

Serves: 8
Hands-on time: 20 minutes
Cooking time: 30 minutes

Del (for Delaware) mar (for Maryland) va (for Virginia) is a corner of the country where three states come together. It's famous for its fresh chicken, apples and cider, and the Lewis Dairy's milk. This dish is everyday easy but also a delicious company feast.

⅓ cup flour
2 teaspoons salt
½ to 1 teaspoon white pepper
2 teaspoons garlic powder
2 teaspoons dried sage
2 pounds boneless, skinless chicken breasts or thighs
3 tablespoons canola oil
4 medium-size unpeeled Granny Smith apples, sliced thinly
2 cups apple cider
1 tablespoon cornstarch
1 cup nonfat milk

Mix the flour, salt, pepper, garlic powder, and sage in a shallow pan. Dredge the chicken through the flour mixture.

Heat the oil in an extra-large heavy skillet or a Dutch oven over medium-high heat; add the chicken pieces and brown each side 5 minutes. Add the apple slices and cider; simmer, uncovered, until the apples are tender, about 20 minutes. The cider should be reduced by half of the original volume.

Remove the apple slices and the chicken to a deep serving platter; cover and keep warm.

Blend the cornstarch into the milk until smooth; pour into a pan with the apple cider sauce. Increase the heat; stir until the sauce thickens. Adjust the sage, garlic powder, and pepper to taste. Pour the sauce over the chicken and apples.

SHOPPING TIP
Look for pasteurized cider to reduce the chance of food contamination.

SERVING SUGGESTION
Serve over rice or barley with a tossed green salad.

NUTRITION NUGGET
Even when you are moderating sodium intake, such as to control blood pressure, you can use some salt in cooking. The key? Use a measuring spoon to keep the amount in check.

NUTRITION PER SERVING	
Serving size	3½ ounces cooked chicken with ½ cup sauce and apples
Calories	230 kcal
Fat	6 g
Saturated fat	0.67 g
Cholesterol	40 mg
Sodium	650 mg
Carbohydrates	25 g
Dietary fiber	2 g
Protein	19 g

Home-Style Meatloaf

Frances Largeman, R.D.

This meatloaf is the masterpiece of Gwen Verhoff, mother of my sweetheart, Thaddeus. Gwen used to make this recipe for him monthly when he was growing up in the Washington, D.C., area. She was happy to share her recipe, but her only request was that I give the exact instructions. When Thaddeus made it for me, he used tomato paste *instead of tomato* sauce. *According to Gwen, that was just not acceptable. (With her permission, I did use some reduced-sodium products.) Thanks, Gwen!*

Serves: 6
Hands-on time: 15 minutes
Cooking time: 70 to 80 minutes

vegetable oil cooking spray
1 medium-size yellow onion, minced
1 cup beef stock, divided
½ cup liquid egg substitute
1½ cups plain bread crumbs
¼ to ½ cup grated Parmesan cheese
1 pound ground sirloin

SAUCE
1 8-ounce can no-salt-added tomato sauce
1 tablespoon reduced-sodium Worcestershire sauce, optional
2 tablespoons vinegar
2 tablespoons packed brown sugar
1 to 2 tablespoons ketchup

Preheat oven to 350°F and spray an 8½-by-4¼-by-2¾-inch loaf pan with the cooking spray.

Sauté the onion in a small nonstick pan with 2 tablespoons beef stock until translucent. Set aside and allow to cool. (Adding hot onions to the egg/meat mixture will cause the egg to begin to cook.)

Combine the egg substitute, bread crumbs, cheese, and beef. Mix until evenly blended.

Pour the remaining beef stock into the pan with the cooling onions to enhance cooling. Add the onions and broth to the meat mixture; blend well. Transfer the mixture to a loaf pan; press down. Bake, uncovered, for 30 minutes. Meanwhile, in a small bowl, combine the tomato sauce, Worcestershire, vinegar, brown sugar, and ketchup; set aside.

Leaving the oven on, remove the meatloaf from the oven after it has baked 30 minutes; spread the sauce evenly over the top. Return to the oven. Bake, uncovered, for 40 to 45 minutes more. Remove from the oven and allow to set for 10 minutes before slicing.

NUTRITION PER SERVING	
Serving size	⅙ of loaf
Calories	330 kcal
Fat	13 g
Saturated fat	4.5 g
Cholesterol	35 mg
Sodium	280 mg
Carbohydrates	31 g
Dietary fiber	2 g
Protein	23 g

Philly Cheesesteak Potato Packets

Deanna Rose, R.D., L.D.N.

Serves: 8
Hands-on time: 20 minutes
Cooking time: 50 minutes

Reminiscent of the Philly cheesesteak, this terrific recipe is great for tail-gating, backyard barbecues, or a warming meal on a cold night. The aroma from the grill will surely attract guests! These cheesesteaks freeze well after cooking, too.

- vegetable oil cooking spray
- 8 medium-size unpeeled russet potatoes, thinly sliced (about 3½ pounds)
- ¼ cup extra-virgin olive oil
- ½ teaspoon black pepper
- ½ teaspoon salt
- 2 large onions, diced
- 1 medium-size green bell pepper, diced
- 1 medium-size red bell pepper, diced
- 8 slices extra-lean deli roast beef, chopped
- 8 ounces shredded part-skim mozzarella cheese, divided

Preheat oven to 400°F or start the outdoor grill. Cut 8 12-inch squares of heavy-duty aluminum foil. Spray each with the cooking oil spray.

Toss the potato slices with the oil, pepper, and salt in a large mixing bowl. Add the onions, peppers, roast beef, and 1 cup of the cheese. Divide the mixture among the foil sheets and top evenly with remaining 1 cup of cheese. Fold the foil packets into tents, leaving space in the tops so the cheese won't stick.

Place directly on the oven racks or grill grates.

Bake or grill for about 50 minutes, or until the potatoes are fork tender.

FOOD TRIVIA
Cheesesteaks were invented in the 1930s at Pat's Steaks, located in the heart of South Philadelphia.

COOK'S TIP
These packets freeze extremely well, so make extra and freeze the left-overs. Freeze after bak-ing by placing the foil packets in a tightly sealed plastic bag or container. Reheat from frozen in a 350°F oven for 20 to 30 minutes.

NUTRITION PER SERVING

Serving size	1 packet
Calories	340 kcal
Fat	13 g
Saturated fat	4 g
Cholesterol	29 mg
Sodium	300 mg
Carbohydrates	41 g
Dietary fiber	4 g
Protein	18 g

Steak Pizziole

Maria Fassano Ruggles, M.S., R.D.

Set this one-pot meal to simmer, as my mom did on many cool nights in our Italian home in New York. While I grew up knowing this dish as "Steak Pizziole," in Italy, it is called Bistecca Pizzaiola, which means "pizza maker's steak." The rich sauce often includes dry white wine (add ½ cup while simmering, if you wish). Serve this meal to guests proudly and they'll think they're in a famous Italian restaurant, and you'll have plenty of time to enjoy their company while it cooks.

Serves: 6
Hands-on time: 15 minutes
Cooking time: 40 minutes

- 3 tablespoons flour
- 2 tablespoons grated Parmesan cheese
- ¼ to ½ teaspoon black pepper
- 1 teaspoon garlic powder
- 1 teaspoon dried oregano
- 1 teaspoon dried basil
- 1 pound round steak, fat removed, cut into 6 pieces
- 1 tablespoon canola oil
- 1 medium-size onion, sliced
- 1 medium-size green bell pepper, chopped
- 1 medium-size red bell pepper, cut into chunks
- 8 ounces sliced mushrooms
- 2 medium-size unpeeled potatoes, cut into bite-size chunks
- 1 29-ounce can Italian-style diced tomatoes

Combine the flour, cheese, pepper, garlic powder, oregano, and basil in a shallow container. Add the steak; toss to coat.

Heat the oil in a Dutch oven or an extra-large skillet over medium-high heat. Add the steak and the onion; brown the steak for 3 to 4 minutes on each side. Stir in the peppers, mushrooms, potatoes, and tomatoes. Cover and simmer 30 minutes, or until the potatoes are fork tender.

To prepare it in the oven, preheat oven to 350°F. Place meat in a glass 3-quart casserole sprayed with vegetable oil cooking spray. Sprinkle with flour, salt, and pepper. Arrange the onion, peppers, mushrooms, and potatoes on top of and around the meat. Sprinkle with the garlic powder, oregano, basil, and cheese. Pour tomatoes over the top. Cover and bake for 1 to 1½ hours, until the meat is tender. Uncover for the final 15 minutes of cooking.

VARIATION

Spice it up by sprinkling crushed red pepper into a flour-Parmesan mixture, and/or add as the dish simmers for the last 30 minutes.

SERVING SUGGESTION

Round out the meal with a tossed salad and crusty Italian bread.

NUTRITION PER SERVING	
Serving size	1½ cups
Calories	290 kcal
Fat	10 g
Saturated fat	3.5 g
Cholesterol	45 mg
Sodium	600 mg
Carbohydrates	30 g
Dietary fiber	4 g
Protein	22 g

German Sauerkraut

Bonnie Athas, R.D.

Serves: 8
Hands-on time: 15 minutes
Cooking time: 1 hour

A boiled dinner is a common dish brought over from the Old World as many immigrants to Pennsylvania did. This German version is based on ham, sauerkraut, and seasonings and is a favorite in our home. Another American favorite is Irish corned beef and cabbage. Although the ingredients are different, the easy preparation and one-dish concept are the same.

1 quart (4 cups) sauerkraut
1 small onion, chopped
¼ teaspoon caraway seed
2 or 3 medium-size apples, cored and sliced
¾ cup Riesling or other white German wine (not too dry)
1 cup reduced-sodium beef broth
2 pounds lean bone-in ham, trimmed of all visible fat
1 teaspoon brown sugar
1 teaspoon celery seed
German mustard to taste

Combine all the ingredients in a large heavy kettle. Bring to a boil; reduce heat, cover, and simmer 1 hour.

Remove the ham; slice and arrange on a platter. Spoon the sauerkraut mixture around the ham with a slotted spoon; discard juices. Serve with the German mustard.

COOK'S TIP

Combine the ham bone with dry great northern beans or lentils, onions, minced garlic, pepper, and water. Simmer to make a delicious soup.

SUBSTITUTION

In place of the wine, use ¾ cup apple cider vinegar plus 2 tablespoons sugar.

NUTRITION NUGGET

Yes, this dish is high in sodium. Balance out the rest of your day by planning lower-sodium meals. Also, remember that you probably don't have meals that are this high in sodium very often, so enjoy! If you are on a sodium-restricted diet for any reason, consult your health care team.

NUTRITION PER SERVING	
Serving size	1 cup sauerkraut mixture plus 3 ounces sliced ham
Calories	290 kcal
Fat	14 g
Saturated fat	5 g
Cholesterol	60 mg
Sodium	1,800 mg
Carbohydrates	14 g
Dietary fiber	6 g
Protein	23 g

Unstuffed Cabbage Casserole

Lori A. Miller, R.D., L.D.

I love to make stuffed cabbage in my northeast Ohio home, but sometimes I just don't have the time for all that stuffing and rolling. This is a quick way to get all the flavors and taste of stuffed cabbage without the tedium of rolling each serving.

Serves: 4
Hands-on time: 15 minutes
Cooking time: 35 minutes

- 1 small cabbage (1 to 1¼ pound)
- vegetable oil cooking spray
- 1 pound extra-lean ground beef
- 1 cup chopped onion
- ½ cup diced celery
- 1 sweet pepper, such as a cubanelle, seeded and finely chopped
- ⅓ cup long grain white rice
- 1 14½-ounce can stewed tomatoes
- ⅓ cup catsup
- ½ teaspoon salt
- ⅛ to ¼ teaspoon ground black pepper

Preheat oven to 350°F.

Slice the cabbage in half vertically; remove the core. Peel off the large leaves only; slit each leaf from the core halfway up. Coat a 2-quart casserole dish with the cooking spray and line it with the large cabbage leaves. Coarsely chop the remaining cabbage to make 3 cups and add to the casserole.

Sauté the ground beef, onion, and celery in a large skillet over medium-high heat. Cook, stirring constantly, until browned, about 10 minutes. Add the chopped pepper, rice, stewed tomatoes, catsup, ⅓ cup water, salt, and pepper to the skillet. Bring to a boil. Spoon the mixture into the cabbage-lined casserole dish. Cover tightly and bake 35 minutes.

SHOPPING TIP
When selecting a sweet pepper for this recipe, look for a cubanelle. It's a big, tapered pepper that can be yellow, orange, or red.

COOK'S TIP
Make sure the casserole dish is tightly covered so steam cooks the rice.

FOOD TRIVIA
Stuffed cabbage, a traditional Hungarian dish, is also known as *Töltött káposzta*. In the United States, it was probably first made somewhere in Pennsylvania.

NUTRITION PER SERVING

Serving size	2 cups
Calories	360 kcal
Fat	11 g
Saturated fat	4 g
Cholesterol	40 mg
Sodium	960 mg
Carbohydrates	39 g
Dietary fiber	7 g
Protein	28 g

Oven Roasted Peppers and Tri-color Rotini

Linda Arpino, C.D.N., M.A., R.D.

Serves: 4 as a main course or 8 as a side dish
Hands-on time: 10 minutes
Cooking time: 40 minutes

New York is not the only, but certainly one of the best, cities in which to find Italian foods. Roasted red peppers are a favorite ingredient, and this recipe is sure to become a favorite way to enjoy pasta.

vegetable oil cooking spray
4 medium-size red bell peppers
2 medium-size yellow bell peppers
8 ounces uncooked pasta, such as rotini
1 tablespoon extra-virgin olive oil
1 tablespoon balsamic vinegar
1 teaspoon dried oregano
1 to 2 cloves garlic, minced
1 teaspoon salt
½ teaspoon pepper
¼ cup minced fresh basil, or 1 tablespoon dried
4 tablespoons shredded or grated Parmesan cheese

Preheat oven to 400°F. Spray a 9-by-13-inch baking dish with the cooking spray. Bake the whole peppers until blackened; about 40 minutes. Cool slightly covered. (Covering makes skins easier to remove.) Meanwhile, cook the pasta according to package directions. Drain and reserve.

When the peppers are cool enough to handle, remove the skins, seeds, and stems, reserving the liquid that drains out of the peppers. Cut the peppers into strips about ½-inch wide, and then dice.

In a small bowl, mix the pepper liquid, olive oil, balsamic vinegar, oregano, garlic, salt, pepper, and basil.

In a medium-size bowl, combine the cooked pasta, peppers, dressing, and Parmesan cheese. Stir well and serve at once.

NUTRITION PER SERVING	
Serving size	2 cups
Calories	370 kcal
Fat	7 g
Saturated fat	2.5 g
Cholesterol	5 mg
Sodium	600 mg
Carbohydrates	66 g
Dietary fiber	6 g
Protein	14 g

Crowd-Pleasing Veggie Sauté

Lauren Swann, M.S., R.D., L.D.N.

We love this dish when the first asparagus pokes out of the Pennsylvania ground in spring as well as any other time asparagus looks good in the market. Mixing grains and vegetables not only makes for a nutritious meal, but they also create great flavor and texture. Whenever you cook brown rice or barley, make a few cups more than you'll use. I love these shortcuts and often freeze leftovers to add to soups and casseroles when I cook in my Philadelphia home.

Serves: 4
Hands-on time: 20 minutes
Cooking time: 20 minutes

2 tablespoons dark sesame oil
2 cloves garlic, minced
1 head broccoli, split into florets (about 4 cups)
1½ cups zucchini, thinly sliced
½ cup reduced-sodium chicken broth, divided
1 cup asparagus, cut diagonally into 1-inch pieces
½ cup sliced mushrooms (4 ounces)
1 10-ounce bag baby spinach leaves
4 cups cooked quick barley or brown rice, hot

Combine the oil and the garlic in an extra-large nonstick skillet over medium heat; cook and stir 3 minutes. Add the broccoli and the zucchini and 2 to 4 tablespoons broth; increase the heat and cook 3 to 4 minutes, stirring constantly. Add the asparagus, mushrooms, and spinach. Add 2 to 3 tablespoons additional broth for stir frying. Cook and stir until the vegetables are crisp tender and the spinach is wilted, about 8 minutes.

Serve over hot barley or brown rice.

NUTRITION PER SERVING	
Serving size	2 cups vegetables plus 1 cup cooked barley; values for rice are similar
Calories	400 kcal
Fat	10 g
Saturated fat	1.5 g
Cholesterol	0 mg
Sodium	105 mg
Carbohydrates	71 g
Dietary fiber	19 g
Protein	15 g

Philly Soft Pretzel Bread Pudding with Chocolate

Deanna Rose, R.D., L.D.N.

Serves: 12
Hands-on time: 15 minutes
Standing time: 1 hour
Cooking time: 55 minutes

I wanted to use one of my favorite hometown staples, the Philadelphia soft pretzel, in a unique way. Since bread pudding is my comfort food of choice, I developed this recipe. I also use Hershey's chocolate products, since the world-famous company is located in Hershey, Pennsylvania, and another food claim to fame in this region. Each serving of this recipe provides a healthy dose of calcium.

vegetable oil cooking spray
6 Philadelphia-style soft pretzels (frozen is okay; thaw first)
1½ cups liquid egg substitute
2½ cups nonfat milk
½ cup chocolate syrup
1 tablespoon vanilla extract
1½ teaspoons cinnamon
½ cup semisweet chocolate chips

Spray a 13-by-9-by-2-inch baking dish with the cooking spray. Poke holes in the soft pretzels with a fork, then cut or break the pretzels into 1-inch pieces and place in the baking dish.

Whisk together the egg substitute, nonfat milk, chocolate syrup, vanilla extract, and cinnamon; mix well. Pour over the pretzels, stir to coat. Let stand for 1 hour to allow the pretzels to absorb some of the liquid mixture.

Preheat oven to 325°F. Cover the baking dish with foil and bake 30 minutes. Uncover. Sprinkle with chocolate chips. Bake an additional 25 minutes or until browned and puffed and the knife comes out clean.

COOK'S TIP

The holes in the pretzels are necessary so the nonfat milk and egg substitute mixture can be fully absorbed, creating the traditional bread pudding texture.

NUTRITION NUGGET

The nonfat milk in this recipe adds calcium to the diet. Chocolate, especially dark chocolate, contains antioxidants and flavonoids, so if chocolate is a favorite of yours, enjoy in small doses.

NUTRITION PER SERVING

Serving size	1⁄12 of pan
Calories	190 kcal
Fat	4 g
Saturated fat	2 g
Cholesterol	0 mg
Sodium	410 mg
Carbohydrates	31 g
Dietary fiber	1 g
Protein	8 g

Must-Have Chocolate Chip Cookies

Kristine Napier, M.P.H., R.D.

The family name for these cookies is "Oatmook Cookies," the name my husband gave them when he was a wee lad of two or three. My mother-in-law managed to sneak in good things like raisins and oats, which he never noticed because of the chocolate. Today, my kids ask for "oatmook cookies," too, even more than chocolate chip cookies, the official state cookie of Pennsylvania.

Serves: 72 (6 dozen)
Hands-on time: 20 minutes
Baking time: 10 minutes (per batch)

- 2 cups raisins
- 1 cup sugar
- 1 stick butter (½ cup)
- 1 cup peanut butter
- 1 cup liquid egg substitute
- 2 teaspoons vanilla
- 2 teaspoons cinnamon
- 1 teaspoon baking soda
- 1 cup flour
- 3½ cups oatmeal (not instant)
- 2 cups semisweet chocolate chips or chunks
- ¼ cup nonfat milk (use as needed)

Preheat oven to 350°F. Combine the raisins and hot water; set aside.

Cream the sugar, butter, peanut butter, egg substitute, vanilla, cinnamon, and baking soda. Add the flour; beat until smooth. Stir in the oatmeal.

Drain the raisins; add to the batter along with the chocolate chips. Stir well by hand. If the batter is stiff, add milk by the tablespoonful.

Drop the batter by teaspoonfuls onto ungreased cookie sheets. Bake 8 to 10 minutes, or just until slightly golden brown. If you like a softer cookie, remove at closer to the 8-minute mark; if you like crunchy cookies, bake closer to 10 minutes.

NUTRITION PER SERVING

Serving size	1 cookie
Calories	100 kcal
Fat	5 g
Saturated fat	2 g
Cholesterol	5 mg
Sodium	35 mg
Carbohydrates	14 g
Dietary fiber	1 g
Protein	2 g

Classic Gingerbread

Kathleen Carozza, M.A., R.D.

Serves: 16
Hands-on time: 15 minutes
Baking time: 40 minutes

Passed down from my great-grandmother, Ella Hoey Wallace of Keyport, New Jersey, this gingerbread is as warm and spicy as Ella herself. Freshly baked gingerbread served with homemade applesauce was a favorite of the Hoey children, who grew up on a farm in Colts Neck, New Jersey (now owned by Bruce Springsteen).

SHOPPING TIP
Look for "first step" puréed prunes that are 100 percent prunes.

- vegetable oil cooking spray
- ¼ cup butter
- ⅓ cup granulated sugar
- 1 2½-ounce jar baby food prunes, or 4 prunes puréed with 1 tablespoon water
- 1 egg
- 1 cup molasses
- 2½ cups all-purpose flour
- 1½ teaspoons baking powder
- 1 teaspoon ground cinnamon
- 1 teaspoon ground ginger
- ½ teaspoon ground cloves
- ½ teaspoon salt
- 1 cup hot water

SUBSTITUTIONS
New Englanders substitute maple syrup for the molasses and southerners use sorghum.

Preheat oven to 350°F. Spray an 8-inch square baking dish with the cooking spray.

Cream together the butter and the sugar; add the eggs, molasses, and prunes, and blend.

Combine the flour, baking powder, cinnamon, ginger, cloves, and salt in a separate bowl, then add to the butter mixture. Add the hot water and mix until smooth.

Bake 40 minutes, or until a toothpick inserted in the middle comes out clean.

COOK'S TIP
Using puréed prunes for part of the butter lowers the fat compared to other gingerbread recipes and also adds a bit of fiber. Best of all, it adds another level of richness.

FOOD TRIVIA
Gingerbread was first made in the Middle Ages by maidens who baked it as a good luck token for knights going into tournaments.

NUTRITION PER SERVING

Serving size	1/16 of loaf
Calories	180 kcal
Fat	3.5 g
Saturated fat	2 g
Cholesterol	20 mg
Sodium	130 mg
Carbohydrates	35 g
Dietary fiber	1 g
Protein	3 g

Sweet Shades of Kwanzaa Bread

Lauren Swann, M.S., R.D., L.D.N.

This bread is attributed to Kwanzaa, the African-American harvest celebration, enjoyed in Philadelphia where I live and also by people throughout the world. The sweet potatoes, carrots, and orange juice contribute not only to the rich orange color, but also to the sweet, robust flavor and an enviable nutrition profile.

Serves: 24
Hands-on time: 20 minutes
Baking time: 45 to 50 minutes

vegetable oil cooking spray
1⅓ cups all-purpose flour
1 cup wheat germ
2 teaspoons baking powder
1 teaspoon baking soda
2 teaspoons cinnamon
1 cup oats (not instant)
1 cup packed brown sugar
1¾ cup cooked, mashed sweet potato
3 eggs, lightly beaten
⅓ cup extra-virgin olive oil
⅓ cup orange juice
1 carrot, grated
1 cup raisins, packed

Preheat oven to 350°F. Spray two 9-by-5-by-3-inch loaf pans with the cooking spray.

Combine the flour, wheat germ, baking powder, baking soda, cinnamon, oats, and brown sugar in a large bowl; set aside.

In a medium bowl, mix the remaining ingredients, then add the wet mixture to the dry ingredients and stir just until combined.

Spoon the batter evenly into the pans. Bake 45 to 50 minutes or until a toothpick inserted in the middle comes out clean.

Cool before cutting into 24 slices.

SUBSTITUTIONS

Instead of cooked sweet potato, you can use one 15-ounce can yams, drained and mashed; 1 pound fresh yams, peeled, boiled, and mashed; or one 15-ounce can pure pumpkin.

VARIATION

Add some crunch by stirring in ½ to 1 cup walnut pieces before baking.

VARIATION

Spoon the batter into 24 muffins cups coated with cooking spray. Bake 30 to 35 minutes, or until a toothpick inserted in the middle of a muffin comes out clean.

NUTRITION PER SERVING	
Serving size	1/24 of loaf
Calories	180 kcal
Fat	5 g
Saturated fat	1 g
Cholesterol	25 mg
Sodium	120 mg
Carbohydrates	32 g
Dietary fiber	2 g
Protein	4 g

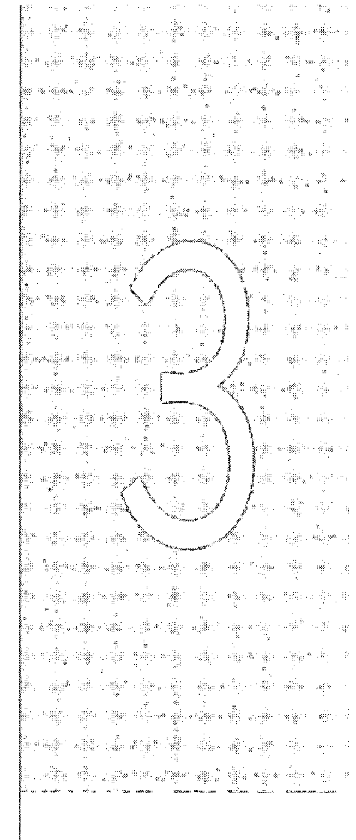

SOUTHERN CUISINE

Smooth Soul Food to Hot 'n' Spicy Cajun Creations

Linda W. Moore, R.D., L.D.N., and Kristine Napier, M.P.H., R.D.

Southern cooking defines comfort food. It speaks of hospitality, leisurely family suppers, and Sunday dinners. Folklore *about* the cooking is as delicious as the food.

While the influences on southern cooking started with Native Americans, followed by English colonists who fanned out from the Jamestown Settlement, these were soon overshadowed by the food culture of African slaves imported to work on rice, cotton, tobacco, and sugar plantations. The African people brought seeds to grow their native foods, as well as recipes and familiar cooking methods. The recipes they developed in their new land acquired names that reveal nothing about the ingredients—"hush puppies," "hoe cakes," and "gut strut"—but much about the culture in which they were created.

Fertile Land, Wealthy Waters

It is no wonder that North American Indians vied for the lands of Virginia, Georgia, Alabama, Kentucky, Tennessee, the Carolinas, Mississippi, and Arkansas. The Mississippi delta offered fertile soil for farming, fields and forests of wild plants for gathering, and lush vegetation with bountiful game. Also, the Mississippi and its many tributaries provided swift passage in addition to plentiful fish. To the east, the treasures of the Atlantic were just a catch away.

Southeast tribes mastered advanced pottery techniques early, crafting sturdy and functional pots that were used over fires and in pits. The Powhaten tribe taught English settlers how to cultivate and cook the local foods: sweet potatoes, squash, pumpkins, and corn. The English settlers brought pigs and seeds for carrots and turnips, foods that have remained important ingredients in southern cuisine. Turnip greens became a very prized southern dish; turnips in the south, in fact, are grown more for their tender, young leaves than for their root. (Carrot Casserole, page 138, Double Apricot Glazed Winter Vegetables, page 30; Pan-Seared Pork Chops with Vidalia Onions, page 160; Sweet and Sour Steamed Greens and Bacon, page 133).

Agricultural Development

First rice and then cotton, sugar, and tobacco grew into significant crops for the South. These industries had a tremendous impact on the food styles that eventually defined southern culture—and still do today. Rice cultivation started in South Carolina in the early 1700s; rice was soon a significant crop in Arkansas, Louisiana, Mississippi, and Texas. Plantation owners became wealthy exporting rice to England by the ton. Rice was cooked into or served with many meals. A coastal area of South Carolina that came to be called the "Low Country" developed a distinct culinary style, which included rice as a staple. In most of the rest of the South, corn bread, grits, and other recipes using cornmeal were the staple. Eventually, rice plantation owners imported slaves from Africa to work the land. Africans brought their history, their culture, and their food to America's South.

Low Country Fare

Charleston lies at the heart of the Low Country, a small section of coastal land richly influenced by the culture and cuisine of Native Americans, as well as the people from France, Portugal, Spain, Barbados, and West Africa who settled there to work the rice fields. It has been described as a cuisine of the water—of the ocean, marshes, ponds, and swamps—and of whatever vegetables are in season.

In the seventeenth century, people who settled there learned to use the figs, pomegranates, and peaches left by Spanish explorers a century before. What people in other parts of the United States call pilaf, those in South Carolina and much of the rest of the South call "pilau," "perloo," "perlau," "plaw," "pilaw." No matter how they spell it, southerners pronounce it *per-low.* The word probably comes from the Turkish *pilau* for rice porridge; indeed, pilau traditionally was any dish of rice cooked with seasoning, possibly meat, possibly beans, and often vegetables. The African culinary influence in the Low Country no doubt influences the development of pilau. In Africa, stews were often served over a starchy base such as rice, cassava, millet, or "fufu" (yams that were boiled and then pounded). As plantation cooks, the African people had a tremendous impact on forming the food ways of the South.

Frogmore Stew (page 144) traces to the town of Frogmore on St. Helena Island. According to legend, a fisherman returned to port with an empty boat. He stewed together the small amount of shellfish he could scrape together—shrimp, clams, and mussels—and boiled them with pork sausage (supposedly from wild boar that roamed the Low Country), potatoes, and corn. Today, it remains a hallmark dish of the Low Country.

African Foods and Cookery Come to America

Some historians say that African cooks saved white slaveholders from nutritional deficiencies. If they did, they accomplished it via culinary knowledge of how to use vitamin- and mineral-rich vegetables, fruits, and grains in their native lands—and the foresight to bring many of these foods with them. To America, they carried:

- Okra, a vegetable native to western Africa. This nutritious vegetable can be fried, boiled, mixed with other vegetables, or used in soups (where it serves as a thickener). While many favorite southern recipes call for frying okra, we offer some fabulous alternatives (Okra Stew, page 140; Okra and Chicken Stew, page 147). Okra is a member of the hibiscus family; like hibiscus, it has large, showy flowers. Its seeds are in the long, green, and tender edible pods.
- Benne, or sesame seeds, which they baked into wafers.
- Sorghum, a grain known today as a powerhouse of nutrition. Its stalks are filled with sweet juice that is boiled down to make a thick syrup called sorghum molasses.
- Black-eyed peas (also called cowpeas), often cooked with greens and a ham bone or pork hock for seasoning (Hoppin' John, page 162, Georgia Caviar, page 137).
- Melons, including watermelon. Historians say watermelon was native to Africa, where it probably has been cultivated for at least four thousand years (Refreshing Cucumber Watermelon Salad, page 243).
- Vegetables, including eggplant. Although the eggplant is really a fruit, it is used as a vegetable.

When African slaves entered plantation houses as cooks, they added their native foods to the slave owners' menus. With phenomenal culinary skills and an abundance of plentiful, fresh ingredients at their fingertips, African slaves brought a whole new meaning to southern cooking. Greens (turnip, collard, dandelion, and others) became a frequent side dish. Sweet potatoes sat next to white potatoes; they were also turned out as dessert in the form of sweet potato pie. Regional fruits and nuts soon became puddings and pies—peach and pecan pies remain southern favorites today.

Thomas Jefferson's Contributions

President Thomas Jefferson, a native Virginian, was an excellent chef and an epicurean. Even before living in Paris as minister to France, he was fascinated with French cuisine. He hired a French chef to train one of his slaves; he subsequently took this man with him to France to study the French culinary arts. When Jefferson returned in 1789, he brought with him many European culinary treasures, including sorrel, dandelion, and other herbs, which he cooked into a delicious array of sauces and stews. Jefferson learned to make ice cream while in France, and one can still see the original recipe he penned in France at the American Treasures exhibit at the Library of Congress. Several of his recipes have been handed through the generations; a total of eight penned in Jefferson's own hand have survived the centuries. They include Jefferson's French rendition of beef stew, *boeuf à la mode* (Jeffersonian Beef Stew, page 143) and a French almond cream, *blanc mange* (try our Swedish Cream, page 412).

Touring northern Italy, President Jefferson saw a picture and plans for a "maccaroni" machine. A holograph drawing and the text (dating to 1787) describing the pasta machine are also visible in the American Treasures exhibit. He was so enamored of the pasta machine, he commissioned his secretary to purchase one in Italy. Because the machine was not very durable, Jefferson made pasta by hand. His pasta dough recipe, *nouilly à macaroni*, penned in his own hand, has survived. Upon returning to America, Jefferson imported Italian olive oil.

JEFFERSON, THE VEGETARIAN?

Well, almost. Mr. Jefferson foresaw today's nutrition advice: enjoy meat in appropriate portions, as a garnish to lots of vegetables, whole grains, and fruits. He said that he ate meat only "as a condiment to the vegetables which constitute my principal diet." True, one cannot call Jefferson a vegetarian as defined today, but he did eat an unusually small amount of meat. He preferred the fruits of his garden, in which he grew more than 250 varieties of herbs and vegetables.

Dessert in the Southern Tradition

Certainly we would never want to rewrite history and erase such fabulous creations—and southern institutions—as sweet potato pie or pecan pie. Such recipes, in fact, remain fabulous holiday treats. But we believe that dessert should be more accessible, nutritionally speaking. In other words, a piece of pie or cake shouldn't break the calorie and fat bank. That's why we've created some delicious desserts that you can enjoy more frequently. Not only are their calorie and fat contents reasonable, but they are also more nutritionally dense. Try Sweet Potato Casserole (page 173) and Sweet Potato Scones or Biscuits (page 118).

The Advent of Soul Food

"Soul food" was given birth in the slaves' far more modest kitchens. There, food did far more than nourish their bodies. It also fed and warmed their souls. Their sparse food rations, in fact, stand in stark contrast to the care and love with which they were transformed into the daily family meal. The slaves' weekly rations of leftover meat (pig's feet, ham hocks, pig ears, and tripe)—the parts the slave owners didn't use—were seasoned with generous amounts of onions, garlic, thyme, and bay leaf. Meager amounts were made to look like more by serving the meat with generous amounts of cooked greens. Most of the weekly cornmeal ration was turned into bread, but the slaves broke the monotony by cooking it into several different types (Moist Corn Bread, page 168). The grains of the remaining cornmeal were mixed with molasses to become dessert. The carefully crafted evening meal became a cherished time for families to be together after long hours of work. The kettles of steaming food became a meal for both body and soul, around which they told and retold the family history. Soon the slaves' cuisine became known as "good times food" or "soul food."

Soul food, too, was born of an ingenious use of food scraps brought back from the plantation owner's home. Leftover fish became croquettes, or fish patties, by adding an egg, cornmeal or flour, and seasonings (Confetti Tuna (or Salmon) Cakes, page 122). Stale bread became bread pudding.

A Southern Eating Glossary

Of all regional cuisine, southern is most in need of a glossary. Let's take a look at some of the terms and recipe names commonly found in southern kitchens.

- *Pot likker.* Juice left in the pot after cooking vegetables. American folklore assigns a magical, nutritive value to pot likker, which was used as gravy or enjoyed as a hot drink.
- *A bowl of wild greens.* Commonly contains leaves of cowslip, cress, dandelion, pigweed, and turnip greens.

- *Collards.* One vegetable referred to as "greens" and commonly eaten with pepper sauce and hot corn bread. Collards are a type of cabbage that does not form a head and are closely related to kale. They are richer in calcium, vitamin C, and beta-carotene than spinach (Sweet and Sour Steamed Greens and Bacon, page 133).
- *Gumbo.* In Africa, another word for okra; in the South, okra is still called gumbo. Gumbo is also the term for a thick stew. Characteristically, gumbos have vegetables (especially okra and tomatoes) and one of several meats and/or shellfish. Okra thickens gumbo; sometimes extra thickening is added in the form of filé, a powder made from sassafras.
- *Red-eye gravy.* Also called red-ham gravy, this traditional southern gravy is made from drippings of fried ham (purists say it must be country-cured ham) with water and, sometimes, hot coffee. There is much debate, in fact, about whether red-eye gravy is good without black coffee. Red-eye gravy is generally served with ham and biscuits or corn bread. There are several stories about the origin of red-eye gravy. The least colorful says the gravy was named because a circle or oval of liquid fat with a reddish cast forms on the surface of the gravy as it thickens. The more colorful version is attributed to General Andrew Jackson's cook, who arrived to prepare breakfast with red eyes after a night of drinking corn whiskey. According to the story, General Jackson asked for country ham and gravy as red as the cook's eyes.
- *Squirrel food.* A southern candy made of pecans, butter, sugar, and eggs.
- *Poke salet (or salett or salat).* The cooked young shoots of the pokeweed plant. When cooked, young pokeweed leaves look like spinach and taste like asparagus. However, most sources, including those at the University of Alabama, say that because the mature pokeweed plant should be considered poisonous (its roots, berries, leaves, and stalks), the shoots should not be eaten. Indeed, folklore says that pokeweed greens are poisonous unless cooked with lots of lard, but this is not documented scientifically. Our recipe for poke salet uses other greens, but cooks them as rural folk once did pokeweed (Poke Salet, page 134).
- *Sweet potatoes versus yams.* Sweet potatoes are the roots of a vine that is a member of the morning glory family and is native to the Caribbean. There are both white and yellow sweet potatoes, but the yellow is considered more desirable. Yams and sweet potatoes are not related botanically, but are often confused. Yams have a more watery flesh than sweet potatoes, which is why they are not as

widely used. Yams are native to Africa and do not grow well in the United States.

Cornmeal Creations

Extensive use of cornmeal probably resulted from the fact that very little wheat was grown in the South. Cornmeal was crafted into a number of wonderful creations:

- *Johnnycakes.* Probably the country's first pancakes. Made of cornmeal instead of flour, most were cooked on the griddle (thus, their other name, griddle cakes) and others were baked.
- *Hoecakes.* Apparently made from much of the same batter as johnny-cakes. Hoecakes were quick breads created from corn bread batter heaped onto a spade or a hoe that was then held over an open fire.
- *Ashcakes.* A cornmeal mixture baked in an open fire; the baked bread was washed after cooking before serving.
- *Hush puppies.* Small cornmeal dumplings usually served with fried catfish. According to stories handed down, plantation cooks saved cornmeal from the "big" kitchen that was used to coat catfish for frying and that would have been thrown out. Back in their own kitchens, they added a little milk, egg, and onion and fried it as these dumplings. It is said that they tossed the dumplings at the dogs to keep them quiet while the food was being transferred from the pot to the table, saying, "Hush, puppy! Hush, puppy!"
- *Grits.* In the South grits refers to hominy grits. Hominy grits are coarsely ground corn; they are cooked with water or milk to make cereal or a side dish. In the purest sense, "grits" refers to any coarsely ground grain such as corn, oats, or rice.

It All Started with a Pig

Pork was, and remains, the most frequently used meat in the south, as well as a key industry. Hams from Virginia, for example, are universally recognized to be America's finest. Bacon and salt pork are used to flavor greens and beans. Ham biscuits are a classic accompaniment to breakfast and dinner. Many different parts of the pig were—and still are—used, including:

- *Chitterlings, or chitlins:* the small intestine of a freshly slaughtered pig, first boiled and then barbecued or fried
- *Gut strut:* a big pot of chitlins
- *Cracklin':* bits of pork fat or pork skin fried until crispy

Some Southern Culinary Landmarks

The foods, recipes, and culinary traditions of the South are too many to mention. Here, we note just a few.

Fried Chicken

Of all southern dishes, fried chicken achieved the most popularity outside the region, to the extent that entire fast food chains sprang up serving debased versions. According to many food historians, southern fried chicken may be the ideal all-purpose, all-occasion American food that can be served hot or cold.

We've included one recipe for fried chicken and two for oven-fried versions. As with other traditional foods, we've made this one more accessible to you nutritionally speaking. In showing you how to cook it to delicious perfection without the skin and with less fat, we hope you will enjoy this favorite food more often. (Smoky Holler Fried Chicken, page 152; Inside Out "Fried" Chicken, page 155).

The Cast-Iron Skillet

Food historians claim that the three most important things about soul cooking are:

- A long, slow simmer
- Never leaving the kitchen while food is cooking
- Using a black cast-iron skillet

Cast-iron skillets became popular in the South during hot summers because cooks used them to place a hot meal on the table without firing up the oven. To this day, ask any southerner how to cook corn bread, and you're in for a lecture about needing a properly cured cast-iron skillet. In fact, you'll probably hear that you need a cast-iron skillet to cook just about anything! Fortunately, used in the southern tradition, most foods can be cooked with significantly less added fat.

Self-Serve Grocery Stores

At the turn of the twentieth century, Clarence Saunders revolutionized society from the South when he introduced the first self-serve grocery store. The first Piggly Wiggly opened in Memphis, Tennessee, in 1916. Until that time, shoppers handed their list to the grocer, who collected the items for the customer. The self-service method, unheard of at the time, was eventually franchised (another first). Not only did this method of shopping free up employees to do other things in the store, and of course, allow for less manpower to operate the store, but shoppers also got closer to all the items in the store, which likely increased impulse shopping.

Cajun and Creole

Southern Louisiana gave birth to two major cuisines: Cajun and Creole. On just a single street in New Orleans, one can also study a plethora of culinary fusions. Indeed, whether your preference is Cajun, Creole, French cuisine, or some fusion, you are certain to find a New Orleans restaurant stirring together just the right combination of foods and spices. New Orleans restaurants—some of the best in the country—have been pleasing palates for at least two hundred years. Somewhere around Bourbon Street, Americans first sampled French cuisine, a notably more sophisticated cuisine than had ever been served in the New World.

Let's step back into the eighteenth century, about a hundred years before restaurateurs set up shop on Bourbon Street, and sort out Cajun from Creole cuisine, the French from the Spanish influences.

Country Cookin', City Cuisine

The name "Cajun" stems from a mispronunciation of Acadians, people of French descent who settled in Canada in the seventeenth century. As land in the Americas changed hands from one European crown to another, groups of settlers often found themselves homeless. Such was the case with a group of Acadians living in Nova Scotia, who then wandered for some thirty years after they were kicked out. The Spanish finally recruited them to settle their newly acquired territory in southern Louisiana. Preferring the country to the city, the Cajuns made the bayous their new home. They lived off the land and from the sea. Cajun cooks experimented with local herbs and spices, creating varying degrees of "heat" in their food. Preferring the simple way of life, the Cajun people often cooked one-pot meals in huge iron kettles.

The Creoles, on the other hand, were city folk. The Spanish who governed New Orleans in the eighteenth century called all people of European heritage *Criollo*, a term which later became *Creole*. Two hundred years ago, the Creole label was given to anyone of refined cultural background who had an appreciation for an elegant lifestyle. Their cuisine was a fusion of the French, African American, Choctaw Indian, and Spanish foodways that merged very quickly as their cultures overlapped and intertwined. After the Civil War, a touch of Italian cuisine further shaped Creole cookery.

The French who settled in what is now New Orleans traveled from

France with Jean Baptiste La Moyne in the early eighteenth century. They continued cooking traditional, elegant French recipes, preferring to linger long in the kitchen fussing over the finest of culinary details. Their African American slaves introduced okra and the deliciously thick gumbos into which it was simmered. The Choctaw Indians taught the European settlers and their slaves how to use indigenous plants, including bay leaf, corn, and filé powder. The Choctaw, say food historians, are the first people to use filé, which soon became a Creole-essential seasoning to thicken and flavor gumbos. Made by grinding dried sassafras leaves into a fine powder, filé has a woodsy flavor that tastes somewhat like root beer.

The Spanish signature in Creole cuisine is found in the mixing of fish and meat in one dish, such as the shrimp and sausage in jambalaya. Rice is the focal point of jambalaya, although most people who have had the pleasure of eating jambalaya don't realize it. The rice absorbs flavors from the lively combination of ingredients, transforming them into another level of fabulous flavor. Jambalaya may be made with beef, pork, chicken, duck, shrimp, oysters, crayfish, sausage, or any combination. The Jambalaya Cook-Off Contest folks in Gonzales, Louisiana (the self-proclaimed Jambalaya Capital of the World), say that no two bowls of jambalaya are the same.

HOW JAMBALAYA GOT ITS NAME

Folklore surrounds the origin of the word *jambalaya,* but most believe the name comes from the French word for ham—*jambon,* a main ingredient of eighteenth-century jambalaya. While more difficult to confirm, some native Louisianians grew up learning that the "ya" in jambalaya is from the African *ya* for rice. They'll also tell you that the Acadian language added the *a la,* which means "everything." John Mariani, in *The Dictionary of American Food and Drink,* relates a more colorful origin of the name for jambalaya. When a man stopped into a New Orleans inn late one night, he found nothing left from the dinner offering. The innkeeper asked the cook, whose name was Jean, to *balayez,* which means "mix some things together" in Louisiana dialect. The satisfied guest called the delicious dish created from leftovers "Jean Balayez," which later became known as jambalaya.

Jambalaya aside, Spanish chefs served almost everything over rice, and their love of hot peppers added a kick to a few Creole dishes. The Italian influence in Creole food is readily identified when red tomato sauce is added to a dish, or when pasta replaces rice.

It is a New Orleans tradition to have red beans and rice on Monday (Red Beans and Rice, page 165). This started because Monday was laundry day and women could put a pot of beans on the stove and let them cook all day while they did the laundry. Most people added the bone from the traditional Sunday ham dinner to flavor the beans. The Monday tradition of eating Red Beans and Rice still continues in many restaurants and family meals in New Orleans.

WHAT *KIND* OF RED BEANS FOR RED BEANS AND RICE?

While many people use red kidney beans when making this classic washday one-pot meal, purists say their flavor is too strong. Instead, they argue, small South Louisiana red beans are the *only* bean to use.

The choice of ham, too, is one of great debate. Traditionalists argue for a baked ham bone, rather than a country or smoked ham bone.

Canned beans in red beans and rice? No, say purists! Given today's time constraints (and a faster method of doing laundry), though, we've cooked up a quicker version calling for canned beans (Easy One-Pot Red Beans and Rice, page 166).

Cajun vs. Creole: Basic Differences

While jambalaya is a classic Creole dish, Cajun versions developed over time. Depending on where you stop in Louisiana, you could end up with a bowl of Creole or Cajun jambalaya. Would you know the difference? Here's how to tell:

- Creole jambalaya uses red tomato sauce (Creole Jambalaya, page 156), and could have pasta instead of rice.
- The Cajun version skips the tomato sauce, but browns the rice—creating a brown, spicier dish; you'll *never* find pasta in Cajun jambalaya.

Fat Tuesday and Other Religious Culinary Traditions

The culinary traditions of Fat Tuesday are many and colorful. King Cake is just one delightfully fun example that spans the Christmas season and Lent (King Cake, page 171). Also known as Twelfth Night Cake, King Cake is a common sight in New Orleans bakeries between the Twelfth Night (January 6) and Ash Wednesday.

French settlers to New Orleans continued a custom dating to twelfth-century France, when a similar cake was made to celebrate the coming of the three wise men bearing gifts twelve days after Christmas. You might also know the Twelfth Night as the feast of Epiphany or King's Day.

The traditional King Cake was round, which portrayed the circular route taken by the wise men to confuse King Herod, who was trying to follow them so that he could find and kill the Christ child.

A figurine symbolizing baby Jesus (or a bean or pea) is baked into the cake, a secondary tradition that started in the nineteenth century to help choose the queen of Mardi Gras. The young woman who was served the slice of cake holding the hidden prize became queen. Even if you're not vying to be Mardi Gras queen, it is considered good luck to get the prized slice—and you also have the honor of holding the next King Cake party.

Since 1872, King Cake icing has been tinted purple (for justice), green (for faith), and gold (for power).

Turkey Sausage

Joanne Milkereit, M.H.S.A., R.D., C.D.E.

Serves: 6
Hands-on time: 10 minutes
Cooking time: 10 minutes

Serve this delightfully seasoned sausage for a breakfast that complements a healthy lifestyle. Americans are known for loving turkey, so why not start the day with it! Here in the Carolinas, we're serious about turkey; North Carolina raises more turkeys than any other state, and we're not far behind in South Carolina.

1 tablespoon seasoning mix (see below)
1 pound extra-lean ground turkey (16 ounces)

SEASONING MIX
1 teaspoon fresh lemon zest or dried lemon peel
½ teaspoon salt
¼ to ½ teaspoon ground black pepper
¼ teaspoon ground coriander
¼ teaspoon ground marjoram
¼ teaspoon ground sage
¼ teaspoon ground thyme

In a small bowl, prepare the seasoning mix by stirring together the lemon zest, salt, pepper, coriander, marjoram, sage, and thyme.

Place the turkey in a medium-size bowl. Add the seasoning mix and combine thoroughly. Shape into 12 patties. Place the patties and ¼ cup water in a large heavy skillet; cover and steam over medium heat for 5 minutes. Remove from heat and drain liquid. Return to heat and continue to cook until the patties are brown on both sides, or until they reach an internal temperature of 165°F.

COOK'S TIP
Triple the seasoning mix recipe using dried lemon peel and keep on hand for later use. It is great in strata-type dishes.

NUTRITION PER SERVING	
Serving size	2 patties
Calories	115 kcal
Fat	15 g
Saturated fat	2 g
Cholesterol	60 mg
Sodium	250 mg
Carbohydrates	Less than 0.5 g
Dietary fiber	15 g
Protein	13 g

Sweet Potato Scones or Biscuits

Laura Faler Thomas, M.Ed., R.D., L.D.

Serves: 12
Hands-on time: 25 minutes
Baking time: 15 minutes

None other than Martha Washington inspired me to create these melt-in-your-mouth scones. Although my kitchen in Idaho is far from Virginia, where Mrs. Washington stirred up sweet potato biscuits, it was fun to create a tribute to colonial America—and also a way to use leftover Thanksgiving sweet potatoes.

- 2 cups all-purpose flour
- 1 tablespoon baking powder
- ¼ teaspoon salt
- 2 tablespoons brown sugar
- ½ teaspoon ground cinnamon
- ¼ teaspoon ground ginger
- ⅛ teaspoon ground allspice
- 3 tablespoons plus 1 teaspoon chilled butter, cut into small pieces
- ¾ cup buttermilk
- ½ cup cooked, mashed, or puréed sweet potato

Preheat oven to 450°F.

Combine the flour, baking powder, salt, brown sugar, cinnamon, ginger, and allspice in a large bowl. Cut in the butter with a pastry blender or two knives until the mixture resembles coarse meal. Add the buttermilk and the sweet potato. Stir until the dry ingredients are just moistened. Turn out onto a lightly floured surface. Knead gently 4 or 5 times.

Scones

Shape the dough into two flat rounds, about 8 inches in diameter.

Place the rounds on an ungreased baking sheet. Score the top surface of each round into six wedges, being careful not to cut completely through the dough. Bake for about 15 minutes or until golden brown. Let cool on a rack or serve warm.

Biscuits

Roll the dough to ½-inch thickness. Cut the dough with a 2½-inch cutter into 12 biscuits. Place on an ungreased baking sheet and bake for 15 minutes or until golden brown. Let cool on a rack or serve warm.

SUBSTITUTIONS

Canned pumpkin makes a great substitute for the sweet potato. One cup of whole wheat flour may be substituted for 1 cup of all-purpose flour.

VARIATION

Press ¼ cup chopped pecans into the tops of the scones or biscuits before baking.

COOK'S TIP

Be creative with your leftovers. Stir leftover sweet potatoes (or canned pumpkin) into Sweet Potato Soup (page 251).

NUTRITION PER SERVING

Serving size	1 scone/biscuit
Calories	130 kcal
Fat	3.5 g
Saturated fat	2 g
Cholesterol	10 mg
Sodium	190 mg
Carbohydrates	23 g
Dietary fiber	Less than 1 g
Protein	3 g

Southern Deep Chocolate Sauce with Soft Mounded Biscuits

Linda W. Moore, R.D., L.D.N.

In central Arkansas during the 1920s and 1930s, my grandmother would prepare this as a breakfast extender to use over hot buttered biscuits when "the hens weren't laying." She had to feed her husband, herself, and their nine children substantially, because they were farmers and all the kids had chores to do before school. My mother adopted the sauce for a breakfast treat in the 1950s and 1960s that she would use to get us to eat our eggs before going off to school.

Serves: 12
Hands-on time: 20 minutes
Cooking time: 25 minutes

SOFT MOUNDED BISCUITS

vegetable oil cooking spray
2 cups (plus 1 cup) all-purpose flour
1 teaspoon salt
¼ teaspoon baking soda
1 tablespoon baking powder
2 teaspoons sugar
6 tablespoons unsalted butter
1¾ cup reduced-fat buttermilk

DEEP CHOCOLATE SAUCE

1 cup sugar
⅓ cup unsweetened cocoa powder
¼ cup all-purpose flour
dash salt
1 cup nonfat milk
1 teaspoon unsalted butter
6 cups raspberries or sliced strawberries

Preheat oven to 450°F. Coat an 8- or 9-inch pie dish with the cooking spray.

Mix 2 cups of flour with the salt, baking soda, baking powder, and sugar in a large mixing bowl. Cut the butter into the flour mixture with a pastry cutter until the butter looks like peas. Make a well in the center of the flour-butter mixture and pour in the buttermilk. Mix together lightly and allow to sit for 2 or 3 minutes. The mixture will be more like batter than dough.

SERVING SUGGESTION

Refrigerate leftover sauce in an airtight container for up to 7 days. Reheat to use as an ice-cream sauce.

NUTRITION PER SERVING	
Serving size	1 biscuit with ¼ cup sauce
Calories	330 kcal
Fat	8 g
Saturated fat	5 g
Cholesterol	20 mg
Sodium	430 mg
Carbohydrates	62 g
Dietary fiber	7 g
Protein	6 g

Southern Deep Chocolate Sauce with Soft Mounded Biscuits *(continued)*

Pour the remaining 1 cup of flour into a shallow bowl. Drop 12 heaping tablespoons of biscuit batter into the flour in the bowl. Cover the scoop of batter with flour and gently lift it from the bowl, tossing lightly from hand to hand to remove excess flour. Place it in the coated pie dish. Repeat with the remaining batter, placing the biscuits close together. Bake for 20 to 25 minutes or until a toothpick inserted into the center biscuit comes out clean.

While the biscuits are baking, prepare the sauce. Mix the sugar, cocoa, flour, and salt together in a medium-size saucepan. Add the milk and cook over medium-low heat until bubbly and thickened, stirring constantly.

Remove from heat and add the butter. Keep warm until ready to use.

Pour the sauce over hot biscuits; top evenly with fruit.

FOOD TRIVIA

Recently, I researched this sauce to see if I could find any other people who knew of using a chocolate sauce on biscuits. I sent an e-mail to a group of approximately one hundred friends throughout the United States and western Europe to see if they knew of anything similar. There were three people who had heard of this and, interestingly, they were from western Tennessee and central Arkansas and were from families involved in farming.

Cheesy Tomato, Bacon, and Green Pepper Bake

Josephine Totten, R.D.

In the South, we pride ourselves in turning ordinary ingredients into scrumptious dishes. These otherwise plain foods bake into a casserole you'll enjoy for breakfast, lunch, or dinner.

Serves: 4 as a main dish or 8 as a side dish
Hands-on time: 20 minutes
Cooking time: 25 minutes

vegetable oil cooking spray
3 strips bacon, diced
3 slices whole-grain bread, cut into cubes
1 medium-size green bell pepper, chopped
1 medium-size onion, chopped
6 medium-size tomatoes, chopped
1 tablespoon sugar
2 tablespoons flour
1 teaspoon salt
⅛ to ¼ teaspoon black pepper
1 teaspoon dried sage
1 cup shredded sharp cheddar cheese (4 ounces)

Preheat oven to 350°F. Spray a 9-by-13-inch casserole dish with the cooking spray.

Combine the bacon, bread, green pepper, and onion in a large nonstick pan over medium heat. Cook and stir until the bacon is crisp and the bread is brown, about 5 to 7 minutes.

Meanwhile, combine the tomatoes, sugar, flour, salt, pepper, and sage in the casserole dish; stir. Add the sautéed mixture; stir. Top with the cheese. Bake, uncovered, 20 minutes.

NUTRITION PER SERVING	
Serving size	1½ cups, main dish
Calories	260 kcal
Fat	12 g
Saturated fat	7 g
Cholesterol	30 mg
Sodium	890 mg
Carbohydrates	30 g
Dietary fiber	5 g
Protein	11 g

NUTRITION PER SERVING	
Serving size	¾ cup, side dish
Calories	130 kcal
Fat	6 g
Saturated fat	3.5 g
Cholesterol	15 mg
Sodium	440 mg
Carbohydrates	15 g
Dietary fiber	2 g
Protein	6 g

Confetti Tuna (or Salmon) Cakes

Melissa Stevens Ohlson, M.S., R.D., L.D.

Serves: 2
Hands-on time: 10 minutes
Cooking time: 10 minutes

Start with a simple can of tuna, add a few ingredients, and you've got the makings for a great appetizer or entrée. Fish croquettes, a favorite soul food, were born when slaves took leftover fish back to their own kitchens and stirred them together with seasonings, cornmeal, and chopped vegetables. These confetti-colored nibbles, which are reminiscent of croquettes, are pan-fried in a bit of oil and lemon juice to infuse great flavor.

SHOPPING TIP
Select a hearty whole-grain bread for this recipe—you'll bump up the fiber and minerals in this great catch.

- ½ cup liquid egg substitute, or 2 egg whites, slightly beaten
- ⅓ cup fat-free mayonnaise
- ¼ cup plus 1 tablespoon lemon juice
- 1 teaspoon extra-hot horseradish
- ½ teaspoon black pepper
- 2 slices whole-grain bread, torn into small pieces
- 1 6-ounce can albacore tuna, or salmon, drained
- ¼ cup minced green onion
- ½ cup yellow pepper, minced
- ½ cup red pepper, minced
- ¼ cup minced cilantro
- 1 tablespoon olive oil

SUBSTITUTION
Keep frozen chopped green peppers and onions on hand. Thaw 1 cup (measured frozen) and use in place of green onions and chopped fresh peppers.

In a small bowl, stir together the egg, mayonnaise, ¼ cup lemon juice, horseradish, and black pepper. Add the bread and mix with a fork. Add the drained tuna or salmon and mix. Fold in the onion, peppers, and cilantro. Shape into six small cakes by forming 2 to 3 tablespoons of the mixture into patties.

Heat the oil and 1 tablespoon lemon juice in a large skillet over medium heat. Cook the cakes for 7 to 10 minutes, turning once.

NUTRITION PER SERVING

Serving size	3 cakes
Calories	350 kcal
Fat	13 g
Saturated fat	2.5 g
Cholesterol	35 mg
Sodium	850 mg
Carbohydrates	30 g
Dietary fiber	4 g
Protein	31 g

Cajun Lemon Chicken Strips

Linda Arpino, C.D.N., M.A., R.D.

Mix up this lemon-fresh Cajun dish a day ahead. Bump up the cayenne if you like more heat, or increase the amount of basil and paprika if you want a little hint of Italy, too.

Serves: 8
Hands-on time: 10 minutes
Marinating time: 1 hour
Cooking time: 10 minutes if grilling, 20 minutes if baking

vegetable oil cooking spray
1 pound boneless, skinless chicken breasts, cut into strips
3 tablespoons lemon juice
3 tablespoons ketchup
1 tablespoon honey
1 teaspoon black pepper
2 teaspoons paprika
1 teaspoon garlic powder
1 teaspoon dried basil
½ teaspoon cayenne

Spray a 9-inch square dish with the cooking spray. Add the chicken.

Blend the remaining ingredients in a small bowl; pour over the chicken. Turn the chicken to coat both sides. Cover and marinate in the refrigerator for at least one hour, but overnight is fine.

Grill 6 to 10 minutes or until the chicken is cooked through, or bake at 350°F for 20 minutes or until the chicken is cooked through. If grilling, discard the marinade. If baking, the chicken can be baked in the marinade.

NUTRITION PER SERVING	
Serving size	2 to 3 strips
Calories	140 kcal
Fat	1.5 g
Saturated fat	0 g
Cholesterol	65 mg
Sodium	120 mg
Carbohydrates	4 g
Dietary fiber	0 g
Protein	26 g

Spinach-Parmesan Stuffed Tomatoes

Mary Etta Moorachian, Ph.D., R.D., C.C.P., C.F.C.S.

Serves: 6
Hands-on time: 40 minutes
Baking time: 25 minutes

I pick a few sun-ripened tomatoes and a bunch of baby spinach from my South Carolina garden for this recipe. Italian flavors of basil, garlic, and Parmesan cheese infuse the spinach stuffing. Although tomatoes are always best straight from the vine, serve this pretty red and green side dish during the Christmas season, using hothouse tomatoes.

- vegetable oil cooking spray
- ½ cup shredded Parmesan cheese
- ¼ cup Italian bread crumbs
- 1 10-ounce bag fresh baby spinach leaves
- 6 medium-size fresh tomatoes
- 1 tablespoon extra-virgin olive oil
- 1 small onion, chopped
- 1 clove garlic, minced
- 1 tablespoon chopped fresh basil, or 1 teaspoon dried
- ¼ teaspoon black pepper
- 1 tablespoon chopped parsley, optional

Preheat oven to 350°F. Coat a 9-by-13-inch baking pan with the cooking spray.

Combine the Parmesan cheese and the bread crumbs in a small bowl; set aside. Chop the spinach and set aside. Trim ¼-inch off the tops of the tomatoes. Scoop out the tomato and reserve the pulp.

Heat the olive oil in a 10-inch skillet. Sauté the onion, garlic, and reserved tomato pulp. Add the chopped spinach with 2 tablespoons of water and wilt until tender. Stir in the basil, pepper, and parsley if desired.

Spoon the spinach mixture evenly into the tomatoes. Top with cheese and bread crumbs. Place in the prepared baking pan and bake for about 20 minutes.

COOK'S TIP

To use frozen spinach, substitute one 10-ounce box of frozen, thawed chopped spinach. Add to a skillet with an onion, garlic, and tomato pulp (do not add water); sauté. Stir in spices and follow the remaining instructions.

NUTRITION PER SERVING

Serving size	1 stuffed tomato
Calories	110 kcal
Fat	5 g
Saturated fat	1.5 g
Cholesterol	5 mg
Sodium	230 mg
Carbohydrates	12 g
Dietary fiber	2 g
Protein	6 g

Scalloped Tomatoes

Mary Etta Moorachian, Ph.D., R.D., C.C.P., C.F.C.S.

In the South, tomatoes are abundant during the summer, and extras are often stewed and canned. Sugar was traditionally added to many vegetables, such as my grandmother's stewed tomatoes—which I vividly remember eating with soda crackers. My grandmother and her stewed tomatoes were the inspiration for this recipe.

Serves: 4
Hands-on time: 10 minutes
Baking time: 35 minutes

2½ cups stewed tomatoes, drained (reserve liquid)
1 medium-size green bell pepper, chopped
1 small onion, chopped
¼ teaspoon salt
⅛ to ½ teaspoon black pepper
1 tablespoon brown sugar
1 bay leaf
1 tablespoon butter
2 tablespoons flour
½ cup bread or cracker crumbs

Preheat oven to 350°F.

Combine the tomatoes, pepper, onion, salt, black pepper, brown sugar, and bay leaf in a medium-size bowl. Spoon into a 1-quart baking dish.

Melt the butter; stir in the flour until smooth. Add ½ cup of reserved tomato liquid. Pour over the tomato mixture. Top with bread crumbs. Bake, uncovered, for 35 to 40 minutes. Remove the bay leaf before serving.

NUTRITION PER SERVING	
Serving size	1 cup
Calories	160 kcal
Fat	3.5 g
Saturated fat	2 g
Cholesterol	10 mg
Sodium	710 mg
Carbohydrates	29 g
Dietary fiber	4 g
Protein	4 g

Roasted Beet, Blue Cheese, and Pecan Salad

Diane A. Welland, M.S., R.D.

Serves: 6
Hands-on time: 20 minutes
Baking time: 40 minutes

In Virginia, we grow Detroit Dark Red and Ruby Queen beets. This easy-to-make but gourmet-in-flavor salad is a hit with any kind of beet—you don't even have to know the variety!

6 beets, peeled and chopped (about 5 cups)
2 medium-size onions, quartered
1 tablespoon extra-virgin olive oil
½ teaspoon black pepper
2 teaspoons dried basil
¼ cup balsamic vinegar
2 tablespoons honey
8 cups mesclun mix
1 cup (4 ounces) crumbled blue cheese
¼ cup pecan pieces

Preheat oven to 425°F.

Combine the beets and onions in a 9-by-13-inch baking dish. Whisk together the oil, pepper, basil, and vinegar. Pour over the vegetables; mix well. Cover tightly and bake for 30 to 40 minutes, or until the beets are fork tender. Drizzle the vegetables with honey; mix. Let the vegetables cool to room temperature.

Line a serving platter with mesclun greens. Top evenly with the beet mixture. Sprinkle with the cheese and pecans.

SERVING SUGGESTION

Stir up this red and green salad for Christmas—not just for the color, but also to add a new flavor to holiday meals.

NUTRITION PER SERVING	
Serving size	1 cup beet mixture plus 2 cups greens
Calories	190 kcal
Fat	12 g
Saturated fat	4 g
Cholesterol	20 mg
Sodium	330 mg
Carbohydrates	17 g
Dietary fiber	4 g
Protein	7 g

Barbara's Black and White Bean Salad

Josephine Totten, R.D.

From my Tennessee neighbor, this bean salad is sure to become one of your favorites—not only because of the taste, but because prepared salsa makes it so easy. If you like a little more spice, look for hot salsa.

Serves: 12
Hands-on time: 15 minutes

1 15½-ounce can great northern beans, or any white bean, rinsed and drained
2 15½-ounce cans black beans, rinsed and drained
2 tomatoes, chopped
1 large red pepper, diced
2 cups frozen yellow corn, thawed
1 bunch green onions, cleaned and sliced
1 cup commercial salsa
¼ cup red wine vinegar
⅓ to ½ cup chopped fresh cilantro
¼ teaspoon ground black pepper

In a large bowl, *gently* stir the beans and tomatoes together. (Be careful not to mash the beans.) Combine the red pepper, corn, and green onions and stir into the bean mixture. Set aside.

In a small bowl, combine the salsa, vinegar, cilantro, and black pepper. Stir with a wire whisk until well blended. Pour over the vegetable mixture and toss gently.

SUBSTITUTION
Substitute any color bell pepper for the red, or a combination of colors.

SERVING SUGGESTION
Place 1½ cups salad on a bed of mixed greens for a main dish salad.

NUTRITION PER SERVING	
Serving size	½ cup
Calories	90 kcal
Fat	1 g
Saturated fat	0 g
Cholesterol	0 mg
Sodium	290 mg
Carbohydrates	19 g
Dietary fiber	5 g
Protein	5 g

Vineyard Rice Salad

Diane A. Welland, M.S., R.D.

Serves: 4
Hands-on time: 15 minutes

Virginia-grown grapes have made this a favorite salad in our home. Enjoy it with grapes from anywhere in the country for a main dish salad that is sure to become a hit in your home.

- 1 tablespoon extra-virgin olive oil
- 3 tablespoons apple cider vinegar
- 1 teaspoon sugar
- ¼ teaspoon black pepper
- ½ teaspoon salt
- 3 cups cooked rice
- 2 cups red seedless grapes, quartered
- 5 green onions, chopped
- ½ cup chopped pecans

Stir together the oil, vinegar, sugar, pepper, and salt in a large bowl. Add the rice and mix well to thoroughly combine. Add the grapes, onions, and pecans; stir gently. Serve immediately or refrigerate. Serving at room temperature enhances the flavor.

SUBSTITUTION
Substitute an equal amount of your favorite type of chopped nuts for the pecans.

COOK'S TIP
Instant rice—white or brown—is a great time-saving product to have on hand.

NUTRITION PER SERVING	
Serving size	1¼ cups
Calories	380 kcal
Fat	15 g
Saturated fat	1.5 g
Cholesterol	0 mg
Sodium	300 mg
Carbohydrates	58 g
Dietary fiber	3 g
Protein	5 g

Classic Baked Beans

Regan Miller Jones, R.D., L.D.

Leave it to us southerners to have a secret ingredient like the cola in these baked beans. These beans will be such a hit that you'll have to pass along the recipe—and reveal your secret.

Serves: 5
Hands-on time: 10 minutes
Baking time: 1½ hours

- 1 28-ounce can vegetarian baked beans
- ¼ cup packed brown sugar
- 1 onion, chopped
- ¼ cup ketchup
- ½ cup cola soda
- 1 teaspoon dried mustard
- 1 teaspoon Worcestershire sauce
- 1 teaspoon red wine vinegar
- salt and pepper to taste
- 2 slices bacon

Preheat oven to 350°F.

Combine all the ingredients, except the bacon. Place in a medium-size baking dish. Top with the bacon slices. Bake, uncovered, for 1 to 1½ hours, or until the sauce is thickened and the bacon is cooked.

SERVING SUGGESTION

Serve these baked beans as the main course (the beans provide plenty of protein), accompanied by a tossed green salad and melon chunks.

NUTRITION PER SERVING	
Serving size	⅔ cup
Calories	320 kcal
Fat	2 g
Saturated fat	1 g
Cholesterol	3 mg
Sodium	270 mg
Carbohydrates	61 g
Dietary fiber	10 g
Protein	10 g

Broccoli with Rice

Mary Etta Moorachian, Ph.D., R.D., C.C.P., C.F.C.S.

Serves: 4 as a main dish or 8 as a side dish
Hands-on time: 40 minutes
Baking time: 20 minutes

Here's an updated version of a classic. It's high in whole grains and lower in sodium than the traditional dish. A few shakes of hot sauce lets others know that this recipe comes from a southern home. Serve it as a meatless meal or as a side dish.

- vegetable oil cooking spray
- 16-ounce bag frozen broccoli florets, thawed
- 1 medium-size yellow onion, chopped
- 1 rib celery, chopped
- 1 10½-ounce can reduced-sodium cream of chicken or cream of mushroom soup
- ½ cup water
- 1½ cups hot cooked brown rice
- hot sauce to taste (3 to 5 dashes)
- black pepper to taste
- 1 cup (4 ounces) shredded sharp cheddar
- 32 reduced-sodium thin wheat crackers, broken coarsely

Preheat oven to 350°F. Spray a 9-inch square pan with the cooking spray.

Combine all the ingredients (except the cheese and the crackers) in a large bowl; mix gently. Transfer to the baking pan. Top with the cheese and then the crackers. Bake 30 minutes.

COOK'S TIP
To use fresh broccoli, separate into small florets; steam in the microwave or on the stove-top until crisp tender. Drain and follow the recipe as directed.

NUTRITION PER SERVING

Serving size	1½ cups
Calories	410 kcal
Fat	16 g
Saturated fat	8 g
Cholesterol	35 mg
Sodium	580 mg
Carbohydrates	51 g
Dietary fiber	7 g
Protein	16 g

NUTRITION PER SERVING

Serving size	¾ cup
Calories	205 kcal
Fat	8 g
Saturated fat	4 g
Cholesterol	17 mg
Sodium	290 mg
Carbohydrates	26 g
Dietary fiber	4 g
Protein	8 g

Mom's Potato Salad

Regan Miller Jones, R.D., L.D.

Admittedly, there are some southern recipes that require "portion control" as the only way to make them "lighter." Mom's Potato Salad is a great example. My mother swears you can only make her potato salad using regular mayonnaise. After trying multiple variations substituting reduced-fat and low-fat mayonnaise, I have to agree. I always enjoy the great taste—just a little less of it on my plate.

Serves: 8
Hands-on time: 15 minutes
Cooking time: 20 minutes

6 to 8 medium-size red potatoes, scrubbed and unpeeled (2½ pounds)
¾ cup regular mayonnaise
¼ cup finely chopped onion, optional
1 tablespoon brown mustard, optional
¼ teaspoon salt
1 teaspoon celery seed
½ teaspoon dried dill
¼ teaspoon pepper
1 2-ounce jar pimientos, drained and chopped
½ cup chopped green bell pepper
2 boiled eggs, chopped

SUBSTITUTION
Substitute 1 finely chopped medium-size red bell pepper for the pimientos.

Place the potatoes in a large saucepan; cover with water. Bring to a boil; cook 20 minutes or just until tender. Drain well and cool slightly. Cube the potatoes.

Combine the mayonnaise, onion, mustard, salt, celery seed, dill, pepper, and pimientos in a large bowl; stir well. Fold in the potatoes, bell peppers, and eggs. Cover and refrigerate at least 2 hours before serving.

NUTRITION PER SERVING

Serving size	½ cup
Calories	220 kcal
Fat	18 g
Saturated fat	2.5 g
Cholesterol	60 mg
Sodium	240 mg
Carbohydrates	10 g
Dietary fiber	5 g
Protein	5 g

Mawmaw Ween's Green Beans

Regan Miller Jones, R.D., L.D.

Serves: 6
Hands-on time: 5 minutes
Cooking time: 1 hour, 30 minutes

Virtually everything I know about cooking I learned from my grandmother, Mawmaw Ween. She was one of the best southern cooks I've ever known. When we'd visit my grandparents, she'd always make my favorite—green beans—no matter what else she was serving. Admittedly, her green beans are different from your average recipe, but our family loved them. Mawmaw is gone now, and while I'm glad I have the recipe, I know they'll never taste quite as good as they did at her house.

SHOPPING TIP
Find pickled peaches online to enjoy this recipe as we do in the South.

- 1 pound fresh green beans, trimmed
- 2 tablespoons sugar
- 2 tablespoons apple cider vinegar
- 1 small onion, finely chopped
- ¼ teaspoon salt
- ⅛ to ¼ teaspoon ground black pepper
- ¼ teaspoon garlic powder
- pickled peaches, or fruit salsa or fruit chutney

COOK'S TIP
Substitute a one-pound bag of frozen green beans for the fresh. Reduce cooking time to one hour.

Combine the green beans, sugar, vinegar, ¼ cup water, onion, salt, pepper, and garlic powder in a large saucepan. Bring to a boil over medium-high heat; reduce heat and simmer, covered, for 1 hour and 30 minutes. Serve with pickled peaches or fruit salsa.

NUTRITION PER SERVING

Serving size	1 cup, without fruit
Calories	60 kcal
Fat	0 g
Saturated fat	0 g
Cholesterol	0 mg
Sodium	100 mg
Carbohydrates	14 g
Dietary fiber	3 g
Protein	1 g

Sweet and Sour Steamed Greens and Bacon

Kristine Napier, M.P.H., R.D.

When I lived in Tennessee, we ate greens just about every day. This was our Sunday-best recipe—a treat I still make in my Wisconsin home, and not just on Sundays.

Serves: 6
Hands-on time: 15 minutes
Cooking time: 10 minutes

- 3 slices bacon, chopped
- 1½ tablespoons flour
- 2 tablespoons white vinegar
- 3 tablespoons sugar
- 1 teaspoon black pepper
- ⅛ teaspoon salt
- 12 cups greens (collards, tender young dandelion, spinach, beet, or any combination), washed, trimmed of stems, and chopped coarsely

Cook the bacon in a large kettle until crisp. Remove the bacon, but leave the bacon grease in the kettle. Cover the bacon and set aside. Whisk the flour into the bacon grease over medium heat; the mixture will be very dry.

Combine the vinegar, ⅓ cup water, sugar, pepper, and salt; whisk into the flour mixture. The mixture will thicken slightly. Reduce heat to low.

Add the greens, one handful at a time, stirring well to coat after each addition. Cover and allow to steam for about 10 minutes, stirring frequently. The greens will give up liquid to aid in steaming.

Transfer to a serving dish and garnish with the bacon.

FOOD TRIVIA
Collards (also called collard greens) are a variety of cabbage that don't form a head. Choose crisp green leaves with no sign of yellowing.

NUTRITION NUGGET
Collards are an excellent source of vitamin A, vitamin C, calcium, and iron.

NUTRITION PER SERVING	
Serving size	½ cup
Calories	90 kcal
Fat	2 g
Saturated fat	0.5 g
Cholesterol	5 mg
Sodium	200 mg
Carbohydrates	17 g
Dietary fiber	3 g
Protein	3 g

Poke Salat

Regan Miller Jones, R.D., L.D.

Serves: 6
Hands-on time: 15 minutes
Cooking time: 25 minutes

Poke greens grow wild in the south. This recipe, my Aunt Anita's, embodies everything old southern cooking is about: eating from the land. Many southerners, like me, grew up eating poke salat as well as garden greens such as turnip and collard. My grandfather always liked plenty of cooked onions in his poke salat, which he added to scrambled eggs. He ate this "messuh" eggs and poke salat with a thin slice of cornbread or Johnny-cakes, buttermilk, and a big piece of raw onion on the side.

- 12 cups poke salat greens, and/or mustard greens, spinach, kale, or chard
- 1 tablespoon butter
- 1 tablespoon olive oil
- 1 medium-size onion, chopped
- ¼ teaspoon salt
- ¼ teaspoon black pepper
- hot pepper sauce to taste
- vinegar to taste

In a large saucepan, cook the greens in boiling water 5 minutes; drain thoroughly.

Heat the butter and the olive oil in a large skillet over medium heat, and cook the onion 3 to 5 minutes or until lightly golden. Add the greens to the onion in the skillet. Cover and reduce heat to low; simmer 20 minutes. Add 1 tablespoon water to the skillet if the cooking liquid evaporates. Season with the salt and pepper. Serve with hot pepper sauce and vinegar.

NUTRITION NUGGET
Like other cruciferous vegetables—such as cabbage, cauliflower, broccoli, turnips, and others—kale and Swiss chard get attention for their strong cooking aroma, their nutrient content (beta-carotene, vitamin C, and fiber), and their cancer-fighting potential, in part from their phytonutrients.

FOOD TRIVIA
An old wives' tale warns that if you don't parboil (cook quickly in boiling water) poke leaves, they are poisonous. While this is indeed just an old wives' tale, it is very important to pick poke greens while they're very young (shoots coming up out of the ground no more than 24 inches), as they can develop poisonous chemicals as they age.

NUTRITION PER SERVING	
Serving size	¾ cup
Calories	80 kcal
Fat	4.5 g
Saturated fat	1.5 g
Cholesterol	5 mg
Sodium	170 mg
Carbohydrates	8 g
Dietary fiber	3 g
Protein	3 g

Fire and Ice

Mary Etta Moorachian, Ph.D., R.D., C.C.P., C.F.C.S.

Fire and Ice, a favorite southern recipe, will become a favorite anywhere fresh tomatoes, peppers, and onions are in abundance. Recently the catchy title has been placed on other recipe concoctions, such as watermelon salsa, cocktails, and pineapple-containing chili.

Serves: 6
Hands-on time: 20 minutes
Cooking time: 2 minutes
Chill time: 2 hours

- 2 large red onions, sliced into rings
- 6 large fresh summer tomatoes, diced
- 1 large green bell pepper, diced
- ¾ cup apple cider vinegar
- 2 teaspoons celery seed
- 1½ teaspoons mustard seed
- ½ teaspoon salt
- 2 tablespoons sugar
- ½ teaspoon cracked black pepper
- 1 dash hot sauce

Combine the red onions, tomatoes, and bell pepper in a large bowl.

Mix the vinegar, celery seed, mustard seed, salt, sugar, black pepper, and hot sauce in a small saucepan (1 to 1½ quart); bring to a boil for 1 minute. Pour the boiled sauce over the chopped vegetables. Chill for several hours prior to serving.

FOOD TRIVIA
Onions are related to the lily.

COOK'S TIP
Store leftover chopped onions in a tightly sealed container up to 4 days.

NUTRITION PER SERVING	
Serving size	1 cup
Calories	90 kcal
Fat	1 g
Saturated fat	0 g
Cholesterol	0 mg
Sodium	220 mg
Carbohydrates	19 g
Dietary fiber	3 g
Protein	3 g

Fresh Cauliflower Gratin

Beth P. Witherspoon, M.P.H., R.D.

My mother-in-law, Frances Witherspoon, and my husband's aunt Anna Lee Edwards, from South Carolina, have been pleasing family and friends with this side dish for years.

Serves: 6
Hands-on time: 10 minutes
Cooking time: 10 to 15 minutes

- vegetable oil cooking spray
- 2 teaspoons salt
- 1 whole head cauliflower, trimmed and washed
- 2 tablespoons reduced-fat mayonnaise
- 4 tablespoons honey mustard or stone ground mustard
- ¼ teaspoon cayenne pepper
- 1 cup shredded sharp Cheddar cheese (4 ounces)

Preheat oven to 350°F. Coat a 2-quart ovenproof casserole dish with the cooking spray.

Bring 3 quarts water to a boil; add the salt and the cauliflower. Reduce heat to medium and simmer about 10 minutes or until the cauliflower is fork tender.

Combine the mayonnaise, mustard, and cayenne pepper in a small bowl; set aside.

Remove the cauliflower with a large slotted spoon and fork. Place in the prepared casserole dish and separate the cauliflower florets slightly. Cover with the mustard mixture and top with the shredded cheese.

Bake, uncovered, for 10 to 15 minutes, or until lightly browned on top.

VARIATION

Replace the fresh cauliflower with 1 pound frozen cauliflower florets. Omit the salt and cook in a microwave according to label directions. Drain and continue as directed, except finish in the microwave on high for 1 to 2 minutes.

COOK'S TIP

Prepare this dish one day ahead but do not bake. Keep refrigerated until ready to bake.

NUTRITION PER SERVING

Serving size	¾ cup
Calories	120 kcal
Fat	7 g
Saturated fat	4 g
Cholesterol	15 mg
Sodium	970 mg
Carbohydrates	11 g
Dietary fiber	2 g
Protein	6 g

Georgia Caviar

Mary Etta Moorachian, Ph.D., R.D., C.C.P., C.F.C.S.

Texans may serve this inland "caviar" for good luck at the New Year, but in Georgia it's a treat all year over fresh greens.

Serves: 12
Hands-on time: 15 minutes

- 2 15-ounce cans black-eyed peas, drained and rinsed
- 1½ cups low-fat vinaigrette dressing
- 1 7-ounce jar roasted red pepper, diced
- 1 small onion, diced (about ¾ cup)
- ¼ cup diced jalapeños, seeds and ribs removed
- ½ cup black olives, sliced
- ½ cup sliced mushrooms
- 1 clove garlic, minced
- ¼ to ½ teaspoon black pepper
- 2 10-ounce bags mixed or mesclun greens

Mix all ingredients except greens. Serve over greens.

VARIATION

To use dried peas, soak ½ pound dried black-eyed peas in 1 quart water overnight. Drain and combine in a large saucepan with 1 quart chicken or vegetable broth. Bring to a boil; reduce heat, cover, and simmer 30 to 40 minutes or until tender.

COOK'S TIP

Always wear protective gloves when handling jalapeño or other hot peppers. Wash the cutting surface well after use or use a disposable cutting surface.

NUTRITION PER SERVING	
Serving size	⅓ cup bean mixture over 1 cup greens
Calories	220 kcal
Fat	15 g
Saturated fat	2 g
Cholesterol	0 mg
Sodium	520 mg
Carbohydrates	14 g
Dietary fiber	5 g
Protein	5 g

Carrot Casserole

Mary Etta Moorachian, Ph.D., R.D., C.C.P., C.F.C.S.

Serves: 6
Hands-on time: 20 minutes
Baking time: 15 minutes

Southern church dinners were a tradition during my childhood, and some of my favorite recipes have been inspired by what was shared at those dinners. Vegetable casseroles were always a hit. Here's one that treats carrots in an entirely new way.

2 bunches fresh carrots, scrubbed and stalks removed (about 12 carrots)
vegetable oil cooking spray
½ cup reduced-fat mayonnaise
1 tablespoon minced onion
1 tablespoon horseradish
½ teaspoon salt
¼ teaspoon white pepper
⅓ cup fine cracker crumbs
1 tablespoon butter
⅛ teaspoon paprika
1 tablespoon chopped fresh parsley

SHOPPING TIP
When buying carrots with the greens attached, choose those with moist, bright green leaves.

Cook the carrots whole. Reserve the liquid.

Preheat oven to 375°F. Coat a 13-by-9-inch oven-safe baking dish with the cooking spray.

Cut the cooked carrots lengthwise into ¼-inch strips. Arrange in the baking dish.

Combine ¼ cup of the reserved cooking liquid with the mayonnaise, onion, horseradish, salt, and white pepper in a small bowl. Pour over the carrots; toss to coat. Sprinkle the cracker crumbs evenly over the top. Dot with the butter. Sprinkle the entire casserole with paprika.

Bake uncovered for 15 minutes, or until the crumbs are lightly browned. Garnish with parsley before serving.

COOK'S TIP
Avoid storing carrots next to apples in the refrigerator. Apples give off a gas that carrots absorb, giving the carrots a bitter taste.

NUTRITION PER SERVING

Serving size	1 cup
Calories	90 kcal
Fat	1 g
Saturated fat	0 g
Cholesterol	0 mg
Sodium	410 mg
Carbohydrates	20 g
Dietary fiber	4 g
Protein	2 g

Peanut Soup

Ann A. Hertzler, Ph.D., R.D., L.D.N.

Forget about peanut butter and jelly sandwiches. This rich and creamy soup from the South takes peanut butter to a whole new level. Cayenne adds a kick of flavor.

Serves: 7
Hands-on time: 15 minutes
Cooking time: 40 minutes

- 2 ribs celery, chopped
- 1 small onion, chopped
- 3 carrots, (chopped; 1 grated)
- 3 14-ounce cans reduced-sodium chicken broth, divided
- 1 cup smooth peanut butter
- 1 teaspoon salt
- ½ teaspoon cayenne pepper
- 1 tablespoon fresh lemon juice
- ¼ cup light sour cream, optional
- 2 tablespoons finely chopped fresh chives, optional

Combine the celery, onion, chopped carrots, and 1½ cans of the chicken broth in a large nonstick saucepan. Bring to a boil; reduce heat and simmer, covered, 30 minutes, or until the carrots are tender.

Transfer the soup to a food processor or blender. Process on high until smooth. Return the purée to the saucepan. Turn heat to medium low. Stir in the peanut butter, salt, cayenne, and the remaining 1½ cans broth. Heat just until the mixture starts to simmer.

Stir in the lemon juice before serving. Garnish with grated carrots, if desired, also garnish with sour cream and chives.

SERVING SUGGESTION
Serve with a salad and crusty multi-grain bread.

NUTRITION PER SERVING

Serving size	½ cup
Calories	290 kcal
Fat	21 g
Saturated fat	4.5 g
Cholesterol	5 mg
Sodium	340 mg
Carbohydrates	17 g
Dietary fiber	4 g
Protein	14 g

Okra Stew

Mary Etta Moorachian, Ph.D., R.D., C.C.P., C.F.C.S.

Serves: 6
Hands-on time: 5 minutes
Cooking time: 30 minutes

Okra Stew is a favorite in our southern area and a healthier alternative to typical southern fried okra.

- 1 tablespoon extra-virgin olive oil
- 1 large onion, chopped
- 2 cloves garlic, minced
- 1 14½-ounce can stewed tomatoes
- 1 16-ounce package frozen cut okra, thawed

Heat the oil in a medium-size saucepan over low heat. Cook the onion and the garlic 3 minutes or until soft.

Add the tomatoes; bring to a boil. Add the okra and cook, covered, 10 minutes. Uncover; simmer 20 minutes or until the okra is tender.

VARIATION

Use 1¼ pounds fresh okra in place of the frozen. Choose firm, brightly colored pods that are not more than 4 inches long. Increase cooking time to 35 minutes, or until the okra is tender.

NUTRITION PER SERVING	
Serving size	¾ cup
Calories	70 kcal
Fat	2.5 g
Saturated fat	0 g
Cholesterol	0 mg
Sodium	30 mg
Carbohydrates	12 g
Dietary fiber	3 g
Protein	2 g

Beaufort Stew

Beth P. Witherspoon, M.P.H., R.D.

My husband's mother, Frances Witherspoon, and his aunt Anna Lee Edwards introduced me to a similar version of this South Carolina Low Country family favorite when we were dating. Since then, it's been a favorite, easy one-pot meal that's good enough to serve company.

Serves: 4
Hands-on time: 10 minutes
Cooking time: 20 to 30 minutes

- 4 teaspoons black pepper
- 1 to 2 tablespoons Old Bay seasoning
- 4 medium-size red potatoes (1 pound)
- 2 large carrots, each cut into 3 large chunks
- ⅓ pound favorite smoked link sausage, cut into 2-inch pieces
- 4 ears corn, shucked and broken in half
- ½ pound raw shrimp in shell

Boil 1 gallon water, pepper, and Old Bay seasoning in a large saucepot. Add the potatoes, carrots, and sausage; reduce heat and simmer 10 to 15 minutes.

Add the corn; cook 5 to 10 minutes. Add the shrimp; cook 3 to 5 minutes or until pink. Drain and serve immediately.

SUBSTITUTION

To make the meal lower in fat, use low-fat sausage or half low-fat and half regular sausage.

SERVING SUGGESTIONS

Serve with a green salad, cocktail sauce for the shrimp, and desired condiments for the corn and potatoes. For more people, just increase the amount of potatoes, sausage, corn, and shrimp according to the size of your crowd.

NUTRITION PER SERVING	
Serving size	2 cups
Calories	290 kcal
Fat	12 g
Saturated fat	4.5 g
Cholesterol	110 mg
Sodium	1,010 mg (with 1 tablespoon Old Bay); 1,450 (with 2 tablespoons Old Bay)
Carbohydrates	26 g
Dietary fiber	7 g
Protein	22 g

Butternut Squash Soup

Mary Etta Moorachian, Ph.D., R.D., C.C.P., C.F.C.S.

Serves: 4 as a main dish or 8 as a side dish
Hands-on time: 20 minutes
Cooking time: 35 minutes

A little zesty, a little gentle, here is a southern version of a delightfully beautiful and healthful dish.

- 1 tablespoon butter
- 1 large onion, chopped
- 1 medium-size butternut squash, peeled and diced (about 2½ pounds)
- 1 large cooking apple, diced (peel on)
- 3 tablespoons all-purpose flour
- 1½ teaspoons curry powder
- ⅛ teaspoon ground nutmeg
- 2 14-ounce cans reduced-sodium chicken broth
- 1 cup nonfat milk
- 1 tablespoon orange zest
- ¼ cup orange juice
- ¼ teaspoon white pepper
- ¼ cup freshly chopped parsley, optional
- 1 tablespoon orange zest, optional

Melt the butter over medium heat in a 3- or 4- quart large saucepan. Sauté the onion until tender, about 5 minutes. Add the squash and the apple; sauté an additional 5 minutes. Stir in the flour, curry powder, and nutmeg; cook 5 more minutes. Stir in the broth, milk, orange zest, orange juice, and white pepper. Cover and simmer 20 minutes, or until the squash is fork tender.

Purée the soup in a blender or a food processor (a blender works best) in small batches (about 1½ cups at a time) until smooth. Garnish the soup with parsley and orange zest, if desired.

COOK'S TIP

Substitute two 12-ounce boxes of frozen winter squash (thawed) for the fresh. Stir in the squash after puréeing the other ingredients. Heat 5 to 7 minutes, or until piping hot.

NUTRITION PER SERVING

Serving size	4, main course
Calories	270 kcal
Fat	5 g
Saturated fat	2.5 g
Cholesterol	15 mg
Sodium	160 mg
Carbohydrates	51 g
Dietary fiber	11 g
Protein	9 g

NUTRITION PER SERVING

Serving size	8, side dish
Calories	130 kcal
Fat	2.5 g
Saturated fat	1.5 g
Cholesterol	5 mg
Sodium	80 mg
Carbohydrates	25 g
Dietary fiber	5 g
Protein	5 g

Jeffersonian Beef Stew

Kristine Napier, M.P.H., R.D.

Thomas Jefferson was quite the gourmet. Among his many signature dishes served in his Virginia home was beef stew. "Boeuf a la mode," the recipe penned in his own hand, is still preserved. President Jefferson loved tomatoes and fresh herbs, which flavor this stew so nicely.

Serves: 6
Hands-on time: 20 minutes
Cooking time: 65 minutes

- 2 tablespoons all-purpose flour
- ½ teaspoon black pepper
- 2 teaspoons beef bouillon granules (2 cubes)
- 1 pound round steak, trimmed of all visible fat, and cut into cubes
- 2 tablespoons canola oil
- 2 large onions, cut into wedges
- 3 cloves garlic, chopped
- 2 14½-ounce cans stewed tomatoes
- ½ cup red wine, optional
- 1 pound unpeeled red potatoes, scrubbed and cut into bite-size pieces
- 4 large carrots, scrubbed and cut into 1-inch chunks
- 1 tablespoon chopped fresh oregano, or 1 teaspoon dried
- 1 tablespoon chopped fresh basil, or 1 teaspoon dried

Blend the flour, pepper, and bouillon granules in a plastic bag; add the meat and shake until coated.

Heat the oil in a heavy 3-quart kettle or a Dutch oven over medium-high heat. Brown the meat on all sides, about 3 to 4 minutes. Reduce heat to medium. Add the onions, garlic, tomatoes, wine, potatoes, and carrots. If using dried herbs, add now. Stir well. Cover and simmer for 30 minutes.

Uncover, stir in the fresh herbs. Simmer gently an additional 30 minutes, or until the liquid thickens, stirring occasionally.

VARIATIONS

Use ⅓ cup red wine or balsamic vinegar in place of the wine; also stir in 2 teaspoons sugar.

NUTRITION NUGGET

Using no-salt-added tomatoes reduces the sodium in this recipe to 300 mg.

NUTRITION PER SERVING

Serving size	1¼ cups
Calories	390 kcal
Fat	10 g
Saturated fat	2 g
Cholesterol	70 mg
Sodium	430 mg
Carbohydrates	42 g
Dietary fiber	5 g
Protein	32 g

Frogmore Stew

Mary Etta Moorachian, Ph.D., R.D., C.C.P., C.F.C.S.

Serves: 8
Hands-on time: 10 minutes
Cooking time: 10 minutes

In Louisiana, we enjoyed shrimp and crawfish boils. When we moved to South Carolina, we were soon introduced to Frogmore Stew, one of many types of Low Country seafood boils. When partaking of this delicious stew, flatware and chairs are not necessary, although napkins are a must.

SHOPPING TIP

The number of shrimp per pound is based on their size. In general, 1 pound yields 21 to 24 jumbo, 26 to 30 extra large, 31 to 35 large, 43 to 50 medium, or 51 to 60 small shrimp.

VARIATION

Substitute equal amounts of any type of shellfish for the shrimp, or mix it up and use a combination of different types.

3 tablespoons shrimp or seafood boil seasoning, such as Old Bay
1 tablespoon salt
1½ gallons chicken or seafood broth
2 pounds red potatoes, whole, skin on
1 pound smoked sausage, cut into 16 slices
4 ears corn, shucked and broken into 3- to 4-inch pieces
4 pounds large shrimp in shells

Combine the seasonings, salt, and broth in a large stock pot; bring to a boil. Add the potatoes and boil just until tender, about 5 to 10 minutes. Add the sausage and corn and cook 5 minutes (begin timing immediately—do not wait until the water begins boiling again). Add the shrimp and cook 3 minutes. Drain immediately.

Serve outdoors with a variety of fresh hot breads on tables draped with paper cloths (or newspapers).

NUTRITION PER SERVING

Serving size	15 to 17 shrimp, 2 slices sausage, 2 or 3 pieces corn, 2 or 3 potatoes
Calories	520 kcal
Fat	22 g
Saturated fat	7 g
Cholesterol	385 mg
Sodium	850 mg
Carbohydrates	24 g
Dietary fiber	5 g
Protein	58 g

Southern Corn Chowder

Mary Etta Moorachian, Ph.D., R.D., C.C.P., C.F.C.S.

I have lived in six different Southern states and all of them claim corn as a favorite ingredient. Although there are many different varieties of corn, all are good in chowder.

Serves: 6
Hands-on time: 20 minutes
Cooking time: 45 minutes

- 3 tablespoons butter
- 1 medium-size onion, chopped
- 1 stalk celery, diced (¼ cup)
- 1 pound medium-size baking potatoes, diced (peel on)
- 1 14-ounce can reduced-sodium chicken stock
- ¼ teaspoon nutmeg
- ¼ cup all-purpose flour
- 3 cups nonfat milk, divided
- 3 cups fresh corn kernels, blanched, or 1 20-ounce bag frozen corn, thawed

Melt the butter in a Dutch oven over low heat. Sauté the onion and celery for 3 to 5 minutes. Add the potatoes, chicken stock, and nutmeg. Cover and simmer until the potatoes are tender.

Combine the flour and the milk in a small bowl; whisk until smooth. Add to the potatoes and stir until thickened. Stir in the corn, heat through, and serve.

COOK'S TIP

Spice it up by adding hot sauce (such as tabasco) if you like a little more kick to your chowder.

NUTRITION NUGGET

Using a small amount of butter in this recipe lends a rich flavor, but adds only 7 grams of fat per serving, an excellent cost-to-benefit ratio.

NUTRITION PER SERVING	
Serving size	1 cup
Calories	260 kcal
Fat	7 g
Saturated fat	4 g
Cholesterol	20 mg
Sodium	180 mg
Carbohydrates	45 g
Dietary fiber	5 g
Protein	11 g

French Market Soup

Mary Etta Moorachian, Ph.D., R.D., C.C.P., C.F.C.S.

Serves: 8
Soaking time: 3 hours or more
Hands-on time: 10 minutes
Cooking time: 2½ to 3½ hours

Bean packets sold in the French Market in New Orleans inspired the name of this soup. Beans provide both taste and nutritional value. Although I grew up on some form of beans every week, it wasn't until living in Louisiana that I learned to add multiple layers of flavors to beans. My brother and I laugh as we have actually added hot sauce to veggie and bean soups for years before I started seeing it in printed recipes.

4 cups bean mixture (see below)
2 cups diced lean ham
1 tablespoon salt
2 bay leaves or a bouquet garni bag
2 medium-size onions, chopped
3 cloves garlic, chopped
1 tablespoon extra-virgin olive oil
2 boneless, skinless chicken breasts, cooked and cubed
3 14½-ounce cans stewed tomatoes
3 stalks celery, sliced thinly
hot sauce (to taste)

Bean Mixture

Combine 1 cup each of any combination of the following:

speckled lima beans	green peas
great northern beans	lentils
navy beans	pinto beans
black beans	fava beans
red kidney beans	green split peas
chick peas	black-eyed or crowder peas

Wash and drain the beans and the peas. Cover with cold water and soak for at least 3 hours.

Rinse the beans. Add 5 quarts water and the ham, salt, and bay leaves or bouquet garni bag. Simmer, covered, for 2 to 3 hours.

Sauté the onions and garlic in olive oil. Add to the beans with the chicken, tomatoes, celery, and hot sauce. Simmer 20 minutes.

VARIATION

Omit the ham and chicken to make a vegetarian dish.

NUTRITION PER SERVING

Serving size	1 bowl
Calories	490 kcal
Fat	7 g
Saturated fat	2 g
Cholesterol	50 mg
Sodium	410 mg
Carbohydrates	71 g
Dietary fiber	21 g
Protein	39 g

Okra and Chicken Stew

Mary Etta Moorachian, Ph.D., R.D., C.C.P., C.F.C.S.

For those of us who live in the South, cooking with okra is commonplace. When you cook okra, it may surprise you that it becomes somewhat slippery, but this is what helps thicken the stew. Look for fresh okra in the produce section or buy it frozen. Southerners learn early that a gumbo always begins with a good roux, but I've learned to make it with a little less fat.

Serves: 8
Hands-on time: 20 minutes
Cooking time: 40 minutes

3 tablespoons canola oil
3 tablespoons flour
2 medium-size onions, chopped
4 green onions, chopped
1 medium-size red bell pepper, chopped
½ cup chopped fresh parsley
2½ pounds cut okra, fresh or frozen
2 14½-ounce cans stewed tomatoes
3 14-ounce cans reduced-sodium chicken broth
1½ pounds cooked chicken (skinned and boned)
hot sauce to taste
filé powder to taste

In a large heavy kettle or Dutch oven, make a dark roux by combining the oil and the flour over low heat. Cook and stir, about 10 to 15 minutes. The roux will darken to a caramel color with continued heating.

Add the onions, peppers, parsley, okra, tomatoes, and broth. Stir to combine. Bring to a boil, stirring. Cover, reduce heat, and simmer 20 minutes, or until the vegetables are tender. Add the chicken and the hot sauce; stir and simmer.

Serve over rice, sprinkle with filé powder.

FOOD TRIVIA

The Choctaw Indians from the Louisiana bayous taught settlers how to use the ground dried leaves of the sassafras tree to season foods. Filé powder is especially popular in Creole cooking, especially to flavor gumbos. Adding a woodsy flavor, filé must be stirred into food after it is removed from the heat; otherwise, the filé becomes tough and stringy.

SHOPPING TIP

Buy filé powder in the spice or gourmet section of large supermarkets; alternatively, order it online.

SUBSTITUTION

Substitute 1½ pounds cooked shrimp for the chicken.

COOK'S TIP

Store filé powder in a cool, dark place for not more than 6 months.

NUTRITION PER SERVING

Serving size	1 to 1½ cups
Calories	340 kcal
Fat	11 g
Saturated fat	2 g
Cholesterol	80 mg
Sodium	400 mg
Carbohydrates	27 g
Dietary fiber	7 g
Protein	36 g

Vegetable Stock

Mary Etta Moorachian, Ph.D., R.D., C.C.P., C.F.C.S.

Serves: 16
Hands-on time: 15 minutes
Cooking time: 1 hour, 30 minutes

Fruit (my southern secret) adds a nice touch of sweetness to this vegetable stock, which is especially delicious as a base for vegetable soups. As a side note, it freezes well, so make the full gallon and divide it into portions.

½ lemon, juiced
1 gallon plus 2 cups cold water
½ pound fresh fruit, peeled and chopped (such as pears or apples)
1½ pound onions, or parsnips, chopped
3 ribs celery, chopped
½ pound turnips, peeled and diced
½ pound leeks, chopped, white parts only
½ pound carrots, chopped
½ pound tomatoes, chopped
1 bay leaf
2 sprigs fresh thyme, or ⅛ teaspoon dried thyme
6 whole black peppercorns
6 whole cloves
1 cup white wine, optional

Mix the lemon juice with 2 cups water in a large bowl. Add the fruit to the water; set aside.

Drain the fruit; combine in a stockpot with the onion, celery, turnips, leeks, carrots, and tomatoes. Cook the vegetable mixture over medium heat 15 minutes. Add the bay leaf, thyme, peppercorns, and cloves. Add white wine, if desired, when entire mixture is warm. Reduce heat; simmer 30 minutes, or until liquid is reduced by half. Add 1 gallon water; return to a simmer and cook 45 minutes.

Strain in large colander. Cool the stock quickly and refrigerate, or freeze it in small batches.

VARIATION

To intensify the flavor, after straining stock, return to the stockpot and simmer over low heat to reduce the liquid and concentrate the flavor and color.

NUTRITION PER SERVING

Serving size	1 to 1½ cups
Calories	70 kcal
Fat	0 g
Saturated fat	0 g
Cholesterol	0 mg
Sodium	15 mg
Carbohydrates	14 g
Dietary fiber	3 g
Protein	1 g

Cajun Salmon over Polenta

Regan Miller Jones, R.D., L.D.

Polenta is a close cousin to grits, a dish that many southerners consider a staple. Polenta is also a favorite around my house. Since a southern kitchen is always stocked with cornmeal for corn bread, preparing polenta is an easy way to dress up our humble grain. Although my husband loves this recipe, he still insists that we're eating "grits for dinner." Steamed broccoli or asparagus are excellent accompaniments.

Serves: 2
Hands-on time: 5 minutes
Cooking time: 20 minutes

2 5-ounce salmon fillets
1 to 2 tablespoons Cajun seasoning (recipe follows)
1 tablespoon butter
1 tablespoon canola oil
¼ cup nonfat milk
¼ teaspoon salt
½ cup medium-grind or stone-ground cornmeal
2 tablespoons grated Parmesan cheese

Preheat oven to 400°F.

Coat the salmon with Cajun seasoning; set aside.

Heat a medium-size ovenproof skillet over medium-high heat for about 2 to 3 minutes. Add the butter and the oil. Let the butter melt until foam subsides. Sear the salmon, skin side up, about 3 to 4 minutes. Turn the salmon over. Transfer the skillet to the oven. Bake, uncovered, about 6 to 8 minutes, or until the salmon is moist and slightly pink in the center.

In a medium-size saucepan, heat 1½ cups water, the milk, and salt to boiling. Gradually whisk in the cornmeal, a little at a time, whisking constantly. Reduce heat and simmer, stirring occasionally, about 5 minutes or until thickened. Remove from heat. Stir in the cheese. Serve the salmon over the polenta.

CAJUN SEASONING

Mix together 1 tablespoon paprika, 1 tablespoon salt, 1 tablespoon garlic powder, 2 teaspoons black pepper, 1 tablespoon onion powder, 1 tablespoon cayenne pepper, 2 tablespoons dried oregano, 1 tablespoon dried thyme.

SHOPPING TIP

Instead of making your own polenta with the water, milk, cornmeal, salt, and Parmesan cheese, purchase polenta in a tube, slice, and heat as directed on the package.

COOK'S TIP

To save time, sprinkle the salmon with your desired amount of Cajun seasoning and bake in a 425°F oven for 10 to 15 minutes, or until the salmon flakes easily with a fork.

NUTRITION PER SERVING	
Serving size	1 salmon fillet and ⅔ cup polenta
Calories	480 kcal
Fat	25 g
Saturated fat	7 g
Cholesterol	100 mg
Sodium	900 mg
Carbohydrates	29 g
Dietary fiber	3 g
Protein	34 g

Shrimp or Crawfish Clemenceau

Julienne T. Stewart, M.S., R.D., L.D.N.

Serves: 4
Hands-on time: 20 minutes
Cooking time: 60 minutes

Clemenceau is a Creole style of cooking that uses potatoes and peas. Generally, Clemenceau-style recipes include Louisiana seafood, such as crawfish. Chicken and other types of fish can be used instead.

vegetable oil cooking spray
2 large baking potatoes, scrubbed and diced
½ pound fresh mushrooms, quartered
1 pound crawfish tails, or peeled shrimp, or some combination totaling 1 pound
2 cloves garlic, minced
1 10-ounce box frozen petite peas, thawed
½ cup white wine
¼ cup fresh lemon juice
1 tablespoon butter, cut into 3 pieces
⅛ teaspoon salt
black pepper to taste
hot sauce to taste
5 green onions, chopped, green part only

Preheat oven to 400°F. Coat the diced potatoes with the cooking spray, place in a baking dish, and bake until soft, about one-half hour.

Meanwhile, coat a large skillet with the cooking spray. Add the mushrooms and cook for 2 to 3 minutes. Add the crawfish, garlic, and peas; stir. (If using shrimp, add the garlic and peas when the shrimp turn pink.) Add the wine and lemon juice to the pan and simmer over low heat to reduce the liquid by one-half, about 15 minutes.

SUBSTITUTION

Instead of using shrimp or crawfish, slice 1 pound of skinless, boneless chicken breasts into bite-size pieces. Sauté the chicken with the mushrooms, adding 2 tablespoons canola oil, over medium-high heat. Cook until the chicken is slightly browned and no longer pink in the middle, about 4 to 6 minutes.

FOOD TRIVIA

Crawfish are very popular in the coastal South, particularly in the Gulf Bayou region of Louisiana, Alabama, Mississippi, and Florida. The majority of crawfish in the United States are harvested from the waters of the Mississippi basin. Coastal crustaceans, such as spiny or rock lobster, are sometimes mistakenly called saltwater crawfish. Although they are not the same species, they can be substituted for the freshwater variety. The names *crayfish*, *crawfish*, and *crawdads* are used interchangeably.

NUTRITION PER SERVING

Serving size	1 cup
Calories	300 kcal
Fat	5 g
Saturated fat	2 g
Cholesterol	180 mg
Sodium	330 mg
Carbohydrates	30 g
Dietary fiber	6 g
Protein	31 g

Add the butter pieces one at a time until the sauce is creamy and slightly thickened. Season with the salt, pepper, and hot sauce.

Place the cooked potatoes on a serving platter. Pour the seafood mixture over the potatoes. Top with the chopped green onion.

FOOD TRIVIA

Georges Clemenceau was a French statesman (1841–1929) who led France during WWI and was the chief of the French delegation to the Paris Peace Conference in 1919. He played a key role in negotiating the Treaty of Versailles. This Creole dish was named for him.

Smoky Holler Fried Chicken, Mashed Potatoes, and Gravy

Kristine Napier, M.P.H., R.D.

Serves: 4
Hands-on time: 20 minutes
Cooking time: 20 minutes

In a beautiful little hollow of Tennessee—called smoky because of the fog that rose from the ground like smoke every morning—my husband's distant cousins fried chicken every Sunday. A favorite part of this meal was the gravy, made with milk. Enjoy!

4 to 6 unpeeled red potatoes (about 1 pound)
⅓ cup flour
3 teaspoons chicken bouillon granules
½ teaspoon black pepper
¼ teaspoon garlic powder
4 skinless bone-in chicken breast halves (about 1½ pounds raw)
1 tablespoon butter
1 tablespoon canola oil
3 tablespoons reduced-fat cream cheese
1 tablespoon butter
½ to 1 teaspoon white pepper
¼ teaspoon salt
2¾ cups nonfat milk, divided

Scrub the potatoes and cut them into small pieces that will boil quickly. Place in a kettle with enough water to cover, plus 1 inch. Cover and bring to a boil. Reduce heat and simmer until fork tender.

Meanwhile, blend the flour, bouillon, pepper, and garlic powder in a large plastic bag; add the chicken, seal the bag, and shake to coat the chicken.

Heat the butter and the oil in a large skillet over medium-high heat. Add the coated chicken; brown each side about 3 to 4 minutes. (Reserve the remaining flour mixture for making gravy later.) Reduce heat, add 2 tablespoons water, cover, and simmer until the chicken is cooked through, about 10 minutes. Do not overcook.

Remove the chicken from the pan; cover and keep warm. Increase heat under the pan; whisk in the remaining flour mixture. The mixture will be very dry. Slowly add 2 cups milk, whisking as you do; the mixture will thicken. Remove from heat, place the chicken in the gravy, cover, and keep warm.

COOK'S TIP
Cooking chicken with the bone in can make it moister and more flavorful.

NUTRITION PER SERVING

Serving size	1 piece chicken plus ¾ cup potatoes plus ¼ cup gravy
Calories	480 kcal
Fat	6 g
Saturated fat	6 g
Cholesterol	100 mg
Sodium	1,020 mg
Carbohydrates	46 g
Dietary fiber	3 g
Protein	39 g

Drain the potatoes and return them to the coo[illegible]
Add the cream cheese, butter, white pepper, salt, and [illegible]
ing 3/4 cup nonfat milk. Cover and heat over low heat, just [illegible]
until all ingredients are hot (do not boil). Mash by hand with [illegible]
a masher or an electric beater or mixer.

king pot.
remain-

hicken

ted chicken rivals its deep-fried traditional
crunch, taste, and texture without the fat and
n thighs, dipped in buttermilk and coated with
n, are delicious and nutritious!

oil cooking spray
ed Parmesan cheese
eat germ
oon dried rosemary leaves, crushed
poon onion powder
spoon garlic salt
aspoon dried thyme
easpoon ground black pepper
cup buttermilk
skinless chicken thighs, rinsed and dried

Preheat oven to 350°F. Spray a baking sheet with the cooking spray.

Combine the Parmesan cheese, wheat germ, rosemary, onion powder, garlic salt, thyme, and pepper in a shallow bowl; set aside. Pour the buttermilk in a separate shallow bowl.

Dip the chicken in the buttermilk, then roll in the wheat germ mixture and place on a baking sheet. Bake for 50 minutes or until tender.

COOK'S TIP
The baking time can be reduced by replacing chicken thighs with chicken tenders.

NUTRITION NUGGET
For a healthier meal, trim any visible fat before beginning.

NUTRITION PER SERVING	
Serving size	1 thigh
Calories	80 kcal
Fat	3 g
Saturated fat	1 g
Cholesterol	5 mg
Sodium	135 mg
Carbohydrates	5 g
Dietary fiber	2 g
Protein	9 g

Inside-Out "Fried" Chicken

Lisa C. Peterson, M.S., R.D., C.D.N.

Transferring the cooking oil to the "inside," under the breading, means lots of flavor, less time over the stove, and less fat. In my Connecticut-shore home, I like to formalize the dish by serving it with a chunky fruit salsa in the summer, roasted tomato marinara in the winter, or caper-herb vinaigrette anytime.

Serves: 4
Hands-on time: 15 minutes
Cooking time: 40 minutes

- vegetable oil cooking spray
- 8 pieces skinless bone-in chicken, breasts, thighs, or drumsticks
- ¼ cup canola oil
- ½ cup seasoned dried breadcrumbs
- ½ cup yellow cornmeal
- ½ teaspoon black pepper
- ½ teaspoon salt
- 1 teaspoon garlic powder, optional
- ¼ teaspoon cayenne, optional

Preheat oven to 400° F. Spray a large sheet pan with cooking spray.

Place the chicken in a bowl large enough to hold all of it. Pour the oil over the chicken and rub it into all pieces. Set aside.

Combine the breadcrumbs, cornmeal, and seasonings in a separate large bowl. Dredge the chicken through the breadcrumb mixture. Arrange the chicken on a prepared pan so the pieces don't touch. Bake about 40 minutes, turning once halfway through the cooking. The internal temperature of the chicken should reach 165°F. Serve hot.

SHOPPING TIP

Try different flavors of seasoned bread crumbs such as Italian, cheese, garlic, and herb-seasoned to see which you most prefer.

COOK'S TIP

Use only bone-in chicken pieces for this recipe since they retain their moisture and flavor best.

NUTRITION PER SERVING	
Serving size	2 pieces
Calories	310 kcal
Fat	10 g
Saturated fat	1.5 g
Cholesterol	95 mg
Sodium	445 mg
Carbohydrates	6 g
Dietary fiber	1 g
Protein	41 g

Creole Jambalaya

Maria C. Alamo, M.P.H., R.D., L.D.

Serves: 6
Hands-on time: 15 minutes
Cooking time: 55 minutes

The Spanish contributions to Creole cuisine include mixing fish and meat in one dish, as well as serving meat dishes over rice. Hence the shrimp, sausage, and rice jambalaya. The Spanish also cook with hot peppers, which add a kick to a few Creole dishes.

- ½ pound chopped andouille sausage
- 1 large onion, chopped
- 2 ribs celery, chopped
- 1 large green bell pepper, chopped
- 2 cloves garlic, chopped
- 2 8-ounce cans no-salt-added tomato sauce
- 1 28-ounce can diced tomatoes
- 1 teaspoon dried basil
- 1 teaspoon dried thyme
- 1 teaspoon paprika
- 1 bay leaf
- ¼ to 1 teaspoon hot sauce
- 1 cup uncooked brown rice
- ½ pound cooked, peeled shrimp

Combine the sausage, onion, celery, green pepper, and garlic in a large heavy kettle over medium heat. Cook and stir until the meat is browned, about 8 to 10 minutes. Add the tomato sauce, tomatoes, 1 cup water, basil, thyme, paprika, bay leaf, and hot sauce. Increase heat and bring to a boil. Add the rice, reduce heat, cover, and simmer 45 minutes.

Remove from heat; stir in the cooked shrimp. Remove the bay leaf before serving.

SUBSTITUTION
Substitute ½ pound uncooked boneless, skinless chicken cut in bite-size pieces for the shrimp. Brown with the sausage in the first step.

NUTRITION PER SERVING

Serving size	1¾ cups
Calories	380 kcal
Fat	14 g
Saturated fat	4.5 g
Cholesterol	85 mg
Sodium	840 mg
Carbohydrates	42 g
Dietary fiber	5 g
Protein	20 g

Cajun Jambalaya

Julienne T. Stewart, M.S., R.D., L.D.N.

Recipes for jambalaya usually use leftover meat seasoned with ham or sausage. My favorite ingredients are chicken or shrimp. Browning the meat in the pot gives the jambalaya nice color.

Serves: 8
Hands-on time: 15 minutes
Cooking time: 50 minutes

½ pound chopped ham, tasso, andouille sausage, or smoked sausage
1 large onion, chopped
2 ribs celery, chopped
1 large green bell pepper, chopped
2 cloves garlic, chopped
1½ cups uncooked rice
2 14-ounce cans reduced-sodium chicken broth
1 teaspoon seasoned salt
1 bay leaf
½ pound cooked chicken, cut into bite-size pieces
¼ to 1 teaspoon hot sauce

Brown the ham or the sausage in a heavy 3-quart kettle, over high heat for about 5 to 7 minutes. Reduce heat to medium. Add the onion, celery, green pepper, and garlic. Cook and stir until the vegetables are lightly browned and wilted, about 5 minutes.

Add the dry rice and stir for about 5 minutes, until the rice has some color. Add the chicken broth and stir to loosen any scrapings from the bottom of the pot. Add the seasoned salt and bay leaf. Bring to a boil. Reduce heat and cook on low for 25 minutes, or until all the liquid is absorbed.

Remove the bay leaf; fluff the rice. Stir in the chicken and the hot sauce.

SHOPPING TIP
Tasso is a Cajun spiced ham; andouille sausage is Cajun seasoned smoked pork sausage.

FOOD TRIVIA
Creoles make red tomato sauce jambalaya (sometimes with pasta) while the Cajuns make a brown spicy jambalaya with rice.

NUTRITION PER SERVING	
Serving size	1¾ cups
Calories	320 kcal
Fat	12 g
Saturated fat	4 g
Cholesterol	45 mg
Sodium	520 mg
Carbohydrates	32 g
Dietary fiber	2 g
Protein	21 g

Natchitoches Meat Pies

Stephanie Green, R.D.

Serves: 8
Hands-on time: 30 minutes
Cooking time: 50 minutes

SUBSTITUTION
Substitute one 16-ounce can of black or pinto beans for one type of meat—or for both—to add more fiber and reduce the fat.

Comfort food at your service, direct from Natchitoches, Louisiana, the oldest permanent settlement in the Louisiana Purchase.

- vegetable oil cooking spray
- ½ pound extra-lean ground beef
- ½ pound pork sausage, casing removed
- 4 cloves garlic, chopped
- 3 ribs celery, finely chopped
- 2 medium-size onions, finely chopped
- 2 tablespoons Cajun seasoning (recipe follows)
- 2 9-inch refrigerated pie crusts
- 2 egg whites

Preheat oven to 350°F. Coat a sheet pan with the cooking spray.

Cook the ground beef, sausage, and garlic in a large skillet over medium-high heat for about 8 to 10 minutes or until no pink remains. Remove the meat from the skillet and set aside, draining off grease. Add the celery, onion, and Cajun seasoning to the skillet and cook, stirring frequently, until tender, about 15 to 20 minutes. Combine the meat and celery mixture in a large bowl. Let cool.

Cut the pie crust sheets into quarters. Place a small portion of the meat filling on one half of each piece of pie crust, leaving a ½-inch border around the outer 2 sides. Brush the edge with egg white and fold the dough into a triangle. Press down with a fork to seal in the meat filling. You should have 4 triangles from each pie crust. Brush the tops with egg white. Place on the prepared sheet pan and bake for 15 to 20 minutes or until golden.

Cajun Seasoning

Blend 1 tablespoon paprika, 2 teaspoons salt, 1 tablespoon garlic powder, 1 tablespoon onion powder, 2 teaspoons cayenne (or more if you like it hotter), 1 teaspoon black pepper, and 2 tablespoons dried oregano. Mix well and store in an air-tight container in the refrigerator or freezer.

NUTRITION PER SERVING

Serving size	1 pie
Calories	290 kcal
Fat	17 g
Saturated fat	4 g
Cholesterol	20 mg
Sodium	760 mg
Carbohydrates	23 g
Dietary fiber	2 g
Protein	12 g

Louisiana Shepherd's Pie

Barbara J. Alvarez, M.P.H., R.D., L.D.N.

Hailing from Louisiana, this version of Shepherd's Pie uses gravy—and a unique one at that!

Serves: 6
Hands-on time: 30 minutes
Cooking time: 30 minutes

vegetable oil cooking spray
2 pounds unpeeled potatoes, washed and diced
½ cup nonfat milk
8 ounces reduced-fat sour cream
½ teaspoon pepper
1 teaspoon salt
1 medium-size onion, chopped
1 pound extra-lean ground beef
1 stalk celery, sliced thinly
2 cloves garlic, minced
1 14-ounce can reduced-sodium beef stock
2 tablespoons all-purpose flour
½ cup old-fashioned oats
1 tablespoon Worcestershire sauce
1 cup frozen green beans
1 cup frozen corn
½ cup shredded sharp cheddar cheese (2 ounces)

Preheat oven to 350°F. Spray a 3-quart casserole dish with the cooking spray.

Boil the potatoes in a large saucepan until fork tender. Drain off any remaining water. Mash the potatoes with the milk, sour cream, pepper, and salt.

While the potatoes are cooking, sauté the onion, beef, celery, and garlic in a large nonstick skillet until the beef is cooked through and the onions are translucent. Remove from the skillet; set aside.

Combine the beef stock, flour, oats, and Worcestershire sauce in skillet to make the gravy. Heat to boiling, stirring until thickened.

Place the beef mixture in the bottom of the prepared casserole dish. Top with the green beans and the corn. Pour the gravy over the top. Spoon the mashed potatoes on top of the gravy layer. Bake, uncovered, 30 minutes. Top with cheese; return to the oven and bake 10 to 15 minutes, or until the cheese bubbles.

NUTRITION PER SERVING	
Serving size	1½ cups
Calories	420 kcal
Fat	15 g
Saturated fat	7 g
Cholesterol	65 mg
Sodium	600 mg
Carbohydrates	45 g
Dietary fiber	4 g
Protein	25 g

Pan-Seared Pork Chops with Vidalia Onions

Regan Miller Jones, R.D., L.D.

Serves: 4
Hands-on time: 20 minutes
Cooking time: 40 minutes

Vidalia onions are one of the best tasting crops to come out of the southern soil. I developed this recipe one spring when my Georgia kitchen was full of Vidalias. This recipe also calls for "brining" the pork chops—a southern tradition. Given the tenderness of pork, brining isn't a necessity, but it does add to the juiciness. You can choose the method that works for you: skip the brining, or try it out for old southern time's sake. I recommend you cook all four onions—they cook down considerably and they're just down-home great!

SERVING SUGGESTION
Serve over mashed potatoes.

- 4 1-inch-thick rib pork chops (about 1½ pounds with bone)
- ¼ cup salt
- ¼ teaspoon ground black pepper
- ¼ to ½ teaspoon ground sage
- 1½ tablespoons canola oil, divided
- 2 to 4 large Vidalia or other sweet onions, cut into thin slices
- ⅔ cup dry white wine
- 2 tablespoons chopped fresh thyme, or 1 teaspoon dried
- 2 tablespoons chopped fresh parsley

FOOD TRIVIA
In the south, Vidalias are the prevailing sweet onions. The Northwest boasts the WallaWalla, and in Maui you'll find the Maui Sweet.

To Brine the Chops

Boil 1 quart water and the salt until the salt dissolves. Cool. Immerse the chops in the water. Cover tightly and refrigerate at least 8 hours.

When ready to cook, remove the pork chops from the brine and pat dry with paper towels.

If Not Brining

Season the pork chops with the pepper and sage. Heat ½ tablespoon canola oil in a large nonstick skillet over medium-high heat. Brown the pork chops in the pan for 8 minutes on each side. Remove the pork chops from the pan, place on a platter, and cover with foil.

Add the remaining 1 tablespoon canola oil and the onion slices to the skillet. Cook over medium-high heat 10 to 15 minutes or until golden. Reduce heat to medium low. Add the wine, scraping to loosen the browned bits on the bottom of the pan. Simmer until the liquid is slightly reduced and thickened, about 5 to 10 minutes. Stir in the thyme.

NUTRITION PER SERVING

Serving size	1 pork chop and ½ cup onions
Calories	460 kcal
Fat	29 g
Saturated fat	8 g
Cholesterol	100 mg
Sodium	706 mg
Carbohydrates	7 g
Dietary fiber	2 g
Protein	35 g

Return the pork chops to the skillet, pouring any juices that have accumulated on the platter back into the pan; spoon the onions over the chops. Continue cooking until the pork chops are done, about 7 to 10 minutes, or until the interior temperature reaches 165°F.

Sprinkle the parsley evenly over the pork chops.

Hoppin' John

Mary Etta Moorachian, Ph.D., R.D., C.C.P., C.F.C.S.

Serves: 8
Hands-on time: 15 minutes
Cooking time: 25 minutes

Having grown up in Tennessee and having lived in Louisiana and now in South Carolina, I have enjoyed many variations of Hoppin' John. I prefer it made with lean ham and a vegetable stock.

1½ cups dried black-eyed peas
1 teaspoon vegetable oil
1 medium-size onion, chopped
2 14-ounce cans vegetable broth
hot sauce
1 teaspoon salt
freshly ground black pepper to taste
2½ cups cooked rice
4 medium-size tomatoes, diced
½ cup minced green onions, including tops
3 tablespoons minced parsley
1 cup lean diced ham, or 8 strips crisply cooked turkey bacon, crumbled

Clean and rinse the peas. Cover with three cups water and let stand overnight.

Drain the peas; discard the water.

Heat the oil in a medium-size saucepan over medium heat; add the onion and cook 5 to 7 minutes, or until the onion is translucent. Add the peas and the broth; bring to a boil. Lower heat and simmer 20 minutes or until the peas are tender and a small amount of cooking liquid remains. If the liquid is absorbed too quickly, add additional broth, ¼ cup at a

FOOD TRIVIA
Hoppin' John is thought to be a variation of "pois a pigeon," a dish brought to America from Africa.

NUTRITION PER SERVING	
Serving size	½ cup, with ham
Calories	250 kcal
Fat	3.5 g
Saturated fat	1 g
Cholesterol	15 mg
Sodium	750 mg
Carbohydrates	42 g
Dietary fiber	5 g
Protein	15 g

NUTRITION PER SERVING	
Serving size	½ cup, with turkey bacon
Calories	250 kcal
Fat	4.5 g
Saturated fat	1 g
Cholesterol	10 mg
Sodium	930 mg
Carbohydrates	42 g
Dietary fiber	5 g
Protein	13 g

FOOD TRIVIA
There is much lore about how this dish was named, including: (1) Family members gathered around the table; when the dish was served, everyone hopped around the table before sitting down to the feast; (2) A custom that children must hop around the table before the dish is served; (3) A man named John who came "a-hoppin" when his wife took the dish from the stove; and (4) It was a southern custom to invite a guest by saying, "Hop in, John."

time. Stir in the hot sauce, salt, and pepper. Cover and simmer 15 minutes.

Place ½ cup rice in each soup bowl; top with peas. Garnish with the tomatoes, green onions, parsley, and ham (or bacon).

FOOD TRIVIA

Black slaves introduced this famous "pea" pilau, closely related to common African and West Indian concoctions, on the rice plantations of the South Carolina Low Country. It is traditionally eaten on New Year's Day, a practice thought to bring good luck; the custom probably stemmed from the superstitions of ancient Egypt and Africa.

Hoppin' John (Variation)

Mary Etta Moorachian, Ph.D., R.D., C.C.P., C.F.C.S.

Serves: 4
Hands-on time: 15 minutes
Cooking time: 5 minutes

Try this time-saving version!

- 4 strips crisply cooked bacon, crumbled
- 1 teaspoon vegetable oil
- 2 cloves garlic, chopped
- 1 medium-size onion, chopped
- 1¼ cups instant rice
- 1 14-ounce can chicken broth
- ⅛ teaspoon black pepper
- hot sauce to taste
- 1 15- or 16-ounce can black-eyed peas, drained and rinsed
- 4 medium-size tomatoes, diced
- ½ cup minced green onions, including tops
- 3 tablespoons minced parsley

Cook the bacon in a large saucepan; remove to paper towels to drain. Wipe out the pan with a paper towel, but do not wash. Set the bacon aside.

Add the oil, garlic, and onion to the saucepan; cook 5 to 7 minutes over medium heat, or until the onion is translucent. Add the instant rice and the broth; bring to a boil. Reduce heat and simmer, covered, for 5 minutes.

Stir in the pepper, hot sauce, and peas. Cover and let stand 5 minutes. Fluff with a fork. Garnish with the tomatoes, green onions, parsley, and bacon (crumbled).

SUBSTITUTION
When fresh tomatoes are not in season, use one 15-ounce can of no-salt-added stewed tomatoes.

NUTRITION PER SERVING	
Serving size	½ cup
Calories	260 kcal
Fat	6 g
Saturated fat	2 g
Cholesterol	10 mg
Sodium	600 mg
Carbohydrates	39 g
Dietary fiber	7 g
Protein	14 g

Red Beans and Rice

Julienne T. Stewart, M.S., R.D., L.D.N.

This recipe for red beans and rice is a classic rendition. If you want a quick version, skip ahead to the recipe on page 166.

Serves: 4
Hands-on time: 30 minutes
Cooking time: 2½ to 3 hours

½ pound ham, tasso, andouille sausage, or smoked sausage
1 pound dry red kidney beans
1 large onion, chopped
3 cloves garlic, chopped
2 ribs celery, chopped
1 green bell pepper, chopped
1 teaspoon seasoned salt
1 bay leaf
2 to 5 drops hot pepper sauce
2 cups hot cooked brown rice

Brown the sausage in a heavy 4-quart kettle, about 5 to 7 minutes. Add 8 cups water and the onion, garlic, celery, green pepper, seasoned salt, and bay leaf. Bring to a boil; simmer covered for 1 to 1½ hours, or until the beans begin to crack.

Uncover and cook for another hour or until the beans are very tender and creamy, adding water if needed.

Add hot sauce to taste. Serve over hot rice.

SHOPPING TIP

The common brand of red beans used in New Orleans is Camellia. They are very young and pink in color. If you can't find this brand, look for young, light-colored beans instead of larger, burgundy-colored beans, which will not get as tender and creamy.

SHOPPING TIP

Tasso is a Cajun spiced ham; andouille sausage is Cajun seasoned smoked pork sausage.

COOK'S TIP

There is a debate in New Orleans on whether to soak beans overnight. This recipe does not require the beans to be soaked, especially if they are young and tender. Beans that have not been soaked just take longer to cook.

NUTRITION PER SERVING	
Serving size	1 cup beans over ½ cup rice
Calories	460 kcal
Fat	170 g
Saturated fat	19 g
Cholesterol	7 mg
Sodium	1,270 mg
Carbohydrates	48 g
Dietary fiber	11 g
Protein	22 g

Easy One-Pot Red Beans and Rice

Maria C. Alamo, M.P.H., R.D., L.D.

Serves: 4
Hands-on time: 15 minutes
Cooking time: 45 minutes
Standing time: 10 minutes

This is an easy, one-pot version of the famous New Orleans dish.

½ pound andouille sausage
1 large onion, chopped
3 cloves garlic, chopped
2 ribs celery, chopped
1 14½-ounce can diced tomatoes with liquid
1 15-ounce can kidney beans, drained and rinsed
½ teaspoon salt
¼ to 1 teaspoon black pepper
2 teaspoons ground thyme
2 teaspoons dried sweet basil
1 to 2 teaspoons cayenne
1 tablespoon paprika
2 to 5 drops hot pepper sauce
1 bay leaf
1 cup uncooked brown rice
1 green bell pepper, chopped

Brown the sausage with the onion, garlic, and celery for about 4 to 6 minutes. Add the tomatoes, kidney beans, 2 cups water, salt, pepper, thyme, basil, cayenne, paprika, hot sauce, bay leaf, and rice. Bring to a boil. Add the rice, decrease heat, cover, and simmer 45 minutes. Remove from heat.

Add the green pepper, stir well, cover, and let stand 10 minutes. Stir before serving.

NUTRITION PER SERVING	
Serving size	2 cups
Calories	515 kcal
Fat	20 g
Saturated fat	0.426 g
Cholesterol	0 mg
Sodium	720 mg
Carbohydrates	65 g
Dietary fiber	13 g
Protein	21 g

Zucchini Pie

Diane A. Welland, M.S., R.D.

Bisquick has been a staple in America's kitchens since the early 1930s. An executive from General Mills got the idea for creating a convenient biscuit mix after he was served fresh, hot biscuits on a train. When he asked the chef how the biscuits were baked so quickly, he learned that the chef had premixed the flour, lard, baking powder, and salt. This recipe shows that today's biscuit mix can do a lot more than just make great biscuits—including making this buttery-flavored dish with all of the zucchini from my Virginia garden.

Serves: 8 as a main dish or 16 as a side dish
Hands-on time: 15 minutes
Baking time: 45 to 50 minutes

- vegetable oil cooking spray
- 2 tablespoons canola oil
- 2 cups liquid egg substitute
- 1 cup reduced-fat Bisquick
- 2 cups (8 ounces) shredded Monterey Jack cheese
- 3 medium-size unpeeled zucchini, shredded
- 1 medium-size onion, diced
- 2 cloves garlic, minced
- 8 ounces sliced fresh mushrooms
- ½ cup chopped fresh parsley

Preheat oven to 350°F. Spray a 9-by-13-inch baking pan with the cooking spray.

Beat together the oil and the egg substitute in a large bowl; stir in the Bisquick. Add the cheese and stir well; set aside.

Combine the zucchini, onion, garlic, mushrooms, and parsley; toss gently to mix. Pour the vegetables into the bowl with the baking mixture; fold gently.

Spoon the mixture evenly into the prepared baking pan. Bake 45 to 50 minutes, or until a knife inserted in the middle comes out clean and the top is golden brown.

COOK'S TIP

Add 1 red pepper, minced, to the mushrooms for a colorful dish.

NUTRITION PER SERVING	
Serving size	main course, ⅛ of casserole
Calories	270 kcal
Fat	15 g
Saturated fat	6 g
Cholesterol	25 mg
Sodium	440 mg
Carbohydrates	17 g
Dietary fiber	2 g
Protein	18 g

NUTRITION PER SERVING	
Serving size	side dish, 1/16 of casserole
Calories	135 kcal
Fat	8 g
Saturated fat	3 g
Cholesterol	15 mg
Sodium	220 mg
Carbohydrates	8 g
Dietary fiber	Less than 1 g
Protein	9 g

Moist Corn Bread

Corrina Riemann, R.D.

Serves: 6
Hands-on time: 10 minutes
Baking time: 20 minutes

Stir up southern-inspired corn bread anywhere in the country to add some variety to your meals. Have it for breakfast or for dinner with a bowl of Checkerboard Chili (page 259).

vegetable oil cooking spray
1 cup all-purpose flour
½ cup cornmeal
⅓ cup sugar
1 tablespoon baking powder
1 teaspoon salt
1 tablespoon canola oil
1 egg, lightly beaten
1 cup nonfat milk
1 teaspoon melted butter

Preheat oven to 375°F. Spray an 8- or 9-inch square baking pan with the cooking spray.

Stir together the flour, cornmeal, sugar, baking powder, and salt.

Combine the canola oil, egg, and milk. Add to the dry mixture and mix just until moist. Pour into the prepared pan and bake for 20 minutes.

Brush with melted butter to keep the top soft.

SHOPPING TIP
Choose a coarser ground cornmeal if you like a corn bread with more texture.

VARIATION
Stir 1 cup of thawed frozen corn into the cornmeal for a heartier version with added texture.

NUTRITION PER SERVING	
Serving size	⅙ of 8-inch or 9-inch square pan
Calories	220 kcal
Fat	5 g
Saturated fat	1.5 g
Cholesterol	40 mg
Sodium	660 mg
Carbohydrates	39 g
Dietary fiber	1 g
Protein	6 g

Grandmother Gibson's Chocolate Pie

Regan Miller Jones, R.D., L.D.

This recipe was given to me as part of a Christmas present: a collection of family recipes assembled by my Aunt Anita. It originated from my uncle's grandmother, Grandmother Gibson, and has become one of my own family's favorites, prepared for just about every holiday. This chocolate pie recipe is simple, uses few ingredients, and tastes great. More important, it always serves to remind me of what a treasure family recipes really are.

Serves: 8
Hands-on time: 15 minutes
Cooking time: 30 minutes

1 cup plus 6 tablespoons sugar
¼ cup all-purpose flour
3 tablespoons unsweetened cocoa powder
dash salt
2 cups 2% milk
3 egg yolks, lightly beaten
1 9- or 10-inch prebaked pie shell
3 egg whites, at room temperature
¼ teaspoon cream of tartar

Preheat oven to 275°F.

Combine 1 cup sugar and the flour, cocoa, and salt in a large heavy saucepan; gradually whisk in the milk. Bring to a boil over a medium-high heat, stirring constantly with a whisk, until the mixture becomes slightly thick and bubbly.

Gradually, add ⅓ cup of the hot milk mixture to the beaten egg yolks; stir well. Return the egg mixture to the pan. Cook 2 minutes or until the mixture becomes very thick, stirring constantly. Pour the filling into the prebaked pie shell.

Using clean, dry beaters, beat the egg whites and the cream of tartar in an electric mixer at high speed until foamy. Add 6 tablespoons sugar, 1 tablespoon at a time, beating until stiff peaks form. Spread evenly over the filling, sealing to the edge of the crust. Bake for 20 minutes or until the meringue is lightly browned.

NUTRITION NUGGET

This recipe works well with 2% milk, which has just enough fat to make it rich and creamy. While you can make the pie with nonfat milk, the final product isn't quite as good.

NUTRITION PER SERVING

Serving size	⅛ of pie
Calories	220 kcal
Fat	4 g
Saturated fat	1.5 g
Cholesterol	85 mg
Sodium	85 mg
Carbohydrates	43 g
Dietary fiber	Less than 1 g
Protein	5 g

Lemon Ice Box Pie

Regan Miller Jones, R.D., L.D.

Serves: 10
Hands-on time: 10 minutes
Cooking time: 1 hour

Everyone knows barbecue is well loved in the South, but my favorite offering at most barbecue joints is the Lemon Ice Box Pie. I searched for years for a recipe, but "Lemon Meringue Pie" kept turning up in cookbooks instead. Ultimately, I found that Lemon Ice Box Pie was a closer match to Key Lime Pie. This recipe is the result of the marriage between the two in my kitchen.

SUBSTITUTION
To save time, instead of making the pie crust yourself, substitute a prepared 9- or 10-inch reduced-fat graham cracker pie crust.

CRUST
- ¼ cup butter
- 1¼ cups graham cracker crumbs
- ¼ cup sugar

FILLING
- 3 egg yolks, lightly beaten
- 1 14-ounce can fat-free sweetened condensed milk
- ½ cup freshly squeezed or bottled lemon juice

MERINGUE
- 3 egg whites, at room temperature
- ¼ teaspoon cream of tartar
- 4 tablespoons sugar

Place the butter in a 9-inch pie plate; melt in the oven while it preheats to 325°F. Remove from the oven. Combine the crumbs and ¼ cup sugar; sprinkle over the melted butter. Mix with a fork until uniform in texture; press firmly on the bottom and sides of the dish. Prebake the pie crust in a 325°F oven for 5 minutes; let cool.

Combine the egg yolks and the sweetened condensed milk; stir in the lemon juice. Pour into the cooled pie crust. Bake at 325°F for 30 minutes. Remove from the oven and reduce oven temperature to 275°F.

Beat the egg whites and cream of tartar in an electric mixer at high speed until foamy, using clean, dry beaters. Add 4 tablespoons sugar, 1 tablespoon at a time, beating until stiff peaks form. Spread evenly over the filling, sealing to the edge of the crust. Bake at 275°F for 20 minutes or until the meringue is lightly browned.

NUTRITION PER SERVING	
Serving size	1/10 of pie
Calories	260 kcal
Fat	7 g
Saturated fat	3.5 g
Cholesterol	80 mg
Sodium	125 mg
Carbohydrates	43 g
Dietary fiber	0 g
Protein	6 g

King Cake

Julienne T. Stewart, M.S., R.D., L.D.N.

King Cakes are traditionally served throughout the Mardi Gras season, which begins on the Epiphany (January 6) and culminates on Mardi Gras Day (the eve of Ash Wednesday). King Cake parties are held in homes and offices weekly in south Louisiana, where people gather to share the cake. The person who gets the piece of cake containing the baby is crowned king or queen and must host the next party. Cakes are round (representing a crown) and are decorated in Mardi Gras colors of purple, green, and gold.

Serves: 20
Hands-on time: 20 minutes
Standing time: 2 hours
Baking time: 20 minutes

CAKE

2 packages active dry yeast
1 cup nonfat milk
4 tablespoons unsalted butter
4 tablespoons fat-free cream cheese
½ cup sugar
1 teaspoon salt
1 cup liquid egg substitute
1 teaspoon lemon or orange zest
4½ cups all-purpose flour
1 tablespoon canola oil

FILLING

8 ounces reduced-fat cream cheese, brought to room temperature
8 ounces fat-free cream cheese, brought to room temperature
2 cups sifted confectioners' sugar
1 tablespoon lemon or orange zest
vegetable oil cooking spray

ICING

1⅓ cups sifted confectioners' sugar
3 tablespoons lemon or orange juice (depending on what type of zest is used)
2 tablespoons unsalted butter, softened to room temperature
2 tablespoons fat-free cream cheese, softened to room temperature
2 tablespoons nonfat milk
1 teaspoon vanilla extract
plastic baby doll (can substitute ½ pecan instead)
purple, yellow, and green sugar

SHOPPING TIP

If you purchase dry active yeast in a jar, use 1 tablespoon for each packet.

NUTRITION PER SERVING	
Serving size	1/20 of cake
Calories	280 kcal
Fat	7 g
Saturated fat	3.5 g
Cholesterol	15 mg
Sodium	270 mg
Carbohydrates	46 g
Dietary fiber	Less than 1 gram
Protein	9 g

King Cake *(continued)*

Sprinkle the yeast into 1/4 cup warm water; stir well. Set aside.

Scald the milk; whisk in the butter, cream cheese, and sugar. Whisk until the sugar is dissolved. Remove from heat. Whisk in the salt, egg substitute, zest, and 1/2 cup of flour. Whisk in the yeast mixture, and then the remaining flour, one cup at a time. Drizzle the oil around the side of the bowl as you mix the dough. The dough will be very sticky. Cover the dough with a damp towel and let rise 1 hour, or until doubled in volume.

Meanwhile, blend the cream cheeses, confectioners' sugar, and zest for the filling.

Preheat oven to 375°F. Coat a baking sheet with the cooking spray.

After the dough has risen, punch it down and knead it on a floured board for 5 minutes. Roll the dough into a large rectangle, about 30 inches long and 6 inches wide.

Spread the filling across the entire length of the dough. Fold in half lengthwise so that the resulting product is 30 inches long and 3 inches wide. Seal the edges by pinching the dough together. Place the dough on the prepared baking sheet. Shape into a circle and pinch the edges together. Cover and let rise 1 hour, or until approximately doubled in size. Bake for about 20 minutes or until lightly golden brown.

After baking, hide the baby in the baked cake by making a slit in one side. Prepare the icing while the cake cools. Combine all icing ingredients except the colored sugar in a medium-size bowl. Whip with an electric mixer or a whisk until smooth. The icing should be the consistency of pancake batter. Spread the icing evenly over the cooled cake. Sprinkle the colored sugar over the cake in stripes, alternating purple, green, and yellow.

Sweet Potato Casserole

Mary Etta Moorachian, Ph.D., R.D., C.C.P., C.F.C.S.

There are so many delicious variations of this traditional southern casserole, which is just a step away from another regional treat, sweet potato pie. Whatever you call it, it's a crowd pleaser.

Serves: 10
Hands-on time: 15 minutes
Baking time: 1 hour, 20 minutes

vegetable oil cooking spray
4 to 5 large sweet potatoes
¼ cup brown sugar
2 eggs
¾ teaspoon nutmeg
¾ teaspoon cinnamon
½ cup fat-free milk, warmed

TOPPING
1 cup chopped pecans
¼ cup brown sugar
¼ cup flour
3 tablespoons butter, melted

Preheat oven to 350°F. Coat a 2-quart casserole dish with the cooking spray. Bake the potatoes for 50 minutes or until fork tender. Leave the oven on. Peel, removing strings, and mash; add the sugar, eggs, nutmeg, cinnamon, and milk; stir to combine. Pour into the prepared casserole dish.

Combine the pecans, brown sugar, flour, and melted butter in a medium-size bowl; spread the topping over the potatoes.

Bake, uncovered, for 30 minutes, or until the topping is golden brown.

VARIATION
Make this dish without the topping for a less sweet side dish.

NUTRITION PER SERVING	
Serving size	⅔ cup
Calories	250 kcal
Fat	13 g
Saturated fat	3 g
Cholesterol	50 mg
Sodium	30 mg
Carbohydrates	31 g
Dietary fiber	2 g
Protein	4 g

4

THE FLORIBBEAN

Big, Bold Tropical Flair

Kristine Napier, M.P.H., R.D.

The flavors of south Florida's foods are as big and bold as its Latin-influenced salsa, calypso, and soca music. The marriage of colorful and spicy Caribbean cooking with traditional Florida standbys has created a relatively new cuisine called "Floribbean" food. While the term is new, centuries worth of collective influences on Florida's foods are not. It reflects rich tribal culture, as well as European and Asian recipes left there—and on the nearby Caribbean islands—over centuries. Spanish, French, Dutch, African, and Filipino culinary highlights stand out distinctively in this delightfully daring yet naturally light cuisine.

Freshness is key, with an abundance of lusciously lean fruits, vegetables, and seafood. Traveling farther into the Caribbean to Puerto Rico, tropical foods are even more central on the menu and in recipes. In other parts of Florida, food reflects and becomes a fusion of several nearby Caribbean cuisines, including the Deep South, Cajun, and Creole. Let's take a look at the foods and recipes that have collected on the Florida table.

The Caribbean's First Inhabitants and Their Food

The Arawak Indians probably greeted Christopher Columbus. The Arawaks' route to the Caribbean was a circuitous one. Historians believed the first Americans crossed the Bering Strait from Asia into Alaska, wound south to the Andes and then followed the Amazon. They traveled north to the coast of Venezuela and eventually spread out into the Antilles. Some ventured into the Florida Keys, probably at about the same time the Spanish first explored there. Historians know less about them in their South Florida home, but know they grew corn much as did their relatives in northern South America.

In the Caribbean, the Arawak were known as the Taino, the same name for their language. Columbus heard the Taino refer to corn as *mahiz*, a word that would become *maize* in Spanish and subsequently other European languages. Corn is believed to have been domesticated from now-extinct wild varieties in southern Mexico somewhere between 8000 and 7000 B.C. From there, it probably spread south into Central America; it entered the United States both via a northern route from Mexico and roundabout through Central and South America and across the Caribbean.

The Spanish described the sweet potatoes they first ate in the Caribbean as cooked roots that tasted like chestnuts (Whipped Swirled Orange and White Sweet Potatoes, page 190). A splendid variety of beans, fish, and shellfish offered a smorgasbord of protein choices. Fruits were not just eaten fresh, but also fermented into alcohol. In Cuba, the Spanish found cassava bread, made from the manioc root, and added it enthusiastically to their culinary repertoire. Later, the French and the Portuguese would become cassava aficionados.

Of all the foods Columbus first tasted in the Caribbean, corn would be the most important throughout history. He wrote about how delicious corn was boiled, roasted, or ground into flour. He carried seeds back to Spain, from where they traveled around the Mediterranean and subsequently criss-crossed Europe. Ferdinand Magellan is credited with taking maize to the Philippines, from where it went to China and became a life-saving crop for the migrants forced from the over-populated Yangtze delta. Portuguese explorers carried maize to Africa, where it grew rapidly and easily.

Corn's nutrition profile was augmented by other Central and South American indigenous foods: tomatoes, avocados, beans (lima beans, kidney beans, butter beans, and others), sweet peppers, hot peppers, and fish. The Caribbean and Latin people seem to have had a glimpse into the science of nutrition that would develop some four hundred years later. They somehow knew to create recipes containing both beans and corn—foods that together make a complete protein. Tomatoes, peppers, and other vegetables supplied vitamins not found in corn.

Chile peppers then, as now, were focal ingredients in Caribbean soups, stews, sauces, and vegetable preparations. Often, several varieties were combined to create the desired flavor profile and just the right amount of heat (Caribbean Soup, Sancocho, page 193). Food experts estimate that there were over forty varieties of chili peppers by the seventeenth century; today, they number over ninety. Columbus also found rhubarb and cinnamon on his first trip to the Caribbean, although food historians trace the origins of both to the ancient Chinese.

Columbus and other explorers learned about barbecuing on their first visits. Barbecuing as a cooking method originated on northern Hispaniola. Early pioneers there learned from the Carib tribe how to smoke-dry meat on wood lattices made from green sticks—called *barbacoa*—built over a fire of animal bones and hides.

North Florida Native Americans

North Florida offered rich farming land—probably a reason why the first Spanish explorers found so many different tribes there in the sixteenth century. The Apalachee and the Timucua tribes, the most widespread, built communities near reliable food and freshwater sources. They grew the ancient agricultural trio: the three sisters of corn, beans, and squash (Zucchini-Corn Casserole, page 188). The climate was good and the ground was high and dry. In addition, the fresh and brackish water spilled forth rich catches of fish and shellfish and the forests held plenty of game.

International Contributions to Floribbean Food

Global influences on the foodways of Florida and the Caribbean islands were multifaceted in origin. For one, worldwide visitors brought many different foods from their homelands, as well as the other lands they had explored. Also, people from many lands settled in Florida and a number of islands (at least temporarily), leaving cultural—including culinary—handprints that are still visible today. Certainly, agriculture and world trade—particularly the sugar industry—drove much of the population movement through the area.

Spanish

From his Spanish port of call, Columbus brought to the Caribbean European vegetable seeds (especially root vegetables), wheat, chickpeas, and sugarcane. The first oranges imported to Florida were small and sour. Seminole Indians sliced the tops off, made a hole, and filled them with honey before eating them. Ponce de Léon could have brought oranges as early as 1513, probably under a Spanish order to explorers to carry citrus seeds and plant them wherever they went, so that citrus would be available as a cure for disease (later recognized as scurvy). People from the Spanish Balearic Islands influenced the use of peppers in many recipes. The peppers combined well in the Caribbean with other typical Spanish ingredients: green peppers, garlic, and onions. Cooked together just so, they become "sofrito," the seasoning for many Floribbean foods (Ropa Vieja—Sofrito and Beef, page 198).

Classic Spanish recipes are still very much a part of Floribbean cuisine, including gazpacho, a spicy, cold, tomato-based soup, rich with vegetables (Gazpacho, page 192); and paella, a vibrantly colored spicy combination of rice, chicken, pork, seafood, peppers, and peas.

Portuguese

Compared to the Spanish kitchen, the Portuguese one produced spicier and richer foods. Portuguese sailors left their recipes for soups and stews, such as Portuguese Stew (page 194), much heartier versions than those simmered on Spanish stoves. Cumin and coriander-spiced foods typify Portuguese cuisine.

Either the Spanish or the Portuguese carried coconuts to the Caribbean from Asia, and breadfruit from the Far East; both remain key ingredients to Caribbean foods (Floribbean Chicken Bites, page 183; Spicy Breadfruit, page 187).

African

The African influence is strong throughout the area—so strong today that specialty stores and restaurants boast "African-Caribbean" food and products. When slaves from West Africa were brought to the Caribbean to work in the plantations and sugar mills, they brought seeds to grow their native food staples—okra, eggplant, and sesame seeds—as well as classic recipes for their use. Many regional specialties trace to the African influence, including black-eyed peas and okra, a dish simmered with salt pork.

Asian and Indian

During the eighteenth and nineteenth centuries, people from China, the Philippines, and India were brought to the Caribbean to work in the sugar industry, and, later in the ginger industry that blossomed. They left their imprints on the cuisine, such as curried dishes, stir-fry recipes, and the use of sweet coconut with hot spices.

New Englanders Head South

In the early nineteenth century, New Englanders headed south to Florida, much as others traveled west to try new lands. Simple New England food fused with piquant Spanish flavors and foods to produce what was called "cracker cooking" or "country cooking." It is often described as the Florida version of soul food. A fusion of New England, Floridian, and Caribbean foods emerged as northerners modified traditional recipes to use the foods available in their new home. Stone crab, for example, was used in New England clam chowder; apple pie was made with mangoes (Apple-Mango Crisp, page 207).

Cuban and Other Recent Caribbean Influence

The 1950s brought a wave of Cuban migration to South Florida. Spanish-influenced culinary themes became stronger in Florida. Lime-marinated grilled fish and seafood became popular, as did salads with tropical fruits and vegetables. Traditional Spanish ingredients—tomatoes, garlic, onions, and peppers—are combined with plantains (the cooking banana), coconut, guava, mango, and conch to create tropical masterpieces.

An excellent example of fusion cooking is "jerk food," a mixture of native Caribbean cuisine, influenced by Asian, African, European, and East Indian foodways. Cooking food slowly in pits was probably introduced to the islands by the Maroons—runaway African slaves—who coated meat with spice mixtures and cooked it in pits to preserve it. Today, jerk cooking is a popular Floribbean method of preparing chicken, pork, and seafood. Jerk seasoning is either a wet paste or a dry rub. Usual ingredients are ginger, tamarind, nutmeg, thyme, green onions, allspice, and chiles (especially Scotch bonnet ones). After the spice, the key secrets of jerk cooking are a long marinating time (at least several hours, up to two days) and long, slow cooking.

Mango and Ricotta Stuffed Omelet

Kristine Napier, M.P.H., R.D.

Serves: 2
Hands-on time: 5 minutes
Cooking time: 15 minutes

Light yet rich and creamy, gentle yet slightly bold in taste and color, the tenets of Floribbean cooking come alive in this easy for a quick breakfast but "fancy" enough for a company dish. The green onions cook into what becomes the outside of the omelet to create that Floribbean culinary sizzle in sight alone.

- 1 teaspoon extra-virgin olive oil
- 4 green onions, finely chopped
- ½ cup liquid egg substitute
- ¼ teaspoon black pepper
- ¼ teaspoon salt
- ½ cup part-skim ricotta cheese
- ½ cup chopped mango

Heat the oil over low heat in a medium-size nonstick pan. Add the onions and sauté just until wilted, about 3 to 4 minutes.

Pour the egg substitute over the onions; sprinkle with the salt and pepper. Cover and cook over low heat 5 minutes.

Meanwhile fold the mango into the ricotta. Spoon the ricotta mixture onto one-half of the omelet. Cover pan and cook 5 minutes, or until the cheese is warmed through.

Slide from the pan, covering the cheese with the other half of the omelet.

SUBSTITUTION
No mangoes available? Substitute ½ cup canned pineapple tidbits (drained well and patted dry).

SERVING SUGGESTION
Serve with a side of Gingered Papaya-Mango Orange Breakfast Salsa (page 181).

NUTRITION PER SERVING	
Serving size	½ omelet
Calories	200 kcal
Fat	9 g
Saturated fat	4 g
Cholesterol	20 mg
Sodium	480 mg
Carbohydrates	13 g
Dietary fiber	2 g
Protein	15 g

Gingered Papaya-Orange Breakfast Salsa

Kristine Napier, M.P.H., R.D.

Floridian and Caribbean fruits are all present and accounted for in this gentle-enough-for-breakfast, yet bold-enough-for-dinner salsa.

Serves: 12
Hands-on time: 20 minutes
Standing time: 8 hours

- 1 medium-size fresh papaya, peeled, seeded, and chopped
- 1 medium-size fresh mango, peeled and chopped
- 1 medium-size fresh Florida orange, peeled and divided into segments, and each segment cut into fourths
- 1 medium-size fresh pink grapefruit, peeled, membranes removed and chopped
- 4 ounces sugared crystallized ginger, chopped finely
- ¼ cup sugar
- ½ teaspoon salt
- 1 cup chopped fresh cilantro

Combine all ingredients in a glass or plastic bowl; cover tightly and allow to stand for at least 8 hours before serving.

SHOPPING TIP

Look for sugared, crystallized ginger in the ethnic food section of the grocery store.

COOK'S TIP

Store up to 5 days (covered tightly) in the refrigerator.

SERVING SUGGESTIONS

Serve on bagels with cream cheese; layer with vanilla low-fat yogurt for a breakfast parfait, or serve with eggs (such as the Mango and Ricotta Stuffed Omelet, page 180).

NUTRITION PER SERVING	
Serving size	⅓ cup
Calories	80 kcal
Fat	0 g
Saturated fat	0 g
Cholesterol	0 mg
Sodium	105 mg
Carbohydrates	21 g
Dietary fiber	1 g
Protein	1 g

Coconut Banana Bread Pudding

Kristine Napier, M.P.H., R.D.

Serves: 8
Hands-on time: 10 minutes
Cooking time: 1 hour

Combining two great Floribbean ingredients—coconut and bananas—this bread pudding is great hot or cold. You can also serve it for dessert with the Balsamic Vanilla Sauce (from the Broiled Strawberries with Balsamic Vanilla Sauce recipe on page 52).

- vegetable oil cooking spray
- 3 just ripe bananas
- ¼ cup sugar
- 6 slices whole wheat bread, broken or cut into 8 to 10 pieces each
- ⅔ cup shredded sweetened coconut
- 1 tablespoon vanilla extract
- 1 cup liquid egg substitute
- 1 13½-ounce can lite coconut milk

Preheat oven to 350°F. Spray a 9-inch square baking dish with the cooking spray. Slice the bananas into the pan and sprinkle with the sugar; toss. Add the bread and coconut; toss.

Combine the vanilla, egg substitute, and coconut milk in a medium-size bowl; pour over the bread mixture. Stir well; press down with a rubber spatula. Bake for 60 minutes, or until the mixture doesn't jiggle in the middle.

NUTRITION NUGGETS

Using whole wheat bread boosts fiber intake. This recipe is also a great example of using a creative combination of ingredients to moderate fat intake. Choosing an egg substitute and lite coconut milk allows the generous addition of texture-enhancing shredded coconut.

NUTRITION PER SERVING

Serving size	1 cup
Calories	220 kcal
Fat	6 g
Saturated fat	4 g
Cholesterol	5 mg
Sodium	210 mg
Carbohydrates	33 g
Dietary fiber	3 g
Protein	8 g

Floribbean Chicken Bites

Lori A. Miller, R.D., L.D.

A tasty appetizer that combines all the tropical zesty flavors of south Florida—lime, herbs, chilies, and coconut. Serve this any time of the year for a Caribbean theme party.

Serves: 12 as an appetizer
Hands-on time: 30 minutes
Cooking time: 30 minutes

vegetable oil cooking spray
1½ pounds boneless and skinless chicken breasts
1 14-ounce can reduced-sodium chicken broth
1 7-ounce package sweetened coconut
1 cup reduced-fat mayonnaise
2 tablespoons fresh lime juice
1 teaspoon lime zest
½ to 1 teaspoon diced chipotle pepper
1 teaspoon ground cumin

Preheat oven to 400°F. Coat a 13-by-9-inch pan with the cooking spray.

Place the chicken and broth in a medium-size skillet; bring to a boil. Cover, reduce heat, and simmer for about 10 to 15 minutes.

Place the coconut in the prepared pan; toast 7 to 10 minutes, stirring occasionally.

Combine the mayonnaise, lime juice, lime zest, chipotle pepper, and cumin in a large bowl. Cut the chicken into ½-inch cubes and add to the mayonnaise mixture; stir gently to coat. Transfer the mayonnaise-coated cubes to the coconut pan. Toss gently.

Refrigerate or serve at once on individual lettuce-lined plates or on toothpicks as an appetizer.

COOK'S TIP

Toast the coconut, prepare the chicken, and make the seasoned dip the day before serving and assemble when ready to serve.

NUTRITION PER SERVING	
Serving size	4 bites
Calories	170 kcal
Fat	7 g
Saturated fat	6 g
Cholesterol	35 mg
Sodium	240 mg
Carbohydrates	12 g
Dietary fiber	Less than 1 g
Protein	14 g

Sesame Honey Glazed Curried Vegetable Kabobs

Kristine Napier, M.P.H., R.D.

Serves: 8
Hands-on time: 20 minutes
Cooking time: 25 minutes

Inspired by the African and Filipino culinary contributions to the cuisine of Florida and the Caribbean, these appetizers are sure to be a big hit.

- 3 carrots, peeled and sliced into ½-inch pieces
- 1 teaspoon curry powder
- 1 teaspoon cumin seed
- ¼ teaspoon ground turmeric
- ¼ teaspoon cayenne pepper
- 3 tablespoons lemon juice
- 1 tablespoon extra-virgin olive oil
- 1 green sweet bell pepper, cut into 1-inch squares
- 1 red sweet bell pepper, cut into 1-inch squares
- 1 tablespoon honey
- 1 tablespoon toasted sesame seeds
- party toothpicks

Combine the carrots, 1 cup water, curry, cumin, turmeric, cayenne, lemon juice, and oil in a medium-size nonstick skillet. Simmer covered for 15 minutes. Add the peppers; stir. Cover and simmer 5 minutes, or until the carrots are fork tender (the peppers should be crisp-tender). Remove the vegetables with a slotted spoon into a plastic or glass container.

Add the honey to the pan and simmer uncovered, stirring occasionally around the edges with a heat-stable rubber spatula until the liquid reduces by at least one-half.

Drizzle the sauce over the vegetables; sprinkle with sesame seeds and toss. Chill.

Place one piece each of red pepper, carrot, and green pepper on each toothpick (in that order for optimal presentation).

VARIATION

To spice it up or down, adjust the cayenne.

COOK'S TIP

This keeps well in the refrigerator up to five days in a tightly sealed glass or plastic container.

NUTRITION PER SERVING	
Serving size	about 3 kabobs
Calories	50 kcal
Fat	2.5 g
Saturated fat	0 g
Cholesterol	0 mg
Sodium	20 mg
Carbohydrates	8 g
Dietary fiber	2 g
Protein	1 g

South Beach Mango Scallop Kabobs

Lori A. Miller, R.D., L.D.

Experience the culinary sizzle of the warm Caribbean with this festive dish. Hot, spicy, and zesty fresh flavor—what a great alternative to the typical barbecue fare! This is our favorite way to barbecue scallops, shrimp, and halibut kabobs in our northeast Ohio home. Save some of this spirited sauce for dipping at the table.

Serves: 8 (3 to 4 kabobs each)
Hands-on time: 25 minutes
Cooking time: 15 minutes

- 1 mango, peeled and coarsely chopped (at least 1 cup)
- 4 teaspoons seeded and chopped Serrano pepper
- 2 tablespoons canola oil
- 1 tablespoon finely chopped fresh ginger
- 2 teaspoons chopped garlic
- ½ cup rice wine vinegar
- ½ cup pineapple preserves
- 1 teaspoon salt, optional
- 1 pound small scallops
- 2 Florida oranges, peeled and divided into segments, each segment cut into thirds
- wooden kabob skewers
- 2 medium-size green bell peppers, cut into 1-inch squares

Preheat oven to 350°F.

Combine the mango, pepper, oil, ginger, garlic, vinegar, pineapple, and salt in a blender or food processor; process until smooth. Reserve ½ cup of the sauce to brush on kabobs just before serving.

Thread 2 green pepper squares, 2 orange pieces, and 1 scallop on each skewer (starting with a green pepper and ending with one; the scallop should be in the middle). Baste the kabobs with sauce.

Bake until done, about 15 minutes, basting frequently with more sauce. Baste with the reserved sauce just before serving.

VARIATION

Spice it up or down by adjusting the amount of Serrano peppers added.

SERVING SUGGESTION

Use this as an excellent dipping sauce for tortilla chips or seafood nachos, or serve it over grilled or baked fish.

COOK'S TIP

Keep separate sauce for basting and sauce for using after cooking to help prevent food-borne illness.

NUTRITION PER SERVING	
Serving size	3 to 4 kabobs
Calories	120 kcal
Fat	3.5 g
Saturated fat	0 g
Cholesterol	10 mg
Sodium	270 mg
Carbohydrates	15 g
Dietary fiber	Less than 1 g
Protein	6 g

Chunky Tropical Avocado Salsa

Mona R. Sutnick, Ed.D., R.D.

Serves: 4
Hands-on time: 10 minutes

Caribbean inspired, this creamy-with-a-kick salsa is great on fish, chicken, or as a dip.

1 medium-size ripe avocado
1 tablespoon lemon juice
2 tablespoons finely chopped red onion
1 to 3 teaspoons white horseradish
⅛ teaspoon salt
1 cup jarred pink grapefruit sections, each cut into 5 small pieces
1 kiwi, sliced into ½-inch slices, slices quartered

Peel and chop the avocado; place in a nonmetal medium-size bowl. Add the lemon juice and toss gently. Add the remaining ingredients; fold gently.

VARIATION

Stir in ¼ cup chopped fresh cilantro or parsley.

SERVING SUGGESTION

Serve with reduced-fat whole wheat crackers.

NUTRITION PER SERVING	
Serving size	¼ cup
Calories	110 kcal
Fat	7 g
Saturated fat	1.5 g
Cholesterol	0 mg
Sodium	80 mg
Carbohydrates	13 g
Dietary fiber	5 g
Protein	2 g

Spicy Breadfruit

Stacy Haumea, R.D.

This recipe is a must-try if you can find breadfruit in your market. Breadfruit is a vegetable native to the Pacific, but a common menu item in the Caribbean. Enjoy it ripe uncooked or unripe cooked.

Serves: 4
Hands-on time: 10 minutes
Cooking time: 55 minutes

1 medium-size breadfruit
1½ teaspoons salt, reserving ½ teaspoon to garnish
2 to 4 crushed hot chili peppers, seeded and diced
4 garlic cloves, minced
1 tablespoon butter

Place the breadfruit in a small heavy saucepan and cover with water. Bring to a boil. Add the salt, hot chili peppers, and garlic. Cook until a sharp knife pierces the skin easily, about 50 minutes.

Remove the breadfruit and cool; reserve the cooking liquid. Cut the breadfruit into quarters; remove and discard the skin, center rib, and seeds. Slice the quarters into ¼-inch thick pieces.

Add the butter to the reserved cooking liquid; bring to a boil. Return the breadfruit to the boiling water and simmer 5 minutes.

Drain the breadfruit slices, transfer to a serving platter, and sprinkle with the remaining ½ teaspoon salt.

SHOPPING TIP
Look for breadfruit in Latin and specialty produce markets. A medium-size breadfruit weighs two to four pounds.

COOK'S TIP
Spice it up by leaving the seeds in the hot peppers to give more heat to your dish.

FOOD TRIVIA
In Hawaii, breadfruit is called ulu.

NUTRITION PER SERVING

Serving size	¾ cup
Calories	150 kcal
Fat	3 g
Saturated fat	2 g
Cholesterol	10 mg
Sodium	880 mg
Carbohydrates	31 g
Dietary fiber	5 g
Protein	2 g

Zucchini-Corn Casserole

Kristine Napier, M.P.H., R.D.

Serves: 4
Hands-on time: 15 minutes
Cooking time: 40 minutes

Even if the three sisters of corn, squash, and beans hadn't been such a natural agricultural and nutritional combination of our Native American predecessors, we'd still combine them for their flavor tango. Caribbean inspired, this dish is a favorite in my Wisconsin home.

vegetable oil cooking spray
1 tablespoon butter
1 medium-size onion, chopped
2 cloves garlic, minced
1 medium-size unpeeled zucchini, thinly sliced
½ teaspoon salt
¼ teaspoon pepper
⅛ to ½ teaspoon cayenne, divided
½ cup nonfat milk
¼ cup all-purpose flour
1 10-ounce package frozen corn, thawed
1 medium-size red bell pepper, chopped
½ cup corn flake cereal, crushed

Preheat oven to 350°F. Coat a 9-inch square casserole dish with the cooking spray.

Melt the butter in a large skillet; add the onion, garlic, zucchini, salt, pepper, and cayenne to taste over medium heat. Cook and stir 5 to 8 minutes, or until the onion is soft. The zucchini may still be crunchy.

Combine the milk and flour; stir until smooth. Pour into a skillet and increase heat; stir until the mixture thickens. Pour the zucchini mixture into the prepared casserole dish; stir in the corn.

Combine the red bell pepper and crushed cereal; add cayenne to taste. Sprinkle over the top of the casserole. Bake for 30 minutes, or until the casserole bubbles.

VARIATION

Increase the pan size to a 13-by-9-inch casserole. Stir one 15-ounce can of black beans (drained and rinsed) into the cooked zucchini mixture. Follow the remainder of the instructions.

SERVING SUGGESTION

Double the serving size and enjoy this dish as a main course.

NUTRITION PER SERVING

Serving size	1 cup
Calories	180 kcal
Fat	3.5 g
Saturated fat	2 g
Cholesterol	10 mg
Sodium	320 mg
Carbohydrates	33 g
Dietary fiber	4 g
Protein	6 g

Tropical Salad with Strawberry Balsamic Dressing

Laura Faler Thomas, M.Ed., R.D., L.D.

We love the taste of tropical food in Idaho, especially in the winter. This salad is picture perfect—right out of a Caribbean travel guide. Enjoy it wherever you are.

Serves: 4
Hands-on time: 15 minutes

SALAD
1 10-ounce bag prewashed spinach
1 orange, sectioned and sections halved, or 1 11-ounce can mandarin oranges in juice, drained
1 cup sliced strawberries
1 papaya, sliced (if not available, add an additional cup of strawberries)
2 kiwis, peeled and sliced
2 hard-cooked eggs, thinly sliced
¼ cup freshly shredded Parmesan cheese (1 ounce)

STRAWBERRY BALSAMIC DRESSING
1 cup sliced strawberries
2 tablespoons extra-virgin olive oil
2 tablespoons balsamic vinegar
2 teaspoons sugar
freshly ground black pepper to taste

Divide the spinach evenly onto 4 plates. Top evenly with the orange segments, strawberry slices, papaya, kiwi, and egg slices, alternating the fruits and egg slices in a circle for color.

For the dressing, combine the strawberries, olive oil, vinegar, and sugar in a food processor and whirl until smooth. Or, mash the strawberries by hand and whisk in the oil, 1 tablespoon of the vinegar, and sugar.

SERVING SUGGESTION
Double your portion for a complete meal.

NUTRITION PER SERVING	
Serving size	2 cups
Calories	280 kcal
Fat	12 g
Saturated fat	3 g
Cholesterol	110 mg
Sodium	180 mg
Carbohydrates	37 g
Dietary fiber	6 g
Protein	9 g

Whipped Swirled Orange and White Sweet Potatoes

Kristine Napier, M.P.H., R.D.

Serves: 4
Hands-on time: 15 minutes
Cooking time: 25 minutes

Sweet potatoes are native to the tropical parts of the United States. While there are many varieties, the two most widely grown are a creamy white one and an orange one. The two have distinctly different flavors that you'll appreciate even more side by side.

- 1 large orange sweet potato, scrubbed well and cubed (about ½ pound)
- 1 large white sweet potato, scrubbed well and cubed (about ½ pound)
- 2 tablespoons butter
- ½ teaspoon ground cinnamon, divided
- 3 tablespoons nonfat milk, divided
- 2 tablespoons fat-free cream cheese
- ¼ teaspoon ground ginger
- 1 teaspoon brown sugar

Place the sweet potatoes in separate medium-size saucepans, cover with water, and bring to a boil. Reduce heat, cover, and simmer until fork tender, about 35 minutes.

Drain the potatoes and return to their respective pots. Add the butter, ¼ teaspoon cinnamon, and 1½ tablespoons milk to the cooked white sweet potato. Cover and allow the butter to melt.

Add the cream cheese, ginger, and remaining 1½ tablespoons milk to the orange sweet potato; allow the cream cheese to soften.

Whip the potato mixtures separately by hand, with an electric mixer, or in a food processor. Place the whipped white sweet potato in a medium-size serving bowl. Place the whipped orange sweet potato on top, and swirl. Stir together the brown sugar and remaining ¼ teaspoon cinnamon; sprinkle on top.

FOOD TRIVIA
Contrary to popular belief, the orange sweet potato is not a yam.

COOK'S TIP
Sweet potatoes do not store very well. Place in a cool, dark place (but not the refrigerator) and use within a week of purchase.

NUTRITION NUGGET
Enjoy the sweet potato skins and boost fiber intake.

NUTRITION PER SERVING

Serving size	¾ cup
Calories	130 kcal
Fat	6 g
Saturated fat	1.5 g
Cholesterol	15 mg
Sodium	50 mg
Carbohydrates	18 g
Dietary fiber	2 g
Protein	2 g

Curried Caribbean Rice Pilaf

Kristine Napier, M.P.H., R.D.

Curry, tomatoes, sweet bell peppers, garlic, and onion meld together to make this Caribbean delight a rice to remember. Serve it with baked chicken, roasted halibut, or all by itself with a few walnuts sprinkled on top. You'll hear the Caribbean tropics beckoning you.

Serves: 6
Hands-on time: 15 minutes
Cooking time: 25 minutes

1 tablespoon canola oil
1 large onion, chopped
4 cloves garlic, chopped
1 cup long grain white rice
1 14-ounce can chicken broth
1 tablespoon curry powder
1 cup cherry tomatoes, halved
1 red bell pepper, minced
1 green bell pepper, minced
1 yellow bell pepper, minced

Heat the oil in a large heavy kettle over medium heat; add the onion and the garlic. Cook and stir 3 to 5 minutes, or until the onion is soft. Do not burn the garlic.

Add the rice, broth, and curry. Bring to a boil. Reduce heat, cover, and cook 15 minutes, or until the rice is tender.

Remove from heat, stir in the tomatoes and bell peppers; cover and let stand 10 minutes. Fluff with a fork and serve.

FOOD TRIVIA

Curry powder is the key spice in all curry dishes; the term curry comes from the South Indian word "kari" which literally means sauce. The powder contains up to 20 different spices, including cardamom, chili pepper, cinnamon, and cloves.

NUTRITION NUGGET

Use long-grain brown rice instead of white rice and increase fiber by 1 gram per serving.

NUTRITION PER SERVING	
Serving size	1½ cups
Calories	180 kcal
Fat	4 g
Saturated fat	0.5 g
Cholesterol	0 mg
Sodium	290 mg
Carbohydrates	33 g
Dietary fiber	2 g
Protein	4 g

Gazpacho

Golda E. Ewalt, R.D., L.D.

Serves: 8
Hands-on time: 20 minutes
Chill time: 2 hours

Here is a northerner's version of this traditional Spanish cold soup that is very popular in Florida and a perfect way to use fresh summer vegetables anywhere.

3 large tomatoes, coarsely chopped
1 green bell pepper, seeded and chopped
1 cucumber, chopped
1 ripe avocado, peeled, seeded, and coarsely chopped
½ medium-size red onion, coarsely chopped
¼ cup chopped Kalamata olives (about 4 to 6 olives)
3 tablespoons chopped fresh cilantro
2 tablespoons chopped fresh basil, or 2 teaspoons dried
2 tablespoons chopped fresh parsley
1 tablespoon chopped fresh dill, or 1 teaspoon dried
2 cloves garlic, minced
2 tablespoons extra-virgin olive oil
2 tablespoons apple cider vinegar
1 teaspoon hot sauce
1 46-ounce can reduced-sodium tomato juice
¼ to ½ teaspoon freshly ground black pepper
croutons or bread sticks

Combine all the ingredients in a large bowl, stirring well. Cover and refrigerate at least 2 hours before serving. Serve with croutons.

SUBSTITUTION
Substitute an equal volume of vegetable juice (regular or spicy) for the tomato juice.

NUTRITION PER SERVING	
Serving size	1 cup
Calories	190 kcal
Fat	13 g
Saturated fat	2.5 g
Cholesterol	0 mg
Sodium	440 mg
Carbohydrates	17 g
Dietary fiber	5 g
Protein	5 g

Caribbean Soup (Sancocho)

Jim McGowan, R.D.

This soup is our version of a Caribbean classic. I extend my heartiest thanks to Samuel Gonzalez and Heriberto Cordero for helping to develop this recipe on our base in Puerto Rico. Yautia, or malanga, is a root vegetable similar in size to a potato but with a papery skin.

Serves: 16 as an appetizer or 8 as a main course
Hands-on time: 30 minutes
Cooking time: 41 minutes

1½ pounds lean pork meat with bone, rinsed and cut into 1-inch cubes
1½ tablespoons salt, divided
1 large onion, chopped
1 small chili pepper, trimmed, seeded, and chopped
3 quarts water
½ pound white yautia (malanga), peeled and diced
½ pound yellow yautia (malanga), peeled and diced
½ pound pumpkin or squash, peeled and diced
½ pound unpeeled potatoes, scrubbed and diced
½ pound unpeeled ñame, scrubbed and diced (ñame = yam)
½ pound unpeeled sweet potatoes, scrubbed and diced
1 medium-size tomato, coarsely chopped
1 medium-size green bell pepper, trimmed, seeded, and coarsely chopped
½ cup chopped fresh cilantro
1 cup frozen or fresh corn
½ cup tomato sauce
1 large green plantain, peeled and quartered
1 large ripe plantain, peeled and quartered

Place the meat, bone, 1 tablespoon of the salt, onion, chili pepper, and 3 quarts water in a stockpot. Bring to a boil; reduce heat and simmer, covered, for 10 minutes. Add the yautia, pumpkin, potatoes, ñame, and sweet potatoes and simmer 20 minutes longer.

Add the tomato, green pepper, cilantro, corn, and tomato sauce. Rinse the green plantain rapidly in water containing the remaining ½ tablespoon salt; drain. Add both the green and ripe plantains to the stockpot; simmer, covered, for 10 minutes or until the ripe plantain is soft.

Remove the pieces of green plantain; mash, shape into balls, and return to the stockpot. Increase heat and boil rapidly for 1 minute. Serve hot.

SUBSTITUTIONS

If you cannot find ñame, double the sweet potatoes. Where malanga (yautia) are not available, use ½ pound of potatoes (unpeeled) and an additional ½ pound of pumpkin or squash.

SHOPPING TIP

Ñame is a term used in some Latin American cuisines for the starchy vegetable yam. True yams should not be confused with American sweet potatoes even though they are frequently labeled as yams. In the United States you're likely to find real yams only in Latin American specialty stores.

NUTRITION PER SERVING	
Serving size	3 cups
Calories	310 kcal
Fat	4.5 g
Saturated fat	1.5 g
Cholesterol	35 mg
Sodium	1,390 mg
Carbohydrates	58 g
Dietary fiber	6 g
Protein	15 g

NUTRITION PER SERVING	
Serving size	1½ cups
Calories	155 kcal
Fat	2 g
Saturated fat	0.8 g
Cholesterol	17 mg
Sodium	690 mg
Carbohydrates	29 g
Dietary fiber	3 g
Protein	8 g

Portuguese Stew

Lisa C. Peterson, M.S., R.D., C.D.N.

Serves: 8
Hands-on time: 30 minutes
Cooking time: 20 minutes

This recipe, created by my friend and local chef Jeff Renkl, captures the delicious nuances of traditional New England coastline cooking. It's a favorite menu specialty at Café Routier, Renkl's "Yankee bistro." Given the world's shipping history, you could have found a version of this on the Florida seacoast hundreds of years ago, too. Sea scallops may be used in place of the cod, and littleneck clams can be substituted for the mussels.

1 tablespoon olive oil
6 ounces Portuguese linguica or chourico sausage, sliced
2 medium-size onions, coarsely chopped
1 green bell pepper, coarsely chopped
1 red bell pepper, coarsely chopped
2 celery ribs, coarsely chopped
4 garlic cloves, peeled and minced
1 tablespoon chopped fresh thyme leaves or 1 teaspoon dried
¼ teaspoon ground allspice
¼ teaspoon sweet paprika
pinch cayenne pepper
¼ cup white wine
4 cups fish stock
1 15-ounce can stewed tomatoes
2 pounds Yukon gold or red bliss potatoes, halved lengthwise, and cut into ¼-inch slices
salt and pepper to taste
3 pounds cod fillets
2 pounds cultured mussels, beards removed

Heat the oil in a large stockpot; sauté the sausage over medium heat for 5 minutes. Add the onions, peppers, celery, garlic, thyme, allspice, paprika, and cayenne; sauté 5 minutes, or until the vegetables are just tender. Add the wine, stock, tomatoes, potatoes, salt, and pepper; bring to simmer. Cook 5 minutes, or until the potatoes are just tender; turn off heat and set aside.

Separately, sauté the cod in a lightly oiled or nonstick sauté pan until lightly seared on each side; add the mussels and a few ladles of the vegetables and broth. Simmer gently for about 3 minutes or until the cod is just cooked through and the mussels have opened.

To serve, arrange the cod in serving bowls. Ladle the vegetables and the broth over the cod and arrange the mussels around the edge. Serve immediately.

FOOD TRIVIA
This dish purportedly originates with the Portuguese, who called it Fishermen's Stew.

COOK'S TIP
Restaurant-style recipes like this one are most successfully prepared when the ingredients are prepped before cooking rather than during. In this process, called *mise en place*, the diced, chopped, measured, sliced, etc., ingredients are arranged near the cook-top and used as the recipe requires. This assures even cooking and more precise timing for the recipe.

NUTRITION PER SERVING

Serving size	1 to 1½ cups
Calories	480 kcal
Fat	14 g
Saturated fat	4 g
Cholesterol	120 mg
Sodium	940 mg
Carbohydrates	35 g
Dietary fiber	3 g
Protein	52 g

Jamaican Chili

Diane Werner, R.D.

Colorful and boldly flavored, the recipe is just as much at home in our Wisconsin kitchen as it is in Jamaica.

Serves: 8
Hands-on time: 15 minutes
Cooking time: 30 minutes

- 1 tablespoon extra-virgin olive oil
- 3 yellow bell peppers, chopped
- 1 large onion, chopped
- 2 garlic cloves, minced
- 1 tablespoon ground cumin
- 1 tablespoon paprika
- 1 tablespoon chili powder
- 2 teaspoons sugar
- 2 14½-ounce cans stewed tomatoes
- 1 15-ounce can kidney beans, rinsed and drained
- 1 15-ounce can cannelini or white kidney beans, rinsed and drained
- 1 15-ounce can black beans, rinsed and drained
- 2 tablespoons tomato paste
- 2 tablespoons balsamic vinegar
- minced fresh cilantro or parsley, optional

In a Dutch oven or a large saucepan, heat the oil over medium heat and sauté the peppers, onion, and garlic until tender. Add the cumin, paprika, chili powder, and sugar and cook for 1 minute. Stir in the tomatoes, beans, and tomato paste. Bring to a boil, cover, reduce heat, and simmer for 20 minutes.

Stir in the vinegar just before serving. Garnish with cilantro or parsley if desired.

SUBSTITUTION

Use any combination of beans you enjoy (e.g., kidney, black, white, or navy); use two 15-ounce cans or about 2½ cups.

FOOD TRIVIA

Paprika is made by grinding sweet red pepper pods into a fine powder. The spice can be mild to hot, bright orange-red to deep blood-red.

NUTRITION PER SERVING	
Serving size	1 cup
Calories	240 kcal
Fat	3 g
Saturated fat	0 g
Cholesterol	0 mg
Sodium	410 mg
Carbohydrates	44 g
Dietary fiber	12 g
Protein	11 g

Citrus-Infused Salmon

Mona R. Sutnick, Ed.D., R.D.

Serves: 4
Hands-on time: 10 minutes
Cooking time: 15 minutes

Fresh, easy, and light, you'll have to pinch yourself to believe you're not in the Caribbean enjoying this delightful—and easy—salmon.

- vegetable oil cooking spray
- 6 tablespoons fresh orange juice
- 2 tablespoons fresh lemon juice
- 1 tablespoon grated lemon zest
- 1 tablespoon grated fresh ginger, or 1 teaspoon ground ginger
- ½ teaspoon salt
- ⅛ teaspoon white pepper
- 1 pound fresh salmon (1⅓ pounds if with skin)
- 1 teaspoon cornstarch
- 1 green bell pepper, seeded and sliced into thin strips
- 1 red bell pepper, seeded and sliced into thin strips

Preheat the oven to 375°F. Line a baking dish with foil; spray the foil with the cooking spray.

Combine the orange and lemon juices, lemon zest, ginger, salt, and pepper.

Place the salmon in prepared pan and pour the juice mixture over it. Bake for approximately 10 minutes per inch of thickness of the salmon, until the fish flakes easily—about 10 to 15 minutes. Remove the salmon from the oven, transfer to a serving dish, and keep warm.

Pour the cooking liquid into a large saucepan; bring to a boil.

Blend the cornstarch into ¼ cup cold water until smooth; pour into a saucepan while stirring constantly. Stir until the mixture thickens slightly. Remove the pan from heat. Place the pepper strips in the sauce, stir to coat, cover and steam 5 minutes, just until crisp-tender.

Pour the sauce and the pepper strips over the salmon; arrange the pepper strips.

COOK'S TIP

Steep leftover ginger in hot water for 20 minutes. Strain and enjoy hot or chilled over ice.

COOK'S TIP

Peel fresh ginger with a paring knife or vegetable peeler. Then grate with a fine grater or place peeled ginger in a mini food processor.

NUTRITION PER SERVING

Serving size	3 ounces cooked salmon plus ½ cup sauce
Calories	190 kcal
Fat	7 g
Saturated fat	1 g
Cholesterol	60 mg
Sodium	340 mg
Carbohydrates	8 g
Dietary fiber	1 g
Protein	23 g

Pan-Seared Grouper with Warm Tomato-Olive Jam

Maureen Callahan, M.S., R.D.

To a native Floridian, there's just something special about Florida-grown tomatoes, particularly when they come from the west coast town of Ruskin. Ruskin is located just south of Tampa Bay. The agricultural climate is just right for growing tomatoes. Here, those tomatoes are cooked and paired with the popular Florida whitefish called grouper. If you can't find grouper, cod or any firm-textured whitefish makes a fine substitute.

Serves: 4
Hands-on time: 15 minutes
Cooking time: 5 minutes

1 tablespoon canola oil, divided
¼ cup finely chopped shallot or red onion
1 large tomato, chopped (about 1½ cups)
½ cup tomato juice
1 tablespoon balsamic vinegar
¼ teaspoon salt, divided
¼ teaspoon pepper, divided
3 to 5 kalamata olives, finely chopped (about 1 tablespoon)
½ teaspoon capers, rinsed and drained
1 tablespoon finely chopped fresh basil, or 1 teaspoon dried
4 5-ounce grouper fillets, or any firm-textured whitefish fillets
4 basil leaves for garnish, optional

Heat 2 teaspoons of the oil in a small saucepan over medium heat. Add the shallot or red onion. Sauté 3 minutes or until soft. Add the tomato, tomato juice, vinegar, ⅛ teaspoon of the salt and ⅛ teaspoon of the pepper. Bring the mixture to a boil. Reduce heat and simmer, stirring constantly and scraping down the sides of the pan, for 15 minutes or until thickened. Stir in the olives, capers, and basil. Remove from heat. Cover and keep warm.

Sprinkle the flesh side of the fish (if the fish is not skinned) with the remaining ⅛ teaspoon salt and remaining ⅛ teaspoon pepper.

Heat the remaining 1 teaspoon oil in a large nonstick skillet over medium-high heat. Add the fish to the skillet, flesh side down, and cook for 4 to 5 minutes. Reduce heat to medium; turn the fish over. Cover and continue cooking until the fish is opaque, about 3 to 7 minutes, depending on the thickness of the fish.

Serve the fish on a warmed dinner plate topped with the tomato-olive jam. Garnish with basil, if desired.

SHOPPING TIP
For this recipe, purchase grouper fillets rather than steaks or the whole fish.

FOOD TRIVIA
Some groupers grow to ⅓ ton. Most, though, weigh in at 5 to 15 pounds.

COOK'S TIP
The lean, firm flesh makes grouper versatile: enjoy it baked, broiled, pan-sautéed, poached, or steamed.

NUTRITION PER SERVING

Serving size	4 ounces cooked grouper plus ¼ cup tomato-olive jam
Calories	200 kcal
Fat	7 g
Saturated fat	1 g
Cholesterol	50 mg
Sodium	350 mg
Carbohydrates	5 g
Dietary fiber	Less than 1 g
Protein	28 g

Ropa Vieja (Old Clothes)—Sofrito and Beef

Barbara J. Alvarez, M.P.H., R.D., L.D.N.

Serves: 8
Hands-on time: 1 hour, 45 minutes
Cooking time: 1 hour, 45 minutes

VARIATION

This dish starts with the classic Cuban seasoning called sofrito, which is sautéed onions, garlic, and green peppers. Fine-tune the flavor to your liking by using varying amounts of each.

This authentic Cuban dish may have a strange name, but it also has a flavor you'll want again and again after trying it. The leftovers freeze well, so cook up a batch and freeze for easy meals on a busy night.

- 1 large onion, diced
- 2 medium-size green bell peppers, diced
- 5 to 6 cloves garlic, peeled and diced
- 2 tablespoons extra-virgin olive oil
- 2 pounds flat cut beef brisket, quartered
- 1 15-ounce can tomato sauce
- 1 cup white or red wine
- 2 large bay leaves
- 2 teaspoons sazon completa (found in the international section of most groceries), or 1 tablespoon paprika, 2 teaspoons oregano, ½ to 1 teaspoon cayenne, 1 teaspoon ground cumin, and 1 teaspoon salt
- 8 cups cooked brown rice
- pimientos for garnish, optional

Stove-Top Method

Sauté the onion, bell peppers, and garlic in oil in a heavy 6-quart (or larger) pot over medium-low heat until soft, about 3 to 5 minutes. Add the meat, increase heat to medium-high; brown each side about 4 minutes.

Reduce heat. Add the tomato sauce, wine, bay leaves, and spices. Cover and simmer gently for 1 hour. Remove from heat.

Shred the beef with two forks. Return the meat to the sauce. Simmer, uncovered, 20 to 30 minutes, or until the sauce has thickened. Serve over rice.

Pressure Cooker Method

Place the rack on the bottom of a 6-quart or larger pressure cooker. Add ½ inch water (2 cups for 6-quart size) to the cooker; place the brisket quarters on the rack. Over high heat, bring the pressure cooker to high pressure. Lower the heat to maintain the cooker at high pressure and cook for 45 minutes. Allow the pressure to release naturally, approximately 15 to 20 minutes. Let the meat cool. With two forks, shred the

NUTRITION PER SERVING	
Serving size	¾ cup meat/ sauce plus 1 cup rice
Calories	480 kcal
Fat	14 g
Saturated fat	4 g
Cholesterol	70 mg
Sodium	710 mg
Carbohydrates	55 g
Dietary fiber	6 g
Protein	30 g

meat into strands of muscle fiber, removing fat or large pieces of fascia. Reserve the cooking liquid.

Meanwhile, heat the olive oil in a 6-quart or larger pot. Add the onion, green peppers, and garlic; cover and cook over medium-high heat until the vegetables are tender, approximately 3 to 4 minutes. Add the shredded meat, tomato sauce, wine, bay leaves, seasoning, and black pepper. Cook over low heat for approximately 30 minutes. If necessary, add more tomato juice, wine, or defatted, reserved beef stock. The meat dish should be moist, but not runny. Garnish with pimientos, if desired. Serve with brown or white rice.

Pastelon de Platanos Amarillos (Ripe Plantain Torte)

Jim McGowan, R.D.

Serves: 6
Hands-on time: 65 minutes
Cooking time: 65 minutes

This recipe, like in many others in Puerto Rican cuisine, combines spicy and sweet flavors. For the filling, you can use vegetables, chicken, or beef (or use just cheese). I learned this recipe from natives Samuel Gonzalez and Heriberto Cordera when I was first transferred to a base in Puerto Rico.

SHOPPING TIP

Most supermarkets have plantains, which often are green and much longer than bananas; they may be called cooking bananas. As the plantain ripens, it changes in color to yellow and then brownish black. The brownish-black version is best for this recipe.

FILLING

2 ounces lean ham, diced
1 tablespoon canola oil
¼ green pepper, chopped
1 small sweet chili pepper, chopped
1 medium-size onion, peeled and chopped
1 medium-size tomato, chopped
½ teaspoon crushed oregano
1 clove garlic, minced
5 olives, chopped
2 dried plums, pitted and chopped
1 tablespoon raisins
¼ cup tomato sauce
1 teaspoon vinegar
½ pound extra-lean ground beef

PLANTAIN MIXTURE

6 cups water
1 tablespoon salt
4 or 5 large very ripe plantains, halved
2 tablespoons butter
½ cup all-purpose flour
vegetable oil cooking spray

Brown the ham in a large skillet over high heat, for 4 to 5 minutes, or until slightly browned. Reduce heat to low. Add the oil, green pepper, chili pepper, onion, and tomato; sauté for 5 minutes. Add the oregano, garlic, olives, dried plums, raisins, tomato sauce, vinegar, and ground beef. Mix well, cover, and cook over moderate heat for 10 minutes, stirring occasionally. Uncover and cook for 10 minutes more, stirring occasionally.

NUTRITION PER SERVING

Serving size	⅙ of pie
Calories	300 kcal
Fat	11 g
Saturated fat	4 g
Cholesterol	25 mg
Sodium	1,400 mg
Carbohydrates	42 g
Dietary fiber	4 g
Protein	13 g

Meanwhile, place the water in a large pot; add the salt. Add the unpeeled plantains, halved. Boil over high heat for 15 minutes. Drain, peel, and mash the plantains; mix with the butter. Add the flour and mix.

Preheat oven to 350°F. Spray a 10-inch glass pie plate with the cooking spray.

Place half of the plantain mixture in the prepared pie plate and spread evenly. Top with the filling and cover with the remaining plantain mixture.

Bake for 30 minutes.

Stove-Top Glazed Ham

Maria C. Alamo, M.P.H., R.D., L.D.

Serves: 8 with leftovers
Hands-on time: 1 hour, 15 minutes
Cooking time: 1 hour 20 minutes for ham, 15 minutes for sauce

This is how we make ham in Puerto Rico. We love this for holidays and special occasions, and always serve it with potato salad.

- 5 pounds bone-in cooked ham
- 15 whole cloves, divided
- 1 20-ounce can pineapple rings (packed in juice); reserve juice
- 8 maraschino cherries, drained, divided
- ½ cup red or white wine, optional
- ⅓ cup maple syrup

Trim all visible fat from the ham. Place the ham in a large pot or Dutch oven. With a knife, make 2 diagonal slashes lengthwise and 3 diagonal slashes cross-wise on top of the ham. Arrange 12 cloves around the incisions. Cover the ham with the pineapple slices. Arrange 5 cherries between the pineapple slices. Cover and cook on medium-high heat for ½ hour on one side. Remove the pineapple slices and cherries from the top; set aside.

Using two serving forks, turn the ham to brown the other side. Cook an additional ½ hour.

Combine the pineapple juice, wine if desired, and maple syrup. Add the remaining 3 cloves and 3 cherries to the liquid.

Place the reserved pineapples in the liquid. Cook for about 15 minutes or until the liquid becomes syrupy and the pineapples are caramelized.

Remove the ham from the pot—using the same method with the forks—and place on a platter with the incisions (diagonal slashes) facing up. Keep warm.

To serve, rearrange the pineapple slices, cherries, and cloves on top of the ham. Pour the syrup over the top.

SUBSTITUTION

Use an equal amount of brown sugar if you don't have maple syrup.

COOK'S TIP

Serve leftover sliced ham in sandwiches or chop and use in the Western Egg Casserole on page 215.

COOK'S TIP

Store whole cloves in a tightly sealed container in the freezer to retain flavor longer.

NUTRITION PER SERVING	
Serving size	4 ounces ham plus 3 tablespoons sauce plus 2 pineapple rings
Calories	300 kcal
Fat	16 g
Saturated fat	6 g
Cholesterol	85 mg
Sodium	60 mg
Carbohydrates	13 g
Dietary fiber	0 g
Protein	24 g

Frijoles Negros (Cuban Black Beans)

Barbara Alvarez, M.P.H., R.D., L.D.N.

Rice and beans create a staple in the Cuban—indeed, the Caribbean—diet. They are also a frequent menu item in New Orleans. We've included the traditional cooking method (which takes a bit longer) and a faster version. They're both great!

Serves: 4
Hands-on time: 15 minutes
Cooking time: 15 minutes

Faster Version

- 2 tablespoons extra-virgin olive oil
- 1 large onion, chopped
- 1 large green bell pepper, finely chopped
- 6 cloves garlic, minced
- 1 tablespoon ground cumin
- 3 tablespoons white vinegar
- 2 bay leaves
- 2 tablespoons sazon completa (found in the international section of supermarkets) or
  - 1 tablespoon paprika
  - 2 teaspoons oregano
  - ½ to 1 teaspoon cayenne
  - 1 teaspoon ground cumin
  - 1 teaspoon salt
- 1 15-ounce can black beans, drained and rinsed
- 3 cups cooked brown rice

Heat the oil in a large nonstick skillet over medium-low heat; add the onion, pepper, garlic, cumin, vinegar, bay leaves, and sazon completa (or other seasonings as noted). Simmer gently, covered, for 15 to 20 minutes, until the onion is tender. Remove the bay leaves.

Add half of the beans whole. Crush the other half gently with the back of a spoon; add the crushed beans to the pan (this thickens the juice).

Serve over cooked rice.

NUTRITION PER SERVING	
Serving size	½ cup bean mixture over ¾ cup rice
Calories	390 kcal
Fat	10 g
Saturated fat	1 g
Cholesterol	0 mg
Sodium	620 mg
Carbohydrates	65 g
Dietary fiber	10 g
Protein	10 g

Frijoles Negros
(continued)

Serves: 8
Hands-on time: 20 minutes
Soaking time: Overnight
Cooking time: 1½ to 2 hours

Longer (Traditional) Version

2 cups dry black beans, picked over and rinsed
2 bay leaves
2 tablespoons extra-virgin olive oil
2 large onions, chopped
2 large green bell peppers, finely chopped
6 cloves garlic, minced
1 tablespoon ground cumin
¼ cup white vinegar
3 tablespoons sazon completa (found in the international section of supermarkets), or
  1 tablespoon paprika
  2 teaspoons oregano
  ½ to 1 teaspoon cayenne
  1 teaspoon ground cumin
  1½ teaspoons salt
6 cups cooked brown rice

Soak the beans overnight in water in a large soup pot, with enough water to cover completely plus 3 inches.

Drain; add 10 cups fresh water and the bay leaves to the beans. Bring to a boil; cover, reduce heat, and simmer 1 to 1¼ hours, or until the beans are very tender.

After the beans have cooked for 45 minutes, heat the oil in a large nonstick skillet over medium-low heat; add the onions, peppers, garlic, cumin, vinegar, and sazon completa (or other seasonings as noted). Simmer gently, covered, for 15 to 20 minutes, until the onions are tender.

Remove 1 cup of cooked beans from the pot; crush gently with the back of a spoon; add the crushed beans back to the pot (this thickens the juice). Add the cooked onion mixture to the beans; cover and simmer gently for 20 minutes (add additional water as needed to ensure there is just enough for the beans to simmer).

Serve over cooked rice.

COOK'S TIP

To make 6 cups cooked brown rice, start with 1½ cups uncooked regular brown rice. In general, 1 cup uncooked brown rice yields 4 cups cooked.

NUTRITION PER SERVING	
Serving size	½ cup beans over ¾ cup cooked rice
Calories	410 kcal
Fat	6 g
Saturated fat	1 g
Cholesterol	0 mg
Sodium	450 mg
Carbohydrates	77 g
Dietary fiber	11 g
Protein	15 g

Margy's Key Lime Pie

Peggy Eastmond, R.D.

This Floribbean delight is a staple at our family gatherings in the western Chicago suburbs—and all the credit goes to my sister-in-law. Just don't tell anyone how easy it is!

1 14-ounce can sweetened condensed fat-free milk
4 egg yolks
½ cup bottled key lime juice, or ½ cup fresh lime juice (juice of 4 limes)
3 to 4 teaspoons grated lime zest
1 prepared graham cracker pie crust

Preheat oven to 325°F.

Whisk together the condensed milk, egg yolks, lime juice, and lime zest until blended and mixture thickens, about 3 minutes. Pour the filling into the pie crust.

Bake 15 to 20 minutes or until the center is set. Chill for at least 2 hours, but up to 4 days.

Serves: 10
Hands-on time: 10 minutes
Cooking time: 15 minutes
Chill time: 2 hours

SUBSTITUTION
Use a reduced-fat pie crust, which cuts 2 fat grams per serving and calories by 18.

COOK'S TIP
Dress it up by topping the cooled pie with a dollop of reduced-fat or fat-free frozen whipped topping.

NUTRITION PER SERVING	
Serving size	1/10 of pie
Calories	260 kcal
Fat	8 g
Saturated fat	2 g
Cholesterol	90 mg
Sodium	180 mg
Carbohydrates	41 g
Dietary fiber	0 g
Protein	6 g

Papaya Boats

Kristine Napier, M.P.H., R.D.

Serves: 2
Hands-on time: 15 minutes
Chill time: 1 hour

So sweet and refreshing by themselves, papayas are also delightfully interesting when combined creatively to make desserts and smoothies. This dish is reminiscent of the time I lived in the Dominican Republic, although we frequently used chopped mango instead of the strawberries and a native cheese (similar to ricotta) instead of the whipped topping. I still prepare this Floribbean dish in my Wisconsin home today.

1 papaya, washed, sliced in half, seeds removed
1 cup fresh strawberries, washed and chopped
¼ cup fat-free whipped topping (thawed if using frozen)
2 teaspoons fresh or bottled lime juice
¼ teaspoon ground cinnamon, optional

Carefully remove the papaya "flesh" from the skin, leaving enough to create a firm "boat." Spritz the boats with lime juice; cover tightly and refrigerate until time to serve.

Chop the papaya flesh; blend with the strawberries and whipped topping. Refrigerate at least one hour.

Fill the boats with the fruit mixture just before serving. Sprinkle with cinnamon, if desired.

SUBSTITUTIONS

Substitute an equal quantity of vanilla, strawberry, or lemon yogurt for the whipped topping. Substitute 1 cup blueberries for the strawberries.

NUTRITION PER SERVING	
Serving size	1 fruit-filled boat
Calories	120 kcal
Fat	0.5 g
Saturated fat	0 g
Cholesterol	0 mg
Sodium	15 mg
Carbohydrates	28 g
Dietary fiber	5 g
Protein	2 g

Apple-Mango Crisp

Kristine Napier, M.P.H., R.D.

Mangos, papayas, and pineapples were the mainstay of fruit on every table in my Dominican Republic town when perinatal research took me there in the mid-1970s. It wasn't until researching this book that I learned that New England colonists who moved south modified traditional recipes—such as apple pie—to accommodate the recipes of their new land. This is my version of their apple-mango pie.

Serves: 18
Hands-on time: 20 minutes
Baking time: 45 minutes
Standing time: 10 minutes

- vegetable oil cooking spray
- ¾ cup all-purpose flour, divided
- ½ cup toasted wheat germ
- ¾ cup old-fashioned oats
- ½ cup dark brown sugar
- ⅓ cup chopped pecans
- 1½ teaspoons ground cinnamon
- ¼ cup unsalted butter, melted (4 tablespoons)
- 4 Granny Smith apples
- 2 red sweet baking apples
- 3 tablespoons lime juice
- 2 mangos, peeled and chopped

Preheat oven to 375°F. Coat a 13-by-9-inch glass or ceramic baking dish with the cooking spray.

Stir together ½ cup flour, the wheat germ, oats, brown sugar, pecans, and cinnamon in a medium-size bowl. Stir in the melted butter; set aside.

Core the apples, chop, and place in a large bowl; spritz with the lime juice; stir. Stir in the remaining ¼ cup flour. Fold in the mangos.

Place the apple-mango mixture in the baking dish. Sprinkle the flour-oat mixture evenly over the top. Bake 45 minutes, or until the apples are tender. Cool slightly and serve warm.

SERVING SUGGESTION

Top each serving with ¼ cup fat-free whipped topping or frozen yogurt.

NUTRITION PER SERVING	
Serving size	1 cup
Calories	140 kcal
Fat	5 g
Saturated fat	2 g
Cholesterol	5 mg
Sodium	0 mg
Carbohydrates	24 g
Dietary fiber	2 g
Protein	2 g

5

THE MIDWEST

America's Breadbasket and Cultural Crossroads

Kristine Napier, M.P.H., R.D.

Imagine a time when you depended on a steamboat or the railroad to bring yeast for making bread—and to give your palate a break from hardtack or sourdough rolls. It's ironic that the region that would one day be called the country's breadbasket would be wanting for bread—but such was life in the Midwest at the beginning of the nineteenth century.

HARDTACK FOR HARD TIMES

Hardtack dough was baked into a hard biscuit that was then dried so that it could be stored for months without refrigeration. Sailors took it on long voyages. Frontier settlers in the central plains depended on it before they could get yeast; they dipped it in coffee, crumbled it into soups, and paired it up with slices of meat and/or cheese. Hardtack is also called ship biscuit or sea bread. To make hardtack, mix together 2 parts flour to not quite 1 part water; add a pinch of salt (if you have it). Knead until the mixture forms a stiff dough and you have the makings of hardtack.

MIDWEST HERBS, FRESH AND DRIED

Central Plains tribes made wise use of the many herbs that grew wild. From basil and horseradish to lavender and parsley, the Native Americans flavored what would have been the same boring soup ingredients with different herbs to create diverse dishes. The frontier settlers did the same; they dried the herbs for use throughout the year as seasonings, and as teas and medicines. Motivated by flavor, Native Americans and pioneers alike also harvested good amounts of phytochemicals via the many herbs they used, no doubt a nutrition boost through lean times.

The hardships that inspired hard work subsequently produced hearty crops. The Midwest—America's heartland—claims another distinction: it is the cultural crossroads of the United States, steeped in European, Middle Eastern, and Asian traditions.

Old and Deep Culinary Roots

The culinary roots of the Midwest—or central plains—run deeper than those planted by easterners moving west in the 1800s in search of better farmland. They're also deeper than those set by Europeans who simply used America's east coast as a stepping stone to reach the fertile soils of the Midwest. Before them, Native Americans worked the land to enjoy prodigious rewards. Midwest crop patterns today, and that region's culinary roots in turn, are reflections of the first inhabitants.

The nomadic Plains Indians lived largely off the buffalo. Not just their food, but their clothes, weapons, cooking containers, farming tools, cooking fuel, and even teepee fabric all came from the buffalo. They augmented their meat diet with fruits and edible roots. Herbs were used fresh and also dried for flavoring soups and for many other uses.

The Ojibwa lived in the forests on the shores of Lake Superior that touched Minnesota and Wisconsin; they also lived on Lake Huron's north shores. To the west, they lived in the Turtle Mountains of North Dakota. They hunted by foot, collected wild rice, and gathered the berries that plumped up so rapidly in the warm months. Wild rice was not only an important food crop (their stockpiles often kept the Ojibwa from starving in the winter), but was also used to barter with French fur traders.

WILD RICE ISN'T RICE

Wild rice (also called Indian rice), first harvested in prehistoric times, is not rice at all, but a long-grain marsh grass. Prized today for its luxurious nutty flavor and chewy texture, it is a bit pricey. Pair it with brown rice or bulgur wheat to make a little go a bit further.

The Ojibwa also grew corn, potatoes, and as many garden crops as would survive the weather. They had to work hard at agricultural pursuits, as they were near the northern limit of where typical North

American Indian agriculture was possible. Anthropologists believe that Ojibwa garden agriculture spread into the upper Mississippi River region.

Living along the Missouri and Mississippi Rivers, the Mandan, Arikara, Hidatsa, Dakota, and Pawnee tribes are thought to have lived almost exclusively on the crops of the three sisters—corn, beans, and squash—as well as sunflower seeds from the massive plants they nurtured. Then as today, the Mississippi was a lifeline, a superfast highway to find food and other essentials.

As important as these crops were to the Native Americans very lives, today they are at least that important to our livelihood. America's cornbelt stretches from Indiana on the east through Illinois, Missouri, and Kansas. Today, corn has more than eight hundred different culinary uses in the United States. On average, each American eats nearly fifty pounds of corn products annually. Three Midwest states contribute critical amounts of beans to the U.S. bean industry: Michigan, North Dakota, and Nebraska. Sunflowers are an important crop in North Dakota.

Frontier Settlers and Food

Life on the frontier was difficult; long, arduous days of making and repairing shelter often left little time for seeking food and then cooking and preserving it. While the central plains Indians learned to live from the land well, there would be a steep learning curve for the settlers to do the same.

In Indiana, the settlers found a wide variety of nuts to sustain them. Hickory nuts, black walnuts, chestnuts, beechnuts, and hazelnuts were paired with other wild foods in season. These included pawpaws, wild cherries, persimmons, wild grapes, plums, crab apples, and berries. Hunting and fishing rounded out the meals when the efforts were successful. When the settlers cleared the fields, corn became the dependable crop; it nourished them in many forms and was also used as their currency. Today, corn remains one of Indiana's main currencies, so to speak.

A BANANA-TASTING BERRY GROWS IN THE MIDWEST?

The pawpaw tree was prized for its edible black berry, which tastes like a cross between a banana and a pear and has a custardlike consistency. Rich in vitamins A and C, the oval berries can reach two to five inches in length. Pawpaws grow on the edge of wooded areas.

A recipe for "Poverty Cake," reported in the Seward Reporter on August 12, 1875, testified to the hard times: two cups of thin cream, two cups of chopped raisins, two cups of sugar, four cups of flour, one teaspoon of soda, salt, and spice.

The Midwest Today: A Cultural Crossroads

The food of the Midwest today reflects not only the early and enduring Native American agricultural contributions, but also the variety of ethnic foods that came in a steady stream starting in the early 1800s. Germans and Eastern Europeans settled in what is now Milwaukee, Chicago, and in

PRESERVING FOOD FOR THE WINTER ON THE FRONTIER

Farmer's almanacs detailed how to store fruits and vegetables for the long winter months on the frontier. Some of the hints included:

- Place cabbages and potatoes in a hole in the ground for storage.
- Do not store squash "down cellar," as the dampness injures them.
- Cut pumpkins, string them, and dry them like apples. To make a pie, boil the pieces with milk first.
- Pack carrots, parsnips, and beet roots in layers of dry sand.
- Hang onions to dry in a cool, dry room.
- Preserve parsley by cutting close to the stalks and then drying in a warm room or in a cool oven on tins.

parts of eastern Missouri. The Swedish and Norwegian settlers are still evident in Minnesota and Door County, Wisconsin, where blond hair coloring predominates. Later, Middle Easterners and Greeks would call Detroit and Cleveland home. Italians settled in Chicago, Cleveland, and many other midwestern towns in their new country.

Midwestern recipes range from genuine German (German Barley Mushroom Casserole, page 308), Czech (Mushroom-Barley Soup, page 255; Upside-Down Lemon Poppy Seed Loaf, page 222), Italian (Italian Beef and Spinach Pie, page 270; Polpettone or Italian Meatloaf, page 276; Fusilli al'Pesto, page 294); Greek (Spinach Pies, page 305), and South Indian (Coriander and Buttermilk Chutney, page 233) cuisines to reflections of Native American roots (Cinnamon Raisin Apple Indian Pudding, page 53). The expansive variety includes fusions of one or more influences, or a fusion of one of them with simply the availability of the day. Cincinnati chili, for example, was born of a Greek chef's ingenuity and the midwestern palate of the day.

Yes, the Midwest is said to be the land of the "meat and potatoes diet." Just by browsing our recipes, we know you'll find a tribute to the early and wise use of the vegetables, herbs, berries, and other fruits of the land.

Cream of Wheat Pongal

Kristine Napier, M.P.H., R.D.

Middle Eastern recipes, found across the country, are a very welcome addition to our country's health. My South Indian cooking expert, Alamelu Vairavan, taught me that hot wheat cereal cooked with cumin and vegetables is a popular breakfast food in her native land. You will find pockets of people from India in many places across our country, including in Milwaukee, Wisconsin, where Alamelu lives.

Serves: 4
Hands-on time: 5 minutes
Cooking time: 4 minutes

- 1 tablespoon canola oil
- 1 teaspoon cumin seeds
- ¼ cup chopped onion
- ½ medium-size tomato, chopped
- 1 cup quick or regular dry hot wheat cereal
- ½ teaspoon finely minced fresh ginger
- 1 chili pepper, chopped, optional
- ½ teaspoon salt
- ½ teaspoon butter
- 2 tablespoons roasted cashew halves, optional
- ¼ cup chopped cilantro

Heat the oil in a skillet over medium heat. When the oil is hot, but not smoking, stir in the cumin seeds; cook until the seeds become brown. Add the chopped onion and tomato and cook for 1 minute. Add the wheat cereal and stir for a minute. Add the ginger, chili pepper, and salt. Stir well.

Add 2 cups of warm water gradually to the mixture while stirring. Cover and cook over low heat, stirring frequently, for about 2 minutes.

Add the butter, cashews, and cilantro and mix well.

SERVING SUGGESTION
Pongal can be served at breakfast, at tea time, or as a snack anytime. It can be served by itself, with Coriander and Buttermilk Chutney (page 233), or with Potato and Eggplant in Lentil Sauce (page 302).

NUTRITION PER SERVING	
Serving size	¾ cup
Calories	230 kcal
Fat	7 g
Saturated fat	1 g
Cholesterol	1 mg
Sodium	300 mg
Carbohydrates	35 g
Dietary fiber	2 g
Protein	6 g

Farmhouse Apple, Bacon, and Egg Casserole

Kristine Napier, M.P.H., R.D.

Serves: 12
Hands-on time: 10 minutes

Enjoy the flavors of an old-fashioned Wisconsin bacon and egg breakfast baked into this delicious casserole. An added bonus, you'll have an easier time achieving your health and nutrition goals!

vegetable oil cooking spray
8 slices whole-grain bread, cubed
2 cups liquid egg substitute
2 cups nonfat milk
2 teaspoons dried sage
1 teaspoon black pepper
½ teaspoon salt
½ pound apple-cured bacon, chopped
3 tart apples, such as Granny Smith
3 red apples, such as McIntosh

Preheat oven to 350°F. Spray a 13-by-9-by-3-inch pan with the cooking spray. Arrange the bread in the pan.

Blend the egg substitute, milk, sage, salt, and pepper; pour over the bread. Mix and push the mixture down with a rubber spatula. Set aside.

Cook the bacon thoroughly, but not crisp. Drain on paper towels; set aside.

Wash, core, and chop the apples (do not peel). Add the apples to the bread mixture; stir well and push down with a rubber spatula. Sprinkle evenly with the bacon.

Bake for 50 to 60 minutes.

VARIATION

Sprinkle 2 cups of shredded sharp cheddar evenly over the top of the casserole after it has baked 30 minutes. Continue cooking until the cheese bubbles, about 20 to 30 minutes.

SERVING SUGGESTION

Create this dish for use as stuffing to accompany a baked ham.

NUTRITION PER SERVING	
Serving size	1⁄12 of casserole
Calories	200 kcal
Fat	7 g
Saturated fat	2.5 g
Cholesterol	15 mg
Sodium	570 mg
Carbohydrates	22 g
Dietary fiber	4 g
Protein	13 g

Western Egg Casserole

Lisa C. Peterson, M.S., R.D., C.D.N.

This hearty dish is reminiscent of skillet eggs made by settlers on move to the West. Best of all, it's a cinch to make.

Serves: 12
Hands-on time: 15 minutes
Chill time: 1 hour
Cooking time: 1 hour

- 1 pound diced baked ham
- 1 tablespoon canola oil
- 1 medium-size green bell pepper, diced
- 1 medium-size onion, diced
- 1 cup sliced mushrooms
- 1 cup liquid egg substitute
- 2 cups nonfat milk
- vegetable oil cooking spray
- 1½ pound loaf whole-grain bread, sliced into 12 to 18 slices
- 1½ cups shredded sharp cheddar cheese (6 ounces)

In a nonstick skillet, heat together the ham and oil until the ham is sizzling; add the pepper, onion, and mushrooms. Sauté until just tender; remove from heat and set aside.

In a medium-size bowl, beat together the egg substitute and milk. Set aside.

Coat a 9-by-13-inch glass baking dish with the cooking spray. Line the casserole with ⅓ of the bread slices; sprinkle with half of the ham/vegetable mixture and sprinkle with ½ cup cheese. Add another layer of ⅓ of the bread slices, the second half of the ham/vegetable mixture and another ½ cup cheese. Top with the remaining bread. Carefully pour the egg mixture over the top; sprinkle with the remaining cheese. Cover tightly with plastic wrap and refrigerate 1 to 24 hours.

Preheat oven to 350°F. Remove the plastic wrap and bake the casserole about 1 hour or until lightly browned and bubbling (the internal temperature should be about 155°F). Serve hot.

SUBSTITUTION

Fresh eggs can be used for all or some of the egg substitute. For each large, whole egg used, decrease the egg substitute by ¼ cup.

COOK'S TIP

To transform this recipe into a *South*western egg casserole, add two tablespoons each of chopped, canned mild green chili peppers and chopped, fresh cilantro. Serve with salsa.

SERVING SUGGESTION

Since the casserole is served straight from the oven, use an attractive baking dish or one that fits into a decorative holder.

NUTRITION PER SERVING	
Serving size	1/12 of casserole
Calories	250 kcal
Fat	9 g
Saturated fat	4 g
Cholesterol	15 mg
Sodium	470 mg
Carbohydrates	31 g
Dietary fiber	5 g
Protein	14 g

Make-Ahead Cinnamon French Toast

Kristine Napier, M.P.H., R.D.

Relax on a Sunday morning while this make-ahead version of a perennial all-American breakfast favorite fills your home with sugar and cinnamon—and everything nice! A touch of butter on this baked version provides a burst of richness—but few calories.

Serves: 4
Hands-on time: 10 minutes
Holding time: 1 hour
Cooking time: 15 minutes

1 16-ounce container liquid egg substitute
2 tablespoons brown sugar
2 teaspoons ground cinnamon
2 teaspoons vanilla extract
8 slices hearty whole-grain bread
vegetable oil cooking spray
4 teaspoons butter

Whisk the egg substitute, sugar, cinnamon, and vanilla in a 13-by-9-by-3-inch pan. Soak the bread in the egg mixture, turning it over to coat both sides; stack the slices as needed. Cover and let sit at least 1 hour or overnight.

Preheat oven to 375°F. Spray one large or two smaller cookie sheets (with a lip) heavily with the cooking spray. Using a large spatula, place the soaked bread on the cookie sheets. Place ½ teaspoon butter on each slice of bread. Bake 15 minutes or until golden brown. Open the oven once to spread the melted butter evenly over tops.

Serve with syrup, fruit, Microwave Applesauce (page 318), or Wild Blueberry Sauce (page 62).

VARIATION

Texas French Toast: purchase a 1½-pound loaf of unsliced whole-grain bread. Cut into 1-inch slices one day ahead. Lay the slices flat on the kitchen counter or on a baker's rack to dry out overnight. Proceed as directed, but stir ¼ cup nonfat milk into the egg mixture before soaking the French toast.

COOK'S TIP

Serve it for dinner: heat small sausage links as directed on the package. Place one link on each slice of French toast, roll, and hold in place with a toothpick.

FOOD TRIVIA

Centuries ago, the English called French toast "poor knights pudding," or "poor knights of Windsor pudding." In France, it was called *pain perdu*, which means "lost bread." The French called it lost bread because the recipe was a way of reviving dried-out French bread.

NUTRITION PER SERVING

Serving size	2 slices
Calories	300 kcal
Fat	10 g
Saturated fat	3.5 g
Cholesterol	10 mg
Sodium	520 mg
Carbohydrates	33 g
Dietary fiber	4 g
Protein	21 g

Buttermilk Chocolate Chip Pancakes

Pamela Aughe, R.D.

Pancakes are an all-American breakfast treat, and this version pairs chocolate chips and fresh bananas for extra goodness. Here in Michigan, where wild berries grow, we love to use blueberry syrup; you can also try them with Wild Blueberry Sauce (page 62).

Serves: 4 to 6
Hands-on time: 10 minutes
Cooking time: 10 minutes

¾ cup all-purpose flour
2 tablespoons sugar
½ cup toasted wheat germ
1 teaspoon baking powder
½ teaspoon baking soda
2 eggs, lightly beaten
1 cup reduced-fat buttermilk
1 banana, mashed
¼ cup semisweet or milk chocolate chips
vegetable oil cooking spray

Combine the flour, sugar, wheat germ, baking powder, and baking soda in a large bowl; set aside. Whisk together the eggs, buttermilk, and banana in a separate medium-size bowl. Pour the wet ingredients over the dry and stir just until mixed. Stir in the chocolate chips.

Spray a skillet with the cooking spray; heat over medium-high heat. Sprinkle a few droplets of water on the surface; the skillet is preheated when water sizzles.

Spoon the batter onto the hot skillet using a ¼-cup measure. When bubbles appear in the center of a pancake, flip it to the other side. Cook both sides to golden brown.

COOK'S TIP

Use an overripe banana for easier mashing and extra sweetness.

NUTRITION NUGGET

Chocolate is rich in phytochemicals, which have been shown to boost your body's serotonin levels. Semisweet chocolate without extra milk fat and sugar is a good choice.

SUBSTITUTION

If you don't have buttermilk, add 1 teaspoon unflavored vinegar to low-fat or skim milk. Swirl gently to mix.

FOOD TRIVIA

Pancakes are one of our oldest forms of bread. They vary in thickness and flavor according to their country of origin. Americans enjoy thicker cakes while the French, for example, specialize in thinner crépes.

NUTRITION PER SERVING	
Serving size	3 small pancakes
Calories	290 kcal
Fat	8 g
Saturated fat	3 g
Cholesterol	80 mg
Sodium	150 mg
Carbohydrates	48 g
Dietary fiber	4 g
Protein	12 g

NUTRITION PER SERVING	
Serving size	2 large pancakes
Calories	200 kcal
Fat	5 g
Saturated fat	2 g
Cholesterol	55 mg
Sodium	100 mg
Carbohydrates	32 g
Dietary fiber	3 g
Protein	8 g

Cinnamon Apple Oatmeal Pancakes

Rebecca Dowling, R.D.

Serves: 6
Hands-on time: 10 minutes
Standing time: 8 hours
Cooking time: 30 minutes

Soul-warming pancakes come in many flavors in our country. Our overnight guests in Illinois often request that my husband make these pancakes, as they are one of his specialties and are very popular. The batter can be made the night before, making breakfast preparation more leisurely.

1½ cups old-fashioned or quick oats (not instant)
¼ cup whole wheat flour
¼ cup all-purpose flour
2 tablespoons sugar
1 teaspoon baking powder
1 teaspoon baking soda
½ teaspoon cinnamon
2 cups buttermilk
½ cup liquid egg substitute
¼ cup unsweetened applesauce
2 tablespoons butter, melted
vegetable oil cooking spray

Mix together the oats, whole wheat flour, all-purpose flour, sugar, baking powder, baking soda, and cinnamon in a large bowl. In a separate bowl, mix the buttermilk, egg substitute, applesauce, and butter. Pour over the dry ingredients and mix well. Cover and refrigerate overnight or up to 3 days.

Coat a large skillet with the cooking spray and place over medium heat. Add ¼ cup of batter at a time to make the pancakes. Cook on one side until tiny bubbles form along the edges. Flip and cook another 3 to 5 minutes per side. Serve immediately.

COOK'S TIP

Double or triple the batch and freeze the extras in a tightly sealed container. Reheat in the toaster until hot, generally one cycle of the toaster. Alternatively, heat in the microwave 1 to 2 minutes, or until piping hot.

NUTRITION PER SERVING

Serving size	3 pancakes
Calories	235 kcal
Fat	7 g
Saturated fat	3 g
Cholesterol	15 mg
Sodium	450 mg
Carbohydrates	35 g
Dietary fiber	3 g
Protein	10 g

Irish Soda Muffins

Kristine Napier, M.P.H., R.D.

The original recipe for these muffins hails from my Irish friend Betty, who baked Irish soda bread in Chicago. Try this version with raisins and also a touch of whole wheat flour to make it just a bit heartier, as well as higher in fiber and minerals. Baking muffins instead of a loaf helps with portion control.

Serves: 24
Hands-on time: 15 minutes
Baking time: 15 to 17 minutes

vegetable oil cooking spray
3 cups all-purpose flour
1 cup whole wheat flour
½ cup sugar
1 teaspoon salt
2 teaspoons baking powder
1 teaspoon baking soda
6 tablespoons cold unsalted butter
1½ cups raisins
⅓ cup egg substitute
1½ cups buttermilk

Preheat oven to 350°F. Coat 24 regular muffin tins with the cooking spray.

Mix the flours, sugar, salt, baking powder, and baking soda together with a wire whisk. Cut in the butter with a pastry blender or two forks. (You will see bits of butter throughout the dough.) Mix in the raisins.

Mix the egg substitute and buttermilk together. Stir all the liquid into the dry ingredients with a spoon just until all are evenly wet, 10 to 15 seconds. Turn onto a surface lightly floured with 2 to 3 tablespoons of flour and knead 6 to 8 times. (The dough will be very soft and sticky. This is okay—no need to add more flour.) Flour your hands liberally.

Drop the batter evenly into the tins. The tins will be nearly full. Bake 15 to 17 minutes or until lightly golden brown. Remove from the muffin tins and cool on a wire rack. Serve hot or warm.

VARIATION

If you want to make these muffins in a more traditional Irish fashion, stir in ¼ cup caraway seeds and use currants instead of raisins.

COOK'S TIP

For muffins, dry ingredients must be well mixed before fat and wet ingredients are added. Use a wire whisk or a sifter.

NUTRITION NUGGET

Stirring some whole wheat flour into baked goods bumps up the fiber and minerals.

NUTRITION NUGGET

Using fat-free, cholesterol-free egg substitute allows the great taste of butter to shine through while still keeping the fat profile within a healthy range.

NUTRITION PER SERVING	
Serving size	1 muffin
Calories	130 kcal
Fat	1 g
Saturated fat	0 g
Cholesterol	0 mg
Sodium	220 mg
Carbohydrates	29 g
Dietary fiber	2 g
Protein	3 g

Hearty Blueberry Muffins

Kristine Napier, M.P.H., R.D.

Serves: 12
Hands-on time: 15 minutes
Baking time: 12 to 15 minutes

These luscious breakfast, snack, or dessert muffins could have originated in Maine where wild blueberries grow or here in northeastern Wisconsin where upper Michigan blueberries are plentiful. Most important, though, they fill your soul with comfort and your body with the essence of health. They also freeze well.

vegetable oil cooking spray
1½ cups all-purpose flour
½ cup toasted wheat germ
⅔ cup sugar
1 tablespoon plus 1 teaspoon baking powder
¼ teaspoon nutmeg
½ cup liquid egg substitute
¾ cup buttermilk
3 tablespoons canola oil
1 teaspoon vanilla extract
1½ cups fresh or frozen blueberries

TOPPING
2 tablespoons quick cooking or old-fashioned oats (not instant)
2 tablespoons ground flaxseed, optional
1 teaspoon cinnamon
1 tablespoon brown sugar
2 tablespoons toasted wheat germ

Preheat oven to 400°F. Spray 12 muffin tins with the cooking spray.

Combine the flour, ½ cup wheat germ, sugar, baking powder, and nutmeg in a large bowl; stir well. Make a hollow in the middle. Place the egg substitute, buttermilk, canola oil, and vanilla in the hollow. Stir gently, just until the dry ingredients are wet. Add the blueberries; fold gently just to mix. Fill the muffin tins evenly with the mixture.

Combine the oats, flaxseed, cinnamon, brown sugar, and wheat germ. Sprinkle on top of the muffins. Bake 12 to 15 minutes, or until a toothpick inserted in the middle comes out clean.

COOK'S TIP
To add some crunch, stir 1 cup milled or ground flaxseed into the dry ingredients.

NUTRITION NUGGET
Flaxseed adds fiber, minerals, phytochemicals, and omega-3s (heart-healthy fats).

NUTRITION PER SERVING

Serving size	1 muffin
Calories	190 kcal
Fat	5 g
Saturated fat	1 g
Cholesterol	0 mg
Sodium	200 mg
Carbohydrates	30 g
Dietary fiber	2 g
Protein	6 g

Banana Bread with Chocolate Chips

Linda Simon, R.D.

What better place than the heartland of America—Wisconsin—to blend chocolate into banana bread to make a breakfast solution? I'm a personal chef in Madison, Wisconsin, with clients who want chocolate-laced comfort food—and the benefits of healthy eating. This recipe is the one that fits both requests. And, yes, it freezes well!

Serves: 12
Hands-on time: 15 minutes
Baking time: 45 to 50 minutes

- vegetable oil cooking spray
- 4 large bananas, peeled
- ¼ cup canola oil
- ½ cup nonfat yogurt
- 1 large egg, lightly beaten
- 1 teaspoon vanilla extract
- 1½ cups whole wheat flour
- ½ cup all-purpose flour
- 1 cup sugar or spoonable sugar substitute
- 1 teaspoon baking soda
- ½ teaspoon salt
- ½ cup mini–chocolate chips

Preheat oven to 350°F. Coat an 8- or 9-inch loaf pan with the cooking spray.

Mash the bananas with a fork. Combine with the oil, yogurt, egg, and vanilla; mix well and set aside.

In a separate bowl, mix the flours, sugar or sugar substitute, baking soda, and salt; mix well.

Combine the banana mixture with the flour mixture and stir just until the dry ingredients are moistened. Fold in the chocolate chips. Pour the batter into the prepared pan. Bake a 9-inch pan for 45 minutes and an 8-inch pan for about 52 minutes, or until a toothpick inserted in the middle comes out clean. Let cool in the pan 10 minutes; remove from the pan.

SERVING SUGGESTION

Spread a slice with peanut or soy nut butter and enjoy with a glass of nonfat milk (or soy milk).

COOK'S TIP

Cool, slice, and wrap each slice individually; freeze. To serve, thaw at room temperature or toast frozen.

NUTRITION PER SERVING	
Serving size	1⁄12 of loaf
Calories	250 kcal
Fat	8 g
Saturated fat	2 g
Cholesterol	20 mg
Sodium	120 mg
Carbohydrates	44 g
Dietary fiber	3 g
Protein	5 g

Upside-Down Lemon Poppy Seed Loaf

Julie Ann Lickteig, M.S., R.D., F.A.D.A

Serves: 24 (2 loaves)
Hands-on time: 10 minutes
Baking time: 50 minutes

Starting in my traditional Czech home in northern Iowa, I learned how to blend poppy seeds and prunes into many bakery treats. This quick bread is an unbelievably moist version of the heavier traditional Czech variety. Freeze individual slices for easy breakfasts and desserts.

- vegetable oil cooking spray
- 1⅓ cups nonfat milk
- ¾ cup egg substitute
- ½ cup unsweetened applesauce
- 1 18¼-ounce box supermoist lemon cake mix
- ½ cup poppy seeds
- 12 ounces pitted prunes, chopped

Preheat oven to 350°F. Coat two 8- or 9-inch loaf pans with the cooking spray.

Combine the milk, egg substitute, applesauce, and cake mix in a large bowl. Beat by hand or with a mixer for 3 minutes. Stir in the poppy seeds and prunes. Pour into the prepared pans.

Bake 45 to 50 minutes, or until a knife inserted in the middle comes out clean. Invert to remove from the pans, so the prunes will be on top.

SUBSTITUTION
Substitute an equivalent amount of chopped dates for the prunes (although this makes it less traditional Czech).

NUTRITION NUGGET
With its good fiber, low fat, and reasonable calorie profile, feel good about starting your day with a slice for breakfast, along with a tall glass of nonfat milk.

NUTRITION PER SERVING	
Serving size	1/12 of loaf
Calories	150 kcal
Fat	3 g
Saturated fat	0.5 g
Cholesterol	0 mg
Sodium	160 mg
Carbohydrates	28 g
Dietary fiber	2 g
Protein	3 g

Pumpkin Bread

Corrina Riemann, R.D.

Enjoy the all-American aroma of pumpkin pie all year long with this delightfully rich and hearty quick bread. In the Native American tradition of using squash (pumpkin is one type) often, we cook and bake pumpkin into many recipes. Pour a glass of nonfat milk to enjoy with a slice at breakfast—and you're ready to start your day.

Serves: 24
Hands-on time: 15 minutes
Baking time: 25 or 50 minutes

- vegetable oil cooking spray
- 2⅔ cups sugar
- ⅓ cup canola oil
- ⅓ cup unsweetened applesauce
- 1 15-ounce can pumpkin
- 4 eggs
- ⅔ cup nonfat plain yogurt
- 2⅔ cups all-purpose flour
- ⅔ cup toasted wheat germ
- 1½ teaspoons salt
- 2 teaspoons baking soda
- 1½ teaspoons baking powder
- 1 teaspoon ground cloves
- 1 teaspoon ground cinnamon
- 1 teaspoon ground nutmeg
- 1½ cups raisins

Preheat oven to 350°F. Spray two 8½-by-4½-by-2½-inch loaf pans or 24 muffin tins with the cooking spray.

Cream together the sugar, canola oil, applesauce, pumpkin, eggs, and yogurt until smooth.

Stir together the flour, wheat germ, salt, baking soda, baking powder, cloves, cinnamon, and nutmeg.

Combine the dry mixture with the wet one; stir until well combined. Fold in the raisins.

Pour into the prepared pans (fill the muffin tins ⅔ full). Bake for 50 minutes (loaves) or 25 minutes (muffins).

SUBSTITUTION

Instead of raisins, substitute sweetened dried cranberries, which lend a tangy taste.

COOK'S TIP

This freezes well as muffins or bread, up to three months. Thaw at room temperature, in the microwave (about 15 seconds per muffin or slice), or in the toaster (slices only).

NUTRITION NUGGET

Applesauce can replace about ⅓ to ½ of the fat in many recipes for baked goods, reducing the overall fat without sacrificing flavor or texture.

NUTRITION PER SERVING	
Serving size	1/12 of one loaf or one muffin
Calories	240 kcal
Fat	4.5 g
Saturated fat	0.5 g
Cholesterol	35 mg
Sodium	300 mg
Carbohydrates	46 g
Dietary fiber	2 g
Protein	4 g

Hearty Bread

Libby Mills, M.S., R.D., L.D.

Serves: 36
Hands-on time: 20 minutes
Baking time: 30 minutes
Rising time: 2 hours

Reminiscent of settlers' kitchens on the western front during the nineteenth century, this hearty whole-grain bread will fill your kitchen with the aroma of great health. Slice the bread when cool and freeze. Toast a slice right from the freezer and warm up your kitchen with a fabulous aroma again.

- 1½ cups warm water
- 2 tablespoons active dry yeast
- ¼ cup full-flavored molasses
- ¼ tablespoon brown sugar
- 1 cup dry oats (not instant)
- 3 tablespoons vital wheat gluten
- 2 cups whole wheat flour
- 1 cup wheat germ
- ¼ cup canola or extra-virgin olive oil
- ½ teaspoon salt
- 2½ to 3½ cups sifted all-purpose flour
- vegetable oil cooking spray
- 1 6-ounce package salted sunflower seeds

Combine the water, yeast, molasses, and brown sugar; mix well to dissolve the yeast. Add the oats; beat for 1 minute. Let stand 5 minutes.

Add the gluten, whole wheat flour, wheat germ, oil, and salt. Beat about 200 strokes by hand or with the wire whisk attachment of an electric mixer.

Add 2 cups all-purpose flour; beat 200 strokes by hand or with the wire whisk of an electric mixer. If using a mixer, switch to the dough hook. Work in the remaining flour 2 tablespoons at a time until the dough is soft, just slightly sticky, and forms a ball. Add the sunflower seeds. Beat with the dough hook about 4 minutes, or knead by hand about 5 to 6 minutes.

Fill a large glass or ceramic bowl with hot water; drain and dry. Spray with the cooking spray. Transfer the dough to the warm bowl. Cover with a clean dish towel and let rise in a draft-free area for about 1 hour, or until the dough has doubled in size.

SHOPPING TIP

Look for vital wheat gluten in the baking aisle of your supermarket.

VARIATION

Omit the sunflower seeds and use 1 cup milled or ground flaxseeds.

COOK'S TIP

Why vital wheat gluten? Whole wheat flour and wheat germ are relatively "heavy" and do not have as much gluten as white flour. As a result, the bread would not rise well without adding vital wheat gluten.

NUTRITION PER SERVING	
Serving size	1/12 of one loaf
Calories	150 kcal
Fat	5 g
Saturated fat	0.5 g
Cholesterol	0 mg
Sodium	70 mg
Carbohydrates	23 g
Dietary fiber	3 g
Protein	5 g

Coat three 9-by-5-by-3-inch loaf pans with the cooking spray. Punch down the dough; divide into three equal pieces, and form each piece into a loaf. Place each piece in a prepared pan. Cover with a clean tea towel. Let rise in a warm, draft-free area for about 45 minutes or until the dough has doubled in size.

Preheat oven to 350°F. Bake about 25 to 35 minutes or until the tops are golden and the loaves sound hollow when tapped. The bread should slide easily from the pans when done. Cool on a wire rack or serve while warm.

Yeast Bread with Flaxseed

Linda Simon, R.D.

Serves: 12
Hands-on time: 30 minutes
Baking time: 40 minutes

What is more welcoming than the smell of baking bread? Ground flaxseeds add a great nutty taste and extra nutrition to this everyday, all-American loaf. Enjoy the luscious aromas again when you pop a slice in the toaster. I grind whole flaxseeds in my coffee grinder and store extras in the freezer to keep it fresh. This bread recipe would have been a welcome addition to the frontier settlers who lived in the midwest, as it is rich in nutrition.

- 2 cups bread flour, divided
- 1 cup reduced-fat, vitamin-and-mineral-fortified plain soy milk (or 1 cup nonfat milk)
- ½ cup finely ground flaxseeds
- 2 tablespoons sugar
- 1 teaspoon salt
- 1 teaspoon yeast
- canola or extra-virgin olive oil

Combine 1 cup flour and the remaining ingredients (except the oil) in a large bowl or bowl of a stand mixer. Beat until smooth, by hand or using a wire whisk attachment. Blend in the remaining flour by hand or using the dough hook of the stand mixer.

Place the dough in a large bowl coated with canola or extra-virgin olive oil; cover. Allow the dough to rise until doubled in bulk, about 40 minutes.

Preheat oven to 350°F about 20 minutes before rising is complete. Coat one 9-by-5-by-3-inch loaf pan with cooking spray.

Bake for 40 minutes or until the loaf sounds hollow when tapped on the bottom.

COOK'S TIP

Use your bread machine. Combine all ingredients in the bread machine and follow the manufacturer's instructions. Alternatively, use only the dough cycle, and then form the bread into loaves of different shapes. You can double the recipe in the bread machine if you use only the dough cycle. Bake two loaves now and freeze one for later.

NUTRITION NUGGET

Did you know that the body cannot "crack into" whole flaxseeds to harvest their goodness? That's why it's important to grind them first (or purchase them already ground or milled).

VARIATION

Adding 1 to 2 teaspoons freshly ground black pepper to the dough mix makes a zingy sandwich bread. I make the pepper bread when fresh tomatoes are in season and use it for BLTs.

NUTRITION PER SERVING	
Serving size	1⁄12 of loaf
Calories	130 kcal
Fat	3 g
Saturated fat	1 g
Cholesterol	0 mg
Sodium	210 mg
Carbohydrates	22 g
Dietary fiber	2 g
Protein	5 g

Feta-Topped Stuffed Grape Leaves (Dolmathes)

Melissa Stevens Ohlson, M.S., R.D., L.D.

This great appetizer can be served warm or cold. It is especially tasty when served warm with a side of hummus and warm pita bread.

Serves: 25
Soaking time: 45 minutes
Hands-on time: 40 minutes
Cooking time: 60 minutes

- 1½ cups uncooked brown rice
- 1 15-ounce can chickpeas, rinsed and drained
- 2 medium-size onions, chopped
- 1¼ cups chopped parsley, divided
- ½ cup chopped fresh mint
- 3 tablespoons extra-virgin olive oil
- freshly ground black pepper to taste
- 75 grape leaves—fresh, jarred, or canned; drain if jarred or canned
- juice of 1 lemon
- ½ cup crumbled reduced-fat feta cheese

Cover the rice with water; soak 45 minutes; drain.

Place the chickpeas in a large bowl; mash slightly with a fork, leaving some large pieces. Add the onions, ½ cup parsley, mint, olive oil, and pepper to taste; stir to combine. Add the rice; stir.

Place 1 to 2 teaspoons of the mixture on each grape leaf, on the side of the leaf where the vein shows, about one-third of the way up the leaf. Fold the sides of the leaves in; roll away from you to close. Layer the stuffed grape leaves in a heavy pot, alternating the direction of the rows. Sprinkle with pepper. Place an inverted saucer on top of the last row of leaves to hold them in place. Cover the stuffed leaves with water, using enough to cover the plate.

Cover the pot and bring to a boil. Reduce heat; simmer for 50 minutes. Let stand 10 minutes.

Remove the plate; add the lemon juice. Sprinkle with the feta cheese and additional fresh parsley.

NUTRITION PER SERVING

Serving size	3 stuffed leaves
Calories	90 kcal
Fat	3 g
Saturated fat	0 g
Cholesterol	0 mg
Sodium	420 mg
Carbohydrates	15 g
Dietary fiber	2 g
Protein	3 g

Tuscan Spring Artichokes with Balsamic Vinaigrette

Barrie Rosencrans, M.S., R.D., L.D.

Serves: 4
Hands-on time: 15 minutes
Cooking time: 40 minutes
Marinating time: 2 hours

While I first made this with just-picked, long-stemmed artichokes from a Florence farmer's market when I lived in Italy, it remains a family favorite in my northeast Ohio home. The rich woodiness of the aged balsamic vinegar brings the delicate flavor of an artichoke to life. Be sure to use extra-virgin olive oil, a favorite in Mediterranean cooking because of its fruity flavor.

1 cup red wine vinegar
4 large artichokes
juice of 2 lemons
1¼ cup aged balsamic vinegar
⅓ cup extra-virgin olive oil
1 teaspoon coarse-grain sea salt
¼ teaspoon black pepper, freshly cracked
½ teaspoon sugar
¼ cup loosely packed fresh basil, chopped
1 tablespoon finely minced garlic (3 to 4 cloves)
½ cup fresh flat-leaf parsley, finely chopped

Fill a 2-quart saucepan with water. Add the red wine vinegar and bring to a boil over high heat.

Wash the artichokes in cold running water; turn them upside down to drain. Cut the prickly tips off each leaf of each artichoke globe, using kitchen scissors. Slice off the stem base with a kitchen knife to create a flat surface. Pour lemon juice over the cut edges of the artichokes to prevent browning. Place the artichokes in the boiling water and boil for 40 minutes or until tender. To ensure even cooking, use tongs to turn the artichokes occasionally. Test doneness by pulling off an outer leaf; if it comes out easily, the artichokes are done.

Place the artichokes upside down in a colander to drain. Gently squeeze out any excess water, then turn them right-side up in a dish that will hold them while they marinate.

SHOPPING TIP

Look for artichokes that have tight, dark green leaves. They may have a tinge of purple color in them. A slight bit of browning on the artichoke's tips won't affect the taste or quality once prepared. Look for large globes in order to get artichokes with the largest tasty hearts inside.

COOK'S TIP

The vinaigrette can be made a day ahead and refrigerated overnight.

NUTRITION PER SERVING	
Serving size	1 artichoke
Calories	300 kcal
Fat	19 g
Saturated fat	2.5 g
Cholesterol	0 mg
Sodium	760 mg
Carbohydrates	31 g
Dietary fiber	9 g
Protein	6 g

Whisk together the balsamic vinegar, olive oil, salt, pepper, and sugar. Add the basil and garlic and whisk again. Divide the vinaigrette in half. Place half in the refrigerator for the second phase of the marinating process. Drizzle the other half of the vinaigrette evenly over all 4 artichokes, making sure the liquid reaches in between the leaves of each artichoke. Close up the leaves and marinate in the refrigerator for 1 hour.

Remove from the refrigerator and distribute the remaining vinaigrette over the artichokes evenly. Marinate for 1 hour or up to overnight. Use the reserved sauce for dipping.

Sprinkle the flat-leaf parsley over the artichokes to garnish, and serve.

SERVING SUGGESTION

Artichokes may be served chilled or at room temperature. When serving as an appetizer, give each person a side bowl for discarded leaves. Serve with French bread to soak up every last bit of vinaigrette.

FOOD TRIVIA

The artichoke is the flower bud of a thistle plant.

Roasted Red Pepper Hummus

Melissa Stevens Ohlson, M.S., R.D., L.D.

Serves: 12 as an appetizer or 6 as a main course
Hands-on time: 15 minutes

I grew up with hummus in our Greek home. This version includes roasted red peppers, which contribute a slightly smoky flavor and vivid red color. Eat hummus by itself, with fresh vegetables, spread on pitas, or as part of a veggie wrap.

- ½ tablespoon extra-virgin olive oil
- 4 cloves garlic, minced
- 1 medium-size onion, diced
- 2 medium-size red bell peppers, roasted, or 1 7-ounce jar roasted red peppers in brine, drained
- 1 16-ounce can chickpeas, drained and rinsed
- ½ cup lemon juice
- 1 tablespoon reduced-sodium soy sauce
- ¼ cup tahini (sesame paste)
- 2 teaspoons hot pepper sauce, or to taste
- ½ teaspoon ground cayenne pepper

Sauté the onion and the garlic in the olive oil until softened, approximately 5 minutes. Set aside.

In a food processor, purée the roasted red pepper, onion, garlic mixture, chickpeas, lemon juice, soy sauce, tahini, hot pepper sauce, and cayenne until you have a smooth, thick paste.

SERVING SUGGESTION

Serve with crackers and raw vegetables.

COOK'S TIP

If making roasted peppers, set the oven to broil. Cut the red peppers in half lengthwise; clean out the pulp and the seeds. Place the pepper halves cut-side down on a baking sheet and broil until the skin becomes blackened. Take out of the oven and carefully place the blackened red peppers into a zip-top plastic bag and let cool. Once cooled, peel away the skin and slice the remaining flesh into strips.

NUTRITION PER SERVING	
Serving size	¼ cup, appetizer
Calories	100 kcal
Fat	4 g
Saturated fat	0.5 g
Cholesterol	0 mg
Sodium	240 mg
Carbohydrates	13 g
Dietary fiber	3 g
Protein	3 g

NUTRITION PER SERVING	
Serving size	½ cup, main course
Calories	200 kcal
Fat	8 g
Saturated fat	1 g
Cholesterol	0 mg
Sodium	480 mg
Carbohydrates	25 g
Dietary fiber	5 g
Protein	7 g

Sylte (Spiced Pork Loaf)

LaDonna Levik, R.D., retired

As part of Minnesota's large Scandinavian population, our family enjoys many traditions from Norway and Sweden. Historically, this recipe was made with a hog's head, but using a pork roast makes it a lot easier.

Serves: 16 to 20
Hands-on time: 30 minutes
Cooking time: 2 to 3 hours
Chill time: 12 hours

- 2 pounds pork loin
- 1 large onion, cut into chunks
- 2 teaspoons salt
- ¾ teaspoon ground cloves
- 1 teaspoon ginger
- ½ teaspoon freshly ground pepper
- 4 envelopes unflavored gelatin
- 4 tablespoons cold water

Place the pork loin and the onion in a large saucepan; cover with cold water. Heat to a gentle boil and then simmer for about 2 hours, until the meat is tender.

Remove the meat from the broth; reserve 2 cups of the liquid. Chop the meat very finely and place in a large bowl. (If you want to use a food processor, pulse only until finely chopped.) Stir in the salt, cloves, ginger, and pepper.

Sprinkle the gelatin over cold water in a small bowl. Stir into the reserved hot broth. Stir the gelatin mixture into the pork mixture.

Line a 9-by-5-by-3-inch loaf pan with aluminum foil. Spoon the pork mixture into the pan, patting it down firmly. Cover and refrigerate overnight.

Remove the sylte from the pan; slice thinly and place on a serving platter. Serve with crackers or as a selection on a cold meat platter.

VARIATIONS

Alter the spices to your personal taste. Adding a couple of bay leaves to the cooking liquid adds a nice flavor. Allspice can be used instead of or in addition to the cloves and ginger.

SERVING SUGGESTIONS

This recipe is part of our Christmas smorgasbord spread. We typically garnish the plate with fresh parsley and cherry tomatoes and serve it with crackers. It's a nice recipe to make ahead and freeze during the hectic holiday season. Leftover sylte makes a nice sandwich filling, too.

NUTRITION PER SERVING	
Serving size	1/16 of pan
Calories	120 kcal
Fat	7 g
Saturated fat	2.5 g
Cholesterol	35 mg
Sodium	320 mg
Carbohydrates	1 g
Dietary fiber	0 g
Protein	13 g

NUTRITION PER SERVING	
Serving size	1/20 of pan
Calories	100 kcal
Fat	6 g
Saturated fat	2 g
Cholesterol	30 mg
Sodium	260 mg
Carbohydrates	1 g
Dietary fiber	0 g
Protein	10 g

Sauerkraut Bites

Julie Ann Lickteig, M.S., R.D., F.A.D.A.

Serves: 4 dozen
Hands-on time: 20 minutes
Baking time: 8 to 12 minutes

These traditional Bohemian crackers, which I learned to make in my Iowa home, can be served as an appetizer or passed in a breadbasket. Challenge your guests to identify the vegetable in the cracker.

1½ cups all-purpose flour
½ cup whole wheat flour
¼ teaspoon salt
1 stick cold butter (4 ounces)
1½ cups Bavarian style sauerkraut (with caraway seeds), drained
6 to 8 teaspoons water
⅛ cup milk
¼ cup caraway seeds
¼ cup poppy seeds

FOOD TRIVIA
Bohemia was in southern Czechoslovakia. Each region of what was once Czechoslovakia had distinctive recipes from the other regions.

Preheat oven to 425°F.

Mix together the flours and salt; cut in the butter until the mixture resembles coarse crumbs. Stir in the sauerkraut; mix until well distributed. Add the water slowly, stirring until a ball forms.

Cut the dough in half. Roll out half the dough on a floured surface to ¼-inch thickness for a crispier texture, or ⅜-inch thickness for a chewier texture. Cut the dough into strips 2 inches long and 1½-inches wide, or into 2-inch squares. Be creative with the shapes, such as using diagonal cuts on the ends. Brush the dough strips with the milk and sprinkle with the caraway seeds, poppy seeds, or a combination of the two.

Place on ungreased cookie sheets and bake for 8 to 12 minutes or until light brown. Repeat with the remaining dough.

NUTRITION PER SERVING

Serving size	1 cracker
Calories	45 kcal
Fat	2.5 g
Saturated fat	1 g
Cholesterol	5 mg
Sodium	60 mg
Carbohydrates	5 g
Dietary fiber	0 g
Protein	1 g

Coriander and Buttermilk Chutney

Kristine Napier, M.P.H., R.D.

I serve this dip with vegetables or use it as a spread for an interestingly different sandwich. It is the original creation of my friend Alamelu Vairavan, an expert on healthy South Indian cooking. Even though it's served cold, the delightful flavors warm up a cold Wisconsin winter day.

Serves: 3 as a sandwich spread or 6 as a dip
Hands-on time: 10 minutes

- 2 cups chopped fresh cilantro
- 1 green chili pepper
- ¼ cup dry roasted peanuts
- 1 teaspoon cumin seeds
- dash salt
- ¼ cup low-fat cultured buttermilk

Place all the ingredients in a blender and grind to a smooth paste. Transfer to a bowl. Cover and refrigerate until serving.

SHOPPING TIP
Cilantro leaves come from the coriander plant; it may be called fresh coriander in some markets.

FOOD TRIVIA
Chutney comes from the East Indian word *chatni.* It can be smooth or chunky, spicy or mild.

NUTRITION PER SERVING	
Serving size	½ cup
Calories	90 kcal
Fat	6 g
Saturated fat	1 g
Cholesterol	0 mg
Sodium	30 mg
Carbohydrates	6 g
Dietary fiber	2 g
Protein	4 g

NUTRITION PER SERVING	
Serving size	¼ cup
Calories	45 kcal
Fat	3 g
Saturated fat	0 g
Cholesterol	0 mg
Sodium	15 mg
Carbohydrates	3 g
Dietary fiber	Less than 1 g
Protein	2 g

Serves: 2 in main dish salads or 4 in side salads or soups
Hands-on time: 5 minutes
Baking time: 10 minutes

NUTRITION NUGGET
Color is not always an indicator of whole-grain bread. Molasses (and other ingredients) can also lend a brown color, but not the nutrition and fiber found in whole-grain bread. Look for the words "whole" or "whole-grain" on the ingredients label. "Wheat flour" or "enriched flour" are not whole grains.

NUTRITION PER SERVING

Serving size	1 cup croutons, or the amount from one slice of bread
Calories	110 kcal
Fat	6 g
Saturated fat	1 g
Cholesterol	0 mg
Sodium	15 mg
Carbohydrates	13 g
Dietary fiber	2 g
Protein	3 g

NUTRITION PER SERVING

Serving size	½ cup croutons, or the amount from ½ slice of bread
Calories	60 kcal
Fat	3 g
Saturated fat	0 g
Cholesterol	0 mg
Sodium	75 mg
Carbohydrates	6 g
Dietary fiber	Less than 1 g
Protein	1 g

Hearty (and Easy!) Croutons

Alice Henneman, M.S., R.D.

The crunch of croutons and the contrast in texture add to the pleasure of any salad and many cream soups. From the heart of America's wheat crops in Nebraska, I advise choosing a hearty whole-grain bread to further enhance the flavor.

vegetable oil cooking spray
2 slices whole-grain or whole wheat bread
2 teaspoons extra-virgin olive oil

Preheat oven to 350°F. Coat a baking sheet with the cooking spray.

Drizzle one side of the bread evenly with the olive oil. Cut into ½-inch cubes.

Spread the cubes in a single layer, oiled side up, on the prepared baking sheet. Bake on the middle shelf of the oven for 10 minutes, or until lightly brown and crisp.

Cool and add to a salad or soup just before serving.

SHOPPING TIP
If you are watching your sodium intake, choose reduced- or lower-sodium bread; you may have to ask your grocer or health food store to order it for you.

COOK'S TIP
While these croutons are at their best when eaten on the day prepared, you can store them in a tightly sealed container for up to four days.

VARIATION
Sprinkle the bread cubes with your favorite dried herbs before baking.

Green Beans with Yellow Split Peas and Ginger

Kristine Napier, M.P.H., R.D.

Try this South Indian favorite way to cook green beans—a prized recipe developed by my friend Alamelu Vairavan who taught me how to make it in her Milwaukee home, just down the road from where I live in Green Bay.

Serves: 4
Hands-on time: 15 minutes
Cooking time: 30 minutes

- ½ cup yellow split peas
- ½ teaspoon turmeric, divided
- 2 tablespoons canola or corn oil
- ¾ teaspoon cumin seeds
- 2 cups green beans, stemmed and diced
- 1 tablespoon minced fresh ginger
- 1 green chili pepper, finely chopped, optional
- salt to taste

Boil 2½ cups of water. Add the split peas and ¼ teaspoon turmeric. Cook over medium heat, uncovered, for 20 to 30 minutes, or until the split peas become tender. Drain and set aside.

Place the oil in a skillet over medium heat. When the oil is hot, but not smoking, stir in the cumin seeds; cook until the seeds become brown. Add the green beans and stir well. Add the ginger and the green chili. Cook, covered, over medium heat for about a minute. Add salt and the remaining ¼ teaspoon of turmeric and 2 tablespoons water; mix well. Cover and cook the beans over low heat for 3 to 5 minutes.

When the beans are tender but still crisp, add the cooked split peas. Stir well. Remove from heat and keep covered until serving time. Be careful not to overcook the beans.

SHOPPING TIP
Choose ginger with smooth skin; wrinkled skin is a tell-tale sign of dryness. Most grocers allow you to break off a piece of ginger from larger ones.

COOK'S TIP
Instead of mincing fresh ginger, grate it using a fine grater.

NUTRITION PER SERVING

Serving size	¾ cup
Calories	170 kcal
Fat	7 g
Saturated fat	0.5 g
Cholesterol	0 mg
Sodium	0 mg
Carbohydrates	21 g
Dietary fiber	2 g
Protein	7 g

Honey Mustard Glazed Brussels Sprouts with Cashews

Roberta L. Duyff, M.S., R.D., F.A.D.A., C.F.C.S.

Serves: 6
Hands-on time: 3 to 5 minutes
Cooking time: 12 to 15 minutes

Brussels sprouts seem so misunderstood. The key to their great flavor, tender texture, and delicate green color is in the cooking: short, uncovered, perhaps with a touch of sweet glaze. Prepared quickly and easily, these flavorful vegetables make a great side dish to complement pork, beef, and lamb. The skeptics in my St. Louis family love brussels sprouts made this way.

- 1 pound bag frozen brussels sprouts
- 2 tablespoons honey mustard
- 1 teaspoon canola oil
- ⅓ cup chopped cashews

Steam the brussels sprouts as directed on the package, until cooked through. Drain excess water from the saucepan.

Drizzle the honey mustard and canola oil over the brussels sprouts in the saucepan. On medium-high heat, cook and stir about 4 to 5 minutes, until nicely glazed. Meanwhile toast the nuts by heating them in a dry skillet over medium heat for 3 to 5 minutes. Shake them often for even toasting.

To serve, top the glazed brussels sprouts with the toasted cashews.

SHOPPING TIP

Fresh brussels sprouts are great in season, but their frozen counterparts are convenient to keep on hand, and they need no prep work.

VARIATION

Top with toasted, Italian-seasoned bread crumbs instead of toasted nuts.

FOOD TRIVIA

Extended cooking, especially with the lid on, intensifies the aroma of cruciferous vegetables and makes the flavor unpleasant. Shirley Corriher, author of *CookWise*, notes that just 5 to 7 more minutes of cooking time for cabbage (another cruciferous vegetable) doubles the amount of strong-smelling compounds that form. So, the advice for cooking cruciferous vegetables is: cook uncovered, for just a short time.

NUTRITION PER SERVING

Serving size	¾ cup
Calories	100 kcal
Fat	5 g
Saturated fat	1 g
Cholesterol	0 mg
Sodium	65 mg
Carbohydrates	10 g
Dietary fiber	3 g
Protein	4 g

Central Plains Succotash

Roberta L. Duyff, M.S., R.D., F.A.D.A., C.F.C.S.

A dish that dates from colonial days, succotash derives from the Eastern Narragansett Indian word msickquatash, *meaning "boiled whole kernels of corn." As a traditional American favorite, enjoyed from New England to the South, succotash is typically a cooked dish, made with lima beans, corn kernels, and perhaps chopped red and green pepper. Regional versions abound: perhaps a southern variation made with okra, a Midwest style combining green beans and corn, or perhaps mom's own version with onion or bacon. A touch of butter and perhaps milk or cream sometimes adds a hint of flavor to this all-American dish.*

Serves: 4
Hands-on time: 10 minutes
Chill time: 1 to 4 hours
Cooking time: 3 minutes

2 tablespoons balsamic vinegar
2 tablespoons cider vinegar
1 tablespoon brown sugar
½ teaspoon ground cumin
½ teaspoon onion powder
1 clove garlic, minced
1½ cups cooked edamame (shelled fresh or frozen soybeans)
1½ cups cooked fresh corn kernels, or drained canned corn, or frozen
½ cup chopped red bell pepper
⅓ cup chopped cilantro

Combine the balsamic and cider vinegars, brown sugar, cumin, onion powder, and garlic in a 1- to 1½-quart saucepan. Heat over medium heat about 3 minutes, or until the sugar dissolves. Remove from heat.

Place the edamame, corn, and red bell pepper in a medium-size bowl. Pour the vinegar mixture over the vegetables. Stir to mix. Cover and refrigerate 1 to 4 hours or until chilled, stirring once.

Stir in the cilantro just before serving. Serve chilled.

FOOD TRIVIA
Soybeans and corn are two of the major crops grown in the Midwest. In fact, 40 percent of the soybeans produced in the United States come from Illinois and Iowa. That's a total of 958 million bushels a year from those two states alone!

SERVING SUGGESTION
Serve grilled chicken or fish fillets over this chilled Central Plains Succotash.

SHOPPING TIP
If you can't find edamame in your supermarket, substitute canned or frozen baby lima or cannellini beans.

NUTRITION NUGGETS
Succotash is a great protein dish, which can be "center plate" in vegetarian meals. Whether this dish is made with soybeans or lima beans, the beans along with the corn provide all the essential amino acids (the building blocks of protein) your body needs.

NUTRITION PER SERVING	
Serving size	¾ cup
Calories	340 kcal
Fat	13 g
Saturated fat	1.5 g
Cholesterol	0 mg
Sodium	10 mg
Carbohydrates	42 g
Dietary fiber	17 g
Protein	25 g

All Year Christmas Rice

Michelle Plummer, M.S., R.D., C.D.

Serves: 8
Hands-on time: 20 minutes
Cooking time: 25 minutes

Giving rice a different face in winter, when fresh vegetables are not as tasty, became easier in my Indiana home with this recipe. While I first made this at Christmastime, my family asks for it all year now.

- 3 cups water
- 1 cup white wine
- 1 tablespoon chicken bouillon granules
- 1 large onion, chopped
- 2 cups long grain rice
- 2 cups shredded Parmesan cheese
- 1 cup frozen peas, thawed
- 1 7-ounce jar roasted red peppers, drained and diced
- 2 cloves garlic, minced
- chopped fresh parsley for garnish, optional

Place the water, wine, chicken base, and onion in a 4-quart saucepan; bring to a boil. Add the rice, reduce heat, cover with a tight-fitting lid, and simmer for 20 minutes.

Remove the lid and fluff the rice. Add the Parmesan cheese, peas, red peppers, and garlic. Stir until the cheese is melted and well incorporated.

Garnish with fresh chopped parsley, if desired.

NUTRITION PER SERVING

Serving size	¾ cup
Calories	310 kcal
Fat	7 g
Saturated fat	4 g
Cholesterol	15 mg
Sodium	680 mg
Carbohydrates	42 g
Dietary fiber	3 g
Protein	13 g

Sweet Potato Poriyal

Kristine Napier, M.P.H., R.D.

My friend Alamelu Vairavan taught me how to cook this South Indian stir-fry dish, an excellent accompaniment to any meal. Enjoy the wonders of Indian cooking wherever you are in the United States, as Alamelu and I do in Wisconsin.

Serves: 6
Hands-on time: 15 minutes
Cooking time: 20 minutes

2 medium-size sweet potatoes
2 tablespoons canola oil
1 teaspoon cumin seeds
½ cup chopped onion
¼ teaspoon turmeric
salt to taste
¼ cup chopped fresh cilantro

Boil, peel, and cut the sweet potatoes into cubes (or mash if you prefer). Set aside.

Place the oil in a skillet over medium heat. When the oil is hot, but not smoking, stir in the cumin seeds; cook until the seeds become brown. Immediately add the onion and cook for 2 to 3 minutes, or until the onion is wilted. Add the turmeric. Stir in the cubed or mashed sweet potato and salt. Cook over medium heat, stirring often, until the potatoes are blended with the seasoning.

Garnish with fresh coriander.

COOK'S TIP

If your eyes water when you chop onions, freeze the onion for 20 minutes before chopping.

NUTRITION PER SERVING	
Serving size	½ cup
Calories	90 kcal
Fat	5 g
Saturated fat	0 g
Cholesterol	0 mg
Sodium	15 mg
Carbohydrates	12 g
Dietary fiber	2 g
Protein	1 g

German Potato Salad

Margaret Pfeiffer, M.S., R.D., C.D.

Serves: 8
Hands-on time: 15 minutes
Cooking time: 35 minutes

Milwaukee, Wisconsin, has a large German population, and German potato salad is common fare. While it's best made the day of serving, don't hesitate to reheat in the microwave.

- 5 unpeeled red-skinned potatoes (about 2 pounds)
- 1 medium-size onion, chopped
- 4 slices bacon or turkey bacon, diced
- ¼ cup sugar or equivalent sugar substitute
- 2 tablespoons all-purpose flour
- ½ teaspoon salt
- ⅛ teaspoon freshly ground pepper
- 1 cup water
- ¼ cup white vinegar
- 1 large egg
- ¼ cup fresh or bottled lemon juice
- ¼ cup chopped fresh chives

Boil the potatoes in a large saucepan for about 20 minutes or until tender (test with a fork). Drain and cool slightly. Slice the potatoes and place in a large serving bowl with the chopped onion and set aside.

Cook the bacon in a medium-size skillet until crisp. Remove from heat and drain on paper towels. Discard all but 2 tablespoons of the bacon fat. Add the sugar, flour, salt, and pepper to the bacon fat in the skillet; stir to combine.

Combine the water, vinegar, egg, and lemon juice in a small bowl; whisk with a fork to blend. Add to the bacon fat mixture in the skillet. Whisk together and cook over medium heat until the mixture starts to boil, stirring frequently. Reduce heat to low and simmer for 5 minutes.

Pour the cooked bacon fat mixture over the potatoes and onions and toss gently. Garnish with chives and serve.

COOK'S TIP
Cook the potatoes a day or two ahead and refrigerate.

NUTRITION NUGGET
Use canola oil instead of bacon fat to lower the saturated fat content.

NUTRITION PER SERVING	
Serving size	½ cup
Calories	120 kcal
Fat	2 g
Saturated fat	0.5 g
Cholesterol	30 mg
Sodium	250 mg
Carbohydrates	23 g
Dietary fiber	4 g
Protein	4 g

Roasted Potato Salad

Michelle Plummer, M.S., R.D., C.D.

A family favorite from Indiana, this roasted version of an American favorite is well worth the time. The familiar tastes and textures of the traditional recipe come through, but are enhanced by heartier, roasted flavors.

Serves: 10
Hands-on time: 30 minutes
Cooking time: 20 minutes

8 red-skinned potatoes, scrubbed, cleaned, and quartered (about 3 pounds)
2 stalks celery, diced
1 large sweet onion, chopped
1 red bell pepper, seeded and diced
2 tablespoons olive oil
4 slices uncooked bacon, chopped
½ cup thinly sliced green onions
¼ cup finely chopped fresh parsley
2 tablespoons finely chopped assorted fresh herbs, such as basil, rosemary, and/or thyme
1 cup reduced-fat sour cream
1 cup reduced-fat mayonnaise
3 tablespoons Dijon mustard
2 tablespoons sugar
2 tablespoons apple cider vinegar or white distilled vinegar
black pepper to taste
1 hard-cooked egg, sliced
2 tablespoons pine nuts, toasted

SHOPPING TIP
For a real time saver, get precut vegetables at your supermarket's salad bar. Look for celery, onions, and bell peppers to help you make this recipe in a snap.

Preheat oven to 400°F.

Toss the potatoes, celery, onion, red bell pepper, and olive oil in a bowl. Spread onto an ungreased 12-by-18-inch baking sheet. Roast for 20 minutes. Remove from oven and cool on the baking sheet on a wire rack.

In a small skillet, cook the bacon over medium heat until crisp; drain on paper towels. Combine the roasted vegetables, bacon, green onions, parsley, and herbs in a large bowl.

Mix together the sour cream, mayonnaise, mustard, sugar, and vinegar in a spouted 2-cup measuring cup. Pour over the roasted vegetable mixture; toss well.

Garnish with the egg slices and pine nuts.

SERVING SUGGESTION
Instead of a loaded baked potato, serve this salad on a bed of greens with fresh fruit slices.

NUTRITION PER SERVING	
Serving size	¾ cup
Calories	250 kcal
Fat	10 g
Saturated fat	3 g
Cholesterol	35 mg
Sodium	410 mg
Carbohydrates	35 g
Dietary fiber	3 g
Protein	6 g

Easy Green Bean Salad with Lemon Vinaigrette

Mary Abbott Hess, L.H.D., M.S., R.D., F.A.D.A.

Serves: 6
Hands-on time: 10 minutes
Cooking time: 1 minute

Summer-garden fresh or chosen from today's wondrously rich produce aisles, this dish can be made all year. I don't wait for special guests to make it, but it's certainly elegant enough to impress. This recipe is a great one in Chicago and other Midwest places where getting fresh vegetables can be a problem in the heart of winter.

1 pound fresh green beans, ends trimmed (or 1 pound frozen cut green beans)
½ pound sliced fresh mushrooms
2 tablespoons fresh chives, cut about ½-inch long

DRESSING
3 tablespoons canola or corn oil
1 tablespoon tarragon or apple cider vinegar
1 tablespoon fresh lemon juice
1 teaspoon grated lemon zest
¼ teaspoon salt
⅛ teaspoon freshly ground pepper

Fill a large bowl with ice and cold water; set aside.

Bring to boil a large pot of water. Add the green beans and boil for 1 minute. Drain the beans and immediately place in the ice water to quickly cool.

Drain the beans and toss with the mushrooms and the chives.

Mix the dressing ingredients in a small bowl. Just before serving, pour the dressing over the beans and toss to mix.

COOK'S TIP

Make this recipe in a snap by using bottled Italian dressing in place of the oil, cider vinegar, salt, and pepper. Use 3 tablespoons low-fat dressing plus 1 tablespoon lemon juice.

NUTRITION PER SERVING	
Serving size	¾ cup
Calories	100 kcal
Fat	7 g
Saturated fat	0.5 g
Cholesterol	0 mg
Sodium	105 mg
Carbohydrates	7 g
Dietary fiber	1 g
Protein	3 g

Refreshing Cucumber Watermelon Salad

Kristine Napier, M.P.H., R.D.

In Wisconsin, cucumbers and watermelon ripen at the same time. This recipe combines both to produce an unexpected, extraordinary salad.

Serves: 4
Hands-on time: 15 minutes
Standing time: 1 hour

2 tablespoons lime juice
2 tablespoons granulated sugar
½ teaspoon salt
¼ cup minced fresh parsley
2 medium unpeeled cucumbers, washed, ends removed, sliced lengthwise then sliced crosswise
3 cups watermelon, cut in 1-inch cubes (about 1 pound)

Combine the lime juice, sugar, and salt in a 2-quart bowl; whisk together. Stir in the parsley. Add the cucumbers; toss with a rubber spatula, coating all cucumber pieces. Add the watermelon; fold in gently. Cover, set aside, and allow the juice from the watermelon to mix with the other juices. Stir gently and let stand at room temperature 1 hour.

SHOPPING TIPS

Choose a watermelon without a flat side and that sounds hollow when you knock on it. Look for a melon with a dull (not shiny) rind free of soft spots, gashes, or blemishes.

NUTRITION PER SERVING	
Serving size	1½ cups
Calories	90 kcal
Fat	0.5 g
Saturated fat	0 g
Cholesterol	0 mg
Sodium	300 mg
Carbohydrates	20 g
Dietary fiber	2 g
Protein	2 g

Cucumber and Mango Salad

Kristine Napier, M.P.H., R.D.

Serves: 4
Hands-on time: 15 minutes
Chill time: 1 hour

This easy yet interestingly delicious salad recipe was given to me by my friend and fellow chef Alamelu Vairavan of Milwaukee. We both grow cucumbers in our gardens. This recipe is a great way to enjoy the extras with a totally new taste sensation.

SHOPPING TIP
To choose a just-ripe mango, select one with thick, yellow-orange skin blushed with red. The fruit should give ever so slightly with a gentle squeeze.

- 2 cups peeled and cubed cucumbers
- 2 cups cubed mango (not too ripe)
- ½ teaspoon ground cumin
- ½ teaspoon black pepper

Place the cut cucumbers and mangos in a bowl. Add the cumin and black pepper. Mix well. Cover and refrigerate at least 1 hour.

NUTRITION PER SERVING	
Serving size	1 cup
Calories	60 kcal
Fat	0 g
Saturated fat	0 g
Cholesterol	0 mg
Sodium	0 mg
Carbohydrates	16 g
Dietary fiber	2 g
Protein	1 g

Wheat Berry Salad with Fresh Herbs

Maggie Green, R.D., L.D., C.C.

Colorful and refreshing, this salad is perfect for either an elegant dinner or a picnic. Whole wheat kernels, or "wheat berries," create a chewy, high-fiber base for this delicious salad.

Serves: 8
Hands-on time: 30 minutes
Cooking time: 50 minutes

- 1 cup uncooked wheat berries (whole wheat kernels)
- 3 cups water
- 1 cup roughly chopped parsley
- 1 head radicchio, torn into small pieces
- ½ cup roughly chopped arugula
- 6 tablespoons extra-virgin olive oil
- 2 tablespoons balsamic vinegar
- 1 clove garlic, minced
- 1½ teaspoons kosher salt
- 1 teaspoon freshly ground black pepper

Combine the wheat berries and water in a 2-quart saucepan. Bring to a boil, stir, and cover. Reduce heat to low and simmer for approximately 50 minutes, until soft but still slightly chewy.

Drain the wheat berries and spread them on a cookie sheet to cool. This will prevent them from sticking together.

Mix together the parsley, radicchio, arugula, olive oil, balsamic vinegar, garlic, salt, pepper, and wheat berries. Stir, tossing to mix well. The salad can be mixed ahead and chilled for up to 3 hours before serving.

SHOPPING TIP

Cooked brown rice, couscous, or pasta may be substituted for the wheat berries.

NUTRITION PER SERVING	
Serving size	½ cup
Calories	200 kcal
Fat	11 g
Saturated fat	1.5 g
Cholesterol	0 mg
Sodium	370 mg
Carbohydrates	21 g
Dietary fiber	2 g
Protein	3 g

Spring Vegetable Sauté

Marjorie Sawicki, M.S., R.D., L.D.

Serves: 6
Hands-on time: 15 minutes
Cooking time: 10 minutes

SHOPPING TIP

If you like the taste of tarragon, look for tarragon vinegar. Use it in this recipe and omit the fresh or dried tarragon to save a step.

COOK'S TIP

Use 1 pound of asparagus and omit the snow peas. The contrasting textures of the mushrooms and the asparagus silently add to the enjoyment of this dish.

Asparagus is the first vegetable to come into Illinois gardens. Fresh or dried, tarragon dances well with the fresh taste of all the vegetables.

- 1 tablespoon canola oil
- 1 clove garlic, minced
- ¼ red onion, cut into slivers
- 1 portabella mushroom, sliced
- 1 pound sugar snap peas, trimmed
- ½ pound fresh asparagus, trimmed and sliced diagonally
- 1 to 2 tablespoons balsamic vinegar
- 1 tablespoon snipped fresh tarragon, or 1 teaspoon dried
- 4 tablespoons slivered almonds, optional

Combine the oil, garlic, and onion in a large nonstick skillet over medium-high heat. Sauté 2 to 3 minutes. Add the mushroom, snap peas, asparagus, and 2 tablespoons water. Sauté 2 to 4 minutes, or until the mushrooms wilt and the peas are crisp tender. Add the vinegar and tarragon; stir. Simmer 2 to 3 minutes, or until liquid reduces.

Sprinkle with the almonds; serve.

NUTRITION PER SERVING	
Serving size	1 cup
Calories	120 kcal
Fat	5 g
Saturated fat	0 g
Cholesterol	0 mg
Sodium	15 mg
Carbohydrates	10 g
Dietary fiber	3 g
Protein	5 g

Potpourri of Vegetables in Balsamic Vinegar

Lana Shepek, R.D., L.D.

By the end of the summer, Illinois gardens have produced all of the ingredients to make this fabulous recipe. Make a batch anywhere, anytime, and enjoy it for several days.

Serves: 8
Hands-on time: 10 minutes
Cooking time: 20 minutes
Chill time: 1 hour

- 2½ tablespoons extra-virgin olive oil, divided
- 3 shallots, thinly sliced
- 1 clove garlic, finely chopped
- 1 bunch beet greens with stems, washed and thinly sliced (2 cups)
- freshly ground black pepper
- ⅓ cup balsamic vinegar
- 2 carrots, halved lengthwise and sliced diagonally into ½-inch pieces
- 2 small turnips, peeled and cut into slices, then diagonally into cubes
- 2 cups small broccoli florets
- 2 small zucchini halved lengthwise and sliced diagonally into ½-inch pieces (about ½ pound)
- 2 small yellow squash, halved lengthwise and sliced diagonally into ½-inch pieces (about ½ pound)

Bring 3 quarts water to a boil in a large covered pot.

In the meantime, heat 1½ tablespoons of the olive oil in a heavy-bottomed skillet over medium heat. Add the shallots and garlic, and sauté for 2 minutes. Stir in the beet greens. Add pepper to taste. Cook the mixture, stirring frequently, for about 7 minutes. Pour the vinegar into the beet mixture. Stir well. Remove the skillet from heat.

Add the carrots to the boiling water and cook for about 1 minute. Add the turnips and broccoli and cook for 2 more minutes. Add the zucchini and yellow squash. Cook all vegetables together about 30 seconds. Immediately drain the vegetables and stop further cooking by rinsing them with cold water. Drain on paper towels.

Transfer the vegetables to a bowl and pour the contents of the skillet over the vegetables. Drizzle the remaining tablespoon of olive oil over the vegetables and toss well. Chill for at least 1 hour. Toss before serving.

SUBSTITUTION

If you don't have shallots, substitute 1 small onion, minced.

NUTRITION PER SERVING	
Serving size	1 cup
Calories	80 kcal
Fat	4.5 g
Saturated fat	0.5 g
Cholesterol	0 mg
Sodium	55 mg
Carbohydrates	8 g
Dietary fiber	2 g
Protein	2 g

Blue Cheese–Yogurt Dressing

Mary Jo Cutler, M.S., R.D., L.D.

Serves: 10
Hands-on time: 5 minutes

Savor the taste of blue cheese in this creamy dressing, but skip the fat. French inspired, but a favorite across the United States. If you haven't tried Iowa's Maytag blue cheese, make a point of it!

1 cup fat-free plain yogurt
¼ cup (1½ ounces) crumbled reduced-fat blue cheese
½ teaspoon dried dill, or 1 tablespoon chopped fresh dill
½ teaspoon dried parsley, or 1 tablespoon chopped fresh parsley
½ teaspoon dried chives, or 1 tablespoon chopped fresh chives

Combine all the ingredients in a medium-size bowl. Stir. Cover and refrigerate at least 1 hour before serving.

VARIATION
Use any combination of fresh or dried herbs to flavor it your way.

NUTRITION PER SERVING	
Serving size	2 tablespoons
Calories	35 kcal
Fat	1 g
Saturated fat	0.5 g
Cholesterol	5 mg
Sodium	65 mg
Carbohydrates	4 g
Dietary fiber	0 g
Protein	2 g

Cauliflower and Tomato Soup

Kristine Napier, M.P.H., R.D.

This thin yet rich, aromatically seasoned soup recipe was given to me by the South Indian culinary expert Alamelu Vairavan. This is easy comfort food at its best, no matter where you are in the United States, any time of the year. Alamelu and I especially enjoy it during the winter months, as it is comforting and warming. We cook it in her Milwaukee, Wisconsin, home where she has taught me South Indian cooking.

Serves: 4
Hands-on time: 20 minutes
Cooking time: 20 minutes

- 2 tablespoons canola oil
- 2 to 3 small pieces cinnamon stick
- ½ bay leaf
- ¼ teaspoon fennel seeds
- ¼ teaspoon cumin seeds
- ½ cup sliced onion, cut lengthwise
- ½ cup chopped tomatoes
- ¼ teaspoon turmeric
- ½ cup tomato sauce
- salt to taste
- ¼ teaspoon cardamom powder, optional
- ½ teaspoon ground cumin
- ½ teaspoon black pepper
- 2 cups 1-inch cauliflower florets
- ¼ cup finely chopped fresh cilantro

Place the oil in a large saucepan and heat over medium heat. When the oil is hot, but not smoking, add the cinnamon stick, bay leaf, fennel, and cumin seeds. Stir until the seasonings are golden brown (about 30 seconds). Add the onion and tomato. Stir. Add the turmeric, tomato sauce, and 4 cups of water. Cook over medium heat for 2 to 3 minutes.

Add the salt, cardamom, cumin, and black pepper; stir well. When the mixture begins to boil, add the cauliflower. Reduce heat and cook, uncovered, until the cauliflower becomes just tender, about 10 minutes. Be careful not to overcook the cauliflower. Add the cilantro and let the soup simmer for a few more minutes.

Remove from heat. Remove the bay leaf before serving.

SUBSTITUTION
Substitute 1 pound of frozen cauliflower for the fresh.

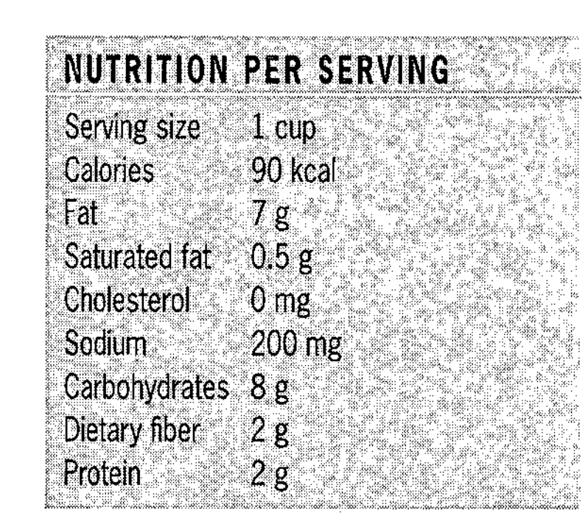

NUTRITION PER SERVING	
Serving size	1 cup
Calories	90 kcal
Fat	7 g
Saturated fat	0.5 g
Cholesterol	0 mg
Sodium	200 mg
Carbohydrates	8 g
Dietary fiber	2 g
Protein	2 g

Bountiful Bean Soup

Beth Ebmeier, M.S., R.D., L.M.N.T.

Serves: 6
Hands-on time: 20 minutes
Soaking time: 1 hour
Cooking time: 1 hour, 40 minutes

This soup could have been made on the westward journey of settlers through Nebraska. We pick up a bag of every kind of dried beans, lentils, and dried peas (about ten in all) and mix them all together to create the bean soup mix called for in the recipe. Store the remaining bean mixture in an airtight container in the freezer.

2 cups mixed dried beans
4 slices bacon, chopped
1 medium-size onion, chopped
6 to 8 cloves garlic, minced
20 baby carrots, cut in thirds
½ pound cubed ham
4 bay leaves
⅛ teaspoon black pepper

Bring 4 cups water and the beans to a boil over high heat in a 4-quart saucepan; boil for 2 minutes. Turn off heat. Cover and let the beans soak for 1 hour. Drain the beans through a large strainer and rinse.

In a skillet, cook and stir the chopped bacon and onion over medium heat for 5 minutes. Add the minced garlic; cook 2 minutes.

Place the drained beans, carrots, bacon mixture, and ham in the skillet; add 6 cups water, the bay leaves, and pepper. Bring to a boil; reduce heat and simmer, covered, for 1½ hours. Remove the bay leaves before serving.

SERVING SUGGESTION

Serve with corn muffins and honey.

COOK'S TIP

To make the mixed beans for soup, combine 10 bags (1 pound each) of an assortment of dried beans, lentils, and dried peas and mix them together in a large container. This may be stored in the freezer. You could also use the premixed packages of dried beans available.

Instead of bringing the water and beans to a boil and soaking for 1 hour, you can substitute this soaking method: Soak the beans with 1 teaspoon of baking soda in 1 quart of water for at least 4 hours. Discard this water and rinse the beans before adding the suggested amount of cooking water. Baking soda eliminates flatulence after eating beans.

NUTRITION PER SERVING	
Serving size	1½ cups
Calories	420 kcal
Fat	16 g
Saturated fat	6 g
Cholesterol	45 mg
Sodium	170 mg
Carbohydrates	44 g
Dietary fiber	14 g
Protein	26 g

Sweet Potato Soup

Cindy Moore, M.S., R.D., L.D., F.A.D.A.

Inspired by a bowl of soup in a Florida French restaurant, this smooth, creamy sweet potato soup is Ohio born. Like its cross-country and cross-cultural roots, this soup is a symphony of flavors.

Serves: 4 as a main course or 8 as an appetizer
Hands-on time: 10 minutes
Cooking time: 30 minutes

2 large sweet potatoes (not yams), washed, peeled, and cubed
2 medium-size onions, quartered
1 14-ounce can reduced-sodium chicken broth
2½ cups fat-free milk
½ teaspoon ground nutmeg
¼ teaspoon white pepper
½ cup heavy cream
nutmeg for garnish, optional

Combine the sweet potatoes, onions, and broth in a heavy 2-quart saucepan over medium heat. Simmer 20 to 30 minutes, or until the sweet potatoes are soft.

Remove the sweet potatoes and onions from the broth, leaving the broth in the saucepan. Combine the sweet potatoes, onions, and milk in a blender and purée, in 3 to 4 batches, until smooth. Return the sweet potato and onion mixture to the saucepan. Stir in the nutmeg, pepper, and heavy cream. Heat thoroughly over low heat, stirring constantly so that the milk and cream do not curdle.

Garnish with additional nutmeg if desired.

COOK'S TIP

Whenever heating milk or cream products, use a low heat and stir constantly to avoid curdling (separation of curds and whey).

NUTRITION NUGGET

Sweet potatoes are a good source of vitamin A. The nonfat milk in this recipe is a significant source of calcium.

NUTRITION PER SERVING	
Serving size	1½ cups, main course
Calories	260 kcal
Fat	15 g
Saturated fat	9 g
Cholesterol	55 mg
Sodium	150 mg
Carbohydrates	24 g
Dietary fiber	3 g
Protein	9 g

NUTRITION PER SERVING	
Serving size	¾ cup, appetizer
Calories	130 kcal
Fat	7 g
Saturated fat	4.5 g
Cholesterol	25 mg
Sodium	75 mg
Carbohydrates	12 g
Dietary fiber	1 g
Protein	4 g

Blue Cheese Vegetable Soup

Cindy Moore, M.S., R.D., L.D., F.A.D.A.

Serves: 4 as a main dish to 8 as an appetizer
Hands-on time: 5 minutes
Cooking time: 15 minutes

Here's a creamy vegetable soup with a couple of twists. The heady flavor from blue cheese stands up to brussels sprouts for a delicious and healthful combination. When fresh sprouts are unavailable in my Cleveland, Ohio, grocery store, I use frozen. This is a great recipe to make in the Midwest, where Maytag blue cheese is so plentiful.

1 pound fresh or frozen brussels sprouts
3 cups nonfat milk, divided
3 tablespoons flour
1 tablespoon butter
1 cup crumbled reduced-fat blue cheese (4 ounces)
¼ to ½ teaspoon ground black pepper

Wash and trim the ends of fresh brussels sprouts; cut in half lengthwise. Steam for 10 minutes. If using frozen brussels sprouts, cook according to the package instructions.

Place the brussels sprouts and 1 cup of the milk in a blender and process until smooth or chunky, whichever you prefer.

Mix the flour and remaining 2 cups milk in a 2-quart saucepan until smooth. Bring the milk mixture just to a simmer. Reduce heat and simmer 5 minutes; stirring constantly until thickened. Add the butter and stir to melt. Add the puréed (or chunky) sprouts, blue cheese, and pepper; stir well. Heat and stir until the cheese is melted.

NUTRITION NUGGET
Brussels sprouts are a member of the cruciferous family of vegetables, noted for having cancer-preventing qualities.

NUTRITION PER SERVING	
Serving size	1¼ cups, main course
Calories	290 kcal
Fat	15 g
Saturated fat	9 g
Cholesterol	50 mg
Sodium	500 mg
Carbohydrates	25 g
Dietary fiber	5 g
Protein	16 g

NUTRITION PER SERVING	
Serving size	¾ cup, appetizer
Calories	140 kcal
Fat	8 g
Saturated fat	4.5 g
Cholesterol	25 mg
Sodium	250 mg
Carbohydrates	12 g
Dietary fiber	3 g
Protein	8 g

Paul Bunyan's Wild Rice Soup

Ingrid Gangestad, R.D., L.D.

Paul Bunyan is a Minnesota legend. With his ox, Babe, he walked around the state, and they created the state's more than 10,000 lakes with their footprints. You'll find statues of Paul Bunyan in Bemidji and Brainerd.

No trip to Minnesota would be complete without eating wild rice! This recipe combines vitamin-rich broccoli, savory Italian sausage, and the wholesome texture of wild rice in a hearty cream soup.

Serves: 7
Hands-on time: 20 minutes
Cooking time: 15 minutes

½ pound reduced-fat mild or hot Italian sausage
2 stalks celery, chopped (about 1 cup)
1 medium-size onion, chopped
⅓ cup all-purpose flour
2 14½-ounce cans reduced-sodium chicken broth
2 cups cooked wild rice
1 large carrot, shredded
1 10-ounce package frozen petite peas
1 cup fat-free milk
¼ to ½ teaspoon ground black pepper

Crumble the sausage into a Dutch oven; add the celery and onion. Sauté over medium-high heat until the sausage is no longer pink and the celery and onion are tender; drain.

Add the flour to the sausage and vegetables and sauté over medium-high heat for 1 minute. Gradually stir in the chicken broth; bring to a boil, stirring occasionally. Stir in the wild rice, carrot, and peas. Reduce heat and simmer 5 minutes.

Stir in the milk and pepper. Reduce heat to low and cook 1 to 2 minutes longer or until the soup is hot (do not boil).

SHOPPING TIP

Try 1 can (14 to 16 ounces) wild rice, drained, instead of cooking your own. Or look for cooked and frozen wild rice in the freezer section of the grocery store.

NUTRITION PER SERVING

Serving size	1 cup
Calories	260 kcal
Fat	12 g
Saturated fat	4.5 g
Cholesterol	30 mg
Sodium	380 mg
Carbohydrates	27 g
Dietary fiber	4 g
Protein	13 g

Potato Mushroom Chowder

Lynnette Jones, M.S., M.B.A., R.D.

Serves: 8
Hands-on time: 40 minutes
Cooking time: 35 minutes

When I was growing up on a farm in Iowa, my family looked forward to the time when the potatoes and dill were freshly harvested from the garden. This recipe takes on the flavor of my family's Czechoslovakian cuisine.

- 2 tablespoons butter
- 1 garlic clove, minced
- 2 tablespoons flour
- 6 cups chicken broth
- 2 pounds unpeeled potatoes, cubed
- 2 ribs celery, sliced
- 1 cup nonfat milk
- 2 cups sliced mushrooms
- 1 tablespoon minced fresh dill
- pepper to taste
- 4 hard-cooked eggs, chopped

Melt the butter in a stockpot over medium heat. Add the garlic; cook and stir until tender but not browned.

Stir in the flour. Reduce heat to low and cook, stirring, for 5 minutes. Pour in the broth. Whisk until smooth. Simmer, stirring often for about 5 minutes. Add the potatoes and celery. Bring to a boil, reduce heat, and simmer until the potatoes are fork tender, about 15 minutes. With a slotted spoon, remove half the potatoes and celery and mash. Return the mashed vegetables to the pot.

Stir in the milk, mushrooms, dill, and pepper to taste. Bring to a boil, cover, reduce heat, and simmer until the mushrooms are soft, about 10 minutes.

Garnish with the chopped eggs.

VARIATION
For a smooth soup, purée the entire contents, in batches.

NUTRITION PER SERVING	
Serving size	2 cups
Calories	200 kcal
Fat	7 g
Saturated fat	3.5 g
Cholesterol	120 mg
Sodium	140 mg
Carbohydrates	26 g
Dietary fiber	2 g
Protein	10 g

Mushroom-Barley Soup

Roberta L. Duyff, M.S., R.D., F.A.D.A., C.F.C.S.

Immigration brought boatloads of central Europeans to the United States in the late 1800s and early 1900s. For many, including my Bohemian (Czech) grandparents, Chicago was their destination. Growing up there, I remember shopping for hearty rye bread, hoska *or* vánočka *(sweet braided bread), poppy seed cake, and apple strudel from Chicago's Bohemian bakeries; for paprika, caraway seed, dill, and other herbs in Czech markets; and for the many unique sausages in local delis. The* svíčková *(marinated beef dish with a rich gravy),* knedlíky *(dumplings), red cabbage, and* bramboráky *(potato pancakes) in local Bohemian restaurants were nearly as good as grandma's! But nothing could be more Czech than a hearty dish, made with mushrooms.*

- 1 medium-size onion, chopped (1 cup)
- 2 tablespoons butter or margarine
- 12 ounces fresh shiitake, crimini, or portabella mushrooms, sliced
- 1 cup diced celery
- ½ cup pearl barley
- 3 14-ounce cans beef broth
- 1 cup diced, unpeeled potatoes
- ½ teaspoon caraway seeds
- 1 clove garlic, minced
- ½ teaspoon dried marjoram
- ⅛ teaspoon black pepper
- 2 tablespoons minced fresh parsley

Serves: 6
Hands-on time: 15 minutes
Cooking time: 1 hour

SHOPPING TIP
For the freshest mushrooms, look for those that are well-shaped, free of spots, and firm in texture. If they appear slimy or moldy, they aren't fresh.

SERVING SUGGESTION
For a Czech-style meal, enjoy this hearty mushroom-barley soup with rye bread, sliced cucumber salad tossed with dill vinaigrette, and a cold glass of milk.

NUTRITION NUGGET
Mushrooms, with their meaty flavor, are low in calories and essentially fat- and sodium-free. They also supply B vitamins, potassium for heart health, and selenium, which is an antioxidant.

NUTRITION PER SERVING

Serving size	1 cup
Calories	270 kcal
Fat	8 g
Saturated fat	4 g
Cholesterol	15 mg
Sodium	140 mg
Carbohydrates	36 g
Dietary fiber	7 g
Protein	12 g

Mushroom-Barley Soup *(continued)*

In a 2-quart saucepan, cook and stir the onion in the butter or margarine over medium heat until the onion is translucent. Add the mushrooms and celery; cook and stir 5 minutes, until tender, not browned. Add the barley. Cook and stir until the barley is light brown, about 5 minutes. Add the beef broth, potatoes, caraway seeds, and garlic. Lower heat; cover and simmer for about 40 minutes until the barley is tender.

Mix in the marjoram and pepper; simmer 5 minutes more. Sprinkle with the parsley and serve.

COOK'S TIP

To properly clean fresh mushrooms, either brush them well with a soft brush or a damp cloth, or rinse them quickly under cool running water. Make sure they're dry before you cook them, as mushrooms absorb water and then become mushy when cooked.

VARIATION

Although this recipe tastes good with ordinary white mushrooms, the unique, rich flavor of portabellas, porcini, and other specialty mushrooms adds an intense flavor. For more convenience, you can use dried mushrooms (sold in specialty stores); just soak them in warm water for about 15 minutes and use the soaking water in the soup.

Cincinnati Chili

Maggie Green, R.D., L.D., C.C.

Hailing from southern Ohio, this chili is quite different from its western cousin. The only resemblance you'll find is the meat, cumin, and chili powder. The mechanics of Cincinnati Chili aren't as complicated as they seem. Serve "2-way" chili with two items: chili and spaghetti. Add grated cheddar cheese and you have "3-way;" "4-way" adds diced onions to the mix; and "5-way" stirs in warmed kidney beans.

Serves: 6
Hands-on time: 15 minutes
Cooking time: 55 minutes

- 1 pound extra-lean ground beef, such as sirloin
- 1 medium-size onion, diced
- 2 cloves garlic, minced
- 1 6-ounce can tomato paste
- 1 tablespoon white vinegar
- 1 tablespoon chili powder
- 1 tablespoon unsweetened cocoa powder
- 1 tablespoon Worcestershire sauce
- 1 teaspoon cinnamon
- 1 teaspoon ground cumin
- ½ teaspoon allspice
- 2 bay leaves
- 1 teaspoon salt
- 1 teaspoon black pepper
- 12 ounces thin spaghetti, cooked

3-WAY

- ¾ cup finely shredded mild cheddar cheese (3 ounces)

4-WAY

- 1 small onion, finely diced

5-WAY

- 1 15-ounce can red or light red kidney beans, rinsed, drained, and heated

NUTRITION PER SERVING	
Serving size	2-way (1 cup)
Calories	260 kcal
Fat	8 g
Saturated fat	3 g
Cholesterol	30 mg
Sodium	520 mg
Carbohydrates	29 g
Dietary fiber	4 g
Protein	20 g

NUTRITION PER SERVING	
Serving size	3-way (1 cup)
Calories	320 kcal
Fat	12 g
Saturated fat	6 g
Cholesterol	40 mg
Sodium	520 mg
Carbohydrates	29 g
Dietary fiber	4 g
Protein	24 g

NUTRITION PER SERVING	
Serving size	5-way (1 cup)
Calories	400 kcal
Fat	13 g
Saturated fat	6 g
Cholesterol	44 mg
Sodium	520 mg
Carbohydrates	44 g
Dietary fiber	10 g
Protein	29 g

Cincinnati Chili
(continued)

COOK'S TIP
This recipe can be easily doubled or tripled, depending on the size crowd you are feeding.

Brown the beef and onion in a large heavy pot (3 quarts or more) over medium-high heat, for about 5 to 7 minutes.

Add 2 cups water and the garlic, tomato paste, vinegar, chili powder, cocoa powder, Worcestershire sauce, cinnamon, cumin, allspice, bay leaves, salt, and pepper. Bring to a boil; cover, and reduce heat to simmer. Cook for 30 minutes, stirring occasionally. Remove the bay leaves before serving. Adjust the cumin and pepper.

Serve over spaghetti. Add ingredients for 3-way, 4-way, and 5-way chili, if desired.

FOOD TRIVIA
Cincinnati Chili was supposedly concocted by a Greek immigrant to Cincinnati who fiddled with a Greek stew to produce the likes of this recipe. Cincinnati has more chili parlors per capita and square mileage than any other city in the United States.

Checkerboard Chili

Corrina Riemann, R.D.

Simple yet pleasing in every way, this Indiana-born chili can be as spicy or as mild as you like it (just adjust the chili powder). Using vegetarian meat crumbles makes this lower in fat, but something to simmer into a meal quickly from the freezer and pantry.

Serves: 6 to 8
Hands-on time: 15 minutes
Cooking time: 1 hour, 45 minutes

1 tablespoon canola oil
1 large red onion, chopped
2 to 3 cloves garlic, minced
2 14½-ounce cans stewed tomatoes
1 15-ounce can kidney beans, drained and rinsed
1 15-ounce can black beans, drained and rinsed
1 15-ounce can white kidney beans (also known as cannellini beans), drained and rinsed
1 10½-ounce can condensed tomato soup plus 1 soup can water
1 12-ounce package vegetarian "meat crumbles"
2 beef or vegetarian bouillon cubes
2 tablespoons brown sugar
2 to 3 tablespoons chili powder
1½ teaspoons ground oregano
1 teaspoon ground cumin
dash cinnamon
1 to 2 teaspoons crushed red pepper, optional
2 tablespoons cornmeal

Heat the oil in a large heavy soup pot. Add the onion and garlic; sauté until the vegetables are softened. Add the tomatoes, beans, soup plus water, crumbles, bouillon cubes, sugar, chili powder, oregano, cumin, cinnamon, and crushed red pepper; bring to a boil. Reduce heat; cover and simmer 1 hour, stirring occasionally.

Remove the lid and stir in the cornmeal. Simmer uncovered 45 minutes.

SHOPPING TIP
Look for vegetarian meat crumbles in the frozen-foods section of your supermarket. One brand is Morningstar Farms.

NUTRITION NUGGET
The vegetarian meat crumbles are an excellent way to work soy into your eating plan.

NUTRITION PER SERVING	
Serving size	2 cups
Calories	430 kcal
Fat	5 g
Saturated fat	0 g
Cholesterol	0 mg
Sodium	1,150 mg
Carbohydrates	70 g
Dietary fiber	16 g
Protein	28 g

Have It Your Way Chili

Pamela Aughe, R.D.

Serves: 6
Hands-on time: 20 minutes
Cooking time: 30 minutes

From Michigan comes this have-it-your-way chili recipe. Make it vegetarian, with ground turkey, or with ground beef. Enjoy the slightly sweet flavor added by the carrot.

- 2 teaspoons canola oil
- 1 pound extra-lean ground beef or extra-lean ground turkey, or 1 10-ounce package frozen meatless crumbles, thawed
- 1 large onion, chopped
- 3 cloves garlic, minced
- 2 ribs celery, chopped
- 1 medium-size green bell pepper, chopped
- 1 medium-size red bell pepper, chopped
- 1 carrot, scrubbed and sliced thinly
- 1 15½-ounce can dark or light kidney beans, drained and rinsed
- 2 14½-ounce cans diced tomatoes
- 1 6-ounce can no-salt-added tomato paste
- 2 tablespoons chili powder
- 1 teaspoon ground oregano
- 1 teaspoon ground cumin
- 1 teaspoon paprika
- ½ teaspoon black pepper
- 3 green onions, sliced thinly, optional
- ½ cup chopped fresh cilantro, optional
- ½ cup fat-free sour cream

Combine the oil, meat (or turkey or meatless crumbles), onion, and garlic in a large pot over medium heat. Cook and stir until the onion is wilted and the meat is lightly browned, about 6 to 8 minutes.

Add the remaining ingredients except the optional ones and the sour cream. Stir well, cover, and reduce heat; simmer gently for 20 minutes. Adjust the chili powder, oregano, and black pepper to taste.

Serve with green onions, cilantro, and/or sour cream.

COOK'S TIP

Double the batch and freeze in individual portions or family-size batches.

NUTRITION PER SERVING

Serving size	1½ cups
Calories	300 kcal
Fat	12 g
Saturated fat	4.5 g
Cholesterol	35 mg
Sodium	540 mg
Carbohydrates	28 g
Dietary fiber	8 g
Protein	23 g

Pork and Butternut Squash Stew

Donna Weihofen, R.D., M.S.

Simmer together the flavors and smells of fall in an unusual liquid—beer—which we love to do here in Wisconsin. Its hops and barley add another layer of rich flavor.

Serves: 6
Hands-on time: 15 minutes
Cooking time: 30 minutes

- 3 tablespoons all-purpose flour
- 1 teaspoon salt
- ½ teaspoon pepper
- 1 teaspoon dried thyme
- 1 pound lean pork loin, cut into 1-inch cubes
- 2 tablespoons canola oil, divided
- 1 large onion, diced
- 12 ounces beer
- 1 teaspoon dried rosemary, crushed
- 1 medium-size butternut squash, peeled and cubed (about 2½ pounds)
- 2 tablespoons cornstarch
- ½ teaspoon salt
- ¼ to ½ teaspoon black pepper
- ¼ cup chopped fresh parsley
- 4 cups cooked egg noodles

Combine the flour, salt, pepper, and thyme in a plastic bag. Add the pork cubes. Close the bag and shake until the meat is coated. Set aside.

Heat 1 tablespoon oil in a large skillet, add the onion, and cook over medium heat until translucent. Remove the onion from the pan and set aside.

Add the remaining 1 tablespoon oil to the pan and add the meat cubes. Cook over medium heat until brown on all sides. Add the beer and stir to deglaze the pan. Return the onion to the pan. Add the rosemary and squash cubes. Cover and gently boil for 25 to 35 minutes, or until the squash is tender. If a thicker broth is desired, mix the cornstarch in ¼ cup cold water and add to the pot. Stir constantly until the mixture thickens. Add salt and pepper to taste and the parsley.

Ladle over the noodles in individual serving bowls.

SHOPPING TIP

Can't find butternut squash? Substitute equal amounts of any winter squash.

SERVING SUGGESTION

This stew is also excellent over mashed potatoes (see page 152 for mashed potato recipe).

FOOD TRIVIA

Stews are thought to have originated with primitive tribes, who simmered foods together for long periods of time. The Amazonian natives used the shells of turtles as their "stew pots."

NUTRITION PER SERVING

Serving size	1 cup stew plus 1 cup noodles
Calories	430 kcal
Fat	11 g
Saturated fat	2 g
Cholesterol	80 mg
Sodium	640 mg
Carbohydrates	57 g
Dietary fiber	8 g
Protein	24 g

Buffalo Stew

Ruth Rauscher, R.D., M.A., L.M.N.T.

Serves: 4 (2 cups) or 6 (1½ cups)
Hands-on time: 15 minutes
Cooking time: 40 minutes

With buffalo meat readily available in many of our mid-continent stores, we can attempt to cook as the early settlers did. If you have an antique Dutch oven, this recipe will really be authentic. Cooked low and slow—this dish will melt in your mouth!

⅓ cup flour
¼ to ½ teaspoon black pepper
1 teaspoon garlic powder
1 pound buffalo meat, cut in chunks
1 tablespoon canola oil
1 29-ounce can stewed tomatoes
2 medium-size onions, quartered
3 small potatoes, scrubbed and cut into bite-size pieces
4 carrots, scrubbed and sliced
2 ribs celery, sliced
1 cup peas, fresh or frozen

Blend the flour, pepper, and garlic powder in a large bowl; add the meat and toss. Set aside.

Heat the oil in an extra-large heavy pot or Dutch oven over medium-high heat. Add the flour-coated meat and brown on all sides; about 4 to 6 minutes. Reduce heat. Add the tomatoes, onions, potatoes, carrots, and celery. Stir, cover, and simmer 30 minutes.

Uncover, stir in the peas. Simmer 10 minutes, or until the peas are cooked through.

COOK'S TIPS

Slice favorite fresh or canned fruit (canned in juice) for dessert. To store celery, leave the ribs attached to the stalk until ready to use. Store in a plastic bag in the refrigerator for up to two weeks.

NUTRITION NUGGET

Buffalo is a very lean meat.

NUTRITION PER SERVING

Serving size	2 cups
Calories	290 kcal
Fat	3.5 g
Saturated fat	0.5 g
Cholesterol	35 mg
Sodium	350 mg
Carbohydrates	44 g
Dietary fiber	6 g
Protein	22 g

Chicken, Cashew, and Apple Stir Fry

Donna Weihofen, R.D., M.S.

Fall in Wisconsin is delightful for many reasons, including bushel baskets of apples. Enjoy the flavor of fall-fresh apples, melded with Asian seasonings, in this easy stir fry all year.

Serves: 4
Hands-on time: 15 minutes
Cooking time: 10 minutes

1 tablespoon canola oil
1 pound boneless, skinless chicken breast, cut into bite-size pieces
½ pound sliced fresh mushrooms
1 large red bell pepper, seeded and cut into strips
2 medium-size apples, cored and sliced

SAUCE
¾ cup apple juice
¾ cup chicken broth
¼ cup reduced-sodium soy sauce
¼ teaspoon cinnamon
½ tablespoon minced fresh ginger
¼ teaspoon ground red pepper
2 tablespoons cornstarch
black pepper to taste
¼ cup cashews or roasted peanuts

SHOPPING TIPS
Choose the best cooking apple: Gala, Rome beauty, McIntosh, or Granny Smith. To save time, purchase sliced mushrooms.

Heat the oil in a large nonstick skillet over medium-high heat. Add the chicken and brown on all sides, about 5 to 7 minutes. Add the mushrooms, pepper, and apples; cook until tender over medium heat, about 5 to 7 minutes.

Meanwhile, combine the sauce ingredients. Mix well, pour into the skillet, and stir constantly until the mixture comes to a boil and thickens to desired consistency. Add additional chicken broth to thin or add additional cornstarch to thicken. Add pepper to taste.

Top with the cashews right before serving.

SERVING SUGGESTION
Serve over brown rice (cook ¾ cup per person).

NUTRITION PER SERVING

Serving size	1 cup
Calories	330 kcal
Fat	11 g
Saturated fat	1.5 g
Cholesterol	65 mg
Sodium	930 mg
Carbohydrates	28 g
Dietary fiber	4 g
Protein	31 g

Pizza Chicken

Kristine Napier, M.P.H., R.D.

Serves: 6
Hands-on time: 10 minutes
Cooking time: 25 minutes

Enjoy the best of two American favorites in this please-every-family-member dish. Reminiscent of Chicago-style pizzas, this dish is Italian-delicious, but moderate in calories and fat. Be sure to try it if you can't get your kids to eat chicken. Spice it up or down with the pasta sauce you choose and be sure to make an extra batch to freeze for another night.

- vegetable oil cooking spray
- 1 pound boneless, skinless chicken breasts, trimmed of all fat and sliced into strips
- 1 medium-size yellow onion, finely chopped
- 1 green bell pepper, cored and thinly sliced
- 1 red bell pepper, cored and chopped
- 1 26-ounce jar favorite pasta sauce
- 1 cup shredded part-skim mozzarella cheese (4 ounces)
- 6 cups cooked favorite family pasta

Spray a large nonstick skillet, Dutch oven, or electric skillet with the cooking spray. Heat to medium high. Add the chicken and onion; brown 3 to 5 minutes.

Reduce heat to medium low. Top the chicken with the peppers, then the pasta sauce. Cover tightly and simmer 20 minutes.

Remove the lid and add the cheese. Replace the lid, remove from heat, and allow the cheese to melt, about 5 minutes.

Serve over pasta.

NUTRITION PER SERVING

Serving size	1 cup chicken and sauce plus 1 cup cooked pasta
Calories	390 kcal
Fat	7 g
Saturated fat	2.5 g
Cholesterol	55 mg
Sodium	880 mg
Carbohydrates	50 g
Dietary fiber	5 g
Protein	30 g

Minnesota Chicken and Wild Rice Casserole

LaDonna Levik, R.D., retired

A potluck supper in Lake Wobegon, or anywhere else in Minnesota, wouldn't be complete without this classic casserole.

Serves: 6
Hands-on time: 15 minutes
Cooking time: 1 hour 10 minutes

- vegetable oil cooking spray
- ½ cup uncooked wild rice
- 1 14-ounce can reduced-sodium chicken broth
- 1 tablespoon canola oil
- 1 pound boneless, skinless chicken breasts, cut into six pieces
- ½ teaspoon garlic salt
- ⅛ to ½ teaspoon black pepper
- ½ pound fresh mushrooms, sliced (about 3 cups)
- 2 medium-size yellow onions, chopped
- 2 ribs celery, diced
- ½ cup uncooked long-grain white or brown rice (not instant)
- 1 10½-ounce can cream of mushroom soup
- 1 10½-ounce can cream of celery soup
- ¼ cup chopped fresh parsley

Preheat oven to 400°F. Coat a 13-by-9-inch baking dish with the cooking spray.

Combine the wild rice and broth in a 1-quart microwave-safe bowl. Microwave on high 5 minutes; stir. Microwave an additional 5 minutes.

Heat the oil in a large nonstick skillet over medium-high heat. Add the chicken; brown 2 to 3 minutes per side. Remove from heat; sprinkle with the garlic salt and pepper; set aside.

Transfer the wild rice with the broth to the baking dish. Add the mushrooms, onions, celery, white or brown rice, and soups; stir. Top with the chicken. Cover tightly and bake 1 hour or until the rice is tender and most of the liquid is absorbed. Let stand 5 to 10 minutes before serving. Sprinkle with the parsley before serving.

SERVING SUGGESTION

Purchase several large serving spoons at a dollar store to take to potlucks. Then if the spoon is missing at the end of the night, you haven't lost a serving piece from your set.

COOK'S TIP

Make an easy side dish or meatless meal by omitting the chicken. Bake as directed.

NUTRITION PER SERVING

Serving size	⅙ of casserole
Calories	335 kcal
Fat	11 g
Saturated fat	2 g
Cholesterol	50 mg
Sodium	1,080 mg
Carbohydrates	36 g
Dietary fiber	3 g
Protein	25 g

Cinnamon-Poached Chicken and Rice

Jackie Newgent, R.D., C.D.N.

Serves: 8
Hands-on time: 20 minutes
Cooking time: 40 minutes

I grew up with cinnamon in savory dishes, not sweet. This savory recipe has gone through some changes over the years. It's now a lighter version, since it no longer has ground beef. My grandmother, straight from Lebanon, served the original version to my mother, who was raised in Peoria, Illinois. A large Lebanese community exists there today. In my Bath, Ohio, home, my mother later served it to me. Now, in New York City, I serve it to my close friends. It's a comforting dish that always "takes me home." This recipe can easily be halved.

- 4 bone-in chicken breast halves, skin removed
- 1 tablespoon sea salt
- ½ cinnamon stick
- 2 cups long-grain white rice, uncooked
- 1 bay leaf
- ½ teaspoon white or black pepper
- ¼ teaspoon ground cinnamon
- ¼ cup plus 2 teaspoons butter
- 1 large white or yellow onion, thinly sliced
- 2 teaspoons extra-virgin olive oil
- ⅛ teaspoon sea salt, or to taste
- ⅛ teaspoon white or black pepper, or to taste
- ¼ cup minced fresh flat-leaf parsley
- ¼ cup toasted pine nuts
- ¼ cup slivered toasted almonds

Place the chicken breast halves in a stockpot. Add 6 cups cold water (or more, if needed to cover the chicken), the salt, and the cinnamon stick. Over medium-high heat, bring just to a boil. Immediately reduce the heat to low and simmer, uncovered, for 20 minutes, or until the chicken is firm and just cooked through. Remove the chicken. Strain the cooking liquid and set aside.

When the chicken is cool enough to handle, shred it into large bite-size pieces. Discard the bones.

In the same stockpot, place the chicken pieces, 4 cups of the strained cooking liquid, the rice, bay leaf, pepper, cinnamon, and ¼ cup butter. Bring to a boil over medium-high heat. Cover, reduce heat to low, and simmer for 15 to 20 minutes. Meanwhile, in small skillet over medium-high heat, sauté the onion in 2 teaspoons butter with the oil, salt, and pepper.

Mix the sautéed onion into the chicken and rice prior to garnishing. Remove the bay leaf. Adjust seasonings to taste. Serve on a large platter garnished with parsley, pine nuts, and almonds.

NUTRITION PER SERVING	
Serving size	1¼ cups
Calories	340 kcal
Fat	13 g
Saturated fat	5 g
Cholesterol	40 mg
Sodium	930 mg
Carbohydrates	40 g
Dietary fiber	2 g
Protein	14 g

Chicken-Vegetable Curry

Madhu Gadia, M.S., R.D., C.D.E.

Chicken curry is the most common way to serve chicken in India, and I still serve it in our Iowa home. The curry sauce tastes great with rice, naan *(an Indian bread), or any kind of bread. Adding the vegetables with the chicken gives it a unique taste and texture. Using boneless, skinless chicken makes this a quick dish. You can also use frozen vegetables for convenience.*

Serves: 4
Hands-on time: 15 minutes
Cooking time: 45 minutes

- 1½ pounds skinless, boneless chicken breasts
- 1 tablespoon vegetable oil
- 1 teaspoon ground cumin
- 1 medium-size onion, finely chopped
- 4 cloves garlic, chopped
- 2 teaspoons chopped fresh ginger
- 1 medium-size tomato, finely chopped
- ½ teaspoon turmeric
- 1 tablespoon ground coriander
- ½ teaspoon cayenne pepper, optional
- 1 teaspoon salt
- ½ cup water
- ¾ cup thinly sliced carrots
- ¾ cup fresh green beans, cut into 1-inch pieces
- ¾ cup thinly sliced mushrooms
- ½ teaspoon garam masala

Cut the chicken into 3- to 4-inch pieces. Cut 2 to 3 slits, ½ inch deep, in each piece of chicken. Set aside.

Heat the oil in a heavy skillet over medium-high heat. Add the chicken pieces in a single layer and sauté for 3 to 5 minutes, turning the pieces over once or twice until they are white. Transfer the chicken to a plate, using a slotted spoon.

Add the cumin, onion, garlic, and ginger to the oil. Sauté for 5 minutes, stirring constantly, until the onion is golden brown. Stir in the tomato, turmeric, coriander, and cayenne (if using). Cook for 2 to 3 minutes until the tomato is soft.

Add the chicken and sprinkle with salt. Stir to coat evenly with the spice mixture. Pour the water evenly over the chicken. Bring to a boil. Cover tightly, reduce heat, and simmer for 10 to 15 minutes. The chicken should be tender to the touch.

Add the carrots, green beans, and mushrooms, stir; cover and simmer for another 8 to 10 minutes until the vegetables are tender. Stir in the garam masala. Transfer to a serving platter. Serve with rice or bread.

VARIATION

Increase the spiciness of the recipe by increasing the garam masala.

NUTRITION PER SERVING	
Serving size	1 cup
Calories	270 kcal
Fat	6 g
Saturated fat	1 g
Cholesterol	100 mg
Sodium	710 mg
Carbohydrates	12 g
Dietary fiber	4 g
Protein	41 g

Chicken Paprikash

Rebecca Dowling, R.D.

Serves: 4
Hands-on time: 15 minutes
Cooking time: 20 minutes

This recipe comes from Katrina Zynda, who was born in Hungary and came to Chicago from Germany in 1951. As you will realize upon taking the first bite of this recipe, she is a fabulous chef. Katrina's rendition of this traditional Hungarian dish is probably the best you'll taste. Katrina is an official Friend Member of the ADA's Food and Culinary Professionals. We are fortunate to have her Hungarian culinary knowledge on board.

4 split chicken breasts, bone in, skin removed (about 1½ pounds)
1 tablespoon reduced-sodium chicken bouillon granules
3 tablespoons butter
2 cloves garlic, chopped
2 medium-size onions, chopped
½ tablespoon sweet paprika
1 tablespoon hot paprika
⅛ teaspoon cayenne
2 tablespoons all-purpose flour
½ cup reduced-fat sour cream

Sprinkle the chicken with the bouillon granules; set aside.

Melt the butter in an extra-large skillet or Dutch oven over medium heat; add the chicken, garlic, and onions and brown, about 3 to 4 minutes per side, making sure the onions are golden brown and soft. Sprinkle the chicken and onions with the paprikas and cayenne; add ½ cup water. Reduce heat, cover, and simmer 10 to 15 minutes, or until the chicken is done.

Adjust the seasoning (cayenne and paprika). Remove the chicken from the pan; set aside and keep warm.

Blend the flour and ¼ cup water until smooth. Increase heat to medium high; stir in the flour mixture and stir until the mixture thickens. Reduce heat to a low simmer; stir in the sour cream until smooth. Place the chicken back in the pan, bone side up. Cover and simmer over low heat 5 minutes.

Serve over spaetzle, pasta, rice, or potatoes.

SUBSTITUTION

If you do not have hot paprika, double the cayenne to ¼ teaspoon.

FOOD TRIVIA

Translated from the German word, *spaetzle* means "little sparrow." It is made up of tiny noodles or dumplings that often includes nutmeg for seasoning.

NUTRITION PER SERVING

Serving size	1 split breast plus ¼ cup sauce
Calories	300 kcal
Fat	13 g
Saturated fat	7 g
Cholesterol	110 mg
Sodium	210 mg
Carbohydrates	14 g
Dietary fiber	1 g
Protein	34 g

Cornish Pasties

Vivian Bradford, R.D.

These hearty meat pasties in their flaky crusts are a favorite dish among our Cornish neighbors in Detroit where I grew up. Years later when I moved to Butte, Montana, I discovered that pasties were a lunch bucket favorite of men working in the mines there. To be sure, though, you don't have to work in the mines to enjoy these rich old-fashioned favorites.

Serves: 8
Hands-on time: 25 minutes
Baking time: 45 minutes

- vegetable oil cooking spray
- ½ pound sirloin steak, cut into ½-inch pieces
- 1 large potato, scrubbed and diced (about 1⅓ cups)
- 1 small onion, finely chopped (½ cup)
- 1 carrot, cut in half lengthwise and then thinly sliced (about 1 cup)
- 1 medium-size rutabaga or turnip, peeled and diced into ¼-inch pieces (about 1 cup)
- ½ teaspoon salt
- ¼ teaspoon black pepper
- ¼ cup chopped fresh parsley
- 2 9-inch pie crusts, each cut into fourths

Preheat oven to 350°F. Coat a large cookie sheet with the cooking spray.

Combine all the ingredients except the pie crust in a medium-size bowl; stir well.

Place a generous ⅓ cup of the meat mixture on each piece of crust. Moisten the edges of the pastry triangle with water; fold the pastry to cover the mixture. Seal by pressing with a fork.

Place the pasties on the cookie sheet and bake for 45 minutes.

SUBSTITUTION
Substitute equal quantities of lean pork for the beef; follow preparation instructions.

COOK'S TIP
Dice all the vegetables equally in size to encourage even cooking.

NUTRITION NUGGET
Leaving the skins on the potato and carrot adds health-important fiber to your nutrient profile.

NUTRITION PER SERVING	
Serving size	1 pastie
Calories	320 kcal
Fat	17 g
Saturated fat	4 g
Cholesterol	13 mg
Sodium	416 mg
Carbohydrates	32 g
Dietary fiber	2 g
Protein	10 g

Italian Beef and Spinach Pie

Donna Weihofen, R.D., M.S.

Serves: 8
Hands-on time: 30 minutes
Cooking time: 30 minutes

Mention Italian beef and thoughts turn to street vendors in Chicago serving sliced beef in a spicy gravy. Most food experts, though, say there is no such dish in Italy; it is instead some vague idea of how Italians might serve beef. Try this wonderful version of beef with an easy and different crust of noodles that you'll use again and again for other casseroles.

CRUST
2 cups dry medium egg noodle noodles (3 ounces)
1 large egg, lightly beaten
vegetable oil cooking spray

TOMATO MEAT SAUCE
½ pound extra-lean ground beef
3 ounces low-fat Italian sausage
1 small onion, chopped
2 cloves garlic, chopped
½ pound fresh mushrooms, sliced
1 medium-size red bell pepper, diced
2 teaspoons Italian seasoning
½ teaspoon salt
¼ teaspoon pepper
1 15-ounce can tomato sauce

SPINACH LAYER
1 10-ounce package frozen chopped spinach, thawed and squeezed dry
⅔ cup fat-free ricotta cheese
1 cup shredded mozzarella cheese, divided

TOPPING
⅓ cup shredded mozzarella cheese
1 large tomato, diced
¼ cup fat-free sour cream

Cook the noodles as directed on the package; drain.

Preheat oven to 350°F. Coat a deep-dish 9-inch pie pan with the cooking spray.

Combine the noodles and egg in the pie pan; mix well. Press into the bottom of the pan. Set aside.

Brown the beef, sausage, onion, and garlic in a large skillet. Cook over medium-high heat until the meat is brown and cooked through, about 5 to 7 minutes. Add the mushrooms, pepper, Italian seasoning, salt, pepper, and tomato sauce; sim-

VARIATION

To spice it up, stir in 1 to 2 teaspoons crushed red pepper when browning the meat.

NUTRITION PER SERVING

Serving size	⅛ of pie
Calories	240 kcal
Fat	12 g
Saturated fat	5 g
Cholesterol	70 mg
Sodium	640 mg
Carbohydrates	19 g
Dietary fiber	3 g
Protein	18 g

mer until the vegetables are tender, about 10 minutes.

Meanwhile, combine the spinach, ricotta, and ⅔ cup mozzarella in a medium-size bowl. Spread the spinach mixture over the noodles. Spoon the meat sauce over the spinach mixture. Bake 35 minutes.

Top with the remaining ⅓ cup mozzarella cheese. Bake 10 minutes, or until the cheese melts. Let stand 10 minutes before cutting.

Garnish with the chopped fresh tomatoes and sour cream.

COOK'S TIP

Make your own Italian seasoning. Use any combination of dried basil, oregano, marjoram, parsley, and/or sage. Store in a tightly sealed plastic or glass container up to 3 months, or up to 1 year if refrigerated.

Mrs. Shim's Chop Chae (Korean Mixed Vegetables with Beef and Noodles)

Rebecca Dowling, R.D.

Serves: 4
Hands-on time: 20 minutes
Cooking time: 40 minutes

Enjoy this authentic, classic Korean noodle-vegetable-meat dish from my Chicago friend, Mrs. Shim. Be sure and use cellophane noodles, which pick up a golden color from the soy sauce and the sesame oil.

SHOPPING TIP
Cellophane noodles are also called bean threads or Chinese vermicelli and are generally made from mung beans. They look like spun threads and are almost clear in appearance.

6 dried shitake mushrooms
4 ounces uncooked cellophane noodles
2 tablespoons dark sesame oil
2 teaspoons soy sauce
2 teaspoons sugar
3 teaspoons toasted sesame seeds, divided
2 teaspoons rice wine
1 clove garlic, minced
⅛ teaspoon pepper
½ pound sirloin beef, thinly sliced
1 tablespoon canola oil, divided
1 cup shredded cabbage
1 medium-size Spanish onion, sliced (1 cup)
1 medium-size carrot, peeled and shredded
2 green onions, chopped
2 cups torn spinach
vegetable oil cooking spray
2 egg whites

Soak the mushrooms in cold water for 20 minutes. Drain and cut into thin strips.

In a large saucepan, cook the noodles in boiling water for 10 minutes. Drain and rinse in cold water. Cut into 4- to 5-inch lengths.

In a medium-size bowl, mix the sesame oil, soy sauce, sugar, 2 teaspoons sesame seeds, rice wine, garlic, and pepper. Add half of the mixture to the sirloin in another bowl; mix and set aside. Reserve the other half of the sauce.

NUTRITION PER SERVING

Serving size	1¼ cups
Calories	400 kcal
Fat	19 g
Saturated fat	45 g
Cholesterol	35 mg
Sodium	180 mg
Carbohydrates	42 g
Dietary fiber	3 g
Protein	16 g

Heat 1 teaspoon canola oil in a large skillet or wok over medium-high heat, and sauté the cabbage, Spanish onion, carrot, and green onions, stirring frequently, for 10 minutes or until the onions are opaque. Add the spinach and sauté for 1 minute. Add the mushrooms and noodles and remove from heat. Mix well and put in a large serving bowl. Set aside.

Heat the remaining 2 teaspoons of canola oil in the skillet. Add the sirloin and cook until done, stirring frequently. Add to the vegetables and noodles; mix well. Add the remaining half of the sauce; mix well.

Coat a small skillet with the cooking spray. Cook the egg whites, making an omelet. Remove from the pan and cut into thin strips. Add on top of the noodle mixture and garnish with the remaining sesame seeds. Serve immediately.

FOOD TRIVIA
Chap Chae is the Korean term for stir-fried mixture.

Hungarian Goulash

Rebecca Dowling, R.D.

Serves: 4
Hands-on time: 10 minutes
Cooking time: 2 hours

Savor this authentic Hungarian dish again and again, as we do in our Chicago home, thanks to this recipe handed down from, Katrina Zynda, one fabulous Hungarian chef. In Hungary, goulash is called gulyas. *As with many authentic goulash recipes, use only paprika to season this Hungarian stew. For a quick, Americanized version, see Twenty-Minute Stove-Top Goulash on page 275.*

1 tablespoon canola oil
2 medium-size onions, thinly sliced
1 teaspoon salt
3 or 4 cloves garlic, minced
5½ teaspoons sweet paprika, divided
1 pound lean beef (such as chuck, rump, or round), trimmed of fat and cubed
⅛ teaspoon hot paprika

Heat the oil in a large heavy pan; add the onions, salt, and garlic. Sauté until the onions are transparent, about 3 to 5 minutes. Stir in 1½ teaspoons sweet paprika and the beef. Simmer, covered, for 1 hour.

Add 4 teaspoons sweet paprika and enough water to just cover the meat. Simmer, covered, 1 more hour or until tender, adding more water if necessary.

Stir in the hot paprika. Remove from heat and let stand 5 minutes. Adjust the hot paprika. Serve over spaetzle, rice, pasta, or potatoes.

SHOPPING TIP
Most supermarkets carry paprika, which is the sweet or mild version. Specialty markets carry the hot or pungent variety.

VARIATIONS
You can make this goulash with lamb instead of beef. Spice it up by adding more garlic and/or hot paprika.

FOOD TRIVIA
Paprika is made by grinding sweet red pepper pods.

NUTRITION PER SERVING	
Serving size	¾ cup
Calories	220 kcal
Fat	9 g
Saturated fat	2 g
Cholesterol	70 mg
Sodium	660 mg
Carbohydrates	9 g
Dietary fiber	2 g
Protein	26 g

Twenty-Minute Stove-Top Goulash

Bonnie Athas, R.D.

Try this quick version of an old-time Hungarian favorite for a one-pot dinner in a hurry.

Serves: 6
Hands-on time: 10 minutes
Cooking time: 25 minutes

- 2 cups macaroni
- 1 pound extra-lean ground beef
- 1 medium-size onion, chopped
- 1 clove garlic, minced
- 1 teaspoon salt
- 1 medium-size green pepper, chopped
- 8 ounces fresh mushrooms, sliced
- 1 cup frozen corn
- 1 10¾-ounce can undiluted cream of tomato soup

Cook the macaroni according to the package directions.

In a Dutch oven or electric skillet over medium heat, cook the beef, onion, garlic, and salt until the beef is brown and cooked through, about 8 to 10 minutes. Stir in the green pepper, mushrooms, corn, and tomato soup; simmer for 15 minutes. Serve over the macaroni.

VARIATION

Make it meatless by eliminating the beef and following the rest of the recipe as indicated.

NUTRITION PER SERVING

Serving size	1½ cups meat mixture, ¾ cup macaroni
Calories	340 kcal
Fat	8.6 g
Saturated fat	3 g
Cholesterol	26 mg
Sodium	730 mg
Carbohydrates	44 g
Dietary fiber	2.6 g
Protein	22 g

Polpettone (Italian Meat Loaf)

Mary Abbott Hess, L.H.D., M.S., R.D., F.A.D.A.

Serves: 6
Hands-on time: 15 minutes
Baking time: 45 minutes

This Italian-style spicy meat loaf created in my Chicago home is delicious served hot but is even better chilled and thinly sliced. It can be prepared ahead, travels well for picnics or buffets, and makes great sandwiches. The hand-formed loaf allows fat to drain and the pan liner makes cleanup easier.

- 1 pound extra-lean ground sirloin
- ¼ pound (or 2 links) hot Italian turkey sausage, removed from casing
- ¾ cup bread crumbs
- ¼ cup grated or shredded Parmesan cheese
- 3 egg whites
- 2 tablespoons chopped fresh parsley
- 1 tablespoon dried basil
- 1 teaspoon crushed dried rosemary (or 1 tablespoon chopped fresh)
- 1 teaspoon fennel seeds
- ½ teaspoon salt
- ½ teaspoon crushed red pepper
- 2 hard-cooked eggs, peeled

Preheat oven to 425°F. Line a shallow roasting pan with heavy-duty foil or a nonstick pan liner.

Mix together the ground beef, sausage, bread crumbs, Parmesan cheese, egg whites, parsley, basil, rosemary, fennel seeds, salt, and red pepper in a medium bowl. Hand form the meat mixture into a firm loaf, about 8½ inches long, 3½ inches wide, and 2½ inches high, on the lined pan.

Slice the hard-cooked eggs lengthwise into quarters. Cut a slit about 1½ inches deep the length of the meat loaf. Insert the egg slices into the slit and press the meat back into a loaf to enclose the egg.

Bake for 15 minutes. Reduce heat to 350°F and bake for an additional 30 minutes or until a thermometer inserted into the meat loaf registers 160°F.

Remove the meat loaf from the pan and discard the drippings. Serve hot or chilled.

VARIATION

Adjust the red pepper to make the loaf milder or spicier.

NUTRITION PER SERVING	
Serving size	⅙ of loaf
Calories	280 kcal
Fat	14 g
Saturated fat	5 g
Cholesterol	130 mg
Sodium	550 mg
Carbohydrates	11 g
Dietary fiber	Less than 1 g
Protein	26 g

Confetti Sloppy Joes

Beth Ebmeier, M.S., R.D., L.M.N.T.

You'd never know after eating this mouth-watering, kid-friendly sandwich that Sloppy Joes originated during financially tough war times in the 1940s as a way of stretching precious and expensive beef.

Serves: 6
Hands-on time: 10 minutes
Cooking time: 20 minutes

- vegetable oil cooking spray
- 1 pound extra-lean ground beef
- 1 small green bell pepper, diced
- 1 small red bell pepper, diced
- 1 small onion, diced
- 1 tablespoon white vinegar
- ¾ cup catsup
- 2 tablespoons prepared mustard
- 6 whole-grain or mixed-grain sandwich buns
- 1 sweet onion, thinly or thickly sliced, optional

Spray a medium skillet with the cooking spray.

Combine the ground beef, diced peppers, and onion in the skillet. Cook on medium heat until the beef is thoroughly cooked, 8 to 10 minutes.

Mix the vinegar, catsup, and mustard together and add to the beef mixture; simmer 10 to 15 minutes.

Scoop one portion onto each sandwich bun. Top with a slice of sweet onion.

FOOD TRIVIA

Sloppy Joes were once called "loose meat" sandwiches; the word "sloppy" was coined rather appropriately because the filling is messy and tends to drip off the bun. The term "Sloppy Joe" was also used to describe any cheap restaurant or lunch counter serving cheap food quickly.

NUTRITION NUGGET

Beef is a good source of iron, and the vitamin C in peppers (and tomato products) enhances absorption of iron.

NUTRITION PER SERVING

Serving size	¾ cup meat mixture plus 1 sandwich bun
Calories	270 kcal
Fat	6 g
Saturated fat	2 g
Cholesterol	47 mg
Sodium	650 mg
Carbohydrates	33 g
Dietary fiber	2 g
Protein	21 g

Beef Stroganoff

Annette Hinton, M.S., R.D., L.D.N., C.E.C.

Serves: 6
Hands-on time: 10 minutes
Cooking time: 20 minutes

Although the origins of Beef Stroganoff are French and Russian, this recipe adds a bit of this and a touch of that to make it all-American delicious. After all, that's what Americans are noted for—adding our own ingenuity to something good to make it something great!

- ¼ cup all-purpose flour
- 2 teaspoons sweet paprika
- 2 teaspoons ground nutmeg
- ½ teaspoon salt
- ¼ to ½ teaspoon black pepper
- 2 tablespoons canola oil
- 1 pound beef tenderloin or sirloin, trimmed and cut into 1-by-2-inch strips
- 4 shallots, minced, or 1 cup minced onion
- 3 cloves garlic, minced
- ½ cup beef broth, divided
- ½ cup red wine
- ½ pound sliced mushrooms
- 2 tablespoons chopped fresh dill weed, or 2 teaspoons dried dill weed, divided
- 1¼ cups reduced-fat sour cream
- ¼ cup catsup
- cooked noodles

Stir together the flour, paprika, nutmeg, salt, and pepper; add the beef strips and toss lightly to coat; set aside.

Heat the oil in a Dutch oven over low heat; add the shallots and garlic. Cook and stir 5 minutes. Increase heat to high. Add 2 tablespoons of the broth and the floured beef. Brown the beef for 4 to 5 minutes, turning frequently. Reduce heat to medium.

Add the wine, mushrooms, remaining 6 tablespoons broth and 1 tablespoon dill; stir well. Cover and simmer until the beef and mushrooms are tender, approximately 10 minutes.

Stir in the sour cream and catsup. Serve over cooked noodles. Garnish with the remaining 1 tablespoon dill weed.

SHOPPING TIP
Although they look more like garlic than onions, shallots are a very mild type of onion. Choose firm and plump shallots with dry skin. Avoid those that are wrinkled or that have begun to sprout. Pinot, Burgundy or Cabernet are all good red wine choices. For the mushrooms, use any combination of button, shitake, straw, and/or crimini mushrooms.

FOOD TRIVIA
Stroganoff was created by a French chef but named after the nineteenth-century Russian diplomat Count Paul Stroganov.

NUTRITION PER SERVING

Serving size	¾ cup (strogonoff only)
Calories	330 kcal
Fat	19 g
Saturated fat	8 g
Cholesterol	65 mg
Sodium	450 mg
Carbohydrates	16 g
Dietary fiber	1 g
Protein	20 g

Sweet and Tangy Marinated Flank Steak

Kristine Napier, M.P.H., R.D.

What could be easier than doing the lion's share of tomorrow's dinner while clearing up tonight's, as I love to do in my Wisconsin home. This is an especially great idea when you anticipate a busy day. Change the sauce to meet your tastes by changing the proportion of ingredients—just be sure and taste before you add the beef.

Serves: 8
Hands-on time: 10 minutes
Marinating time: 4 hours to overnight
Cooking time: 10 minutes

- ¼ cup lite soy sauce
- 3 tablespoons honey
- 2 cloves garlic, minced
- ¼ cup wine vinegar or wine
- ¼ cup olive oil
- 2 pounds lean flank steak, trimmed of all fat
- 4 sweet onions, quartered (such as Vidalia, Walla Walla, or Maui Sweet)

Blend the soy sauce, honey, garlic, vinegar, and oil. Pour over the meat and onions in a tightly sealing glass or plastic container and marinate for at least 4 hours, but overnight is better.

Heat the broiler or start the outdoor grill.

Remove the meat from the marinade; discard the marinade. Grill or broil the meat to desired doneness and the onions until just soft, about 5 to 10 minutes.

COOK'S TIP

Discard unused marinade after removing the uncooked meat, as leftover meat, fish, and poultry marinade has the same food poisoning risk as does raw meat. Also, use a clean plate for the cooked meat, not the one used before cooking.

NUTRITION PER SERVING	
Serving size	1 3½-ounce cooked slice plus ½ grilled onion
Calories	390 kcal
Fat	22 g
Saturated fat	7 g
Cholesterol	80 mg
Sodium	390 mg
Carbohydrates	14 g
Dietary fiber	1 g
Protein	33 g

Uncle Bob's Sauerbraten

Rebecca Dowling, R.D.

Serves: 20 (freezes well)
Hands-on time: 15 minutes
Marinating time: 5 to 7 days
Cooking time: 4 hours

This German specialty replicated here in Chicago is made by marinating beef for two to seven days (depending on the chef) before browning and then simmering it. The result is worth waiting for—an extremely tender roast and a delicious sauce.

8 cups vinegar
6 cloves garlic
1½ cups red wine
2 teaspoons salt
2 onions, sliced
12 ginger snaps
2 to 4 bay leaves
2 teaspoons brown sugar
12 peppercorns
5 to 6 pounds beef roast

Heat all the ingredients except the meat to boiling. Cool. Place the meat in a large container and pour cooled marinade over the top. Cover and refrigerate 5 to 7 days.

Preheat oven to 375°F. Remove the meat and onions from the marinade and put in a roasting pan. Strain and reserve the marinade. Roast for 20 minutes. Add a small amount of strained marinade to the pan, cover, and bake 3½ hours, basting often and turning twice. Take the liquid out of the pan and continue baking for another ½ hour so the meat will dry out a bit.

FOOD TRIVIA
Sauerbraten is the German word for "sour roast," although the finished product is anything but sour! The turning of the roast may have originated when wood stoves, with their uneven heat, were used.

COOK'S TIP
Sauerbraten is traditionally served with dumplings, boiled potatoes, or noodles.

NUTRITION PER SERVING

Serving size	4 ounces
Calories	210 kcal
Fat	7 g
Saturated fat	2.5 g
Cholesterol	60 mg
Sodium	310 mg
Carbohydrates	6 g
Dietary fiber	0 g
Protein	24 g

Bratwurst and Beer Casserole

Julie Ann Lickteig, M.S., R.D., F.A.D.A.

A German invention brought to Wisconsin, the bratwurst replaces hot-dogs at most summer picnics and football games in the state. This delightfully delicious recipe turns the bratwurst into a hearty but (don't tell them) healthy meal.

Serves: 6
Hands-on time: 15 minutes
Cooking time: 50 minutes

- 1 pound apple-smoked bratwurst, sliced into 1-inch pieces
- 2 medium-size onions, chopped
- 2 stalks celery, thinly sliced (½ cup)
- vegetable oil cooking spray
- 1 cup medium-size barley
- 1 12-ounce can beer
- 8 ounces sliced mushrooms
- ¼ to 1 teaspoon black pepper
- ½ teaspoon marjoram
- ½ teaspoon caraway seeds
- 1 medium-size green bell pepper, chopped
- 1 medium-size red bell pepper, chopped
- 2 tablespoons chopped fresh parsley

Brown the bratwurst, onions, and celery in a medium-size skillet over medium heat, stirring occasionally, about 5 to 7 minutes. The sausage should be browned and the onions golden.

Meanwhile, heat oven to 400°F. Coat a 2-quart casserole dish with the cooking spray. Transfer the sausage mixture to the casserole dish. Add the barley, beer, mushrooms, black pepper, marjoram, and caraway seeds. Stir well. Cover tightly and bake 30 minutes.

Uncover. Stir in the chopped peppers. Bake an additional 15 minutes. Sprinkle with the parsley just before serving.

VARIATIONS

Wisconsinites have a running debate about how to cook bratwurst. One camp believes in browning first and then simmering in beer. The other says first to simmer in beer and then brown. Either way, the alcohol in the beer cooks off, leaving behind wonderfully rich flavors.

FOOD TRIVIA

German immigrants from ten different German regions settled close to Lake Michigan in Sheboygan County, Wisconsin, in the mid 1800s. Sausage making became an industry in this county, including bratwurst. It is made from ground pork and veal and seasoned with a variety of spices including ginger, nutmeg, coriander, and caraway.

NUTRITION PER SERVING

Serving size	2 cups
Calories	370 kcal
Fat	20 g
Saturated fat	7 g
Cholesterol	45 mg
Sodium	440 mg
Carbohydrates	31 g
Dietary fiber	4 g
Protein	15 g

Donna's Honey Apricot Glazed Ham

Donna Weihofen, R.D., M.S.

Serves: 12
Hands-on time: 10 to 20 minutes
Standing time: 2 hours
Cooking time: 1 hour

SHOPPING TIP
Convert the weight to a bone-in ham. Purchase 4 pounds bone-in ham to make this recipe. (In other words, each 1 pound of ham with the bone yields about ¾ pound edible meat.)

COOK'S TIP
The sugars found in the dried fruit, orange juice concentrate, and apricot preserves will create a glaze over the ham; basting will ensure a sweet and moist product, even with the fat trimmed.

NUTRITION NUGGET
Dried fruits, such as apricots and raisins, are a good source of iron and fiber.

NUTRITION PER SERVING

Serving size	4 ounces ham plus 3 tablespoons sauce
Calories	240 kcal
Fat	5 g
Saturated fat	1.5 g
Cholesterol	50 mg
Sodium	1,440 mg
Carbohydrates	19 g
Dietary fiber	1 g
Protein	23 g

The apricot-flavored basting sauce with nutmeg and cloves is a perfect complement to ham. This recipe will definitely be one of your Sunday bests.

½ cup brandy
1 cup dried apricots
½ cup raisins
⅛ teaspoon nutmeg
⅛ teaspoon cloves
⅛ teaspoon ginger
vegetable oil cooking spray
¼ cup frozen orange juice concentrate
¼ cup apricot preserves
3 pounds very lean, fully cooked boneless ham, trimmed of all visible fat

Stir together the brandy, apricots, raisins, nutmeg, cloves, and ginger. Cover tightly with plastic wrap and let stand at room temperature a minimum of 2 hours, overnight is fine.

Preheat oven to 325°F. Coat a small roasting pan with the cooking spray.

Add the orange juice concentrate and apricot preserves to the brandy and fruit mixture; stir well.

Place the ham in the prepared pan and coat with the basting sauce. Cook for 1 hour, basting 4 to 6 times during the cooking period.

Fall Braised Pork Medallions with Apples, Dried Cherries, and Horseradish Sauce

Lana Shepek, R.D., L.D.

The local ingredients—pork, apples, and horseradish—grown in the St. Clair County, Illinois, area are showcased in this easy recipe that you can enjoy all year.

Serves: 4
Hands-on time: 15 minutes
Cooking time: 15 minutes

- 1 pound pork tenderloin
- 2 teaspoons coarsely ground black pepper
- 1 teaspoon crushed dried sage leaves
- 1 teaspoon dried thyme leaves
- 2 teaspoons grated fresh ginger
- 2 tablespoons canola oil
- 1 medium-size onion, chopped
- 1 large Granny Smith apple, cored and cut into ¼-inch slices
- ½ cup apple cider
- ½ cup dried cherries
- 2 tablespoons grated fresh horseradish

Slice the pork crosswise into eight medallions. Mix together the pepper, sage, thyme, and ginger. Coat both sides of the medallions with the spice mixture.

Heat the oil in a large skillet over medium heat. Sauté the pork on both sides until evenly browned, about 8 to 10 minutes. Remove the pork from the skillet and set aside. Cover loosely with aluminum foil to keep warm.

Add the onion and sliced apple to the skillet. Sauté 3 minutes. Add the cider, dried cherries, and horseradish. Return the pork medallions to the skillet. Cover and simmer for 5 minutes.

VARIATION

To spice up this recipe, add more horseradish and/or black pepper.

FOOD TRIVIA

The Granny Smith apple traces to French crabapples that were supposedly tossed out in grandmother Marie Ana Smith's Australian garden. They sprouted, she nurtured them, and thus we have this wonderfully tart apple.

NUTRITION PER SERVING

Serving size	1¼ cups
Calories	300 kcal
Fat	11 g
Saturated fat	2 g
Cholesterol	75 mg
Sodium	65 mg
Carbohydrates	23 g
Dietary fiber	3 g
Protein	25 g

Glazed Pork Tenderloin Medallions

Marjorie Sawicki, M.S., R.D., L.D.

Serves: 4
Hands-on time: 5 minutes
Cooking time: 10 minutes

Not just for company, this quick-cooking and low-fat pork dish is great for families in a hurry—from my home in Illinois to anywhere across the United States. I was given a gift of spring onion jelly, with which I developed this recipe. Substitute your favorite fruit marmalade in place of the spring onion jelly.

1 pound pork tenderloin, trimmed of excess fat
vegetable oil cooking spray
1 teaspoon salt-free lemon pepper
½ cup spring onion jelly, or apricot or orange marmalade
1 tablespoon mirin (sweet rice wine)

Slice the pork into four pieces and season with the lemon pepper.

Coat a large nonstick skillet with cooking spray; heat over medium-high heat. Add the pork and cook 4 minutes on each side or until a thermometer inserted into the pork registers 160°F (the meat will be slightly pink).

Add the jelly or preserves and mirin to the skillet; stir to make a glaze, about 1 minute. Spoon the glaze over the pork.

SHOPPING TIP

Keep 1 pound (per four people, or ½ pound per two people) of pork tenderloin on hand for quick meals. Ask the meat department at your favorite supermarket to package one or two of the size you need to have on hand.

COOK'S TIP

To round out the meal, cook up instant rice and microwave frozen broccoli. Serve canned peaches (packed in juice) for dessert.

NUTRITION PER SERVING

Serving size	1 medallion
Calories	200 kcal
Fat	4 g
Saturated fat	1.5 g
Cholesterol	75 mg
Sodium	170 mg
Carbohydrates	13 g
Dietary fiber	0 g
Protein	24 g

Ham Loaves with Mustard Sauce

Ingrid Gangestad, R.D., L.D.

This recipe is submitted in memory of Irene Johnson Jones, R.D. She was an active member of the ADA for over fifty years. Aside from that, this classy lady was a great cook and my great-aunt. This is one of the recipes she shared with her Minnesota family and now it is a favorite of mine as well.

Serves: 4
Hands-on time: 30 minutes
Cooking time: 1 hour

LOAVES

½ pound ground fully cooked smoked ham (about 1½ cups)
⅓ pound extra-lean ground pork
½ cup dry bread crumbs
1 large egg, lightly beaten
¼ cup apple juice or apple cider
1 small onion, chopped
¼ teaspoon dry mustard
⅛ teaspoon ground black pepper
¼ teaspoon Worcestershire sauce

GLAZE

¼ cup dark corn syrup
3 tablespoons cider vinegar
¾ teaspoon dry mustard

MUSTARD SAUCE

½ cup sugar
1 tablespoon dry mustard
1 teaspoon all-purpose flour
½ cup evaporated skim milk
¼ cup cider vinegar
1 egg yolk

SERVING SUGGESTION

These loaves are elegant enough for entertaining. To pull together an easy dinner party, serve with baked potatoes, a quick-serve salad from a bag, fresh fruit, and crusty rolls. To save time, the potatoes can be cooked in the oven with the loaves.

NUTRITION PER SERVING	
Serving size	1 loaf plus ⅓ cup sauce
Calories	480 kcal
Fat	16 g
Saturated fat	5 g
Cholesterol	165 mg
Sodium	780 mg
Carbohydrates	61 g
Dietary fiber	Less than 1 g
Protein	26 g

Ham Loaves with Mustard Sauce *(continued)*

COOK'S TIP

The loaves may be prepared in advance by mixing and shaping as directed. Wrap each uncooked loaf in plastic wrap; place in a resealable zip-top plastic bag and freeze until ready to cook. Remove the loaves from the freezer and top with the glaze. Bake as directed, adding 30 minutes to the suggested baking time, or until the internal temperature reaches 170°F. The sauce may be prepared and refrigerated up to 3 days in advance.

Heat oven to 300°F.

Combine all the ingredients for the loaves in a large bowl; mix with a spoon or by hand until combined. Shape into 4 loaves. Place in a 13-by-9-inch baking dish.

Prepare the glaze by combining the corn syrup, vinegar and dry mustard in a 1-cup glass measuring cup or small bowl. Microwave on high 1 minute or until heated through and bubbly.

Spoon glaze over the loaves. Bake 1 hour or until internal temperature reaches 170°F.

Prepare the mustard sauce by combining the remaining ingredients in a small saucepan. Bring to a boil over medium-high heat, stirring constantly. Remove from heat; serve warm with the loaves.

Pork Tenderloin, Sweet Red Pepper, and Asparagus Stir-Fry

Donna Weihofen, R.D., M.S.

Asian-inspired cooking spread across this country and became part of the way we cook, including in Wisconsin. It's no wonder, because it is quick, versatile, flavorful, and healthy. This version features pork, peppers, and asparagus, but with a few substitutions, it could just as easily be Chicken, Mushroom, and Broccoli Stir-Fry.

Serves: 8
Hands-on time: 30 minutes
Marinating time: 30 minutes to 2 hours
Cooking time: 35 minutes

- 1 pound pork tenderloin, trimmed
- 2 tablespoons soy sauce
- 6 tablespoons dry sherry, divided
- 1 cup reduced-sodium chicken broth
- 4 tablespoons sesame oil, divided
- 1 tablespoon rice wine or white wine vinegar
- 1 tablespoon cornstarch
- ¼ teaspoon white pepper
- 1 pound fresh asparagus, cut into 2-inch pieces
- 1 large red bell pepper, trimmed, seeded, and thinly sliced
- 1 8-ounce package fresh mushrooms, sliced
- 1 teaspoon minced garlic
- 1 teaspoon minced ginger
- 4 cups cooked brown rice (about 1⅓ cups uncooked)

Cut the pork crosswise into ½-inch slices, and cut the slices into ¼ inch strips. Place in a zip-top plastic bag. Add the soy sauce and 4 tablespoons sherry. Refrigerate for 30 minutes or up to 2 hours.

Combine the chicken broth, 2 tablespoons sherry, 1 tablespoon sesame oil, and the rice wine, cornstarch, and white pepper in a small bowl; set aside.

Heat 2 teaspoons sesame oil in a large skillet over high heat. Add the pork and stir-fry for 3 to 4 minutes until lightly browned. Remove the pork to a dish and keep warm.

Heat the remaining oil in the same skillet over high heat. Add the asparagus and stir-fry 1 to 2 minutes. Add the bell pepper and mushrooms. Stir-fry 1 to 2 minutes until tender. Add the garlic and ginger; stir-fry 1 to 2 minutes. Add the stir-fried pork and the chicken broth mixture. Cook and stir on medium heat until the mixture thickens, about 30 seconds. Serve with the cooked rice.

SHOPPING TIP

Most broth comes in 14-ounce flip-top cans. Open one and measure out what you need; pour the remainder into a storage container and refrigerate. Some broths now also come in resealable paper cartons. You can use it to warm this dish up the next day, to season rice during cooking, or to steam vegetables.

NUTRITION PER SERVING

Serving size	1 cup rice plus 1 cup stir-fry
Calories	250 kcal
Fat	7 g
Saturated fat	1.5 g
Cholesterol	35 mg
Sodium	230 mg
Carbohydrates	30 g
Dietary fiber	4 g
Protein	17 g

Pork Tenderloin with Roasted Asparagus

Raeann Sarazen, R.D.

Serves: 4
Hands-on time: 15 minutes
Cooking time: 20 minutes

Impress guests and family alike with this exquisite pork roast, as I love to do in my Chicago home. Long, thin asparagus spears add an element of elegance to the presentation, as well as rounding out the meal nutritionally. Your guests will never know that you really didn't have to slave over it.

2 tablespoons Dijon mustard
1 tablespoon chopped fresh thyme
1 tablespoon chopped fresh sage
½ teaspoon salt
½ teaspoon freshly ground pepper
1¼ pounds pork tenderloin
1 pound asparagus, trimmed
2 teaspoons olive oil

Heat broiler, placing oven rack about 4 inches from heat source.

Stir together the mustard, thyme, sage, salt, and pepper in a small dish.

Place the tenderloin in the bottom half of a broiler pan lined with aluminum foil. Rub the mustard mixture over the pork. Broil for 8 minutes. Remove from oven; turn over the tenderloin.

Place the asparagus next to the tenderloin, coating it with oil and spices; return to oven. Broil, turning the tenderloin and asparagus once, until an instant-read thermometer inserted in the thickest part of the tenderloin reads 135°F and the asparagus is tender, about 13 minutes. (The pork will be cooked through, but slightly pink in the center.) Remove from oven, cover pan with foil, and let sit 5 minutes or until pork temperature reads 145°F in the thickest part.

NUTRITION NUGGET
Asparagus is an excellent source of folic acid, which helps prevent birth defects and may help in reducing colon cancer risk. It's also extremely low in calories. Ten spears have only 35 calories, but 2.5 grams of fiber and over 200 mg of folic acid—half of an adult's daily need.

NUTRITION PER SERVING

Serving size	4 ounces cooked meat and 8 to 10 asparagus spears
Calories	230 kcal
Fat	8 g
Saturated fat	2 g
Cholesterol	90 mg
Sodium	550 mg
Carbohydrates	6 g
Dietary fiber	3 g
Protein	33 g

FOOD TRIVIA
Dijon mustard, hailing from France, is known for its clean, sharp taste. Choose your favorite version: mild, hot, or somewhere in between.

Grandma Glatz's Hasenpfeffer

Rebecca Dowling, R.D.

This traditional German recipe for rabbit comes from the kitchen of my landscaper and remodeler friend Connie Helms in Wisconsin. Try this easy recipe for a different holiday meal.

Serves: 6
Hands-on time: 30 minutes, divided time
Marinating time: overnight
Cooking time: 1½ hours

- 2 rabbits, cut into stewing pieces
- 2 cups red or white wine
- ½ teaspoon parsley
- 2 cups sliced onions
- 2 bay leaves
- 1 teaspoon pickling spices
- 2 teaspoons salt
- ½ teaspoon coarsely ground pepper
- ¾ teaspoon thyme
- 4 slices bacon
- ¾ cup flour
- 1 teaspoon sugar
- 1 pound small white onions, peeled
- vegetable oil cooking spray

Place the rabbit pieces in a large bowl with the wine and 1 cup water. Add the parsley, onions, bay leaves, pickling spices, salt, pepper, and thyme. Cover and refrigerate overnight, turning occasionally.

Brown the bacon in a large skillet. Remove the bacon, but reserve the drippings in the pan.

Remove the rabbit pieces from the bowl; dry with paper towels. Strain and reserve marinade. Coat the rabbit pieces with the flour. Brown in the bacon drippings over medium-high heat, about 4 to 5 minutes per side. Remove from pan and place on a platter to keep warm.

Pour the strained marinade into the pan. Add the sugar, heat to boiling. Whisk until smooth. Remove from heat. Add the cooked bacon and the onions; set aside.

Preheat oven to 225°F. Coat a large roasting pan with the cooking spray. Place the rabbit pieces in the pan. Pour the sauce over the rabbits. Cover tightly and bake 1 to 1½ hours or until the meat is fork tender. Baste occasionally.

Remove the rabbits to a warm platter and pour the sauce over the top.

SHOPPING TIP

Not frozen, a dressed rabbit should have springy, pinkish white flesh. Look for a rabbit weighing 2 to 2½ pounds to get the most tender meat.

NUTRITION NUGGET

Roasted rabbit meat has just slightly more than 2 grams of fat per ounce, which makes it quite low in fat. It is an excellent source of selenium and vitamin B_{12} and a good source of iron and zinc.

NUTRITION PER SERVING	
Serving size	4 ounces cooked meat plus 3 tablespoons sauce
Calories	330 kcal
Fat	8 g
Saturated fat	2.5 g
Cholesterol	70 mg
Sodium	910 mg
Carbohydrates	24 g
Dietary fiber	3 g
Protein	27 g

Mama Rosa's Pizza

Angela Miraglio, M.S., R.D., F.A.D.A.

Serves: 20
Hands-on time: 15 to 20 minutes
Cooking time: 10 to 15 minutes for sauce
Baking time: 20 to 30 minutes

This is my mother's recipe for pizza, a regular Friday night meal when I was growing up in Chicago. Of course, in those days, Catholics didn't eat meat on any Friday throughout the year so we had cheese pizza and occasionally added anchovies to one for those of us who liked them. My mother learned to make pizza from my grandmother, an immigrant from southern Italy. Since my mother didn't bake her own bread, as my grandmother did, she modernized the recipe to use Pillsbury Hot Roll Mix for the dough. This pizza crust is thicker than most commercial pizzas and thinner than deep-dish pizza.

Tomato Sauce

1 6-ounce can no-salt-added tomato paste
¼ teaspoon freshly ground black pepper
½ teaspoon garlic powder
2 teaspoons dried oregano (or 2 fresh sweet basil leaves)
½ teaspoon baking soda

In a 1-quart saucepan, blend the tomato paste, 1 to 1½ cans water, and the pepper, garlic powder, and oregano. Bring to a boil. Add the baking soda and stir until foaming stops, about 30 seconds. Simmer over very low heat for 10 to 15 minutes.

Dough

1 1-pound box hot roll mix
vegetable oil cooking spray

Follow the directions on the box for mixing pizza dough on a 16-by-12-inch baking sheet sprayed with the cooking spray. Set aside as you prepare the toppings.

NUTRITION PER SERVING	
Serving size	1 piece of basic cheese pizza
Calories	150 kcal
Fat	5 g
Saturated fat	2 g
Cholesterol	10 mg
Sodium	280 mg
Carbohydrates	18 g
Dietary fiber	1 g
Protein	7 g

NUTRITION PER SERVING	
Serving size	1 piece of veggie pizza
Calories	160 kcal
Fat	5 g
Saturated fat	2 g
Cholesterol	10 mg
Sodium	280 mg
Carbohydrates	20 g
Dietary fiber	1 g
Protein	8 g

Toppings

- ¾ pound part-skim low-moisture mozzarella cheese, shredded (8 ounces)
- ¼ to 1 teaspoon dried oregano
- ¼ pound reduced-fat Italian sausage, cooked and drained (4 ounces)
- ½ pound sliced mushrooms (8 ounces), optional
- 1 medium-size onion, coarsely chopped (about 1 generous cup), optional
- 1 large green bell pepper, sliced (about 1½ cups), optional
- 1 can anchovies, optional

When the dough and the sauce are ready, preheat oven to 425°F. Spread the tomato sauce over the entire surface of the dough. Add the grated mozzarella cheese. Sprinkle with the oregano. Add any or all of the optional ingredients.

Bake until the crust is golden brown, about 20 to 30 minutes. Let cool for about 5 minutes. Remove the pizza to a wire cooling rack. Cut into 20 pieces approximately 3½ inches by 3 inches.

COOK'S TIP

It is important to cook the sauce over very low heat or the sauce will "pop" out of the pan. Stir occasionally. If cooked longer, the sauce will become bitter with the herbs whether dried or fresh. Plus it would cook down to the consistency of a paste, not stay as a sauce. And longer cooking would create an overcooked flavor, especially since the pizza is to be cooked again. Note that the baking soda cuts the acid in the tomato sauce.

NUTRITION PER SERVING	
Serving size	1 piece of sausage pizza
Calories	150 kcal
Fat	5 g
Saturated fat	2 g
Cholesterol	10 mg
Sodium	280 mg
Carbohydrates	18 g
Dietary fiber	1 g
Protein	7 g

NUTRITION PER SERVING	
Serving size	1 piece of anchovy pizza
Calories	160 kcal
Fat	5 g
Saturated fat	2 g
Cholesterol	10 mg
Sodium	360 mg
Carbohydrates	18 g
Dietary fiber	1 g
Protein	8 g

Garden-Fresh Tomato Basil Pasta

Kristine Napier, M.P.H., R.D.

Serves: 4
Hands-on time: 15 minutes
Standing time: 4 hours
Cooking time: 10 minutes

In Wisconsin, tomatoes and green peppers come into season at the same time, so I'm always looking for more—and flavorful—ways to use them. This recipe is so easy, and it's great for leftovers, too!

- 2 pounds fresh tomatoes, coarsely chopped (about 6 to 8)
- 1 sweet onion, such as Vidalia, chopped
- 1 medium-size green bell pepper, finely chopped
- ¼ cup extra-virgin olive oil
- 1 tablespoon balsamic vinegar
- 2 tablespoons granulated sugar
- 1 teaspoon salt
- 1 teaspoon black pepper
- 1 teaspoon ground oregano
- 1 cup packed basil leaves, chopped
- 2 to 4 cloves garlic, minced
- 8 ounces uncooked spinach fettuccine
- 4 tablespoons grated Parmesan cheese

Combine all the ingredients except the fettucine and cheese in a large glass or ceramic bowl (not metal); stir well and cover tightly. Allow to sit at room temperature at least 4 hours; or overnight in the refrigerator. If refrigerating, bring to room temperature before serving.

Cook the pasta; drain but do not rinse. Toss the pasta with the fresh tomato sauce; divide among four plates. Sprinkle each serving with up to 1 tablespoon Parmesan cheese.

VARIATION
After tossing the pasta with the sauce, sprinkle a 15-ounce can of garbanzo beans (drained and rinsed) on top.

SERVING SUGGESTION
Serve this dish just slightly warm or at room temperature.

NUTRITION PER SERVING

Serving size	1 cup cooked pasta, 1½ cups sauce, and 1 tablespoon Parmesan cheese
Calories	430 kcal
Fat	18 g
Saturated fat	3.5 g
Cholesterol	5 mg
Sodium	840 mg
Carbohydrates	60 g
Dietary fiber	7 g
Protein	12 g

Mediterranean Couscous with Savory Vegetables

Marjorie Sawicki, M.S., R.D., L.D.

Fresh veggies and mint from my Illinois garden, teamed up with interesting spices, fruit juice, and couscous created this zippy dish.

Serves: 4
Hands-on time: 10 minutes
Cooking time: 10 minutes

1 tablespoon olive oil
1 medium-size zucchini, diced
1 red onion, diced
1 medium-size red bell pepper, diced
1 carrot, diced
1 clove garlic, minced
1 to 2 teaspoons Morocco Ethmix (recipe follows)
¼ teaspoon lemon zest, dry
1 14-ounce can reduced-sodium chicken broth
1 cup uncooked whole wheat couscous
2 medium-size fresh tomatoes, diced
¼ cup lemon juice
⅓ cup chopped fresh mint, or 1 tablespoon dried

Heat the oil in a large heavy skillet or Dutch oven over high heat. Add the zucchini, onion, pepper, carrot, garlic, Morocco Ethmix, and lemon zest. Sauté for 4 minutes or until the vegetables are just tender. Add the chicken broth and bring the mixture to a boil.

Stir in the couscous. Cover the skillet and remove from heat. Let stand 5 minutes or until the broth is absorbed. Fluff the couscous with a fork. Mix in the tomatoes, lemon juice, and mint. Transfer to a serving dish.

FOOD TRIVIA
Couscous is pasta that originates from Africa.

Morocco Ethmix

5 teaspoons ground nutmeg
5 teaspoons ground cumin
5 teaspoons ground coriander
2½ teaspoons ground allspice
2½ teaspoons ground ginger
1¼ teaspoons ground cayenne pepper
1¼ teaspoons ground cinnamon

Mix the spices thoroughly. Store in an airtight container in a cool, dark place. Use within 6 to 8 weeks. Alternatively, store in an airtight container in the freezer up to one year.

NUTRITION PER SERVING	
Serving size	1 cup
Calories	300 kcal
Fat	6 g
Saturated fat	1 g
Cholesterol	0 mg
Sodium	75 mg
Carbohydrates	55 g
Dietary fiber	9 g
Protein	11 g

Barrie's Genovese Fusilli al'Pesto

Barrie Rosencrans, M.S., R.D., L.D.

Serves: 4
Hands-on time: 10 to 15 minutes
Cooking time: 10 to 12 minutes

Preparing this classic aromatic northern Italian pesto from the region of Liguria is as simple as can be. Originally pesto was pounded to perfection with a mortar and pestle. In my Cleveland home, I use a food processor to make the process much easier; you can also use a blender.

- 8 ounces uncooked fusilli pasta
- 1½ teaspoons salt
- 1½ cups loosely packed fresh basil leaves, stems removed and tiny leaves saved for garnish
- 3 cloves garlic
- 2 tablespoons pine nuts (pignoli)
- ½ cup freshly shredded Parmigiano-Reggiano cheese (2 ounces), divided
- 1½ tablespoons extra-virgin olive oil
- 2 teaspoons lemon juice
- ⅛ teaspoon salt
- ⅛ teaspoon cracked black pepper
- 2 cups cherry or grape tomatoes, halved (1 pint)
- 1 yellow bell pepper, very thinly sliced

Cook the pasta in salted water to al dente stage according to the package directions. Drain the pasta and keep warm; reserve ½ cup of the cooking water.

Make the pesto sauce by placing the basil, garlic, pine nuts, all but 2 tablespoons cheese, olive oil and lemon juice in a food processor or blender. Process 2 to 3 minutes until smooth. Add the salt and pepper; process again. Set aside.

Mix the pesto and 1 to 2 tablespoons of the reserved cooking water; pour over the pasta and toss well to coat. Stir in the tomatoes and bell pepper. Garnish with the remaining 2 tablespoons of cheese and tiny basil leaves.

SERVING SUGGESTIONS

Garnish with tiny tomatoes, strips of red or yellow peppers, and a sprinkle of toasted pine nuts. This dish can be a wonderful appetizer, buffet item, or side dish with grilled main courses.

VARIATIONS

A tasty twist on this dish would be to add peas and/or roasted red peppers. If you would like to add a zippy spiciness to this dish, add ⅛ of a teaspoon crushed red pepper flakes to the food processor when making the pesto mixture. Using freshly grated Reggiano Parmesan cheese will give this dish the nutty flavor it deserves. Alternative pasta shapes might be linguini, penne, tagliatelle, orricchette, farfalle (bowties), or gnocchi.

COOK'S TIPS

Pesto must be served raw and unheated. It can be made a day ahead and kept covered in the fridge. Pesto will freeze very nicely in a covered ice cube tray and can be used anytime for pasta sauces or even added to minestrone soup. When freezing, put a fine layer of olive oil on top of each pesto section to keep the pesto from browning in the freezer.

NUTRITION PER SERVING

Serving size	1 cup pasta plus ⅓ cup pesto
Calories	350 kcal
Fat	12 g
Saturated fat	3.5 g
Cholesterol	10 mg
Sodium	1,190 mg
Carbohydrates	46 g
Dietary fiber	4 g
Protein	14 g

Garlic Sautéed Spinach with Parmesan Rotini

Kristine Napier, M.P.H., R.D.

Whether you're in Wisconsin, where I live, Georgia, or Oregon, enjoy this special taste of Italy. Both kids and adults with more sophisticated palates will love it!

Serves: 4
Hands-on time: 15 minutes
Cooking time: pasta cooking time only

8 ounces uncooked tricolor rotini pasta (3 cups)
1 to 2 cloves garlic, minced
2 tablespoons extra-virgin olive oil, divided
2 tablespoons lemon juice (fresh or bottled), divided
1 10-ounce package fresh baby spinach
½ to 1 teaspoon freshly ground black pepper
½ teaspoon salt
¼ cup Parmesan cheese
2 cups grape or cherry tomatoes, quartered

Cook the pasta as directed on the package.

Sauté the garlic in 1 tablespoon oil and 1 tablespoon lemon juice over low heat about 5 minutes, allowing the flavors to fully release in the oil. Add the spinach; stir to coat the spinach with the garlic sauce. Cover and steam over low heat until the spinach is wilted, about 5 minutes.

Drain the cooked pasta, but do not rinse; return to the pan.

Blend the remaining oil and lemon juice, pepper, salt, and cheese in a small bowl; pour over the hot pasta and toss. Add the spinach and toss. Serve at once, garnished with the tomatoes.

SUBSTITUTION

Substitute one 10-ounce package of frozen chopped spinach for the fresh. Thaw and squeeze out excess liquid. Use as directed in the recipe.

NUTRITION PER SERVING	
Serving size	1½ cups
Calories	280 kcal
Fat	10 g
Saturated fat	2 g
Cholesterol	5 mg
Sodium	410 mg
Carbohydrates	39 g
Dietary fiber	2 g
Protein	9 g

White Lasagna with Creamed Mushrooms

Monica L. Ceille, R.D., C.D.

Serves: 9 or 12
Hands-on time: 20 minutes
Cooking time: 45 minutes
Standing time: 15 minutes

Lasagna has come a long way since becoming popular in the United States during the 1960s and 1970s. A move from the typical Wisconsin meat and potatoes my family is used to, this version is a refreshingly different dish. This white lasagna features fresh mushrooms and meatless Italian sausage.

- 9 lasagna noodles
- vegetable oil cooking spray
- 1 tablespoon extra-virgin olive oil
- 1 pound fresh mushrooms, sliced
- 1 medium-size onion, chopped
- 3 cloves garlic, minced
- 1 10-ounce package Italian-flavored meatless sausage
- ¼ cup chopped fresh basil, or 1 tablespoon dried
- ¼ teaspoon cayenne pepper
- 3 cups nonfat milk
- ⅓ cup all-purpose flour
- 1 pound fat-free ricotta cheese (16 ounces)
- ½ pound shredded part-skim mozzarella cheese (8 ounces)
- 1 cup shredded fresh Parmesan cheese (4 ounces)

Cook the noodles as directed on the package; drain.

Preheat oven to 325°F. Spray a 13-by-9-by-2-inch baking dish with the cooking spray.

Heat the oil in a large heavy saucepan over medium-low heat. Add the mushrooms, onion, garlic, and sausage; sauté until the mushrooms and onion wilt, about 5 to 7 minutes. Stir in the basil and cayenne.

Whisk together the milk and flour in a small bowl; pour over the vegetable mixture. Increase heat and bring the mixture to a boil; decrease heat. Stir and cook until thickened.

Spread ⅓ of the creamed mushroom mixture into the bottom of the baking dish. Place 3 lasagna noodles over the mushroom mixture. Spread ⅓ of the ricotta cheese on the noodles. Place ⅓ of the sliced mozzarella cheese on top of the ricotta cheese. Repeat the process until you have three layers of the mushroom/sausage mixture, noodles, ricotta, and mozzarella. Top with Parmesan.

Bake for 45 minutes. Allow the lasagna to rest for 15 minutes before cutting and serving.

SUBSTITUTION
In place of fresh garlic, substitute 2 teaspoons garlic powder. Use an equal amount of fresh or dried oregano in place of the basil, or use both basil and oregano.

NUTRITION PER SERVING	
Serving size	⅑ of casserole
Calories	410 kcal
Fat	17 g
Saturated fat	9 g
Cholesterol	40 mg
Sodium	630 mg
Carbohydrates	34 g
Dietary fiber	3 g
Protein	31 g

NUTRITION PER SERVING	
Serving size	1/12 of casserole
Calories	310 kcal
Fat	13 g
Saturated fat	6 g
Cholesterol	30 mg
Sodium	470 mg
Carbohydrates	26 g
Dietary fiber	3 g
Protein	23 g

Rainbow Penne Pasta

Melissa Stevens Ohlson, M.S., R.D., L.D.

Many of my Cleveland heart patients wanted a heart-healthy recipe that their kids would like, too. From many reports, this fits the bill. Make a great meatless meal with broccoli, pasta, and freshly shredded Parmesan cheese. It's kid-friendly, packed with vitamins and minerals, and bursting with layers of rich flavor.

Serves: 8
Hands-on time: 10 minutes
Cooking time: 10 minutes

8 ounces uncooked penne pasta
2 tablespoons extra-virgin olive oil
2 cloves garlic, minced
1 16-ounce package frozen broccoli florets, thawed
1 16-ounce can garbanzo beans, drained and rinsed
1 medium-size red bell pepper, thinly sliced; slices halved
½ teaspoon salt
¼ cup freshly grated or shredded Parmesan cheese
freshly ground black pepper to taste

Cook the pasta in boiling salted water according to the package directions.

Heat the oil in a large skillet over low heat. Add the garlic and sauté 5 minutes, allowing the flavors to fully release into the oil. Add the broccoli, beans, pepper, 3 tablespoons water, and salt. Cover and adjust heat to medium. Steam, stirring occasionally, 5 to 7 minutes, or until the broccoli is hot and the pepper is crisp tender.

Toss the pasta with the vegetables. Top with the Parmesan cheese and fresh pepper.

SUBSTITUTION

Substitute any vegetables your children (or you) like, varying cooking time as needed.

COOK'S TIP

For a spicier flavor, add more garlic and/or pepper.

NUTRITION PER SERVING	
Serving size	1 cup
Calories	265 kcal
Fat	6 g
Saturated fat	2 g
Cholesterol	2 mg
Sodium	215 mg
Carbohydrates	41 g
Dietary fiber	7 g
Protein	12 g

Donna's Tuscan Pasta Salad with Artichokes and Sun-Dried Tomatoes

Donna Weihofen, R.D., M.S.

Serves: 8
Hands-on time: 20 minutes

Take a lunch or dinner culinary tour to the Mediterranean with this salad, as I love to do on a cold Wisconsin January day. The salad is as fantastically beautiful as it is flavorful.

- 3 tablespoons extra-virgin olive oil
- 2 cloves garlic, minced
- ¼ cup balsamic vinegar
- ½ pound uncooked rigatoni
- 1 14-ounce can artichoke hearts in water, drained and cut into quarters
- ½ cup oil-packed sun-dried tomatoes, drained and chopped
- ¼ cup fresh basil, chopped (pack leaves to measure, then chop)
- ½ cup black olives, chopped
- ¼ pound extra-lean ham, chopped
- 6 ounces tomato-and-basil flavored feta cheese
- 1 10-ounce bag fresh baby spinach
- ¼ cup toasted pine nuts, optional

Combine the olive oil, garlic, and vinegar in a small jar. Shake to blend.

Cook the pasta in salted water according to the package directions until al dente. Drain and set aside.

Combine the cooked pasta, artichoke hearts, sun-dried tomatoes, basil, olives, ham, and feta cheese. Mix well.

Wash the spinach leaves and remove stems. Add the spinach and dressing to the pasta mixture just before serving. Toss gently. Top individual servings with pine nuts, if desired.

SUBSTITUTION
In place of the rigatoni, substitute an equal amount of penne.

FOOD TRIVIA
Pine nuts are found inside pine cones and are extracted by a labor-intensive heating process, which is why they are so expensive.

NUTRITION PER SERVING

Serving size	1½ cups
Calories	260 kcal
Fat	12 g
Saturated fat	4 g
Cholesterol	20 mg
Sodium	515 mg
Carbohydrates	29 g
Dietary fiber	5 g
Protein	9 g

Goat Cheese and Sun-Dried Tomato Topped Salad

Kristine Napier, M.P.H., R.D.

Mix up this unlikely combination of sweet and savory ingredients and you've got a superstar main dish salad. It's created from Wisconsin honey, grapes, and dried cranberries. Hayward, in northwest Wisconsin, is the home of Wisconsin's annual cranberry festival.

Serves: 8
Hands-on time: 15 minutes

- 2 10-ounce bags romaine lettuce
- 2 cups seedless green grapes, halved
- 2 cups seedless red grapes, halved
- 1 cup thinly sliced green onions (tops and bottoms)
- 1 6-ounce package sweetened dried cranberries
- 1 cup raisins
- ⅓ cup sun-dried tomato vinaigrette salad dressing
- 8 ounces crumbled goat cheese
- 1 cup slivered almonds
- 6 cups whole-grain croutons (page 234)
- 1 tablespoon honey

Place the lettuce in a very large salad bowl. Place the grapes, green onions, cranberries, raisins, and salad dressing in a medium-size bowl; stir well. Add to the lettuce and toss.

Top the salad with the goat cheese, almonds, and croutons. Drizzle with honey.

COOK'S TIP

Wash, drain, and dry all lettuce, even bagged varieties that are pre-washed.

NUTRITION PER SERVING	
Serving size	2 cups
Calories	470 kcal
Fat	19 g
Saturated fat	6 g
Cholesterol	15 mg
Sodium	350 mg
Carbohydrates	65 g
Dietary fiber	8 g
Protein	12 g

Black Bean, Wild Rice, and Bell Pepper Salad

Lana Shepek, R.D., L.D.

Serves: 4
Hands-on time: 20 minutes
Cooking time: 45 minutes
Chill time: 1 hour

SHOPPING TIP
Choose shallots that are firm and that have dry skins.

Hearty foods have been standard in Illinois since it was the western frontier for settlers. Today, hearty foods like this salad fuse with America's taste for good health.

- 1 cup uncooked wild rice
- 2¾ cups reduced-sodium chicken broth
- 2 shallots, finely chopped
- 1 red bell pepper, seeded and cut into thin strips, reserving some for garnish
- 1 green bell pepper, seeded and cut into thin strips, reserving some for garnish
- 1 yellow bell pepper, seeded and cut into thin strips, reserving some for garnish
- 1 jalapeño pepper, seeded and finely chopped
- 1 15½-ounce can black beans, drained and rinsed
- 5 green onions, trimmed and thinly sliced
- 2 tablespoons fresh cilantro or parsley, finely chopped

DRESSING

- 1 tablespoon Dijon mustard
- ¼ cup white wine vinegar
- ¼ cup virgin olive oil
- 1 teaspoon chili powder
- 4 to 6 drops red hot pepper sauce or Thai chili pepper sauce
- 1 clove garlic, finely chopped
- 1 tablespoon sugar
- 1 teaspoon dried thyme, optional
- freshly ground black pepper to taste

FOOD TRIVIA
Shallots are mild-tasting onions that are formed more like garlic bulbs than onions.

To prepare the wild rice, bring the broth to a boil in a saucepan. Add the wild rice and shallots; lower the heat to maintain a simmer. Cook the rice, covered, until it is tender and the liquid is absorbed, about 40 to 45 minutes.

Combine the peppers, beans, and onions in a medium-size bowl; set aside.

While the rice is cooking, prepare the dressing. Combine the mustard and vinegar in a small bowl. Whisk in the oil, chili powder, red pepper sauce, garlic, sugar, thyme, and pepper.

Stir the cooked rice into the bean mixture. Pour the dressing over the top; toss. Chill for at least 1 hour.

Garnish with pepper strips.

NUTRITION PER SERVING	
Serving size	1½ cups
Calories	520 kcal
Fat	24 g
Saturated fat	3.5 g
Cholesterol	5 mg
Sodium	190 mg
Carbohydrates	62 g
Dietary fiber	12 g
Protein	18 g

Polenta with Tuscan-Style Vegetables

Melissa Stevens Ohlson, M.S., R.D., L.D.

Using already-prepared polenta made it very easy to include corn—an easy-to-use whole grain—in recipes for my Cleveland heart patients. Topping it with delightfully seasoned sautéed vegetables was the bonus.

Serves: 4
Hands-on time: 20 minutes
Cooking time: 15 minutes

- vegetable oil cooking spray
- 1 16-ounce tube polenta, plain or flavored, sliced into 16 pieces
- ¼ cup chopped fresh parsley
- 1 tablespoon dried oregano
- 1 tablespoon extra-virgin olive oil
- 3 cloves garlic, minced
- 1 medium-size onion, sliced and separated into rings
- 1 red bell pepper, cut into 1-inch strips
- 1 yellow bell pepper, cut into 1-inch strips
- 1 medium-size zucchini, cut diagonally into ¼-inch slices
- 2 large portabella mushrooms, chopped
- 1 cup prepared marinara sauce
- freshly ground black pepper

Spray a large nonstick skillet with the cooking spray; cook the polenta slices over medium-high heat 3 minutes on each side or until the polenta is browned. Sprinkle with the parsley and oregano during the last minute of cooking. Remove from pan and keep warm.

Add the oil and garlic to the skillet; reduce heat to medium. Add the onion; cook 4 minutes. Add the bell peppers, zucchini, and mushrooms; cook 5 to 7 minutes or until both the peppers and the zucchini are lightly browned. Add the marinara sauce and pepper to taste.

Serve the polenta rounds topped with the vegetable mixture.

SUBSTITUTION

Make your own marinara sauce by starting with one 8-ounce can of tomato sauce and adding your favorite herbs and spices.

NUTRITION PER SERVING

Serving size	4 polenta rounds plus 2 cups vegetables and sauce
Calories	175 kcal
Fat	5 g
Saturated fat	0.7 g
Cholesterol	0 mg
Sodium	270 mg
Carbohydrates	29 g
Dietary fiber	4 g
Protein	5 g

Potato and Eggplant in Lentil Sauce

Kristine Napier, M.P.H., R.D.

Serves: 4
Hands-on time: 15 minutes
Cooking time: 50 minutes

This highly aromatic, easy-to-make vegetable dish cooked with cumin in a creamy moong lentil-based sauce was created by my dear friend, Alamelu Vairavan, an expert on health-promoting South Indian cooking. Yellow in color, the split and skinned moong lentils are also known as mung beans. This lentil sauce is best served over cooked basmati or plain rice. This dish can also be served as an accompaniment to any meal or with pita or any Indian bread, such as naan.

½ cup yellow moong lentils (dal)
½ teaspoon turmeric, divided
3 teaspoons canola oil, divided
½ teaspoon cumin seeds
½ cup chopped onion
½ cup chopped tomatoes
1 large unpeeled potato, cubed (about ⅓ to ½ pound)
1 eggplant, cubed
½ teaspoon cayenne pepper
½ teaspoon salt

Boil 3 cups of water in a large saucepan. Reduce heat to medium and add the moong lentils with ¼ teaspoon turmeric and 1 teaspoon oil. Cook, uncovered, for 20 to 30 minutes until the lentils become soft. Set aside.

Place 2 teaspoons oil in a saucepan over medium heat. When the oil is hot, but not smoking, stir in the cumin seeds; cook until the seeds become brown. Add the onion, tomato, potato, and eggplant. Stir well with the seasoning for one minute. Add the remaining ¼ teaspoon turmeric, cayenne, and salt. Mix well.

Add the cooked lentils with 3 cups of warm water to the vegetable mixture and stir well. When the mixture begins to bubble, reduce heat to medium. Cook, covered, until the potato is tender.

SHOPPING TIP
Moong lentils are available in natural food stores and Indian grocery stores.

SUBSTITUTION
Red lentils (also known as Masoor dal) can be used as a substitute for the mung beans.

NUTRITION PER SERVING	
Serving size	1 generous cup
Calories	180 kcal
Fat	4 g
Saturated fat	0.34 g
Cholesterol	0 mg
Sodium	300 mg
Carbohydrates	29 g
Dietary fiber	10 g
Protein	9 g

Lesco (Hungarian Sweet Peppers)

Rebecca Dowling, R.D.

Cooking Hungarian Lesco is easy—especially with a bumper crop of peppers from my Chicago garden. Many thanks to Katrina Zynda for sharing a family recipe.

Serves: 6 as a main dish or 8 as a side dish
Hands-on time: 10 minutes
Cooking time: 35 minutes

- 1 tablespoon extra-virgin olive oil
- 1 14-ounce can reduced-sodium chicken broth
- 3 large onions, chopped
- 3 hot chili peppers, such as jalapeños, finely chopped
- 1 29-ounce can crushed tomatoes
- 1 yellow bell pepper, chopped
- 1 red bell pepper, chopped
- 1 orange bell pepper, chopped
- 1 green bell pepper, chopped
- ½ teaspoon black pepper
- 4 cups cooked brown rice (1⅓ cup uncooked)
- ¼ cup chopped fresh parsley or cilantro

Bring the olive oil and chicken broth to a boil in a large saucepan. Reduce heat to medium and add the onions and chili peppers. Cook, stirring frequently, for 10 minutes or until the onions are transparent. Add the tomatoes and bell peppers; cook 25 minutes or until the peppers are done to your preference, stirring occasionally. Season with black pepper.

Serve over cooked rice and garnish with the parsley or cilantro.

VARIATIONS

Try squash, frozen broccoli, or carrots in place of the peppers. The lesco makes a nice topping for pasta, too.

COOK'S TIPS

To save time, use a food processor to chop the vegetables. Chop the chili peppers first and then add the onions. Remove and then chop the bell peppers.

NUTRITION PER SERVING	
Serving size	1⅓ cups, main course
Calories	280 kcal
Fat	4.5 g
Saturated fat	1 g
Cholesterol	0 mg
Sodium	230 mg
Carbohydrates	55 g
Dietary fiber	8 g
Protein	8 g

NUTRITION PER SERVING	
Serving size	1 cup, side dish
Calories	210 kcal
Fat	3.5 g
Saturated fat	0.5 g
Cholesterol	0 mg
Sodium	170 mg
Carbohydrates	41 g
Dietary fiber	6 g
Protein	6 g

Wheat Berry Stuffed Eggplant

Golda L. Ewalt, R.D., L.D.

Serves: 4
Hands-on time: 20 minutes
Cooking time: 2 hours

In northern Italy, ground beef is used to stuff eggplant instead of the wheat berries that I use in my northern Illinois home. This rich-tasting dish carries you to many parts of the Mediterranean, including Greece.

- ½ cup raw wheat berries
- 2 eggplants
- 1 tablespoon olive oil
- 1 small onion, chopped
- 2 cloves garlic
- ½ cup roasted red peppers from a jar (about 4 pieces)
- 1 cup sliced mushrooms
- 1 14½-ounce can diced tomatoes
- ¼ teaspoon salt
- ground pepper to taste
- 2 tablespoons chopped fresh basil, or 2 teaspoons dried
- 2 tablespoons chopped fresh parsley, or 2 teaspoons dried
- 1 tablespoon chopped fresh oregano, or 1 teaspoon dried
- vegetable oil cooking spray
- 1 cup crumbled reduced-fat feta cheese (4 ounces)

Place the wheat berries in a heavy pot with 2 cups water. Bring to a boil, uncovered; reduce heat, cover, and simmer. Cook for about 1 hour; check occasionally, adding more water if necessary. The wheat berries should be firm, but tender. Drain.

Preheat oven to 350°F.

Cut the eggplants in half lengthwise. Create a ½-inch shell by removing the inside of the eggplant with a sharp paring knife, taking care not to cut the eggplant's skin. Dice the removed eggplant; set aside.

Heat the oil in a large skillet over medium heat; add the onion and garlic and cook 5 minutes, stirring occasionally. Add the diced eggplant, roasted pepper, mushrooms, tomatoes, salt, pepper, basil, parsley, and oregano. Cook for about 10 minutes, stirring occasionally. Stir in the wheat berries.

Spray the eggplant shells on the outside and inside with the cooking spray and place on a baking sheet. Fill each eggplant shell with the wheat berry filling and top each with ¼ cup feta cheese. Bake 45 minutes, or until slightly golden.

SUBSTITUTION

Substitute ¾ cup bulgur or cracked wheat, which cook much faster, for the wheat berries.

FOOD TRIVIA

Wheat berries, which are actually unprocessed wheat kernels, are considered a whole grain.

COOK'S TIP

To use the leftovers, drain and chop the remaining roasted red pepper; stir into reduced-fat sour cream, plain yogurt, or cream cheese for a vegetable dip.

NUTRITION PER SERVING

Serving size	½ of a stuffed eggplant
Calories	250 kcal
Fat	7 g
Saturated fat	2.5 g
Cholesterol	10 mg
Sodium	760 mg
Carbohydrates	39 g
Dietary fiber	11 g
Protein	13 g

Spinach Pies

Melissa Stevens Ohlson, M.S., R.D., L.D.

This gentle yet insistent blend of feta, garlic, nutmeg, lemon, and spinach carries you to the country's greatest Greek restaurants, starting in Cleveland where I've explored most of them with my Greek family.

Serves: 6

Hands-on time: 1 hour, 20 minutes

Cooking time: 22 minutes

CRUST

1¼ cups whole wheat flour, divided
1¼ cups all-purpose flour, divided
1 tablespoon yeast or 1 packet rapid-rise yeast
¾ teaspoon salt
1 cup warm water (approximately 130°F)
2 tablespoons extra-virgin olive oil

FILLING

2 10-ounce boxes chopped frozen whole leaf spinach, thawed
vegetable oil cooking spray
3 cloves garlic, minced
⅔ medium-size onion, chopped
¼ to ½ teaspoon freshly ground black pepper, divided
1 cup egg substitute
½ cup nonfat ricotta cheese
1 cup crumbled feta cheese (4 ounces)
½ teaspoon ground nutmeg
2 tablespoons lemon juice
¼ toasted pine nuts, optional

Preheat oven to 400°F.

Combine 1 cup whole wheat flour, 1 cup all-purpose flour, yeast, and salt in a medium-size bowl. Stir the water and olive oil into the dry ingredients. Add the remaining flour as needed to form a soft dough. Knead on a lightly floured surface until smooth and elastic. Cover with a cloth and let rise 15 to 20 minutes.

Squeeze the spinach to remove as much liquid as possible. Place in a colander to drain the remainder of the liquid; set aside.

SUBSTITUTION

Two 9-inch prepared pie crusts may be used in place of homemade crusts. Pour the spinach mixture evenly into 1 crust; top with the remaining crusts and crimp together the crust edges to seal the pie. Bake in preheated 400°F oven 45 minutes or until inserted knife comes out clean. Cut the pie into 6 slices.

NUTRITION PER SERVING

Serving size	1 individual pie or ⅙ of double-crusted pie
Calories	330 kcal
Fat	13 g
Saturated fat	5 g
Cholesterol	25 mg
Sodium	690 mg
Carbohydrates	37 g
Dietary fiber	5 g
Protein	18 g

Spinach Pies
(continued)

COOK'S TIPS
Thaw the spinach in a microwave 5 minutes on high. Press out the juices using a colander with a spatula or your hands. There will be about 2 cups squeezed spinach.
Prepare dough in a mixer on low speed. Add flour as needed until the dough pulls away from the sides of the bowl. The total amount of flour needed depends on the humidity in your kitchen.

Spray a large nonstick skillet with the cooking spray. Add the garlic and onion; cook over medium-high heat 2 minutes or until the onion is translucent. Add the spinach; reduce heat to medium; cook 5 minutes. Add pepper to taste; set aside to cool.

Combine the egg substitute, ricotta cheese, feta cheese, nutmeg, lemon juice, and pepper in a medium-size bowl. Add the spinach mixture; mix well. Toss in the pine nuts, if desired.

Preheat oven to 400°F. Coat a baking sheet with the cooking spray.

Punch down dough; shape into six 3¼-inch balls. Roll each ball to a 1⁄16-inch-thick pie round. Spoon ½ cup spinach filling into the center of each round. Fold two edges of the dough over the third edge to form a triangle, pinching the edges and using a dab of water to seal, if necessary.

Place the spinach pies, pinched edges up, on the prepared baking sheet. Bake 15 minutes or until the bottom of the crusts are brown. To ensure even browning, switch from upper to lower oven shelves for the last 5 minutes of baking.

Wild Rice with Cranberries and Walnuts

Donna Weihofen, R.D., M.S.

Wisconsin cranberries and Minnesota wild rice team up to create an anywhere favorite. This dish has plenty of protein to serve as a main dish.

Serves: 4 as a main dish or 6 as a side dish
Hands-on time: 10 minutes
Cooking time: 50 minutes
Chill time: 2 hours

- 1 cup wild rice
- 1 14-ounce can chicken broth
- 2 tablespoons extra-virgin olive oil
- ¼ cup white wine vinegar
- 1 teaspoon dried thyme
- 1 teaspoon dried rosemary, crushed
- 1 tablespoon honey
- ⅛ teaspoon salt
- ¼ teaspoon pepper
- 6 green onions, thinly sliced
- 1½ cups sweetened dried cranberries (6 ounces)
- ½ cup walnut pieces

Combine the rice, chicken broth, and 1 cup water in a large saucepan. Bring to a boil. Cover and simmer on very low heat for 50 to 55 minutes or until the rice is tender-crisp.

Combine the olive oil, vinegar, thyme, rosemary, honey, salt, and pepper. Whisk to blend well, making a dressing. Toss the cooked rice and dressing in a large serving bowl. Add the onions and dried cranberries, stir gently. Cover and refrigerate until ready to serve, at least 2 hours.

Top with the walnuts just before serving.

COOK'S TIP

Combining dressing with hot grains or pastas helps the grain or pasta absorb the flavor of the dressing.

NUTRITION NUGGET

Wild rice is a good source of fiber.

NUTRITION PER SERVING	
Serving size	1 cup, main dish
Calories	495 kcal
Fat	18 g
Saturated fat	2 g
Cholesterol	0 mg
Sodium	495 mg
Carbohydrates	76 g
Dietary fiber	7 g
Protein	11 g

NUTRITION PER SERVING	
Serving size	¾ cup, side dish
Calories	330 kcal
Fat	12 g
Saturated fat	1 g
Cholesterol	0 mg
Sodium	330 mg
Carbohydrates	51 g
Dietary fiber	4 g
Protein	7 g

German Barley Mushroom Casserole

Julie Ann Lickteig, M.S., R.D., F.A.D.A.

Serves: 6
Hands-on time: 15 minutes
Cooking time: 10 minutes

Barley, mushrooms, and marjoram are staples in my Wisconsin home as they were in my mom's kitchen in Iowa where I grew up. How beautifully they combine in this German-inspired dish that is a pleasant change from rice for dinner, and it cooks up quickly, thanks to quick-cooking barley.

- 1 cup quick-cooking barley
- 1 tablespoon canola oil
- 1 large onion, chopped
- 2 ribs celery, chopped
- 1 green bell pepper, cut in julienne strips
- 1 red bell pepper, cut in julienne strips
- ½ pound fresh sliced mushrooms
- ½ teaspoon salt
- ½ teaspoon black pepper
- ¼ teaspoon sage
- ½ teaspoon marjoram
- ½ teaspoon basil, optional

Cook the barley as directed on the package.

Meanwhile, heat the oil in a large skillet over medium heat and brown the onion and celery. Add the peppers, mushrooms, and spices; stir. Cover and cook 10 minutes, or until the peppers and mushrooms are soft.

Stir in the cooked barley.

FOOD TRIVIA
Barley is a hardy grain that dates back to the Stone Age. It is used in breads, soups, and cereals.

NUTRITION PER SERVING	
Serving size	1½ cups
Calories	140 kcal
Fat	1 g
Saturated fat	0 g
Cholesterol	0 mg
Sodium	430 mg
Carbohydrates	30 g
Dietary fiber	8 g
Protein	6 g

Blackberry Cobbler

Beth Ebmeier, M.S., R.D., L.M.N.T.

Settlers traveling through Nebraska enjoyed blackberries and other wild berries. With the baking staples they carried, they might have baked a dish similar to this. Serve it for breakfast as well as for dessert. No matter where you live, you can make this cobbler all year with frozen blackberries.

Serves: 10
Hands-on time: 20 minutes
Baking time: 30 minutes

- vegetable oil cooking spray
- ¾ cup sugar, divided
- 3 tablespoons cornstarch
- ¼ cup cold water
- 1½ teaspoons ground cinnamon, divided
- 2 to 3 teaspoons grated orange peel, optional
- 2 16-ounce packages frozen unsweetened blackberries, or 2½ to 3 cups fresh berries
- ¾ cup whole wheat flour
- ¾ cup all-purpose flour
- 2 teaspoons baking powder
- ½ cup nonfat milk
- 3 tablespoons butter, melted

Preheat oven to 400°F. Coat a 2-quart casserole dish with the cooking spray.

Mix ½ cup sugar and the cornstarch in a 2-quart saucepan; stir in the cold water. Bring to a boil; reduce heat and cook, stirring constantly, until the mixture thickens. Remove from heat. Stir in 1 teaspoon cinnamon and the grated orange peel, if using.

Place the blackberries in the prepared casserole dish. Pour the warm sauce over the berries and stir; set aside.

Mix the flour, remaining ¼ cup sugar, baking powder, and remaining ¼ teaspoon cinnamon in a medium-size bowl. Stir in the milk and butter. The dough will be soft and sticky. Drop the dough by 8 spoonfuls onto the fruit mixture. Bake for 25 to 30 minutes or until the topping is golden brown.

SHOPPING TIP
Look for frozen blackberries packaged without added sugar.

COOK'S TIP
Store leftovers in the refrigerator. Microwave a portion for 1 minute to enjoy it hot.

NUTRITION PER SERVING

Serving size	1 cup
Calories	220 kcal
Fat	4 g
Saturated fat	2 g
Cholesterol	10 mg
Sodium	10 mg
Carbohydrates	46 g
Dietary fiber	6 g
Protein	4 g

Carrot Cake

Corrina Riemann, R.D.

Serves: 24
Hands-on time: 15 minutes
Baking time: 45 minutes

Here in Indiana, a hearty carrot cake is popular year-round as "company food." This recipe is so easy that you can make it for family dessert, and so healthy you can have it often.

vegetable oil cooking spray
3 cups grated carrots (4 to 6 large carrots)
1½ cups raisins
1½ cups nonfat plain yogurt
3 eggs, lightly beaten
¼ cup applesauce
⅓ cup canola oil
1 teaspoon vanilla extract
2 cups all-purpose flour
1½ cups granulated sugar
1½ teaspoons baking soda
2 teaspoons ground cinnamon
1 teaspoon ground nutmeg
1 teaspoon ground cloves
1 teaspoon ground allspice
1 teaspoon salt
1 cup chopped walnuts, optional

Preheat oven to 350°F. Coat a 13-by-9-inch pan with the cooking spray.

Stir together the carrots, raisins, yogurt, eggs, applesauce, oil, and vanilla; set aside.

Combine the flour, sugar, baking soda, cinnamon, nutmeg, cloves, allspice, and salt in a medium-size bowl. Add the dry ingredients to the wet; stir well. Stir in the nuts, if desired. Pour into the prepared pan. Bake for 45 minutes or until a toothpick inserted in the middle comes out clean.

If desired, frost with cream cheese icing, using this recipe:

½ cup reduced-fat cream cheese, at room temperature (4 ounces)
3 cups powdered sugar
2 teaspoons lemon juice
1 to 2 tablespoons nonfat milk

Combine all ingredients in a medium-size bowl and whip until smooth.

FOOD TRIVIA
Carrot cake supposedly originated in Scotland.

NUTRITION PER SERVING	
Serving size	1/24 of pan, without frosting
Calories	170 kcal
Fat	4 g
Saturated fat	0.5 g
Cholesterol	27 mg
Sodium	200 mg
Carbohydrates	32 g
Dietary fiber	1 g
Protein	3 g

NUTRITION PER SERVING	
Serving size	1/24 of pan, with frosting
Calories	260 kcal
Fat	8 g
Saturated fat	1.5 g
Cholesterol	30 mg
Sodium	220 mg
Carbohydrates	45 g
Dietary fiber	2 g
Protein	4 g

Apple Cake with Hot Coconut–Brown Sugar Topping

Donna Weihofen, R.D., M.S.

Pick a bag of fresh apples—in Wisconsin on a gorgeous fall day—or in your supermarket any day of the year. Just be sure and stir some into this cake that's perfect for company but healthy enough for breakfast.

Serves: 16
Hands-on time: 15 minutes
Baking time: 30 minutes

- vegetable oil cooking spray
- ¼ cup canola oil
- ½ cup fat-free vanilla yogurt
- ¾ cup sugar
- 1 large egg
- ½ teaspoon baking soda
- ½ teaspoon baking powder
- ½ teaspoon salt
- 1 teaspoon cinnamon
- ¼ teaspoon nutmeg
- ¼ teaspoon ginger
- 1 teaspoon vanilla extract
- 1¼ cups flour
- 3 medium-size unpeeled apples, chopped

TOPPING

- 3 tablespoons butter
- 3 tablespoons brown sugar
- 2 tablespoons nonfat milk
- 1 cup sweetened dried coconut
- 1 teaspoon cinnamon

Preheat oven to 325°F. Coat two 9-inch loaf pans with the cooking spray.

Combine the oil, yogurt, sugar, and egg in a large bowl. Beat well. Add the baking soda, baking powder, salt, cinnamon, nutmeg, ginger, and vanilla. Mix well. Stir in the flour, then the apples.

Spoon into the prepared pans. Bake for 30 minutes or until lightly brown and set in the middle.

While the cake is baking, combine the topping ingredients in a small saucepan. Heat over low heat until the butter is melted. When the cake is done, gently spread the topping evenly over the cake. Place the cake under the oven broiler and broil until the topping is bubbling and lightly browned.

COOK'S TIP

To freeze one loaf for later, cool one cake completely. Reserve half of the coconut mixture; freeze in a tightly sealed container. Spread the coconut mixture evenly over the cake after thawing; place under the broiler until hot and bubbly.

NUTRITION NUGGET

Substitute an equal quantity of spoonable sugar substitute for the sugar to reduce the calories.

NUTRITION PER SERVING	
Serving size	⅛ of one cake
Calories	160 kcal
Fat	7 g
Saturated fat	3.5 g
Cholesterol	15 mg
Sodium	150 mg
Carbohydrates	23 g
Dietary fiber	1 g
Protein	2 g

Bread Pudding with Bourbon Sauce

Michelle Plummer, M.S., R.D., C.D.

Serves: 18
Hands-on time: 30 minutes
Baking time: 1 hour

This recipe has been handed down a long chain of friends in Indiana, each one of us making it slightly better than the last.

½ cup chopped pecans, toasted
1 cup golden raisins
16 slices toasted whole-grain bread
2 cups egg substitute
2 teaspoons vanilla extract
1 teaspoon cinnamon
½ teaspoon mace or nutmeg
4 cups evaporated skim milk
¼ cup bourbon
Bourbon Sauce (recipe follows)

Preheat oven to 350°F.

Sprinkle nuts and raisins in the bottom of a 9-by-13-inch glass baking dish. Cut the toast slices into thirds and layer on top of the nuts and raisins.

Mix the egg substitute, vanilla, cinnamon, mace or nutmeg, milk, and bourbon together until well blended.

Pour the egg mixture over the bread and allow to stand for 30 minutes.

Fill a larger baking dish with 1 inch of hot water; place the pudding dish in the larger pan and bake for 1 hour. Remove and serve warm with Bourbon Sauce.

Bourbon Sauce

1 cup sugar
1 cup evaporated skim milk
2 tablespoons butter
2 tablespoons cornstarch
2 tablespoons bourbon

Combine the first 4 ingredients in a 1-quart mixing bowl and blend well. Microwave on high for 3 minutes. Stir and repeat. Stir in the bourbon. Ladle over the warm bread pudding just before serving.

VARIATIONS

Substitute an equal amount of walnuts for the pecans. For even more color, use a combination of golden and dark brown raisins.

NUTRITION PER SERVING	
Serving size	1⁄18 of pan
Calories	260 kcal
Fat	5 g
Saturated fat	1.5 g
Cholesterol	5 mg
Sodium	250 mg
Carbohydrates	39 g
Dietary fiber	2 g
Protein	12 g

Rhubarb Bread Pudding

Donna Weihofen, R.D., M.S.

Rhubarb comes in early in Wisconsin—sometimes in early May. We enjoy it in a wide variety of baked items and then freeze as much as we can to enjoy until the next spring.

Serves: 12
Hands-on time: 15 minutes
Baking time: 1 hour, 15 minutes

- vegetable oil cooking spray
- 2 cups nonfat milk
- 2 large eggs
- 1⅔ cups sugar
- 2 teaspoons vanilla extract
- ½ teaspoon nutmeg
- ½ teaspoon cinnamon
- 7 slices dry whole-grain bread, cubed
- 5 cups diced rhubarb, fresh or frozen (thawed)

Preheat oven to 350°F. Coat a 2-quart baking dish with the cooking spray.

In a large bowl, combine the milk, eggs, sugar, vanilla, nutmeg, and cinnamon. Beat well. Stir in the bread and rhubarb.

Pour into the prepared baking dish. Bake, uncovered, for 60 to 75 minutes, or until a knife inserted in the middle comes out clean. Using a spatula, press down on the bread a few times during the baking process.

SUBSTITUTIONS

Substitute ½ cup liquid egg substitute for the 2 large eggs. To reduce the calories, substitute ⅔ cup spoonable sugar replacement for ⅔ cup of the regular sugar (retain the remaining 1 cup regular sugar).

FOOD TRIVIA

Rhubarb is a vegetable, although it typically is used as a fruit.

NUTRITION PER SERVING	
Serving size	⅔ cup
Calories	190 kcal
Fat	1.5 g
Saturated fat	0 g
Cholesterol	35 mg
Sodium	120 mg
Carbohydrates	40 g
Dietary fiber	2 g
Protein	4 g

Microwave Chocolate Pudding

Beth Ebmeier, M.S., R.D., L.M.N.T.

Serves: 4
Hands-on time: 5 minutes
Cooking time: 7 minutes

There is no substitute for home-cooked pudding. The microwave eliminates the need to cook and stir the mixture constantly over the stove. Another bonus? Kids anywhere can make it for an after-school treat.

- 3 tablespoons cornstarch
- ⅓ cup sugar
- ½ cup semisweet chocolate chips
- 2 cups nonfat milk
- 1 teaspoon pure vanilla extract

Mix the cornstarch, sugar, and chocolate chips in a medium-size glass bowl; gradually stir in the milk.

Cook, uncovered, in a microwave on high, approximately 6 to 7 minutes, stirring every 2 minutes. Stir in the vanilla.

SUBSTITUTION

Replace the sugar with an equal amount of sugar substitute to reduce the calories by 40 and the carbohydrates by 12 grams.

VARIATION

To make butterscotch pudding, instead of granulated sugar, mix ½ cup plus 2 tablespoons packed brown sugar with the cornstarch and omit the chocolate chips.

NUTRITION PER SERVING	
Serving size	¾ cup
Calories	150 kcal
Fat	4.5 g
Saturated fat	2.5 g
Cholesterol	0 mg
Sodium	45 mg
Carbohydrates	28 g
Dietary fiber	Less than 1 g
Protein	3 g

NUTRITION PER SERVING	
Serving size	¾ cup, with sugar substitute
Calories	110 kcal
Fat	4.5 g
Saturated fat	2.5 g
Cholesterol	0 mg
Sodium	45 mg
Carbohydrates	16 g
Dietary fiber	Less than 1 g
Protein	3 g

Gooey Double Fudge Brownies

Kristine Napier, M.P.H., R.D.

Every cookbook has to have brownies. Who would have thought this all-American favorite was created accidentally as a result of a chocolate cake falling? Brownies get their name for their dark brown color. Yes, this Wisconsin version recipe uses black beans as a substitute for part of the fat. The surprising taste benefit is that they add excellent texture and so much moisture.

Serves: 9
Hands-on time: 10 minutes
Baking time: 25 minutes

vegetable oil cooking spray
1 cup granulated sugar
½ cup liquid egg substitute
⅓ cup cooked black beans, or drained and rinsed canned beans
¼ cup all-purpose flour
¼ cup whole wheat flour
¼ cup butter, melted
2 squares unsweetened baking chocolate, melted and stirred
2 tablespoons vanilla extract
¼ cup semisweet mini chocolate chips
1 tablespoon sifted powdered sugar

Preheat oven to 350°F. Spray a 9-by-9-inch pan with vegetable cooking spray.

Combine the sugar, egg substitute, and beans in a food processor; process until very smooth. Transfer the bean mixture to a medium-size mixing bowl. Stir in the flours, butter, and chocolate until smooth. Add the vanilla and chocolate chips; stir until smooth. Transfer the mixture to the baking pan.

Bake approximately 25 minutes; the middle should be slightly jiggly and wet when removed from the oven. Cool. Sprinkle with powdered sugar just before serving.

SUBSTITUTION

To reduce the calories, use ½ cup spoonable sugar substitute and ½ cup regular sugar in place of the 1 cup regular sugar.

NUTRITION PER SERVING	
Serving size	⅑ of pan
Calories	230 kcal
Fat	10 g
Saturated fat	6 g
Cholesterol	15 mg
Sodium	50 mg
Carbohydrates	34 g
Dietary fiber	2 g
Protein	3 g

Chocolate-Mandarin Ganache Layered Cake

Kristine Napier, M.P.H., R.D., and Linda Simon, R.D.

Serves: 16
Hands-on time: 20 minutes
Cooking time: 5 minutes (plus baking time if you bake angel food cake)
Chill time: 2 hours

Traditional ganache is a rich combination of semisweet chocolate and whipping cream that originated in nineteenth-century Europe. With subtle changes in the proportion of ingredients, as well as the addition of liqueurs, it has myriad uses from frostings to cake fillings to candy truffle centers. Here is a lightened-up version—from two Wisconsin neighbors—infused with orange-flavored liqueur to complement both the angel food cake and the chocolate.

- ½ cup nonfat milk
- 1 tablespoon corn syrup
- ½ cup liquid egg substitute
- 1 cup semisweet chocolate chips
- 3 tablespoons Grand Marnier, or 1 tablespoon vanilla extract and 2 tablespoons orange juice
- 1 tablespoon chopped orange zest, optional
- 1 angel food cake
- 2 cans (11 ounces, undrained weight) mandarin oranges in juice, drained and patted dry

Combine the milk and corn syrup in a heavy medium-size saucepan. Bring to a boil; boil 2 minutes, stirring constantly. Reduce heat; whisk in the egg substitute. Remove from heat; stir in the chocolate until it melts. Stir in the Grand Marnier and orange zest. Place the mixture in a container, cover loosely, and refrigerate at least 2 hours or overnight.

Slice the angel food cake crosswise into thirds. Spread ⅓ of the chocolate mixture on top of the bottom layer; top with a layer of mandarin oranges, placed close together. Drizzle a small amount of chocolate on top of the oranges.

Place the second layer of cake on top of the first layer. Repeat the chocolate-orange process; drizzle the top with chocolate.

Place the third layer on top of the second layer. Repeat the chocolate-orange process; drizzle the top with chocolate. Garnish the plate with the remaining oranges. Refrigerate or serve at once.

COOK'S TIP
Prepare ganache at least 2 to 3 hours before assembling the cake (or the day ahead).

NUTRITION PER SERVING

Serving size	1⁄16 of cake
Calories	140 kcal
Fat	3.5 g
Saturated fat	2 g
Cholesterol	0 mg
Sodium	180 mg
Carbohydrates	25 g
Dietary fiber	Less than 1 g
Protein	3 g

Angel Food Cake

Lynnette Jones, M.S., M.B.A., R.D.

Birthdays were never without my mother's melt-in-your-mouth angel food cake. It's still a favorite in our Illinois home. My mother made this favorite recipe often, and even kept at least one cake in the freezer just in case company dropped in. She was very particular about the pan being grease-free—she washed the pan at least three times before using. She also made sure that the dry ingredients were fluffed so the cake would be light and high, sifting the flour and sugar a minimum of six times.

Serves: 16
Hands-on time: 15 minutes
Baking time: 30 minutes
Cooling time: 2 hours

1¼ cups flour
1¾ cups sugar, divided
1½ cups egg whites (usually, whites from 13 large eggs)
3 teaspoons water
1¼ teaspoons cream of tartar
½ teaspoon salt
1 teaspoon vanilla extract

Preheat oven to 375°F.

Sift the flour and 1 cup sugar at least six times. Set aside.

Beat the egg whites and water until very foamy. Add the cream of tartar and salt to the egg whites and beat until soft peaks form. Beat the remaining ¾ cup sugar and vanilla into the egg white mixture until stiff peaks form.

Fold the flour mixture into the egg whites in four parts, using not more than 15 strokes per addition. Pour evenly into an ungreased angel food cake pan. Remove large air bubbles by slicing through the cake mixture in the pan. Bake for 30 minutes or until the top of the cake is golden brown and the cake springs back when touched.

Invert the cake immediately to cool upside down in its pan to prevent it from sinking. Cool for at least 2 hours. To remove the cake from the pan, gently free the cake from the sides and the center with a knife.

COOK'S TIP

This cake is so moist, it doesn't need frosting. But you could add a dollop of Lemon Sauce (page 414) or Wild Blueberry Sauce (page 62) if you choose.

NUTRITION PER SERVING	
Serving size	1/16 of cake
Calories	130 kcal
Fat	0 g
Saturated fat	0 g
Cholesterol	0 mg
Sodium	120 mg
Carbohydrates	30 g
Dietary fiber	0 g
Protein	4 g

Chunky (or Smooth) Microwave Applesauce

Kristine Napier, M.P.H., R.D.

Serves: 12
Hands-on time: 5 minutes
Cooking time: 7 to 10 minutes

There's nothing like fresh, hot applesauce to spoon on top of pancakes, to eat as a snack, or to have for dessert. Make it easy by not peeling the apples, which also lends more fiber. Make the applesauce to your liking by processing in the microwave as much or as little as you wish. In our Wisconsin home, we like the sauce chunky, and we especially love it when we start with a variety of apples.

- 4 medium-size unpeeled apples, cored and quartered
- 3 packed tablespoons brown sugar
- 1 teaspoon cinnamon
- 1 cup raisins, optional

Combine all the ingredients with 1 cup water in a microwave-safe dish. Stir well.

Microwave on high for 4 minutes. Stir. Microwave on high 3 minutes. The apples should be very soft. If not, microwave in 1-minute increments until soft.

Transfer to a food processor. Pulse just until the mixture reaches desired chunkiness. Serve hot or cold.

COOK'S TIP

Freeze extra applesauce in a tightly sealed container for up to two months; refrigerate up to five days.

NUTRITION PER SERVING	
Serving size	½ cup
Calories	80 kcal
Fat	0 g
Saturated fat	0 g
Cholesterol	0 mg
Sodium	10 mg
Carbohydrates	21 g
Dietary fiber	3 g
Protein	0 g

Frosty Strawberry Fruit Cups

Ingrid Gangestad, R.D., L.D.

One of my cardinal rules for entertaining is to make as much food ahead of time as possible. These fruit cups have become a do-ahead favorite for brunch and light meals. My kids also enjoy them instead of all-sugar ice pops for a frosty treat on a hot Minnesota summer day.

Serves: 20
Hands-on time: 25 minutes
Freezing time: 5 to 7 hours

- ¼ cup sugar
- ¼ cup lemon juice
- 1 6-ounce can frozen orange juice concentrate, thawed
- 1 10-ounce package frozen strawberries in syrup, thawed
- 2 cups sliced fresh strawberries
- 1 20-ounce can pineapple chunks in juice, undrained
- 6 ripe bananas, diced

Stir together the sugar, lemon juice, and orange juice concentrate in a large bowl.

Purée the frozen strawberries in a blender. Stir into the orange juice mixture. Stir in the fresh strawberries, pineapple, and bananas. Spoon into 20 4-ounce soufflé dishes; cover tightly with plastic wrap. Place the dishes in a 13-by-9-inch pan; place in the freezer for 5 to 7 hours, or until frozen.

Remove from the freezer; let stand 30 minutes before serving.

SHOPPING TIP

Disposable clear plastic soufflé cups or footed 4-ounce cups may be purchased at party supply stores.

SUBSTITUTIONS

Frozen raspberries in syrup make a great substitution for the strawberries. When fresh peaches are in season, use only 3 bananas and add 3 chopped fresh peeled peaches.

COOK'S TIPS

Once frozen, the cups can be combined into large sealed containers or bags and stored in the freezer for up to one month.

NUTRITION PER SERVING	
Serving size	1 soufflé cup or 1/20 of recipe
Calories	80 kcal
Fat	0 g
Saturated fat	0 g
Cholesterol	0 mg
Sodium	0 mg
Carbohydrates	21 g
Dietary fiber	2 g
Protein	1 g

Mango Lassi

Madhu Gadia, M.S., R.D., C.D.E.

Serves: 2
Hands-on time: 5 minutes

SUBSTITUTION
Omit the mango; substitute 1 to 2 tablespoons orange juice concentrate.

Lassi is a very popular drink in northern India, especially on a hot summer day. It tastes great on hot days in Iowa, too. When made with mangos, it has an especially refreshing flavor.

1 medium-size mango, peeled and cubed (about 1 cup)
1½ cups fat-free plain yogurt
4 to 6 ice cubes

Place all the ingredients in a blender with ½ cup cold water. Blend until frothy.

Pour into a tall glass and serve immediately.

NUTRITION PER SERVING	
Serving size	1½ cups
Calories	230 kcal
Fat	3 g
Saturated fat	2 g
Cholesterol	10 mg
Sodium	135 mg
Carbohydrates	43 g
Dietary fiber	2 g
Protein	10 g

6

TEX-MEX

Fusing Mexican-Texan and Mexican Cultures

Kristine Napier, M.P.H., R.D.

Birthed in the southernmost corner of what is now the United States, Tex-Mex cuisine fused Texan and Mexican cultures in the mid 1850s. Also called south-of-the-border and Mexican-style food, the Tex-Mex style of cooking has exploded in popularity.

Join us for a ride on the chuck wagon, one of the great symbols of the American cowboy, for a ride through Texas culinary corners. To be sure, poblano, cascabel, and other chilis are sure to be at every rest stop along the way!

Native American Influences

The vast land of Texas—occupying what is now 7 percent of the total area of the United States—was home to a vast diversity of Native American cultures. Many were hunters and gatherers, others farmers, and some both. Their command of the land and its resources paved the way for the next people to walk there. Some of the tribes and their connections to today's culinary atmosphere include:

TEJAS MEANS FRIEND

The early Spanish called a subgroup of the Caddos the Tejas, which eventually became the name of the state. In their tribal language, Tejas means friend.

- The Caddos, of east and northeast Texas, who were successful farmers. They taught the Europeans and Mexicans who followed them how to grow and cook with corn, as well as wild plants. Later, this area of Texas would prove to be a good place to grow wheat.
- The Karankawas, who lived along the Gulf Coast between what are now present Galveston and Corpus Christi, and harvested the fruits of the sea. Texans continue in this very early tradition, yearly harvesting more than 100 million pounds of shrimp, oysters, crabs, and finfish.
- The Coahuiltecan, who lived a sparse existence along the lower Rio Grand in the far south of Texas. Their recipes used the whole paddles or the pads of the prickly pear cactus (*nopalitos* or *nopales*, respectively). Roots and herbs were also important in their diet.
- The Patarabuyres, who farmed the area along more forgiving areas of the Rio Grand and the Apaches and had an important presence from west Texas into present New Mexico and Arizona.

The early Native Americans who migrated from Mexico and Central America into Texas brought their ancient, highly refined technique of making flat corn bread from ground maize. What the Spanish called tortilla, the Native Americans called *tlaxcalli* in the Nahuatl language. Many Texans still make fresh tortillas daily, to eat as bread, use as a plate, or fill to make one of many tortilla-based dishes. Corn bread, too, is a favorite.

Spanish Influences on Texas Food

In search of a shorter route to the Far East in the early sixteenth century, the Spanish explored Texas. They stopped there for some three hundred years, building missions and farming the land. The Spanish blended European foods with the native foods of the region: corn and oats, as well as wild cattle, hogs, and sheep. Flan, for example (Creamy Flan, page 344), traces at least one culinary root to Spain and Portugal, where, in turn, the love of this sweet, caramel-flavored custard is traced to the Moors and

FLAN IN ANCIENT ROME AND IN FIFTEENTH-CENTURY ITALY

The ancient Romans ate two types of flan: sweet and savory. Savory flan could have been made with eel, cheese, spinach, and/or fish; this was also a favorite during Lent in the Middle Ages when meat was forbidden. A mid-fifteenth-century cookbook, doubling as a health book, detailed the health benefits of custard dishes. A dish such as flan was thought to soothe the chest, aid the kidneys and liver, increase fertility, and eliminate urinary tract problems.

before that to the Romans. The word comes from the Old French *flaon* and from the Latin *flado*, both meaning "flat cake." The word *flan* in France and Spain is also used for an egg custard, which is made in a mold, turned out, and eaten cold.

Cattle farming, too, started with the Spanish. Texas cattle ranches were started on land given to Mexican families by the king of Spain. What we know today as Texas longhorns are descendents of wild cattle left by the Spanish in the early fifteenth century. They were the preferred breed for raising in the harsh Texas climate.

The Spanish first encountered the tomato after their conquest of Mexico in the early 1500s; there they learned that Aztec lords combined tomatoes with chili peppers and ground squash seeds for use as a condiment on turkey, venison, lobster, and fish. This combination was subsequently called "salsa."

Spanish cuisine dominated for their three hundred years of possession, but changed sharply when Mexico took control of the region in 1821. Politics affected the region in many ways, including culinary styles. The Mexican government encouraged people from the United States to settle in Texas, which brought the birth of Tex-Mex cuisine. "Northerners" brought chicken, potatoes, and other vegetables. Mexican chilis, blended with Spanish spices such as cumin, flavored the food, as it still does. Beans, in the Mexican tradition, became another staple. Tacos, guacamole (Guacamole, page 329), enchiladas (Squash Enchiladas, page 343), and tortillas (Tortilla Roll-Ups, page 327) became daily fare.

Of Chuck Wagons and Cowboys

After the Civil War, Texas cowboys began to drive cattle from Texas ranges to the Kansas railroad, where they could be shipped to the East Coast and even on to Europe. The cowboys worked from sunup to sundown, with no time for making food. The chuck wagon, originally designed by the Texas cattleman Charles Goodnight as a military supply wagon, rose to the occasion. In cowboy lingo "chuck" meant food; the chuck wagon was a kitchen on wheels. Its tailgate folded down to become a work station, revealing inside storage compartments.

The "cookie" or "coosie" was the chuck wagon's cook (from the Spanish word *cocinero*, meaning "male cook"). But he was much more; he was also the doctor, the barber, and the undertaker. While a cowhand earned a dollar a day, the cookie made twice that. Although the cookie was hired for his ability to drive the wagon and not his culinary skills (cookies were often older cowboys), he had to bring his cooking ability up to speed quickly. Cowboys were hungry, and good food was critical to their mood. A cowboy cuisine emerged, with chili (Texas Chili, page 337), stew, and barbecue at the top of the list.

Essential Tex-Mex Vocabulary

If you have trouble (as we do) understanding the difference between an enchilada and a flauta, you've come to the right place.

- Burrito: Top a flour tortilla with favorite ingredients, roll it up, and then tuck in the ends to make a burrito, which means "little burro" or donkey.
- Chimichanga: A deep-fried version of a burrito.
- Enchilada: Top a corn tortilla with meat, cheese, chili sauce, and/or chorizo sausage, roll it up, and you have an enchilada. The term means "filled with chili."
- Flauta: A white or yellow corn tortilla stuffed with beef, chicken, or pork, folded and then fried until crisp.
- Quesadillas: A flour or corn tortilla is folded in half around a filling (cheese, peppers, chorizo, and so forth) and then toasted or fried. Try our pan-toasted versions on pages 78, 342, and 437.
- Fajitas: Grilled steak, chicken, or fish rolled into a flour tortilla with grilled onions and/or peppers. Fajita comes from the Spanish *faja*, for girdle or strips, and describes the cut of meat itself.
- Tacos: The story of the taco begins with the story of corn and the art of making tacos. The Mexicans often made soft tacos as appetizers, topping fresh tortillas with cooked and shredded meat and then drizzling with a green or red sauce. While crisp taco shells were a Mexican invention, they aren't used as commonly there as they are in the United States today.
- Guacamole: Avocados were abundant in Peru, the Yucatan, and Mexico. The Incas, the Mayas, and the Aztecs, respectively, mashed avocados (with and without onions and tomatoes). The fat (monounsaturated) was extremely important to them nutritionally, as their diets contained little other fat. When the Europeans learned how to make guacamole, they fell into three camps when it came to seasoning: with salt, with sugar, or with both salt and sugar.
- Mole: In the Nahuatl language, mole means a concoction; indeed, this sauce is a mixture of many ingredients. Mole always starts with simmered chili peppers; in the seventeenth century a small amount of bitter chocolate was added.
- Refried beans aren't refried at all. First, pinto beans are boiled and then mashed and fried. *Frijoles refritos* means "well-fried beans." Try Tom 'n' Henry's Refried Beans on page 334.

Eggs Machaca

Elsa Ramirez Brisson, M.P.H., R.D.

In northern Mexico, eggs machaca was a very common breakfast among miners. They would take it to work in a small container with a flour tortilla on top to keep it warm. They made it with leftover roast beef, shredded finely by hand with two forks. This is a much faster version.

Serves: 4
Hands-on time: 15 minutes
Cooking time: 10 minutes

1 tablespoon canola oil
¼ to 1 jalapeño pepper, stem removed and minced
1 medium-size onion, chopped
4 ounces deli thin roast beef, chopped
1 medium-size tomato, chopped
1½ cups liquid egg substitute
8 corn tortillas, warmed

Combine the oil, pepper, onion, beef, and tomato in a large nonstick skillet over medium heat; sauté until the onion is wilted and golden.

Add the egg substitute and stir until the egg is cooked through.

Serve with the warmed tortillas.

COOK'S TIP

Wear gloves when working with peppers. The seeds and veins are the hottest part of jalapeños and other hot peppers. To adjust the heat, adjust how much of them you add to your recipe.

NUTRITION PER SERVING	
Serving size	¾ cup egg mixture and 2 tortillas
Calories	240 kcal
Fat	8 g
Saturated fat	1.5 g
Cholesterol	15 mg
Sodium	510 mg
Carbohydrates	22 g
Dietary fiber	3 g
Protein	20 g

Scrambled Salsa Egg Burritos

Kristine Napier, M.P.H., R.D.

Serves: 4
Hands-on time: 15 minutes
Cooking time: 10 minutes

Seasoned in the Mexican tradition, these breakfast burritos make their own salsa as they cook—saving you one step. They also make for easier eating because they aren't as messy.

- 3 cloves garlic, minced
- 5 green onions, finely chopped
- 1 tablespoon extra-virgin olive oil
- 1 medium-size green sweet bell pepper, finely chopped
- 1 medium-size tomato, chopped
- 1½ cups liquid egg substitute
- ¼ teaspoon salt
- ¼ to ½ teaspoon cayenne pepper
- black pepper to taste
- 4 8-inch flour tortillas

Sauté the garlic and onions in the oil over low heat until wilted, about 3 to 4 minutes, in a large nonstick skillet.

Add the pepper and tomato; cook 5 minutes over medium heat.

Add the egg substitute and stir until the eggs are cooked through.

Season with the salt, cayenne, and black pepper.

Place ¾ cup egg mixture in the middle of each tortilla and fold burrito style.

COOK'S TIP

To fold burrito style, fold up the bottom of the tortilla over the top of the egg mixture. Then fold one end and then the other end toward the middle.

NUTRITION PER SERVING	
Serving size	¾ cup egg mixture and 1 tortilla
Calories	280 kcal
Fat	10 g
Saturated fat	1.5 g
Cholesterol	0 mg
Sodium	570 mg
Carbohydrates	31 g
Dietary fiber	1 g
Protein	17 g

Tortilla Roll-Ups

Brenda Bracewell Valera, R.D.

Tortillas are popular in Texas at just about every meal. This appetizer version is sure to become a party favorite.

Serves: 12
Hands-on time: 20 minutes
Chill time: 4 to 24 hours

- 1 4½-ounce can chopped green chilis, or 1 fresh jalapeño pepper, chopped
- 1 medium-size red bell pepper, minced
- 1 medium-size green bell pepper, minced
- 1 carrot, grated
- 1 to 3 cloves garlic, minced
- 8 ounces light cream cheese, softened (1 cup)
- 4 ounces nonfat sour cream (½ cup)
- ½ teaspoon ground cumin
- ¼ teaspoon cayenne pepper
- 6 10-inch whole wheat or flavored tortillas
- salsa

Combine the chilis, bell peppers, carrot, and garlic in a medium-size bowl; mix well and set aside.

Combine the cream cheese, sour cream, cumin, and cayenne until well blended. Use a fork or a food processor. Fold the vegetable mixture into the cream cheese mixture. Spread the mixture evenly over the tortillas; roll tightly. Wrap in foil or plastic wrap and refrigerate at least 4 hours or up to 24 hours.

Slice each tortilla into 6 pieces. Serve with salsa.

COOK'S TIPS

Wear gloves when working with peppers. For a milder flavor, substitute Anaheim or ancho chilis. Removing the seeds also lessens the heat of chilis.

NUTRITION NUGGET

Salsa is low in calories, yet high in flavor and a wonderful way to add extra vegetables to your diet, especially corn, tomatoes, and onions. If substituting flavored tortillas in this recipe, check the fat content. Often extra fat is used to make the tortillas more pliable.

NUTRITION PER SERVING

Serving size	3 slices
Calories	80 kcal
Fat	1.5 g
Saturated fat	1 g
Cholesterol	5 mg
Sodium	320 mg
Carbohydrates	14 g
Dietary fiber	2 g
Protein	5 g

Tex-Mex Pita Crisps with Salsa and Guacamole

Melissa Stevens Ohlson, M.S., R.D., L.D.

Serves: 12
Hands-on time: 20 minutes
Cooking time: 12 minutes

You can't go wrong serving chips, salsa, and guacamole at a party. Here I've lightened up the festive fare with baked pita crisps instead of chips and stretched the guacamole with peas. This is a favorite party food among my heart patients.

vegetable oil cooking spray
6 whole wheat pita bread rounds, halved
2 tablespoons lime juice
1 tablespoon extra-virgin olive oil
1 teaspoon ground cumin
1 teaspoon chili powder
1 teaspoon garlic powder
½ teaspoon salt

Preheat oven to 400°F. Spray a large cookie sheet with the cooking spray.

Slice open each pita half at the seam. Spray both sides with the cooking spray. Arrange in a single layer, "inside" up, on the cookie sheet.

Combine the lime juice, olive oil, cumin, chili powder, garlic powder, and salt; spread evenly over the pita layers.

Bake for 10 to 12 minutes, or until the edges turn golden brown. Cool slightly, then break into chips.

NUTRITION PER SERVING	
Serving size	3 or 4 pita crisps
Calories	100 kcal
Fat	2 g
Saturated fat	0 g
Cholesterol	0 mg
Sodium	270 mg
Carbohydrates	18 g
Dietary fiber	3 g
Protein	3 g

Salsa

1 lime, peeled
2 cloves garlic
6 scallions
2 tablespoons canned sliced jalapeño pepper, seeded
2 tablespoons chopped fresh cilantro
2 large ripe tomatoes, chopped
2 teaspoons dried oregano
½ teaspoon salt
¼ teaspoon ground cumin
¼ teaspoon freshly ground black pepper

Mince the lime, garlic, scallions, jalapeño pepper, and cilantro; mix thoroughly. Add the tomatoes, oregano, salt, cumin, and pepper; mix well and serve. (If refrigerated, stir well before serving.)

NUTRITION PER SERVING	
Serving size	¼ cup salsa
Calories	10 kcal
Fat	0 g
Saturated fat	0 g
Cholesterol	0 mg
Sodium	125 mg
Carbohydrates	3 g
Dietary fiber	Less than 1 g
Protein	0 g

NUTRITION PER SERVING	
Serving size	3 tablespoons guacamole
Calories	35 kcal
Fat	2 g
Saturated fat	0 g
Cholesterol	0 mg
Sodium	0 mg
Carbohydrates	3 g
Dietary fiber	2 g
Protein	1 g

Guacamole

1 ripe avocado, peeled and quartered
½ cup frozen peas, thawed
2 to 3 cloves garlic
2 tablespoons lime juice
1 large tomato, chopped (reserve juice created from chopping)
½ cup minced red onion
¼ teaspoon Tabasco, or to taste

Place the avocado, peas, garlic, and lime juice in a food processor. Process until smooth. Stir in the chopped tomato and the juice, onion, and Tabasco.

Texas Caviar

Stephanie Green, R.D.

Serves: 8
Hands-on time: 15 minutes
Chill time: 30 minutes

This recipe brings back memories of all those backyard cookouts in the Lone Star State. While all the barbecue meats are a-cookin' up on the grill, this dish is a refreshing way to help beat the heat during those summer gatherings.

2 15-ounce cans black beans, drained and rinsed
4 tomatoes, chopped
2 stalks celery, finely diced
1 large sweet onion, finely diced (about 1 cup)
1 cup mild picante sauce
1 cup finely minced fresh cilantro
1 jalapeño pepper, finely diced
1 tablespoon lemon juice
½ teaspoon salt
4 green onions, chopped, optional, for garnish
1 avocado, thinly sliced, optional, for garnish

Combine all the ingredients except the optional garnish in a large bowl. Mix well. Refrigerate 30 minutes before serving.

Garnish with the green onions and avocado slices, if desired.

SHOPPING TIPS

If you can't find sweet onions, such as Vidalia, Walla Walla, or the Grand Canyon, use a red onion. If you'd like to spice up this recipe, use your favorite medium to hot picante sauce. If you need to lower the sodium, choose no-salt-added canned tomatoes.

NUTRITION PER SERVING

Serving size	1 cup with garnishes
Calories	170 kcal
Fat	4.5 g
Saturated fat	0.5 g
Cholesterol	0 mg
Sodium	750 mg
Carbohydrates	25 g
Dietary fiber	9 g
Protein	8 g

Lone Star Caviar

Barbara J. Pyper, M.S., R.D., C.D., F.H.C.F.A., F.C.S.I.

Texans insist that eating Lone Star Caviar on New Year's Day is good luck. I serve this northerner's version all year in Seattle because my guests love it, and I am proud to serve such a nutrition-packed dip.

Serves: 8
Hands-on time: 20 minutes

2 15-ounce cans black-eyed peas, drained and rinsed
1 medium-size red bell pepper, trimmed, seeded, and cut into ¼-inch dice
½ medium-size red or yellow onion, cut into ¼-inch dice
2 green onions, thinly sliced
2 jalapeño peppers, trimmed, seeded, and finely diced, or ⅓ cup canned jalapeño slices, finely diced
3 to 4 cloves garlic, minced
½ teaspoon hot pepper sauce, optional
½ cup reduced-fat Italian salad dressing
½ teaspoon salt, or to taste

Mix the black-eyed peas, peppers, onion, green onion, and garlic. Add the hot pepper sauce and salad dressing; toss lightly. Add salt to taste and stir. Refrigerate until ready to serve.

VARIATION
For additional color in this dip, try adding other types of beans or some frozen corn.

SERVING SUGGESTION
This dip is great served with baked corn chips or baked pita chips.

NUTRITION NUGGET
Black-eyed peas are a good source of protein and fiber.

NUTRITION PER SERVING	
Serving size	½ cup
Calories	110 kcal
Fat	2 g
Saturated fat	0 g
Cholesterol	0 mg
Sodium	590 mg
Carbohydrates	18 g
Dietary fiber	4 g
Protein	6 g

Thai Green Beans in Coconut Milk

Barbara Gollman, R.D.

Serves: 4
Hands-on time: 23 minutes
Cooking time: 15 minutes

It's no secret that Texans love fiery food and this fills a need for spicy veggies. Fresh lemongrass is often found in Asian stores, and the search is well worth the effort. These beans are so flavorful that you may never want traditional green bean casserole again.

4 cups (about 1 pound) small green beans, cut into 2-inch lengths
vegetable oil cooking spray
½ cup chopped red bell pepper
2 tablespoons chopped lemongrass, or grated lemon peel
3 to 4 cloves garlic, minced
1 to 2 teaspoons Thai red or green curry paste
½ cup diced onion
1 cup low-fat unsweetened coconut milk
¼ cup water
1 to 2 tablespoons Thai fish sauce
½ cup sliced fresh basil and/or mint leaves

Steam the green beans for about 10 minutes or until barely tender (or cook, covered, 6 to 8 minutes on high in a microwave); set aside.

Coat a large skillet with the cooking spray and heat over medium-high heat. Add the red bell pepper, lemongrass, garlic, and curry paste; cook and stir until the mixture begins to stick. Add 2 tablespoons water, reduce heat, and simmer, covered, 2 minutes, adding water as necessary.

Stir in the onion; cover and cook for another 2 minutes. Add the coconut milk and water. Simmer, covered, for 2 to 3 minutes. Add the green beans and stir well. Cook, covered, 4 minutes or until the beans are tender. Stir in the fish sauce and basil.

SHOPPING TIPS
Look for lemongrass, curry paste, and Thai fish sauce in the ethnic food section of many supermarkets or an Asian food store. You can also order them online.

SERVING SUGGESTION
Team the beans with blackened fish, seared tuna, or grilled shrimp and brown rice.

NUTRITION PER SERVING

Serving size	1 cup
Calories	60 kcal
Fat	0.5 g
Saturated fat	0 g
Cholesterol	0 mg
Sodium	390 mg
Carbohydrates	13 g
Dietary fiber	5 g
Protein	3 g

Pepito (Jicama) Salad

Angela M. Kirke, R.D., L.D.

Just south of the Texan border jicama is prized for its sweet taste and delicate crunch. Teamed up with the seasoning in this recipe, it makes an out-of-the ordinary salad.

Serves: 6
Hands-on time: 10 minutes
Standing time: 30 minutes

1 tablespoon extra-virgin olive oil
½ cup lime juice
3 tablespoons granulated sugar
¼ to ½ teaspoon cayenne pepper
½ teaspoon salt
1 medium-size jicama, peeled
1 medium-size red bell pepper, minced
½ cup minced fresh parsley

Combine the oil, lime juice, sugar, cayenne, and salt in a large bowl; stir. Set aside.

Chop the jicama and add to the juice mixture (this will prevent browning). Add the pepper and parsley; stir well.

Let stand at room temperature for 30 minutes before serving. Alternatively, make a day ahead and store, covered tightly, in the refrigerator.

VARIATION

Peel the jicama and cut into 2-inch-long thin strips. Marinate in a combination of the remaining ingredients (except the red bell pepper). Serve as an appetizer.

NUTRITION PER SERVING

Serving size	1 cup
Calories	100 kcal
Fat	2.5 g
Saturated fat	0 g
Cholesterol	0 mg
Sodium	200 mg
Carbohydrates	19 g
Dietary fiber	6 g
Protein	1 g

Tom 'n' Henry's Refried Beans

Linda Ferber, M.S., R.D.

Serves: 4
Hands-on time: 6 minutes
Cooking time: 12 minutes

The story of this recipe is almost as good as the taste. Henry's mother was from Guatemala and she married a guy from Mexico who had a ton of relatives. She cooked a lot for the family and made her beans from scratch. But one day, Henry discovered that you could buy the plain pinto beans already cooked, and with a little seasoning have beans ready in no time that were almost as good as his mother's. Henry's friend Tom found that the recipe was equally good when made with black beans.

SHOPPING TIP
Look for Mexican brands of pinto or black beans for authentic flavor.

- 1 teaspoon olive oil
- 1 large or 2 medium-size cloves garlic, minced
- 2 15-ounce cans pinto or black beans, undrained
- ⅛ teaspoon salt, optional
- ⅛ teaspoon ground black pepper

SERVING SUGGESTION
For a quick and satisfying Mexican-flavored meal, buy a whole cooked rotisserie chicken at the market. Cook up a batch of these beans and serve with the heated chicken, fresh salsa, chopped cilantro, and fresh, warm tortillas.

Heat the olive oil in a 10-inch frying pan over medium heat. Add the garlic and sauté for 2 to 3 minutes. Raise the heat to medium-high and gradually add the liquid from the beans, stirring each time until the mixture thickens, about 6 to 7 minutes.

Add 1 can of beans and mash with a wooden spoon. Add the second can of beans, stirring gently.

Cook until blended, about 3 minutes. Season with the salt and pepper. The beans may thicken slightly upon standing. To reheat, add 1 to 2 tablespoons of water if needed.

NUTRITION PER SERVING	
Serving size	½ cup
Calories	200 kcal
Fat	3 g
Saturated fat	0.5 g
Cholesterol	0 mg
Sodium	700 mg
Carbohydrates	33 g
Dietary fiber	10 g
Protein	10 g

Pecan and Sausage Stuffing

Barbara Gollman, R.D.

Southerners, which we sometimes call ourselves here in Texas, favor pecans in our stuffing, while Italians prefer sausage. This recipe transcends culinary boundaries and is excellent in its own right.

Serves: 12
Hands-on time: 10 to 20 minutes
Baking time: 35 to 45 minutes

- olive oil cooking spray
- 1½ cups chopped celery
- 1½ cups chopped onion
- 1 jalapeño pepper, finely minced
- 12 ounces turkey Italian sausage, or other reduced-fat sausage, casing removed
- 3 egg whites
- 1 egg
- 1 to 1½ cups fat-free milk, divided
- 2 to 2½ cups fat-free chicken broth, divided
- 6 fresh sage leaves, finely minced or 1 teaspoon dried sage
- 2 teaspoons poultry seasoning
- ½ teaspoon salt, or to taste
- ¼ teaspoon ground black pepper, or to taste
- 1 14-ounce package dried bread cubes
- 1 6-ounce package corn bread stuffing mix, with seasoning packet, if provided
- 1 14-ounce can mushroom pieces, drained
- ½ cup chopped toasted pecans

Coat a large skillet with the cooking spray. Add the celery, onion, and jalapeño pepper. Cook over medium heat, covered, stirring occasionally. When the vegetables are soft, remove from the skillet and set aside. (This can be done one day in advance and refrigerated).

In the same skillet, crumble the sausage and slowly cook until no longer pink. Use a fork to break the sausage into very small pieces.

Beat the egg whites and the egg with ¾ cup milk and 1 cup chicken broth. Add the sage, poultry seasoning, salt, and pepper.

FOOD TRIVIA
The pecan became the state tree of Texas in 1919. Pecan culture was taught at Texas A&M beginning in 1909.

COOK'S TIPS
Vegetables may be sautéed a day ahead. The ingredients may be combined early and refrigerated till ready to bake. This stuffing recipe freezes very well. Enjoy it later with pork chops or baked chicken.

NUTRITION PER SERVING

Serving size	1⁄12 of pan
Calories	260 kcal
Fat	8 g
Saturated fat	1.5 g
Cholesterol	25 mg
Sodium	870 mg
Carbohydrates	35 g
Dietary fiber	3 g
Protein	12 g

Pecan and Sausage Stuffing *(continued)*

In a large mixing bowl, layer the bread cubes, corn bread mix, cooked vegetables, sausage, mushrooms, and pecans. Add the egg mixture and mix gently, using gloved hands. Continue to add milk and broth until the mixture is quite moist, but not mushy. (This can be done several hours in advance.) Cover and refrigerate.

Preheat oven to 350°F. Coat a 9-by-13-inch baking dish with the cooking spray and add the stuffing. Spray the top with cooking spray before baking. Bake 35 to 45 minutes, until the top is brown and the center is firm.

FOOD TRIVIA

Stuffing in the Middle Ages was known as farce, from the Latin *farcire* (and French *farcir*) meaning to stuff. It was also called forcemeat when chopped meat was used in the mix. In the late nineteenth century, the Victorian upper class did not like the term *stuffing*, and so they called it dressing. While the terms are interchangeable today, people in the South and East prefer the term dressing. In literature, the term *farce* originally denoted a brief, lighthearted play "stuffed" in between acts of a religious play to keep the audience from being bored.

Texas Chili

Stephanie Green, R.D.

Nothing sticks to your ribs like a hearty bowl of Texas chili. It's sure to warm you up on a chilly night!

Serves: 4
Hands-on time: 20 minutes
Cooking time: 40 minutes

1 teaspoon canola oil
1 large white onion, diced (1 cup)
1 pound extra-lean ground beef
2 cloves garlic, minced
2 tablespoons tomato paste
1 14½-ounce can diced tomatoes
1 15-ounce can pinto beans, drained and rinsed
2 tablespoons dark chili powder
1 tablespoon ground coriander
2 teaspoons ground cumin
1 tablespoon paprika
¼ teaspoon crushed red pepper flakes
½ teaspoon kosher salt
¼ teaspoon freshly ground black pepper
1 teaspoon balsamic vinegar
½ cup coffee
1 red onion, finely chopped, optional, for garnish
4 green onions, finely chopped, optional, for garnish

Heat the oil in a large saucepan over medium-high heat. Add the onion and sauté for about 5 minutes. Mix the beef and garlic with the onion. Cook for an additional 5 minutes, stirring frequently until the beef is cooked.

Stir the tomato paste into the mixture and cook for a couple of minutes, mixing well. Stir the tomatoes, with their liquid, and the pinto beans into the mixture. Add the chili powder, coriander, cumin, paprika, red pepper flakes, salt, pepper, and vinegar. Mix well to incorporate the spices into the meat and cook for about 2 minutes.

Reduce heat to simmer. Add the coffee and continue to cook for about 30 to 40 minutes.

Garnish with the diced red onion or chopped green onions, if desired.

SERVING SUGGESTION

For a great presentation, serve the chili in a 6-inch cast-iron skillet with a side of corn bread.

COOK'S TIP

Freeze the leftover tomato paste in a zip-top plastic bag and break off sections for future recipes.

NUTRITION PER SERVING	
Serving size	1¼ cups
Calories	370 kcal
Fat	14 g
Saturated fat	4.5 g
Cholesterol	40 mg
Sodium	810 mg
Carbohydrates	33 g
Dietary fiber	11 g
Protein	31 g

King Ranch Casserole

Brenda Bracewell Valera, R.D.

Serves: 8
Hands-on time: 10 minutes
Baking time: 1 hour

The advent of casseroles made with canned soups in the 1940s and 1950s liberated the lady of the house. Such dishes were considered the height of space-age cuisine—they could not only be made quickly, but they could be frozen for later use. The secret of the Texan staple King Ranch Casserole, say Texans, is that it is boring. Boring? Food writers insist that this creamy, gentle food is the snuggliest of comfort foods.

- vegetable oil cooking spray
- 1 pound boneless, skinless chicken breast, cooked and cubed
- 1 10½-ounce can reduced-sodium cream of chicken soup
- 1 10-ounce can stewed tomatoes with green chilis
- 1 8-ounce container reduced-fat sour cream
- 1 medium-size onion, chopped
- 1 green bell pepper, finely chopped
- 2 ribs celery, finely chopped
- 3 cloves garlic, minced
- 1 teaspoon ground cumin, optional
- 12 6-inch corn tortillas
- 2 cups grated sharp cheddar cheese, divided (8 ounces)

Preheat oven to 350°F. Coat a 13-by-9-inch baking dish with the cooking spray.

Combine the chicken, soup, tomatoes, sour cream, onion, pepper, celery, garlic, and cumin in a large bowl. Mix well.

Place 6 tortillas in the bottom of the prepared dish; they will overlap. Spoon half of the chicken mixture over the tortillas evenly. Sprinkle with 1 cup cheese. Top with the remaining tortillas, which will overlap. Spoon the remaining mixture on top; sprinkle with the remaining cheese.

Cover and bake 45 minutes. Uncover and bake an additional 15 minutes, or until the cheese bubbles and is lightly golden.

VARIATION

Use a combination of Monterey Jack and cheddar, or all Monterey Jack for a different flair.

COOK'S TIPS

Use your leftovers: Chop leftover chicken or turkey for use in this casserole. To spice it up, add chopped hot chilis and/or cayenne pepper.

NUTRITION PER SERVING	
Serving size	1½ cups
Calories	390 kcal
Fat	18 g
Saturated fat	10 g
Cholesterol	90 mg
Sodium	690 mg
Carbohydrates	28 g
Dietary fiber	3 g
Protein	29 g

West Texas Chipotle Chicken Salad Wrap

Lori A. Miller, R.D., L.D.

This trendy southwestern style of chicken salad is a snap made with supermarket rotisserie chickens. Make this the day before serving and let the flavors meld. Wrap in tortillas or serve on a bed of lettuce.

Serves: 6
Hands-on time: 15 minutes

- ½ cup reduced-fat mayonnaise
- ¼ cup light sour cream
- 2 tablespoons fresh lime juice
- 1 jalapeño pepper, seeded and minced
- ½ teaspoon diced chipotle pepper
- ¼ teaspoon salt, optional
- 3 cups cooked chicken, cut in ¾-inch cubes
- 1 cup chopped tomato
- 1 avocado, peeled and chopped
- 3 tablespoons chopped fresh cilantro
- 6 flour tortillas

Combine the mayonnaise, sour cream, lime juice, jalapeño, chipotle peppers, and salt in large mixing bowl.

Place the chicken, tomato, avocado, and cilantro in a bowl with the mayonnaise mixture and toss lightly to coat. Top each of the 6 tortillas evenly with the chicken mixture. Roll.

SHOPPING TIP
The chipotle, a dried roasted jalapeño pepper, is also available in powdered form.

SERVING SUGGESTIONS
This filling can serve as a cold entrée, a wrap sandwich filling, or a tasty pasta salad (add 2 cups cooked orzo and increase the seasonings to taste).

NUTRITION PER SERVING	
Serving size	1 tortilla and ⅙ of chicken mixture
Calories	480 kcal
Fat	20 g
Saturated fat	4 g
Cholesterol	65 mg
Sodium	820 mg
Carbohydrates	48 g
Dietary fiber	4 g
Protein	28 g

Grilled Chicken Fajitas

Josephine Totten, R.D.

Serves: 6
Hands-on time: 15 minutes
Marinating time: 6 to 24 hours
Cooking time: 8 to 10 minutes

Fajitas make terrific party food. This simple marinade for south-of-the-border-inspired fajitas is packed with punch! Marinate the chicken and peppers up to twenty-four hours before serving. Then, set out bowls of salsa, light sour cream, shredded cheese, and chopped fresh cilantro for the buffet table. Heat some tortillas and let your guests serve themselves.

- 1 12-ounce can beer or nonalcoholic beer
- 2 to 6 tablespoons of tequila, optional
- juice of 1½ limes
- 1 teaspoon black pepper
- 1 pound boneless, skinless chicken breasts, sliced into ½-inch strips
- 2 medium-size green bell peppers, thinly sliced
- 1 medium-size yellow bell pepper, thinly sliced
- 1 medium-size red bell pepper, thinly sliced
- 1 onion, chopped
- 2 tablespoons canola oil
- 6 10-inch flour tortillas

Combine the beer, tequila (if using), lime juice, and pepper in a 3-quart glass or plastic container. Stir in the chicken, peppers, and onion. Marinate, covered, in the refrigerator at least 6 hours or up to 24 hours.

Heat the oil in a large pan or grill pan over medium-high heat. Stir-fry the chicken and peppers until the chicken is cooked through and the peppers are slightly browned and soft. Divide the mixture evenly among the 6 tortillas.

SERVING SUGGESTION

Set out bowls of chopped green peppers, reduced-fat sour cream and/or salsa for garnishes.

NUTRITION PER SERVING

Serving size	1 fajita
Calories	360 kcal
Fat	7 g
Saturated fat	2 g
Cholesterol	40 mg
Sodium	380 mg
Carbohydrates	49 g
Dietary fiber	4 g
Protein	23 g

Chuck Wagon Casserole

Melissa Stevens Ohlson, M.S., R.D., L.D.

This Tex-Mex casserole is certain to be a staple in many homes—not only is the flavor high yet gentle enough for most palates, but it's also a great complete meal in one dish. It freezes well, so don't hesitate to make a double batch to have a couple of quick meals on hand. Freeze it in squares to help with portion size.

Serves: 6
Hands-on time: 25 minutes
Cooking time: 30 minutes

vegetable oil cooking spray
½ pound extra-lean ground beef
1 large onion, minced
1 to 3 cloves garlic, minced
1 medium-size red bell pepper, chopped
1 medium-size green bell pepper, chopped
2 tablespoons lime juice
1 teaspoon ground cumin
½ to 1 teaspoon cayenne pepper
1 teaspoon dried basil
1 14½-ounce can no-salt-added diced tomatoes
1 15-ounce can ranch-style black beans
12 6-inch corn tortillas
1½ cups shredded Mexican-style cheese blend or sharp shredded cheddar cheese (6 ounces)

Preheat oven to 350°F.

Coat a large nonstick skillet with the cooking spray; add the beef, onion, and garlic. Sauté over medium-high heat 5 to 7 minutes or until the meat is browned.

Remove the pan from heat; stir in the bell peppers, lime juice, cumin, cayenne, basil, tomatoes, and beans.

Coat a 13-by-9-inch baking dish with the cooking spray; line the bottom of the dish with 6 tortillas. Spoon the beef mixture over the tortillas; cover with the remaining tortillas. Top with the cheese and bake for 30 minutes or until the cheese is melted and the filling is bubbly.

SUBSTITUTION

Use a desired amount of a southwest spice mix in place of the cumin, cayenne, and basil.

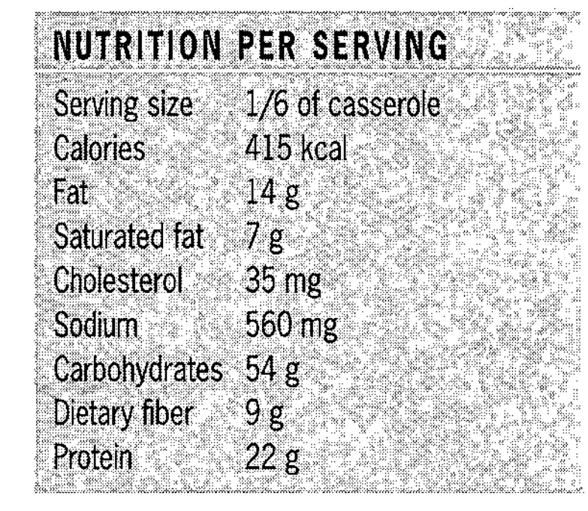

NUTRITION PER SERVING	
Serving size	1/6 of casserole
Calories	415 kcal
Fat	14 g
Saturated fat	7 g
Cholesterol	35 mg
Sodium	560 mg
Carbohydrates	54 g
Dietary fiber	9 g
Protein	22 g

Easy Cheesy Beef Quesadillas

Laura Faler Thomas, M.Ed., R.D., L.D.

Serves: 6 as a main course or 12 as an appetizer
Hands-on time: 10 minutes
Cooking time: 10 minutes

Southwest inspired, these quesadillas take on flavors from around the world—starting in Philadelphia and into the Mediterranean. They require little time in the kitchen, so plan them for busy nights, or serve them as party appetizers and impress the most discerning palate.

- ½ pound extra-lean ground beef
- 1 small zucchini, chopped
- 1 16-ounce can fat-free refried beans
- 6 10-inch flour tortillas
- ½ cup shredded sharp cheddar cheese, and/or Colby or Jack cheese (2 ounces)
- ½ cup salsa
- 1 medium-size tomato, chopped
- 1 medium-size green bell pepper, chopped

Cook the beef and zucchini in a large nonstick skillet over medium-high heat 5 to 7 minutes. Stir in the refried beans; cook 4 minutes or until heated through. Remove the beef mixture from the skillet; do not wash the pan.

Spread ⅓ of the mixture evenly over each of 3 tortillas. Sprinkle evenly with cheese. Top each with another tortilla. Cook each quesadilla in the skillet over medium-high heat for 1 minute per side or until the cheese is melted. Cut each into 4 wedges; serve with the salsa, chopped tomato, and pepper.

VARIATION

Make your own refried beans by mashing 1¼ cups black or pinto beans with your favorite spices, such as cumin and cayenne.

NUTRITION PER SERVING	
Serving size	2 wedges, main course
Calories	420 kcal
Fat	12 g
Saturated fat	2 g
Cholesterol	10 mg
Sodium	820 mg
Carbohydrates	54 g
Dietary fiber	6 g
Protein	20 g

NUTRITION PER SERVING	
Serving size	1 wedge, appetizer
Calories	210 kcal
Fat	6 g
Saturated fat	2 g
Cholesterol	10 mg
Sodium	410 mg
Carbohydrates	27 g
Dietary fiber	3 g
Protein	10 g

Squash Enchiladas

Taiga Sudakin, R.D., L.D.

Squash in Mexican enchiladas? Indeed! This recipe will please even those members of your family who say they don't like squash.

Serves: 6
Hands-on time: 25 minutes
Baking time: 15 minutes

vegetable oil cooking spray
1 12-ounce package frozen winter squash, thawed
¼ teaspoon allspice
1 19-ounce can enchilada sauce, divided
12 6-inch corn tortillas
1 medium-size onion, diced
1½ cups shredded sharp cheddar cheese, divided (6 ounces)

Preheat oven to 450°F. Coat a 9-by-13-inch baking dish with the cooking spray.

Combine the squash and allspice in a medium-size bowl; stir well.

Pour ½ cup enchilada sauce on a plate and ½ cup in the prepared baking pan; spread evenly over the bottom of the pan.

Soak 1 corn tortilla in the sauce on the plate for 30 seconds or until both sides are coated. Remove the tortilla from the sauce and place on a clean plate. Place 1 tablespoon squash, 2 teaspoons onion, and 1 tablespoon cheese in the center of the tortilla. Roll up, burrito-style, and place in the baking pan, seam side down. (The tortilla may split, but it will not matter after the enchiladas are baked.) Repeat this process until all tortillas are filled and placed in the pan.

Cover the enchiladas with the remaining sauce; sprinkle with the remaining cheese. Bake, uncovered, 15 minutes or until the cheese is melted and bubbly.

SUBSTITUTION

Make it from scratch by substituting 1 small butternut squash, cooked and mashed, for the frozen squash.

VARIATION

If you like it spicier, stir cayenne into the squash.

NUTRITION PER SERVING	
Serving size	1/12 of recipe
Calories	150 kcal
Fat	6 g
Saturated fat	2.5 g
Cholesterol	15 mg
Sodium	390 mg
Carbohydrates	20 g
Dietary fiber	2 g
Protein	6 g

NUTRITION PER SERVING	
Serving size	1/6 of recipe
Calories	300 kcal
Fat	12 g
Saturated fat	5 g
Cholesterol	30 mg
Sodium	780 mg
Carbohydrates	40 g
Dietary fiber	5 g
Protein	12 g

Creamy Flan

Maria C. Alamo, M.P.H., R.D., L.D.

Serves: 8
Hands-on time: 20 minutes
Cooking time: 1 hour
Cooling time: 30 minutes
Chill time: overnight

*My abuelo (grandmother) and I share a love for my mother's flan. I have fond memories of sitting around our kitchen table with grandma and my mother, Blanca. We would eat, talk, and celebrate our lives together. Since becoming a dietitian, I adapted her flan recipe by using lower-fat ingredients. The result is a creamy, velvety flan that is just as tasty!*1 12-ounce can fat-free evaporated milk

- ¾ cup plus 1 cup sugar
- 1 12-ounce can fat-free evaporated milk
- ¾ cup fat-free (skim) milk
- 5 large eggs
- 1 teaspoon vanilla extract
- pinch salt
- 1 teaspoon rum, optional

To caramelize the mold, heat ¾ cup sugar and ½ cup water in a small, heavy, flat-bottomed saucepan on medium-high heat until the syrup turns golden brown. Carefully remove from heat and quickly pour the caramel into a 1-quart flan mold or deep 8- or 9-inch round mold, tilting to evenly coat the bottom and about ½ inch up the sides. Set aside.

Preheat oven to 350°F.

Place the milks, eggs, 1 cup sugar, vanilla, salt, and rum (if using) in a blender container. Cover and blend until just mixed. Strain the mixture through a fine sieve, if desired. Pour the mixture into the caramelized mold. Cover with foil, being careful to keep the foil off the liquid surface. Place the mold in a 13-by-9-by-2-inch baking pan. Add hot water to the pan to come up to half the height of the mold.

Bake for 1 hour or until a knife inserted 1 to 2 inches from the center comes out clean (the center will be wiggly and continue to cook out of the oven). Carefully remove the mold from the water; loosen the foil to vent steam, but keep the flan covered. Cool 30 minutes to room temperature. Refrigerate until the flan is well chilled, preferably overnight.

To serve, run a thin knife around the mold edges to loosen. Holding the sides of the mold, gently shake in circular motion back and forth to loosen the flan from the bottom. Place a

SUBSTITUTION

Substitute one 14-ounce can sweetened condensed milk for 1 cup sugar in the mix.

COOK'S TIP

Avoid under- or overcooking the caramel. A light caramel lacks flavor. Caramel continues to darken after removal from heat.

NUTRITION PER SERVING	
Serving size	½ cup
Calories	210 kcal
Fat	0 g
Saturated fat	0 g
Cholesterol	0 mg
Sodium	65 mg
Carbohydrates	50 g
Dietary fiber	0 g
Protein	4 g

serving platter, larger in diameter, over the mold. Holding both together, quickly and gently turn over the mold onto the platter. Allow melted caramel from the mold to bathe the flan. Cut into 8 portions.

Vanilla-Cinnamon Atole

Elsa Ramirez Brisson, M.P.H., R.D.

Serves: 4
Hands-on time: 5 minutes
Cooking time: 10 minutes

This gentle drink is made from a surprising combination of ingredients. We bet the first taste will surprise you with its texture, but with the second taste, this may just become your favorite comfort food. Atole is an ancient Mexican soup and, when thinned (as in this recipe), a hot drink. We've also created a chocolate version—not to be missed!

2 cups nonfat milk
⅓ cup Masa Harina (stone-ground golden cornmeal flour)
2 cinnamon sticks, each broken into 2 pieces
1 teaspoon vanilla extract
⅓ cup plus 1 tablespoon dark brown sugar

Combine the milk and 2 cups water in a heavy medium-size saucepan. Sprinkle in the Masa Harina while whisking; whisk until smooth.

Add the cinnamon stick pieces.

Cook over low heat (the mixture should just barely bubble) for 10 minutes, whisking frequently.

Remove from heat. Stir in the vanilla and sugar. Remove the cinnamon stick pieces.

Serve in a mug.

VARIATION

To make chocolate milk, stir in 3 tablespoons unsweetened cocoa powder.

COOK'S TIP

Other uses for Masa Harina include making tortillas. You can also freeze it for long-term keeping.

NUTRITION PER SERVING	
Serving size	⅔ cup
Calories	170 kcal
Fat	0.5 g
Saturated fat	0 g
Cholesterol	0 mg
Sodium	85 mg
Carbohydrates	35 g
Dietary fiber	Less than 1 g
Protein	6 g

NUTRITION PER SERVING	
Serving size	with unsweetened cocoa powder
Calories	180 kcal
Fat	1 g
Saturated fat	0.5 g
Cholesterol	0 mg
Sodium	85 mg
Carbohydrates	38 g
Dietary fiber	2 g
Protein	7 g

7

SOUTHWESTERN CUISINE

Meso-American Roots Fuse with Trendy Cuisine

Kristine Napier, M.P.H., R.D.

Picture a long string of bright red, fresh chilis tied together and you have a great visual of the heat and liveliness of southwestern cuisine. Southwestern food is influenced less by the Spanish and more by the vast number and rich variety of Native American tribes that lived in the arid deserts of what is now New Mexico and Arizona. It is distinctly different from Tex-Mex cuisine although in many restaurants and homes the two food styles have fused to create yet more variations.

Let's take a look at the roots of these foods that are bold, earthy, rich, smoky—and sometimes even subtle in character. We'll also touch on their fascinating ancient cultural and religious significance.

There are at least six colors of corn in the southwest: red, white, blue, black, yellow, and variegated. Many tribes, including the Zuni, regarded the corn with deep religious respect, as related in "The Zuni Origin Story":

> After eight days where the plumes of a Tchu-e-ton stood, rose seven corn plants, and they were called the seven maidens. The eldest was called yellow corn, of the Northland, the color of the light of winter.

STRINGS OF RED RISTRAS

The inspiration for chili pepper decorative lights dates to hundreds, and possibly even thousands, of years ago. The Aztecs called the long strings of bright red, fresh chili peppers ristras. These many chilis could be used right away or hung to dry and used a year or more later. In Native American lore, families keep one ristra for each family member, in the length equivalent to the person's height.

Native American Roots

The Navajo, Pima, Hopi, Pueblo, and Zuni tribes had the most significant influence on southwestern cuisine. Their basketry technology was so advanced that they could make baskets that were watertight. In these baskets they placed heated rocks and water and boiled their food.

The Pima were also known as the "Papago," or bean people. This notoriety originated with their expertise in growing beans, an agricultural skill they learned from the Hohokam tribe, their ancient ancestors. During the fourth century, the Pima designed a highly effective irrigation system for their crops.

The Navajo, originally an arctic tribe, learned to farm when they moved to the southwest. They modified their traditional nomadic hunting and gathering ways and learned to subsist on farming and gardening.

> Next was blue corn, of the West, the color of the great world of waters. Next was red corn, of the South, the land of everlasting summer. The fourth was white corn, of the East, white like the land whence the sun brings the daylight. Next was speckled corn, of the Zenith, with many colors like the clouds of dawn and sunset. The sixth was black corn, of the Nadir, color of the caves of first humankind. The youngest corn was sweet corn, which remains soft even when ripe. The two clans linked: one gave the people corn in place of wild seeds and the other water to drink. Together they gave life to the people. (Richard I. Ford. "Corn Is Our Mother," in *Corn and Culture in the Prehistoric New World*, edited by Sissel Johannessen and Christine Hastorf. Boulder, Colorado: Westview Press, 1994, pp. 513–525; Evan Jones. *American Food: The Gastronomic Story*, Second Edition. New York: Random House, 1981.)

The Zuni attributed protective powers to corn: they thought they could protect themselves from Spanish conquistadors by sprinkling dried kernels in the path of the invaders. The Zuni also believed that the "corn maiden" gave them corn to sustain life. Indeed, for them and most other tribes, corn was life itself.

The Hopi, thought to have the most profound effect on southwestern cooking, held blue corn in the highest esteem. Because blue corn was the most difficult to cultivate, the Hopi believed it symbolized a difficult but rewarding life.

The Three Sisters Sustain Southwestern Life

Southwestern tribes grew many varieties of the three sisters—corn, beans, and squash—which were native to the area. Pinto beans (and a smaller version, the pinquito) were most commonly used, but there were numerous other types. Today there is a resurgence of ancient varieties of beans, called heirloom beans. One variety, the Anasazi bean, was cultivated at least five hundred years ago. First grown by a tribe with the same name, the beans are mottled black and brown or red and white and are sweet in flavor. One great advantage is that they produce much less intestinal gas than most other beans, so they might be a good choice for those with sensitive stomachs.

Squash was the third of the three sisters. Native American tribes have grown zucchini, yellow summer squash, and many varieties of winter squash. In some areas, this vegetable is still called by its Spanish name, *calabicitas*.

Corn, beans, and squash not only provided excellent nutrition, but they were also easy to dry and store for later, leaner times.

SOUTHWEST TRIBES DISCOVER A NUTRITION SECRET—ACCIDENTALLY

Looking only for more efficient ways to cook corn bread, southwestern–tribes made a critical discovery that no doubt improved their health dramatically. They added wood ash to speed the cooking of corn bread. Little did they know that adding these alkaline (basic) minerals made corn a complete protein food.

Typical Southwest Spices

Blend cumin and cinnamon together with hot chili peppers and basil and you have the start of Southwest cuisine. Other herbs and spices frequently used to spice Southwest food include:

- Achiote, also known as annatto seeds, the seeds of the tropical annatto tree. They are used to flavor food and to color it yellow and orange.
- Cilantro, also called Chinese parsley, used in its many forms in southwestern cuisine. The leaves are chopped fresh and used as an ingredient or garnish; the dried coriander seeds are used whole, or ground as cumin.

TIME TRAVEL ROUTE 66

The Hopis founded the village of Old Oraibi (in Arizona) around 1150. Thought to be one of the oldest continually inhabited towns in the United States, you'll find it on Route 66 near Flagstaff.

- Limon, which is related to the key lime. This Mexican lime is small, round, and yellowish in color.
- Pignones, or pine nuts, harvested from the cones of pine trees growing at high altitudes in the southwest and Rocky Mountains. Pignones are often roasted or ground to lend a distinctive flavor.

EXTRA CHILE FOR YOUR CHILI?

Today, chili with an "i" identifies the state dish of Texas, a combination of meat, beans, and ground chile (with an "e") peppers to spice it and add heat.

Chili peppers are the key ingredient in Southwest cuisine. Chili is a variation of the Aztec word *chil*. Distinct from sweet bell peppers, chilis are pungent, with varying degrees of heat. Some people argue that pungency should be the fifth main taste sensory, after bitter, sweet, sour, and salty.

The chili peppers' pungency comes from phytochemicals called *capsaicins*. Chili pungency is measurable and is expressed in Scoville Heat Units. Developed in 1912, the Scoville Organoleptic test was the first reliable measurement of how hot or pungent each type of chili is; today a machine has replaced the human-conducted study.

Chili pungency depends on the cultivar, weather conditions, growing conditions, and fruit age. Chili growers can stress the plant by depriving it of water to make it even more pungent. As a general rule, leave in the seeds and veins when more heat is desired in a recipe; remove some or all to reduce the amount of heat. The seeds and membranes can contain up to 80 percent of a chili's capsaicin.

Let's take a look at several types of chili peppers you may need to simmer up some Southwestern cuisine:

- Anaheim chili. One of the most widely available chilis in the United States. It is medium green in color, long and narrow in shape, and mostly sweet with a little bite in flavor. The red strain is the Colorado chili from which ristras are made. Buy these chilis fresh or canned.
- Ancho chili. Made from the fresh, green poblano chili, the ancho is the deep reddish brown, dried version. It can be slightly fruity and mild or pungent.
- Cascabel chili. This rich, nutty-flavored chili with medium heat is a dried, plum-shaped, dark blood-red chili that is about 1 to 1½ inches in diameter. It might also be called chile bola.
- Charleston hot chili. Some twenty times hotter than the jalapeño pepper, this one becomes hotter as it ripens. It is least ripe when yellow-green, and most ripe when crimson red.
- Cherry pepper. Also called the Hungarian cherry pepper, it is small, round, and bright red in color. Slightly sweet, it can be mild to medium hot. Buy it fresh or pickled.

- Chilaca chili. Dark green when least ripe and dark brown when fully ripened, this long narrow chili can grow up to 9 or 10 inches in length; it is often twisted in shape. It can be mild or medium hot, and is generally rich-flavored. When dried (usually the way it is found in the United States), it is known as the pasilla. Look for it fresh in farmers' markets.
- Chipotle chili. The very hot dried and smoked jalapeño. Buy this wrinkled, dark brown-skinned chili dried, pickled, or canned.
- Fresno chili. As hot as the jalapeño, the Fresno ranges from light green (less ripe) to bright red (fully mature). Use it in small amounts.
- Habanero chili. This extremely hot chili is small and shaped like a lantern. Buy it fresh or dried; when it is bright orange it is ripest (and hottest!).
- Jalapeño chili. Smooth, dark green (least ripe) or scarlet red (most ripe), these chilis are hot to very hot. They hail from Jalapa, the capital of Veracruz, Mexico. Buy it fresh, canned, or dried (the dried version is called chipotle).
- Pequín chili. Tiny, oval-shaped dried chilis that are bright red-orange in color, they are sweet and smoky, but fiery hot.
- Poblano chili. The dark green, almost black chili is rich and mildly snappy. Choose the darkest ones for the richest flavor. Poblanos are 2½ to 3 inches wide and 4 to 5 inches long and triangular in shape. Dried, they are called ancho or mulatto chilis. Use them to make Baked Chilis Rellenos (page 362).
- Santa Fe Grande chili. Yellow to orange or red in color, this small, cone-shaped chili is medium hot to hot in spiciness.
- Serrano chili. This small, pointed chili is very hot. There are color transitions from bright green (least ripe) to scarlet red, and then yellow (most ripe). Buy it fresh, canned, pickled, or packed in oil. The dried version, chili seco, is available whole or powdered.

FRESH CHILI BUYING TIPS

Buy chilis with bright, vivid colors. Avoid those with shriveling or soft spots. As a general rule, the larger the chili, the milder it is.

NUTRITION IN CHILIS? YES!

Chilis are rich in vitamins, especially vitamin C, and are a good source of folic acid, potassium, and vitamin E.

Phoenix Quiche

Barbara J. Pyper, M.S., R.D., C.D., F.H.C.F.A., F.C.S.I.

Serves: 6
Hands-on time: 15 minutes
Cooking time: 50 minutes

This recipe is from the southwest corner of the country—Yuma, Arizona—and has been a family favorite for years. The blend of Monterey Jack cheese, green chilis, and roasted red bell pepper bursts with southwestern flavor.

COOK'S TIP

To make it spicier, add ¼ to 1 teaspoon cayenne when you add the cumin.

- 1½ cups shredded Monterey Jack cheese, divided (6 ounces)
- 1 cup shredded reduced-fat Cheddar cheese (4 ounces)
- 1 single 9-inch pie crust (purchased or homemade), unbaked
- 1 can (4 ounces) diced green chilis, drained
- 1 medium-size red bell pepper, roasted, or use half a jar (7 ounces) of roasted red bell pepper, drained and chopped
- 1 medium-size yellow bell pepper, finely chopped
- ¾ cup liquid egg substitute
- 1 cup (8 ounces) nonfat milk
- ¼ teaspoon ground cumin

Preheat oven to 350°F. Sprinkle ¾ cup of the Monterey Jack cheese and all of the cheddar cheese evenly in the pie shell. Top with the chilis and peppers. Combine the egg substitute, milk, and cumin in a small bowl. Pour over the peppers and cheese. Top evenly with the remaining cheese.

Bake for 50 minutes or until a knife inserted in the middle comes out clean.

COOK'S TIP

Freeze any remaining slices, individually wrapped in foil and then placed together, in a large tightly sealed bag. Remove from the foil and heat in a microwave for 5 minutes if thawed; if not thawed, heat 10 minutes on 50 percent power followed by 2 to 3 minutes on full power, or until heated through.

COOK'S TIP

Roast the pepper under a broiler, turning until evenly charred, about 5 minutes. Place in a small bowl and cover tightly with plastic wrap; let it stand for 10 minutes. Peel, seed, and chop.

NUTRITION PER SERVING

Serving size	⅙ of pie
Calories	300 kcal
Fat	20 g
Saturated fat	7 g
Cholesterol	30 mg
Sodium	700 mg
Carbohydrates	15 g
Dietary fiber	Less than 1 g
Protein	18 g

Roasted Red Bell Pepper and Spinach Strata

Lori A. Miller, R.D., L.D.

Serve this colorful, Southwest-inspired, delicious casserole for breakfast—and enjoy the leftovers cold the next day. Just don't tell anyone that you've added so many healthy touches—whole-grain bread, spinach, and red peppers!

Serves: 9 for breakfast or 12 as a side dish
Hands-on time: 20 minutes
Cooking time: 45 minutes
Standing time: 4 hours or overnight

nonstick cooking spray
6 slices hearty whole-grain bread, cut into cubes
1 10-ounce package frozen chopped spinach, thawed and liquid squeezed out
1 7-ounce jar roasted red peppers, drained and chopped or 1 red bell pepper, roasted and chopped
1½ cups (6 ounces) Mexican/taco flavored cheese or sharp cheddar cheese
3 cups nonfat milk
1 carton (8 ounces) egg substitute
1 teaspoon garlic powder
1 teaspoon cumin
½ teaspoon black pepper
½ teaspoon salt

Layer the bread in a 9-by-13-inch baking dish coated with the nonstick cooking spray. Sprinkle evenly with the spinach, red peppers, and cheese. Combine the nonfat milk, egg substitute, garlic powder, cumin, black pepper, and salt in a large bowl. Pour over the bread mixture. Cover and refrigerate at least 4 hours or overnight.

Preheat oven to 350°F.

Bake, uncovered, for 45 minutes or until a knife inserted into the center comes out clean. Let stand for 10 minutes before serving.

COOK'S TIP

Roast the pepper under a broiler, turning until evenly charred, about 5 minutes. Place in a small bowl and cover tightly with plastic wrap; let it stand for 10 minutes. Peel, seed, and chop.

VARIATION

For flavor versatility, replace red peppers with 3 plum tomatoes, seeded and diced; for a heartier version, add 1 pound turkey sausage, cooked and drained.

NUTRITION PER SERVING	
Serving size	1/9 of casserole
Calories	280 kcal
Fat	13 g
Saturated fat	7 g
Cholesterol	30 mg
Sodium	810 mg
Carbohydrates	23 g
Dietary fiber	4 g
Protein	21 g

NUTRITION PER SERVING	
Serving size	1/12 of casserole
Calories	140 kcal
Fat	6 g
Saturated fat	6 g
Cholesterol	15 mg
Sodium	400 mg
Carbohydrates	12 g
Dietary fiber	2 g
Protein	10 g

Southwest Black Bean Dip

Jessica Terry, R.D.

Serves: 8
Hands-on time: 5 minutes

Tennessee born, this Southwest-inspired dip spices up or down depending on how many times you shake the ground red pepper jar.

2 tablespoons lime juice
2 teaspoons extra-virgin olive oil
½ teaspoon ground cumin
¼ to ½ teaspoon ground red pepper
¼ teaspoon salt
1¼ cups fresh or frozen corn (thaw and drain if frozen)
¼ cup chopped fresh cilantro
1 15-ounce can black beans, rinsed and drained
1 large red bell pepper, chopped
tortilla chips or dipping vegetables

Mix the lime juice, oil, cumin, ground red pepper, and salt in a large bowl. Add the corn, cilantro, black beans, and red bell pepper; toss. Serve with tortilla chips or vegetables for dipping.

COOK'S TIP
This dip is best served at room temperature, but can be prepared up to three days in advance. Store tightly covered in the refrigerator.

NUTRITION PER SERVING	
Serving size	¼ cup
Calories	70 kcal
Fat	1.5 g
Saturated fat	0 g
Cholesterol	0 mg
Sodium	240 mg
Carbohydrates	10 g
Dietary fiber	3 g
Protein	3 g

Goat Cheese and Roasted Red Pepper Bruschetta

Kristine Napier, M.P.H., R.D.

Southwest colorful and characteristically seasoned, this bruschetta is made just a bit more genteel with creamy goat cheese. Double your portion and make it the featured part of an easy lunch.

Serves: 18
Hands-on time: 10 minutes
Cooking time: 10 minutes

11 ounces goat cheese
1 teaspoon cumin
1 teaspoon cayenne pepper
½ teaspoon salt
1 10-ounce bag frozen yellow corn, thawed
3 medium-size red sweet bell peppers, finely chopped
6 green onions, finely chopped
1 cup fresh cilantro, finely chopped
16 ounces Italian bread, cut in half lengthwise

SUBSTITUTION
Use a 1-pound baguette or 1-pound whole-grain loaf.

Preheat oven to 375°F. Cover a large cookie sheet with aluminum foil. Combine the cheese, cumin, cayenne, and salt in a medium-size bowl; blend with a fork. Add the corn, peppers, onions, and cilantro; stir to combine.

Press the mixture into the cut sides of the bread; spread to cover the edges.

Bake for 10 minutes, or just until the edges turn golden brown. Cool slightly and cut into 36 pieces.

NUTRITION PER SERVING	
Serving size	2 pieces
Calories	140 kcal
Fat	5 g
Saturated fat	3 g
Cholesterol	10 mg
Sodium	280 mg
Carbohydrates	18 g
Dietary fiber	2 g
Protein	6 g

South-of-the-Border Broccoli Bake

Melissa Stevens Ohlson, M.S., R.D., L.D.

Serves: 4 as a main course or 8 as a side dish
Hands-on time: 10 minutes
Cooking time: 35 minutes

Spice up this hearty broccoli casserole with more chili peppers and cayenne, or tone down the heat as you wish. Enjoy this casserole as a one-pot meal or a delicious side dish.

4 thick slices multigrain bread
vegetable oil cooking spray
1 16-ounce package frozen broccoli florets, thawed
1 medium-size onion, chopped
1 4-ounce can chopped chili peppers
1 medium-size red bell pepper, chopped
1 10¾-ounce can reduced-fat, reduced-sodium cream of mushroom soup
¼ teaspoon ground cumin
½ to 1 teaspoon cayenne pepper
1 teaspoon garlic powder
2 cups shredded sharp cheddar cheese (8 ounces)

Preheat oven to 350°F. Toast the bread slices in a toaster or a toaster oven. Cut into cubes; set aside.

Coat a 9-by-13-inch oven-safe baking dish with the cooking spray. Arrange the broccoli in the pan. Top with the onion, chili peppers, bell pepper, and bread cubes. Combine the soup, 1 can of water, cumin, cayenne pepper, and garlic powder in a medium-size bowl; stir. Pour over the broccoli mixture. Top with the cheese.

Bake, uncovered, at 350°F for 35 minutes or until the cheese bubbles.

COOK'S TIPS

Save time by using frozen broccoli and increase the baking time by 5 to 7 minutes. Lay the bread out to dry the night before to omit the toasting step.

NUTRITION PER SERVING	
Serving size	scant 1 cup, side dish
Calories	200 kcal
Fat	12 g
Saturated fat	7 g
Cholesterol	30 mg
Sodium	270 mg
Carbohydrates	16 g
Dietary fiber	4 g
Protein	10 g

NUTRITION PER SERVING	
Serving size	1¾ cup, main course
Calories	400 kcal
Fat	23 g
Saturated fat	13 g
Cholesterol	55 mg
Sodium	540 mg
Carbohydrates	33 g
Dietary fiber	9 g
Protein	21 g

Gazpacho with Garlic Parmesan Croutons

Elsa Ramirez Brisson, M.P.H., R.D.

The Spanish influenced Mexican cuisine in many ways, including gazpacho. This is my version of a classic, which traces its roots to the Andalusia region in southern Spain. This soup just gets better and better with time—so enjoy!

Serves: 4
Hands-on time: 25 minutes
Cooking time: 3 minutes

- vegetable oil cooking spray
- 2 cloves garlic, divided
- 2 tablespoons extra-virgin olive oil
- ¼ cup (2 ounces) freshly grated Parmesan cheese
- 4 slices whole-grain bread
- 3 ripe tomatoes, chopped and divided
- 1 medium-size green bell pepper, chopped and divided
- 1 medium-size cucumber, chopped and divided
- 1 medium-size sweet yellow onion, cut into chunks
- ½ teaspoon salt
- ¼ teaspoon ground black pepper
- 3 tablespoons balsamic vinegar

Preheat oven to 400°F. Coat a baking sheet with the cooking spray.

Mince 1 clove of garlic; combine with the oil and cheese. Spread the mixture over the bread. Toast the bread for 3 minutes, or until golden brown. Let it cool; cut into croutons and set aside.

Reserve ¼ cup each of tomato, bell pepper, and cucumber for garnish; refrigerate until ready to serve. Combine the remaining garlic, tomato, bell pepper, cucumber, onion, salt, pepper, and balsamic vinegar in a food processor or blender. Pulse until blended or until the gazpacho reaches the desired consistency. Refrigerate until ready to serve.

Pour the gazpacho into four soup bowls; top with the reserved vegetables and croutons.

COOK'S TIPS

Make a double or triple batch of croutons. Cool them and freeze for later use. Cut vegetables into quarters. Place in a food processor in batches and pulse until the desired consistency is achieved.

NUTRITION PER SERVING	
Serving size	1 cup
Calories	210 kcal
Fat	10 g
Saturated fat	2 g
Cholesterol	5 mg
Sodium	530 mg
Carbohydrates	26 g
Dietary fiber	5 g
Protein	7 g

Roasted Carrot and Beet Soup

Elsa Ramirez Brisson, M.P.H., R.D.

Serves: 8 as an appetizer or 4 as a main course
Hands-on time: 15 minutes
Cooking time: 1 hour, 15 minutes

Although it is an unconventional California-born combination, beets and carrots unite to produce a flavor that is exceptionally interesting and comforting. There's just enough "kick" from the onion and black pepper, but if you want more, add a few dashes of cayenne.

- vegetable oil cooking spray
- 5 large carrots, peeled and sliced (3 cups)
- 2 celery ribs, thinly sliced (1½ cups)
- 1 large onion, quartered (2 cups)
- 1 tablespoon extra-virgin olive oil
- 2 tablespoons brown sugar
- 2 teaspoons ground cinnamon
- 1 teaspoon ground ginger
- ½ teaspoon nutmeg
- ¼ teaspoon black pepper
- 1 15-ounce can beets, rinsed and drained
- 3 14-ounce cans reduced-sodium chicken broth
- ¼ cup reduced-fat sour cream for garnish
- snipped fresh chives for garnish

Preheat oven to 400°F. Coat a 9-by-13-inch baking dish with the cooking spray. Combine the carrots, celery, and onion in the dish. Drizzle with the olive oil and sprinkle with the sugar, cinnamon, ginger, nutmeg, and pepper. Toss. Cover the dish tightly with aluminum foil and bake for 1 hour, or until the carrots and the celery are fork tender.

In a food processor or blender, purée the roasted vegetables and beets with the broth in batches until smooth. Combine the batches in a heavy 2-quart kettle. Heat on medium-low until warmed through. Garnish with the sour cream and chives.

SUBSTITUTION

Substitute 1 pound of fresh beets for canned. Peel and chop; roast with other vegetables before puréeing.

NUTRITION PER SERVING

Serving size	2 cups, main course
Calories	220 kcal
Fat	8 g
Saturated fat	2 g
Cholesterol	10 mg
Sodium	440 mg
Carbohydrates	32 g
Dietary fiber	6 g
Protein	8 g

Lime Chicken with Black Bean Sauce

Diane Werner, R.D.

America's neighbors to the southwest continue to inspire our cooking because we love the popular flavors of lime, fresh cilantro, beans, and a bit of cayenne. Those flavors are showcased here in a simple grilled chicken breast and salsa (or sauce). Marinate the chicken breast overnight for a quick-to-the-table, zesty entrée that is low in fat. Partner with Spanish rice and a garden salad for a healthy, enjoyable meal.

Serves: 4
Hands-on time: 15 minutes
Marinating time: 1 hour or overnight
Cooking time: 10 minutes

Lime Marinated Chicken

- ⅓ cup lime juice
- ¼ cup olive or canola oil
- 3 cloves garlic, minced
- ¼ teaspoon cayenne red pepper
- ⅓ cup chopped fresh cilantro, divided
- ¼ teaspoon salt
- ¼ teaspoon ground black pepper
- 1 pound boneless, skinless chicken breast halves

Mix together the lime juice, oil, garlic, red pepper, all but 1 tablespoon cilantro, salt, and pepper in a small bowl. Add the chicken and marinate for at least 1 hour in the refrigerator, turning occasionally.

Grill the chicken breasts about 5 to 7 minutes on each side over a medium-hot grill. The chicken should be firm to the touch and the juices should run clear. Discard the leftover marinade.

Serve the grilled chicken topped with Black Bean Sauce (recipe follows) garnished with the remaining cilantro and additional chopped red peppers and onions, if desired.

COOK'S TIP

The chicken and marinade may be stored in the refrigerator in a tightly sealed plastic bag up to 3 days.

COOK'S TIP

Broil the chicken instead. Preheat the broiler; coat the broiler pan with cooking spray. Broil the chicken 5 to 7 minutes per side, or until cooked thoroughly.

NUTRITION PER SERVING

Serving size	3½ ounces cooked chicken with ¼ cup sauce
Calories	250 kcal
Fat	2.5 g
Saturated fat	0 g
Cholesterol	65 mg
Sodium	550 mg
Carbohydrates	22 g
Dietary fiber	7 g
Protein	33 g

Lime Chicken with Black Bean Sauce *(continued)*

Black Bean Sauce

1 15-ounce can black beans, rinsed and drained
1 medium-size red bell pepper, trimmed, seeded, and minced
1 small yellow onion, minced
½ cup orange juice
2 tablespoons balsamic vinegar
2 cloves garlic, minced
¼ teaspoon salt
⅛ teaspoon ground black pepper

Mash the black beans with a fork in a medium-size bowl. Add the bell pepper, onion, orange juice, balsamic vinegar, garlic, salt, and pepper. Mix until fully blended. Chill the sauce until ready to serve or if desired, heat it before serving.

Santa Fe Turkey Breast Panini

Susan Kell Peletta, R.D.

This slightly zippy, definitely smooth and comfort-food-in-nature sandwich is easy enough to enjoy often by yourself, but most definitely excellent enough to enjoy in the company of others. Many thanks to my mentor Jonathan Rose, Chef at Stanford University, under whom I developed this recipe.

Serves: 8
Hands-on time: 15 minutes
Marinating time: 4 hours or overnight
Cooking time: 10 minutes
Standing time: 1 hour

- 1 5½-ounce can vegetable juice cocktail or tomato juice
- ¼ cup lime juice
- 2 tablespoons extra-virgin olive oil
- 1 teaspoon sugar
- ¼ teaspoon cayenne pepper
- ½ teaspoon ground coriander
- ½ teaspoon dried oregano
- ¼ teaspoon chili powder
- ½ teaspoon black pepper
- 1 teaspoon salt
- 1 pound boneless, skinless turkey breasts, cut into strips
- 1 16-ounce loaf French bread or a baguette
- 1 avocado, chopped
- 2 tablespoons prepared salsa, chunky style
- 2 tablespoons chopped fresh cilantro (stems removed first)
- 1 medium-size cucumber, diced (unpeeled)
- 2 cups fresh spring mix (lettuce mix)

Combine the vegetable juice, lime juice, oil, sugar, cayenne, coriander, oregano, chili powder, black pepper, and salt in a plastic or glass shallow container. Add the turkey breast strips. Marinate at least four hours; overnight is fine.

Remove the turkey and discard the marinade. Grill, bake, or broil the turkey approximately 4 to 5 minutes on each side, or until cooked through (juices should run clear).

Slice the loaf of bread lengthwise in half, but leave the two halves attached. Open the loaf to expose both inner sides. From each side, scoop out some of the bread.

Stir together the avocado, salsa, cilantro, and cucumber. Fold in the spring mix. Press the avocado/spring mix into the bread hollows. Top with the turkey slices.

NUTRITION PER SERVING	
Serving size	⅛ of sandwich
Calories	300 kcal
Fat	10 g
Saturated fat	2 g
Cholesterol	30 mg
Sodium	440 mg
Carbohydrates	35 g
Dietary fiber	4 g
Protein	18 g

Baked Chilis Rellenos

Barbara J. Pyper, M.S., R.D., C.D., F.H.C.F.A., F.C.S.I.

Serves: 4 as a main dish or 8 as an appetizer
Hands-on time: 20 minutes
Cooking time: 25 minutes

Traditional Southwest chilis take on a delightfully different flavor in this recipe that uses canned tuna in a richly flavored stuffing. Serve them for dinner or as appetizers.

8 large mild green chilis such as poblano or Anaheim
vegetable oil cooking spray
1 6-ounce can water-packed tuna, drained and flaked
½ cup nonfat ricotta cheese
1 cup (4 ounces) shredded cheese, such as Monterey Jack or pepper jack, divided
1 cup frozen corn, thawed and drained
1 medium-size onion, minced
1 egg, lightly beaten
¼ teaspoon ground black pepper
salsa for garnish, optional

Preheat oven to 425°F. Wash and dry the chilis; cut a slit lengthwise in each one. Remove the stems, seeds, and membranes. Place on a baking sheet coated with the cooking spray.

Stir together ⅔ cup tuna and the ricotta cheese, shredded cheese, corn, onion, egg, and black pepper; mix well. Stuff each chili with about ¼ cup of the tuna and cheese mixture. Top with the remaining ⅓ cup of the shredded cheese. Bake, covered, for 20 to 25 minutes or until the chilis are tender and the filling is hot. Garnish with the salsa, if using.

SUBSTITUTION

Use canned whole green chilis for ease of preparation.

COOK'S TIPS

Wear gloves when handling fresh chilis. Also, do not touch your face or eyes while handling chilis; wash your hands thoroughly in soapy water after handling. Don't waste your leftover ricotta cheese! Spread it on toast or bagels and top with your favorite jam or marmalade for an easy, delicious breakfast.

NUTRITION PER SERVING

Serving size	2 stuffed chilis
Calories	240 kcal
Fat	13 g
Saturated fat	7 g
Cholesterol	100 mg
Sodium	810 mg
Carbohydrates	8 g
Dietary fiber	2 g
Protein	23 g

Southwest Style Flank Steak

Stephanie Green, R.D.

At my local farmers' market in Phoenix I love to show people what to do with those not-so-familiar vegetables. Swiss chard is one of them, which is a shame because it tastes great. When working beside my organic farmer friend Frank, I use it to stir up something that's fast, fresh, and flavorful, such as this favorite dish of mine.

Serves: 4
Hands-on time: 10 minutes
Cooking time: 10 minutes

1 tablespoon canola oil
1 pound (16 ounces) flank steak, thinly sliced
1 bunch Swiss chard, sliced into 1-inch ribbons, discard the stalks
1 tablespoon honey
1 tablespoon ginger root, finely grated
salt and pepper to taste
toasted sesame seeds

Place a teaspoon of oil into a large skillet and heat to medium-high. Add the flank steak and cook over medium-high heat for about 2 minutes. It's okay for the meat to be slightly pink. Remove the steak from the pan and keep warm.

Add the remaining oil to the pan and heat to medium-high. Place the Swiss chard in the pan, stirring frequently over medium-high heat for about 1 to 2 minutes. Add the honey and ginger and stir well to coat.

Add the meat to the center of the pan and warm thoroughly. Season with salt and pepper. Be careful not to overcook the Swiss chard. The carryover heat will finish cooking it for you.

Garnish with the toasted sesame seeds.

FOOD TRIVIA

Swiss chard belongs to the beet family. It is basically a beet that is all tops. It is a very hardy vegetable and grows up until the first frost. There are many different colors of Swiss chard from red to orange to yellow. Swiss chard is also used in savory pies and casseroles.

SHOPPING TIP

Always look for bright, shiny leaves when purchasing Swiss chard. If you can get it from a farmers' market, it will last much longer than the standard two days in the refrigerator.

COOK'S TIP

This recipe can be served as a vegetable side dish by leaving out the beef.

NUTRITION NUGGET

Swiss chard is a good source of vitamin A and calcium. Save the stalks and use in a soup or a casserole.

NUTRITION PER SERVING

Serving size	1 cup cooked Swiss chard plus 3½ ounces cooked meat
Calories	240 kcal
Fat	13 g
Saturated fat	4.5 g
Cholesterol	50 mg
Sodium	410 mg
Carbohydrates	11 g
Dietary fiber	3 g
Protein	22 g

Southwest Pasta with Sun-Dried Tomato Sauce

Roberta L. Duyff, M.S., R.D., F.A.D.A., C.F.C.S.

Serves: 4
Hands-on time: 20 minutes
Refrigeration/standing time: 5 minutes (or overnight)
Cooking time: 30 minutes

America does fusion cooking well. The inspiration for this make-ahead casserole comes from the variety of healthful Southwest, Mediterranean, and Asian ingredients in today's kitchens, including my own. Enjoy this creative way to fit vegetables, tofu, and dairy foods into your family meals. For convenience, prepare Southwest Pasta with Sun-Dried Tomato Sauce today, refrigerate, and bake it tomorrow.

- 12 ounces uncooked tri-color rotini or penne pasta
- ½ cup salsa
- 1 tablespoon extra-virgin olive oil
- 12 ounces edamame (shelled fresh or frozen soybeans)
- 1 medium-size red bell pepper, cut into thin strips
- 1 medium-size green bell pepper, cut into thin strips
- 2 cloves garlic, minced
- 1 cup Mexican blend shredded cheese, divided (4 ounces)
- ½ cup chopped sun-dried tomato
- 6 ounces soft tofu, puréed
- ¾ cup evaporated nonfat milk (6 ounces)
- 1 4-ounce can chopped green chili peppers
- ¼ cup chopped fresh cilantro or parsley
- 2 tablespoons soy sauce
- 1 tablespoon lemon juice
- ¼ teaspoon black pepper
- dash hot sauce

Preheat oven to 350°F. Cook the rotini or penne pasta according to the package instructions. Drain. Add the salsa. Set aside.

Heat the oil in a medium wok or skillet. Add the edamame, red and green bell peppers, and garlic. Cook and stir over medium heat for 4 to 5 minutes until the peppers are tender-crisp. Set aside.

Combine ¾ cup of the cheese, and the sun-dried tomatoes, tofu, milk, green chilis, cilantro, soy sauce, lemon juice, pepper, and hot sauce in a large mixing bowl; stir until blended.

Blend the edamame mixture into the pasta. Pour into a shallow 9-by-13-inch ovenproof pan. Sprinkle the remaining ¼ cup of cheese evenly over the dish. Bake uncovered for 30 minutes, or until heated through and lightly browned.

SUBSTITUTION

If your store doesn't sell edamame, substitute a 15-ounce can of red kidney beans, soybeans, or almost any canned beans (drained) on your pantry shelf.

SHOPPING TIP

Supermarkets sell many different types of tofu. Because it keeps its shape, buy firm or extra firm regular tofu for grilling or pan frying. Use soft silken tofu with its creamy texture in sauces, dips, spreads, and smoothies. For more variety, look for flavored tofu: try the lemon pepper, barbecue, Oriental, and Thai flavors.

FOOD TRIVIA

You can freeze tofu. When frozen, creamy-white tofu turns yellow. Once thawed, its creamy-white color returns.

NUTRITION NUGGET

For more soy benefits (see pages 586–590), look for soy pasta in your supermarket to use in place of traditional pasta.

NUTRITION PER SERVING	
Serving size	2 cups
Calories	460 kcal
Fat	14 g
Saturated fat	5 g
Cholesterol	20 mg
Sodium	560 mg
Carbohydrates	63 g
Dietary fiber	7 g
Protein	25 g

Sweet Corn Pudding Pie

Kristine Napier, M.P.H., R.D.

Serves: 10
Hands-on time: 10 minutes
Cooking time: 1 hour

While corn pudding is served frequently in Mexico and the Southwest as a side dish, here it's made just a bit sweeter—and accented with vanilla—to make a wonderful dessert. The extras freeze well and also make a great breakfast. The dry cornmeal cooks up into its own crust.

- vegetable oil cooking spray
- ¼ cup white cornmeal
- 4 large eggs, beaten slightly
- 1 cup nonfat milk
- 1 cup sour cream
- ½ cup sugar
- ¼ teaspoon salt
- 1 tablespoon vanilla extract
- 29 ounces canned white hominy, drained

Preheat oven to 350°F. Spray a deep pie dish with the cooking spray. Sprinkle the dry cornmeal evenly over the bottom of the pan.

Mix the eggs, milk, sour cream, sugar, salt, and vanilla in a medium-size bowl. Stir in the hominy.

Pour the mixture over the cornmeal. Bake for 1 hour, or until the mixture doesn't jiggle in the middle.

SUBSTITUTIONS

Where blue cornmeal is available, substitute that for the white, and create a blue piecrust.

NUTRITION PER SERVING

Serving size	⅒ of pie
Calories	200 kcal
Fat	8 g
Saturated fat	4 g
Cholesterol	95 mg
Sodium	280 mg
Carbohydrates	27 g
Dietary fiber	2 g
Protein	6 g

Papaya Cheesecake

Kristine Napier, M.P.H., R.D.

Serves: 12
Hands-on time: 20 minutes
Standing time: 12 hours
Cooking time: 50 minutes

Who would have guessed you could make a cheesecake without the crust? In so doing, we've created one that is nutrient-rich but lighter on calories. It's also southwest colorful and oh-so-delicious!

32 ounces nonfat plain yogurt, strained into yogurt cheese
vegetable oil cooking spray
8 ounces low-fat cream cheese
8 ounces fat-free cream cheese
½ cup liquid egg substitute
¾ cup plus 1 tablespoon sugar
1 tablespoon vanilla extract
3 tablespoons cornstarch
1 fresh papaya, peeled, seeded, and chopped
2 fresh kiwis, peeled and chopped

The day or night before, set the yogurt to strain into yogurt cheese (see the "Cook's Tip").

The next day, preheat oven to 325°F. Spray a 9-by-9-inch baking dish with the cooking spray.

Combine the yogurt cheese, cream cheeses, egg substitute, ¾ cup sugar, vanilla, and cornstarch in a food processor; blend until smooth. Stir in half of the papaya. Pour into the treated dish; bake for 50 minutes, or until a knife inserted into the middle comes out clean. Chill.

Combine the remaining papaya, kiwis, and 1 tablespoon sugar; chill. Serve the cheesecake squares topped with the papaya and kiwi mixture.

SUBSTITUTION

Use 2 cups sliced strawberries in place of the papaya and kiwis, but don't stir any into the batter. Use all for garnish.

COOK'S TIP

To make yogurt cheese, line a mesh strainer with a coffee filter and place over a medium-size bowl. Transfer 1 quart of yogurt into the strainer. Cover with plastic wrap or foil; place in the refrigerator overnight. The liquid will strain off, leaving a thick yogurt cheese.

NUTRITION PER SERVING

Serving size	1/12
Calories	220 kcal
Fat	4 g
Saturated fat	2.5 g
Cholesterol	15 mg
Sodium	230 mg
Carbohydrates	34 g
Dietary fiber	Less than 1 g
Protein	10 g

8

FROM THE ROCKY MOUNTAINS TO THE PACIFIC NORTHWEST

Kristine Napier, M.P.H., R.D.

The fruits of the Pacific Rim—the states of Washington, Oregon, and Alaska—unite and simmer into a cuisine that is in striking contrast to the survival cuisine that has remained standard fare in the Rocky Mountains. Bridging them, though, is one of the most fertile dryland crop-growing areas in the world, the Palouse. From the French word for green lawn, the Palouse circles the eastern corners of Washington and Oregon and the northwest corners of Idaho and produces economically significant amounts of lentils, dry beans, wheat, barley, oats, canola, mustard, and Walla Walla sweet onions.

Let's take a closer look at this little-known neck of the woods and its critical significance to our nation's economy, nutrition, and culinary life. Then we'll examine the kitchens on either side of it.

The Palouse Region

The wind-blown, volcanic soil of the Palouse is incredibly rich and productive. The striking landscape formed of contoured, rolling hills is in stark contrast to the flatter farmland of the central plains. A moderate, Mediterranean-type climate combined with warm summer days and cool summer nights ensures abundant crop yields.

Lentils became a significant crop in the area because of religion-based dietary preferences. A Russian-German Seventh Day Adventist minister introduced lentils to the Palouse. Minister Schultz purportedly gave a good quantity of lentil seeds to J. J. Wagner of Farmington, Washington, to plant in his garden. Realizing great success with his first lentil crop and recognizing an economic opportunity, Wagner started producing lentils for the Seventh Day Adventist community, who needed it for one of their main protein sources. Even today, the Palouse produces a significant percentage of the nation's lentils (Montana and North Dakota also grow lentils). Stop by the annual Lentil Festival in Pullman, Washington, next summer. Don't miss their lentil pancake breakfast, and a Lentil Lane food court where you can even find lentil ice cream.

Wheat is also produced in abundance in the Palouse, especially soft white wheat. The first wheat farmers started here in the 1870s. Wheat farming, fortunately, has changed dramatically since then. Back then it took dozens of workers as much as a month to harvest each farm. Those first harvest crews used horse-drawn implements to cut the wheat, and then fed it by hand into the stationary threshers. Other workers bagged the grain in the field and loaded it onto a wagon to bring it to a warehouse. In the spirit of the Texas chuck wagon, Palouse cook wagons cooked and served lunch in the fields. A typical meal in this premechanical era included meat, potatoes, gravy, homemade bread, vegetables, and pies. These meals were large and caloric in order to energize the workers. Today, some farms harvest ten times the acreage with just two people and in half the time. Rather than stopping for lunch, the wheat farmers eat a quick lunch in the cabs of their air-conditioned combines.

Ethnic Diversity in the Palouse

The Palouse has a rich and diverse history of settlers from many countries. A striking one-third of the settlers were foreign-born. Irish, British, Chinese, Japanese, Germans, Swiss, Norwegians, Swedes, Volga and Black Sea Germans, Greeks, and Italians made the Palouse their home in different waves.

The local cookbooks reflect these diverse ethnicities. The German people brought recipes for stuffed cabbage, apple bread, date-filled cookies, sauerkraut, and hot potato salad. Scandinavian culinary habits are reflected in the many recipes for dessert cream (Swedish Cream, page 412), flatbread, lutefisk, Swedish meatballs, pea salad, and fruit cake.

Rocky Mountain Culinary Roots

The culinary heritage of the Rocky Mountain states was founded on survival. Foods and cooking methods were often dictated by the geography, flora, and climate. Pioneers on the grueling Oregon Trail learned from the Native Americans how to make soup from locusts, or how to fry the insects when there was nothing else to eat. Examining their strategies for food choices is a study in contrast to today's nutrition strategies.

The Salish (Flathead) tribes of the Bitterroot Valley in Montana learned to rely on the starchy roots of the succulent Bitterroot plant (this plant, with its strikingly beautiful small, pink blossoms, later became the Montana state flower). The Salish shared this survival secret with Captain Clark of the Lewis and Clark expedition and with other explorers.

NATIVE PLANTS USED BY NEVADA INDIANS

- Cattails. These lovely reeds provided food in many ways: the roots were used raw in salads and cooked in other dishes; the young flowering shoots were eaten raw (and considered a delicacy).
- Joshua Tree flower buds. These were eaten hot or cold after being roasted. They were considered "candy" because they are so sweet.
- Yucca flowers. These were eaten and the stalks cooked. They were a source of energy because they are high in sugar.

Survival on the Trail: A Study in Contrasts

Learning to cook on the trail was a necessary survival skill. Over a century later, we fall back to the pioneers' preferred methods of cooking meat, but for different reasons. The pioneers and trappers preferred roasting meat to frying it. The only necessary equipment was a tree branch and a fire; no pots or other equipment was required. Frying was used only when there was no other choice, because it dried out the meat. Today, we prefer roasting to frying for nutritional reasons, primarily because roasted meat has less fat than fried.

Berries, roots, and other herbs complemented the meat. The pioneers ate the fruits of the land fresh when available. But they also had to think of food for the next week, the next month, or even the next year, never knowing what was around the corner for them. They dried as many of these foods as possible in the sun, creating stashes for leaner days ahead. Today our practices mimic these early patterns but for different reasons. We recommend planning food in advance to round out nutrition. For example, if you want a piece of our Triple Chocolate Cake (page 415), then think about how you can eat today and tomorrow to accommodate those extra calories.

In the past, eating just the right amount of calories was key to getting through a long day on the trail, covering the maximum amount of ground possible. Eating enough was often difficult, and was a predictor of survival. In contrast, today we strive to balance energy intake with output. Our caloric balance is difficult because food is available abundantly and with virtually no physical work on our part.

The Pacific Northwest: Salmon to Apples, Berries to Shellfish

As in every other part of the country, we learned many culinary treasures from the Pacific Northwest Native Americans. One of these is the potlatch. From the Chinook word for "gift," a potlatch also describes a ceremonial feast. For the Chinook, the feast was probably connected with native rituals or a significant event. These traditional potlatches included a cornucopia of seasonal foods, each dish contributed by a family. The potlatch is an American tradition; we know it as a potluck meal.

Fusion Cuisine Rooted in Cultural Diversity

The rich land of the Palouse and the Gold Rush of the mid-1800s brought a huge influx of people from other countries, especially from Asia. These settlers from the other side of the Pacific add another level of meaning to the term Pacific Rim cuisine; indeed, both sides of this rim are represented. Much of the bounty of the Pacific is the same on its shores in different continents, including salmon and many varieties of shellfish.

People from China introduced their traditional cooking methods to the Pacific Northwest. The Japanese planted oyster species that would become the most common varieties available in this region. Thai, Korean, Filipino, and Vietnamese people brought their favorite native ingredients and shared their treasured food combinations with the area. For example, they brought fresh cilantro, bok choy, bitter melon, mustard greens, and ginger to the region over a century ago, and these ingredients remain prominent in Asian cuisine. This rich cultural diversity has given rise to fusion cooking, which comprises a significant part of Pacific Northwest cuisine.

Hunting for Mushrooms

From October through December, the recreational hunt for wild forest mushrooms in Oregon and Washington State is a popular sport.

Chanterelles, boletus, matsutake, and dozens of other varieties appear during this time when temperatures cool and the fall rains start.

The art of mushroom hunting is just that: an art. Ask any "shroom hunter," and you'll learn that there are many dos, musts, and don'ts to mushroom gathering. Some enthusiasts don't start foraging until two weeks after the first heavy rainfall.

Some of the popular finds include:

- Yellow chanterelles. Their apricot fragrance, subtle flavor, and firm texture make them a prized ingredient in many recipes.
- Boletes, one variety of which is the porcino mushroom (also called cepes). They are pale brown in color and can weigh just an ounce or half a pound. They have a pungent, woodsy flavor.
- Matsutake. This dark brown mushroom has a dense, meaty texture and a nutty, fragrant flavor.

IS IT POISONOUS?

If you don't know with absolute certainty whether the mushroom you have just found is poisonous, assume it is. Identifying mushrooms by looking at pictures in books isn't even safe, say mushroom foraging enthusiasts. Learn from a seasoned expert, and exert extreme caution.

IS THERE A DIFFERENCE BETWEEN A MUSHROOM AND A TOADSTOOL?

Not really, say mycologists (people who study mushrooms and other fungi). The two different terms arose at some unknown date in history when mushroom hunters started referring to the edible varieties as mushrooms and the poisonous ones as toadstools.

PRESERVING MUSHROOMS FOR TOMORROW

According to the Washington State Department of Natural Resources, mushroom hunters can help ensure there will be mushrooms in years to come by respecting some rules, which include:

- Harvest mushrooms at least 50 feet away from streams, lakes, or other bodies of water.
- Cut or pull mushrooms from the soil; don't rake them.
- Leave broken and very ripe mushrooms where they are, as they still may be spreading spores (which means more mushrooms for next year).

Alaska: Tlingits, Twenty-Pound Cabbages, and Sourdoughs

Long before the Klondike Gold Rush of 1897–1898, the Tlingit Indians called the southern area of Alaska home. Their communities hugged the coast; the sea provided most of their sustenance.

Twenty Hours of Sunlight

Hundreds of years later, in the 1930s depression era, farmers from Michigan, Wisconsin, and Minnesota moved near one of the Tlingit's homes: the

Matanuska Valley near Anchorage. The soil was fertile and growing conditions were outstanding. Although the growing season is short—from July to September—vegetables grow to enormous proportions in the Land of the Midnight Sun. With twenty hours of sunlight for several weeks in the summer, a cabbage can grow to twenty pounds. Compare that to the average three-pound cabbage bought in the lower forty-eight states! Zucchini, cucumbers, tomatoes, and other common vegetables grow to three or four times the size they do in the continental United States.

Klondike Gold Rush

In between the Tlingits and the depression-era transplanted farmers came the Klondike Gold Rush of 1897–1898. After Skookum Jim and William Moore located the pay dirt that started the gold rush, people descended upon Alaska from the south and east. Life on the trail to the gold mines and in the camps surrounding them was grueling even on the best days. Traveling and living in extreme conditions meant learning to live off the land. But the settlers were also masters of invention: they learned to make yeast from scratch. They also became experts at transporting it and keeping the yeast starter alive even in the most extreme conditions.

In more mild conditions, Alaskan prospectors added enough flour to make a ball of dough. They then tucked the ball deep into sacks of flour. When they arrived, they would tear off a piece of the dough to keep the starter alive. In very cold weather, the prospectors placed the ball of dough under their clothes next to their skin to keep the starter alive. A pinch of sugar or a drizzle of honey provided food for the starter. Today, people keep sourdough starter in crocks, and speak of their starter as crocking. To give someone crocking is considered giving the gift of life.

WALK THE SOURDOUGH TRAIL

Klondike Gold Rush National Historical Park in and around Skagway, Alaska, celebrates the Klondike Gold Rush of 1897–1898. In Skagway's Historic District, you can meander through fifteen restored buildings. Then, set out on the Chilkoot Trail or the White Pass Trail.

Fruited Bulgur Breakfast

Anita Crook, R.D., C.D.

Start the day with a warm breakfast of cooked bulgur. With nuts and fruit, this Palouse Region–inspired bulgur recipe makes a satisfying and nutritious start to the day. Vary the fruit depending on what is in season. For a great nutty flavor, toast the bulgur before simmering.

Serves: 4
Hands-on time: 10 minutes
Cooking time: 30 minutes

1 cup uncooked bulgur
½ teaspoon salt
¼ teaspoon ground cinnamon
⅓ cup chopped, dried apricots
⅓ cup dried cranberries
2 ripe nectarines, each cut into 10 wedges
1 cup fresh blueberries
¼ cup pecans, chopped
8 teaspoons brown sugar
1 cup calcium fortified vanilla soy milk or cow's milk, optional

Heat a heavy bottomed nonstick medium skillet (9½ inch) on medium heat. Rinse the bulgur in a strainer. Put the bulgur in the dry, heated skillet, stirring occasionally while the bulgur is wet. As the bulgur dries, stir often, and toast until dry, lightly browned, and fragrant. Pour in 3 cups water and add the salt, cinnamon, apricots, and cranberries. Bring the mixture to a boil, then turn the heat down to medium-low, cover, and let simmer for 20 minutes or until the water is absorbed.

Remove from the heat and pour into 4 bowls. Arrange 5 nectarine slices on top of each bowl of bulgur, spoke-fashion. Sprinkle ¼ cup blueberries between the nectarines. Put 1 tablespoon of chopped pecans in the center. Sprinkle 2 teaspoons of brown sugar over the top. If desired, pour ¼ cup of milk over the top.

COOK'S TIPS

Cook the bulgur and fruit mixture the night before and store it overnight in the refrigerator. In the morning reheat it with some milk in the microwave and then top it with the fruits, nuts, and sugar. Use roasted nuts on top for more flavor.

VARIATION

Try finishing the bulgur with different seasonal fruits. For example, in fall and winter cook the bulgur with dried pears and currants or dried apples and raisins. Top with fresh pear slices and chopped apples and sprinkle with walnuts. Substitute pure maple syrup or honey for sugar.

NUTRITION PER SERVING	
Serving size	1 bowl
Calories	320 kcal
Fat	6 g
Saturated fat	0.5 g
Cholesterol	0 mg
Sodium	300 mg
Carbohydrates	64 g
Dietary fiber	11 g
Protein	6 g

Dried Cherry Scones

Martha Marino, M.A., R.D., C.D.

Serves: 8
Hands-on time: 25 minutes
Cooking time: 15 to 20 minutes

For more than twenty years, I have lived in Washington, one of the nation's top cherry-producing states. During fresh cherry season, my kids and I shop at our local farmers' market for sweet Bing cherries and yellow Rainier cherries. This recipe uses dried tart cherries, but you can also use dried sweet cherries or dried cranberries.

½ cup dried tart cherries or cranberries
2 tablespoons apricot nectar, peach nectar, or apple juice
2 cups all-purpose flour
3 tablespoons sugar
1 tablespoon baking powder
¼ teaspoon salt
6 tablespoons cold butter
¼ cup sliced almonds, toasted
1 egg, beaten
⅓ cup plus 2 teaspoons half-and-half, divided
2 teaspoons pearl sugar or granulated sugar

Preheat oven to 375°F. Soak the cherries in the nectar or juice in a shallow bowl, such as a soup bowl, for 15 minutes. Do not drain.

Combine the flour, 3 tablespoons sugar, baking powder, and salt. Cut in the butter with a pastry blender or two knives until the mixture looks like coarse cornmeal. Stir in the almonds.

Combine the egg and ⅓ cup half-and-half. Add this to the cherry mixture. Add the egg-cherry mixture to the dry ingredients. Stir just until moistened.

Gather the dough into a ball and turn it onto a floured surface. Knead it 10 to 12 times. Pat it into a circle ¾ inch thick and 8 inches in diameter. Cut the dough into 8 wedges. Place the wedges 1 inch apart on an ungreased baking sheet. Brush the tops of the scones with 2 teaspoons half-and-half; sprinkle with pearl sugar or granulated sugar. Bake for 15 to 20 minutes or until golden. Remove the scones from the baking sheet and cool them on a wire rack for 5 minutes. Serve warm.

COOK'S TIP

I like to use pearl sugar to top these scones. Pearl sugar is a coarse sugar that remains bright white when baked.

SHOPPING TIP

You'll find pearl sugar in Scandinavian food stores (called parlsocker) and other specialty food stores.

SUBSTITUTION

The recipe is equally delicious when using granulated sugar.

COOK'S TIPS

To toast the nuts, preheat oven to 350°F. Place the nuts in a single layer on a baking sheet. Bake for 5 to 10 minutes, stirring or shaking the pan once or twice so that the nuts toast evenly. Watch closely toward the end of toasting so that the nuts don't scorch.

NUTRITION PER SERVING	
Serving size	1 scone
Calories	280 kcal
Fat	12 g
Saturated fat	6 g
Cholesterol	55 mg
Sodium	270 mg
Carbohydrates	38 g
Dietary fiber	1 g
Protein	5 g

Greek Brunch Bake

Taiga Sudakin, R.D., L.D.

Dill, feta, tomatoes, and spinach blend together to create this Greek dish that is a favorite in our Oregon home. You can serve it proudly as a vegetarian lunch or dinner.

Serves: 12 as an appetizer or 6 as main dish
Hands-on time: 15 minutes
Cooking time: 30 minutes

1 10-ounce package frozen chopped spinach, thawed
vegetable oil cooking spray
1 16-ounce container egg substitute
1 14½-ounce can diced tomatoes, drained
2 packages (3.5 ounces each) crumbled reduced-fat feta cheese
3 green onions, white and green parts finely chopped
1 tablespoon chopped fresh dill
dash ground black pepper

Defrost and drain the spinach in the refrigerator up to 24 hours before using. (When ready to use, squeeze out any excess liquid.)

Preheat oven to 400°F. Spray a 9-by-13-inch baking dish with the cooking spray.

Beat the egg substitute with an electric mixer at medium speed in a large bowl until foamy and until it doubles in volume. Add the spinach, tomatoes, feta cheese, onions, dill, and pepper to the egg substitute. Stir until well blended.

Pour the mixture into a prepared baking dish and bake 30 to 35 minutes or until a knife inserted near the center comes out clean. Let stand for a few minutes before cutting and serving.

SUBSTITUTION
Substitute 2 ripe fresh tomatoes (chopped) when tomatoes are abundant.

VARIATION
If you like dill, try doubling or tripling the amount of fresh dill you add to the casserole.

NUTRITION PER SERVING	
Serving size	⅙ of casserole
Calories	150 kcal
Fat	6 g
Saturated fat	3 g
Cholesterol	10 mg
Sodium	700 mg
Carbohydrates	7 g
Dietary fiber	2 g
Protein	18 g

Herbed Cheese Roll

Laura Faler Thomas, M.Ed., R.D., L.D.

Serves: 5
Hands-on time: 15 minutes
Chill time: at least 2 hours

With so many great breads and crackers to accompany cheese rolls, they are a great combination with a chilled summer wine—here in Idaho or anywhere in the country.

4 ounces low-fat cream cheese, softened
1 cup shredded, part-skim mozzarella cheese
2 tablespoons finely chopped sun-dried tomatoes (not oil packed)
2 cloves garlic, minced
6 tablespoons finely chopped fresh basil leaves

Mix the cream cheese, mozzarella cheese, and tomatoes until smooth. Shape the cheese mixture into a log. Roll it in plastic wrap and chill until firm, at least 20 minutes. Roll the chilled log in fresh basil, then rewrap. Chill.

Cut it into 20 slices and serve it with slices of roasted garlic bread.

VARIATION

Substitute ½ cup of low-fat ricotta cheese for the mozzarella. The cheese roll will be softer. If desired, shape it into a ball, cover it with fresh herbs, and chill. Serve it with a cheese spreader and breads or crackers.

NUTRITION PER SERVING

Serving size	4 slices
Calories	120 kcal
Fat	8 g
Saturated fat	5 g
Cholesterol	25 mg
Sodium	17 mg
Carbohydrates	4 g
Dietary fiber	0 g
Protein	8 g

Green Chili Cheese Roll

Laura Faler Thomas, M.Ed., R.D., L.D.

What's better than choice, especially when it comes to food? The green chili version can be as hot or as mild as you like, while the gently bold blue is just plain distinctly fabulous.

- 4 ounces low-fat cream cheese, softened
- 1 cup shredded, reduced-fat sharp cheddar cheese
- 2 tablespoons canned, diced green chilis, dried with a paper towel
- 1 teaspoon dehydrated minced shallots
- 3 tablespoons finely chopped cilantro leaves
- 3 tablespoons finely chopped chives

Mix the cream cheese, cheddar cheese, and chilis until smooth. Shape the cheese mixture into a log. Roll it in plastic wrap and chill until firm, at least 20 minutes. Roll the chilled log in a mixture of the fresh cilantro and chives, then rewrap. Chill.

Blue Cheese Roll

- 4 ounces low-fat cream cheese, softened
- ½ cup blue cheese crumbles
- ¼ cup finely chopped dates
- ¼ cup chopped walnuts

Mix the cream cheese and blue cheese until smooth. Shape the cheese mixture into a log. Roll it in plastic wrap and chill until firm, at least 20 minutes. Roll the chilled log in a mixture of the dates and walnuts; then rewrap. Chill.

Cut it into 20 slices and serve with crackers.

VARIATION

Substitute ½ cup of low-fat ricotta cheese for the cheddar cheese. The cheese roll will be softer. If desired, shape it into a ball, cover it with fresh herbs, and chill. Serve it with a cheese spreader and breads or crackers.

NUTRITION PER SERVING	
Serving size	4 slices, green chili cheese roll
Calories	90 kcal
Fat	6 g
Saturated fat	3.5 g
Cholesterol	15 mg
Sodium	210 mg
Carbohydrates	3 g
Dietary fiber	0 g
Protein	8 g

NUTRITION PER SERVING	
Serving size	4 slices, blue cheese roll
Calories	160 kcal
Fat	12 g
Saturated fat	5 g
Cholesterol	25 mg
Sodium	260 mg
Carbohydrates	9 g
Dietary fiber	1 g
Protein	6 g

Smoked Salmon Spread

Melissa Stevens Ohlson, M.S., R.D., L.D.

Serves: 8
Hands-on time: 15 minutes

Salmon and dill are a timeless combination in this easy, lightened-up spread that is Alaskan-inspired. For optimal flavor, use fresh lemon juice and fresh dill. Need a do-ahead recipe that does double duty during the holidays? This Smoked Salmon Spread makes elegant appetizers atop cocktail rye bread or cucumber slices. Garnish the plate with a few wispy sprigs of dill. In the morning, serve it on bagels with fresh tomatoes, which is one of my favorite ways to serve this spread.

- 8 ounces low-fat cream cheese, room temperature
- ¼ cup nonfat plain yogurt
- 4 green onions, thinly sliced
- 1 medium-size red bell pepper, minced
- 2 tablespoons chopped fresh dill (or 2 teaspoons dried)
- 1 tablespoon fresh lemon juice
- dash Tabasco sauce or to taste
- 4 ounces smoked salmon, finely chopped
- 16 slices party rye bread

Mix the cream cheese and yogurt in a mixing bowl. Stir in the green onions, red pepper, dill, lemon juice, and Tabasco sauce thoroughly. Gently fold in the smoked salmon, leaving shreds of the salmon whole. Spread on the party rye bread.

SERVING SUGGESTION
Hollow out a loaf of French bread; spoon in the dip. Chill and slice.

NUTRITION PER SERVING

Serving size	⅓ cup spread, 2 slices party rye
Calories	170 kcal
Fat	7 g
Saturated fat	3.5 g
Cholesterol	20 mg
Sodium	480 mg
Carbohydrates	19 g
Dietary fiber	3 g
Protein	10 g

Smoked Salmon Pizza

Roberta L. Duyff, M.S., R.D., F.A.D.A., C.F.C.S.

With one topping or another, who doesn't like pizza? Made with smoked salmon, this recipe was inspired by the delicious pizza my family enjoyed from a small bakery-deli on the Northwest coast. The salmon was caught and smoked by a local Native American fisherman. The whole wheat crust was bakery fresh; the tomatoes were picked from the bakery-deli's backyard garden; and it was topped with flavorful Walla Walla sweet onions. Our pizza picnic was made even more remarkable by its wonderful setting: a magnificent beach on Washington's Olympic Peninsula.

Serves: 6
Hands-on time: 20 minutes
Cooking time: 15 to 20 minutes

- 1 12-inch unbaked pizza crust, preferably whole wheat
- 2 tablespoons dill mustard
- 2 medium-size tomatoes, thinly sliced
- 1½ cups flaked, smoked salmon
- 1 cup caramelized onions
- 1 cup shredded Swiss cheese (4 ounces)

Preheat oven to 425°F. Place the pizza crust on a pizza or baking pan. Spread the mustard on the crust. Arrange the tomatoes, salmon, onions, and shredded cheese on top. Bake for 15 minutes, or until the crust is golden brown.

COOK'S TIP

To caramelize the onions, melt 2 tablespoons butter or margarine in a medium-size frying pan. Cook and stir 2 medium-size, thinly sliced onions uncovered over medium heat until their moisture evaporates and their natural sugars turn them golden (but not black around the edges), usually 15 to 20 minutes. For convenience, caramelize onions ahead and freeze them.

FOOD TRIVIA

Onions taste sweeter when they're cooked. Some other vegetables, such as bell peppers, carrots, fennel, and sweet potatoes do, too. Just a touch of brown sugar or other sweetener or a sweet seasoning (cinnamon, ginger, mint, nutmeg) in your carrot or sweet potato recipe enhances the sweetness even more.

SHOPPING TIP

If you can't find smoked salmon in your seafood department, use canned (smoked or not) salmon instead. The benefit? Convenience. With the ingredients on hand, you can create a flavorful salmon pizza at a moment's notice.

SERVING SUGGESTION

Serve this pizza with a tossed garden salad, made with a mesclun (gourmet salad mix) of young, small salad greens, sliced pears, and honey vinaigrette.

SUBSTITUTION

For their smoked flavor, Canadian bacon or deli ham make great substitutes for smoked salmon.

NUTRITION PER SERVING	
Serving size	1 slice
Calories	300 kcal
Fat	13 g
Saturated fat	6 g
Cholesterol	35 mg
Sodium	690 mg
Carbohydrates	29 g
Dietary fiber	2 g
Protein	17 g

Chicken Breast Roll-ups with Fruited Sauce

Naomi Kakiuchi, R.D., C.D.

Serves: 8
Hands-on time: 30 minutes
Cooking time: 45 minutes

Seattle born, this dish makes a great appetizer or a main course. Your taste buds will be delightfully surprised by this concert of flavors.

1 pound boneless, skinless chicken breasts
⅓ cup crumbled blue or Roquefort cheese
2 green onions, sliced
1 tablespoon extra-virgin olive oil
½ teaspoon salt
¼ to ½ teaspoon black pepper
1 17-ounce can fruit cocktail in its own juice
2 tablespoons butter
1 tablespoon cornstarch
2 teaspoons prepared mustard
2 teaspoons chicken bouillon
¼ cup chopped fresh parsley
1 tablespoon lemon juice

Preheat oven to 350°F. Cut the chicken breasts in half. Flatten them slightly by pounding. Sprinkle the chicken with the cheese and onions. Roll up and (if necessary) skewer.

Place the chicken in a shallow baking pan. Brush with the oil; sprinkle with salt and pepper. Bake for 30 to 45 minutes or until the meat reaches 165°F.

Meanwhile, drain the fruit cocktail, saving the juice. Add enough water to the juice to make 1 cup of liquid. Blend the fruit cocktail in a food processor or blender lightly. Do not purée.

Place the butter in a saucepan; stir in the cornstarch. Heat until bubbly. Stir in the mustard, bouillon, and juice mixture. Cook and stir until the mixture is thickened.

Five minutes before serving, add the fruit, parsley, lemon juice, and 2 tablespoons of drippings from the pan in which the chicken was baked to the sauce mixture and heat. Remove the skewers from the chicken; slice each chicken roll-up into 4 pieces. Place the sauce in a bowl alongside the sliced chicken roll-ups.

SERVING SUGGESTION
To serve chicken roll-ups as a main dish, do not slice them after baking. Serve the chicken on a bed of rice.

NUTRITION PER SERVING	
Serving size	2 to 3 slices
Calories	160 kcal
Fat	7 g
Saturated fat	3.5 g
Cholesterol	45 mg
Sodium	300 mg
Carbohydrates	9 g
Dietary fiber	Less than 1 g
Protein	15 g

Roasted Red Bell Pepper Wasabi Sauce and Dip

Lori A. Miller, R.D., L.D.

Roasting the red bell peppers provides a concentrated sweet pepper flavor, which, embellished with the fiery zing of Asian-inspired wasabi, make a tantalizing accompaniment for sandwiches and chips or vegetables anywhere in the country.

Serves: 8
Hands-on time: 30 minutes

- 1 red bell pepper, halved, cored, and seeded
- 1 teaspoon wasabi powder (dried horseradish powder)
- 1 clove garlic, coarsely chopped
- ¼ cup reduced-fat sour cream
- ¼ cup reduced-fat mayonnaise
- 2 ounces nonfat or reduced-fat Neufchatel cheese, softened

Broil the peppers, cut-side down, for 5 minutes. Turn over and repeat.

Place the broiled peppers in a paper bag for 10 minutes. Peel the cooled peppers and coarsely chop.

Mix 2 teaspoons water and the wasabi powder. Set aside for 10 minutes to rehydrate.

Place the peppers and the garlic in a food processor; purée 2 minutes. Add the sour cream, mayonnaise, cheese, and wasabi. Purée 2 minutes longer, or until the mixture is smooth. Scrape down the sides of the bowl as needed to make a smooth dip.

COOK'S TIP

So versatile, this cold dipping sauce can be used as a dip for raw vegetables or shrimp, a sauce topping for seafood, or a topping for sandwiches such as the North Pacific Seafood Wrap (page 401).

NUTRITION PER SERVING	
Serving size	2 tablespoons
Calories	70 kcal
Fat	4.5 g
Saturated fat	2 g
Cholesterol	9 mg
Sodium	86 mg
Carbohydrates	5 g
Dietary fiber	Less than 1 g
Protein	2 g

German Salad Dressing

Bonnie Athas, R.D.

Serves: 26
Hands-on time: 10 minutes

Germans frequently serve a side salad of thinly sliced cucumber, tomatoes, chopped fresh onions, and grated carrots. This dressing is a typical accompaniment for that salad. Try it with fresh greens, too, as we do in Utah.

- 1 cup cider vinegar
- 1 cup sugar
- 1½ tablespoons dried onion flakes (or 1 small yellow onion, minced)
- 2 teaspoons garlic powder or 1 large clove garlic, minced
- 1½ teaspoons dried thyme leaves or 1 teaspoon ground thyme
- 1½ teaspoons dried basil leaves
- ½ teaspoon dried rosemary leaves
- 1 teaspoon chopped dill weed (or ½ teaspoon dried dill weed)
- 2 teaspoons capers plus 1 teaspoon caper juice
- ½ cup orange juice
- ¼ cup lemon juice
- ½ cup extra-virgin olive oil
- dash salt

Mix the vinegar and sugar in a quart jar until dissolved; add the onion, garlic, herbs, capers plus caper juice, orange juice, and lemon juice. Stir in the olive oil; mix thoroughly. Add salt as needed. Keep refrigerated until ready to use.

SERVING SUGGESTION
You will need to shake the dressing vigorously before serving as it settles quickly. Try serving it in a pitcher with a spoon so that each person can stir the dressing before using it.

NUTRITION PER SERVING

Serving size	2 tablespoons
Calories	80 kcal
Fat	4.5 g
Saturated fat	0.5 g
Cholesterol	0 mg
Sodium	5 mg
Carbohydrates	9 g
Dietary fiber	0 g
Protein	0 g

Green Peas and Red Pepper Salad with Lime-Ginger Dressing

Anita Crook, R.D., C.D.

Here is a salad that uses both sugar snap peas and green split peas, both available in the Palouse region. The red pepper adds a bright contrast to the green hues. The lime-ginger dressing adds a zesty complement to the vegetables and rice.

Serves: 6 or 12
Hands-on time: 30 minutes
Cooking time: 30 minutes (to simmer rice and split peas)

- 1 cup jasmine rice
- ½ teaspoon sea salt
- ½ cup green split peas
- 2 cups sugar snap peas
- 1 cup sweet red pepper, cut into ½-inch squares

DRESSING

- 2 tablespoons canola oil
- 1 teaspoon toasted sesame oil
- 2 tablespoons fresh lime juice
- 2 tablespoons rice vinegar
- 1 tablespoon mellow white miso
- 1 tablespoon sugar
- 1 teaspoon grated fresh ginger

Bring the rice, 2 cups water, and sea salt to boil in a medium-size saucepan. Turn the heat to low, cover, and simmer rice for 20 minutes or until done.

Bring the split peas and 1½ cups water to boil in a medium-size saucepan. Turn the heat down to medium-low, partially cover, and simmer for 25 to 35 minutes or until the peas are tender but not mushy. Drain the excess water. (Split peas tend to froth easily and boil over. Keep the pan partially covered with the lid one-half inch away from the edge of the pan to avoid boiling over.)

Bring ⅓ cup of water to boil in a small saucepan. Add the sugar snap peas. Turn the heat down to medium, cover, and cook for 3 minutes until the peas are bright green and crisp-tender. Remove from heat, pour off the cooking water, and immediately plunge the sugar snap peas in ice-cold water to shock them. Drain and set aside.

Whisk together the canola oil, sesame oil, lime juice, rice vinegar, miso, sugar, and ginger to make the dressing.

Combine the cooked rice, cooked split peas, cooked sugar snap peas, and red pepper in a large bowl. Pour the dressing over the vegetables and rice. Stir to combine, and serve.

SHOPPING TIP
Look for sugar snap peas that are stringless—otherwise you will need to "de-string" them.

VARIATION
Scatter ½ cup of roasted coarsely chopped almonds or cashews on top just before serving.

FOOD TRIVIA
Thomas Jefferson grew thirty different types of peas in his Monticello garden.

NUTRITION PER SERVING

Serving size	1¼ cups
Calories	270 kcal
Fat	6 g
Saturated fat	0 g
Cholesterol	0 mg
Sodium	280 mg
Carbohydrates	46 g
Dietary fiber	3 g
Protein	8 g

Pacific Northwest Tuna Salad

Lori A. Miller, R.D., L.D.

Serves: 4
Hands-on time: 15 minutes

In this Pacific-Northwest-inspired recipe, pickled ginger and wasabi add an Asian influence to seafood salad.

- 2 teaspoons wasabi powder
- 2 6-ounce cans white albacore tuna, drained
- 1 green onion, thinly sliced
- ¼ medium-size red bell pepper, minced
- 2 tablespoons (about 10) finely diced water chestnuts
- ¼ cup reduced-fat mayonnaise
- 2 to 4 tablespoons minced pickled ginger
- 2 cloves (1 teaspoon) minced garlic
- 8 cups romaine lettuce or other mixed greens

Combine the wasabi powder and 1 tablespoon water; set aside for 10 minutes. Toss together the tuna, onions, bell pepper, and water chestnuts in a small mixing bowl. Blend together the mayonnaise, pickled ginger, wasabi, and garlic until fully blended. Add the dressing to the tuna mixture and stir to coat.

Chill and serve on a generous bed of romaine lettuce or mixed greens.

VARIATIONS

If you're tired of tuna, substitute canned salmon or try the dressing as an accompaniment to sushi.

COOK'S TIP

Blend all the ingredients except the greens, and store in the refrigerator up to 2 days ahead. Stir the salad before spooning it onto a bed of lettuce.

NUTRITION NUGGET

If you're looking for the most omega-3s, reach for albacore tuna. Another advantage of albacore is that it's always water packed to sidestep extra fat grams.

NUTRITION PER SERVING

Serving size	2 cups romaine plus ½ cup tuna salad
Calories	170 kcal
Fat	3 g
Saturated fat	0.5 g
Cholesterol	35 mg
Sodium	780 mg
Carbohydrates	13 g
Dietary fiber	4 g
Protein	23 g

Summer Fresh Tomato, Grain, and Bean Salad

Anita Crook, R.D., C.D.

Savor fresh-from-the-vine summer tomatoes and sun-drenched basil in this quick salad that is the Palouse region's answer to Middle Eastern tabbouleh. Crunchy fennel adds interesting flavor, too. Serve this as a main dish salad or in smaller portions for a refreshing side dish.

Serves: 6
Hands-on time: 30 minutes
Standing time: 60 minutes (to soak bulgur)

1 cup bulgur
1½ cups chopped tomatoes
½ cup coarsely chopped fresh basil
½ cup chopped scallion
½ cup chopped fennel bulb
1 15¼-ounce can 50% less sodium kidney beans, rinsed and drained

DRESSING
3 tablespoons extra-virgin olive oil
2 tablespoons sherry vinegar
2 tablespoons lemon juice
1 teaspoon sea salt
½ teaspoon freshly ground black pepper

Pour 2 cups boiling water over the bulgur in a large bowl. Let it sit until the water is absorbed and the bulgur is tender, about 60 minutes. Pour off any excess water.

Whisk together the dressing ingredients.

Combine the tomatoes, basil, scallion, fennel, and kidney beans with the bulgur. Add the dressing, fold in to combine, and serve immediately. If desired, sprinkle more freshly ground black pepper on individual servings.

SERVING SUGGESTION

Serve with warm pita bread, hummus, and an assortment of olives from the olive bar at your local grocery store.

COOK'S TIP

Avoid storing fresh tomatoes in the refrigerator unless they are overripe. Refrigeration makes tomatoes lose their flavor and makes their texture mealy. If you do not have a garden to grow your own tomatoes, get some wonderful ones at the farmers' market.

NUTRITION PER SERVING	
Serving size	1 cup
Calories	220 kcal
Fat	8 g
Saturated fat	1 g
Cholesterol	0 mg
Sodium	440 mg
Carbohydrates	32 g
Dietary fiber	11 g
Protein	8 g

Cucumber Salad

Ellen Hird, M.B.A., R.D.

Serves: 4
Hands-on time: 15 minutes
Standing time: 15 minutes

Pluck a garden-fresh cucumber from your backyard or look for English cucumbers in the produce section of your supermarket for the freshest tasting salad. With our long Colorado winters, we certainly need both options.

- ½ cup Chinese pea pods (about 1½ ounces), cut in half
- 1 rib celery, diced
- 1 medium-size cucumber, peeled and diced
- 1 large tomato, diced
- 3 green onions, thinly sliced
- ¼ cup rice vinegar or white distilled vinegar
- 2 teaspoons toasted sesame oil or hot sesame oil
- 1 tablespoon minced fresh or 1 teaspoon dried dill
- ¼ teaspoon sugar
- ¼ teaspoon salt (optional)

Bring 2 quarts of water to a boil; prepare a large bowl of ice water. Add the pea pods to the boiling water; blanch for 1 minute. Remove with a slotted spoon and immediately plunge into the ice water.

Repeat the procedure with the celery, blanching 1½ to 2 minutes before plunging into the ice water. Drain the pea pods and celery; pat them dry with a paper towel.

Combine the pea pods, celery, cucumber, tomato, and onions in a medium-size salad bowl. Toss the vegetables with the vinegar, sesame oil, dill, sugar, and salt, if desired. Refrigerate for at least 15 minutes or up to 1 hour before serving.

SUBSTITUTION

Dill is a traditional accompaniment to the cucumber's crunch, but you may enjoy a substitution of 2 tablespoons of minced cilantro for an Asian-inspired twist.

COOK'S TIP

This recipe may be assembled up to one day in advance by preparing all the vegetables and the dressing separately. Toss the salad with the dressing 15 minutes before serving.

NUTRITION PER SERVING	
Serving size	1 cup
Calories	50 kcal
Fat	2.5 g
Saturated fat	0 g
Cholesterol	0 mg
Sodium	15 mg
Carbohydrates	6 g
Dietary fiber	2 g
Protein	2 g

The Best Potato Salad

Naomi Kakiuchi, R.D., C.D.

Salad trends come and go, but potato salad never goes out of style. What summer picnic would be complete without potato salad? Here's a great recipe I grew up with in our Seattle Chinese-American home—although I've lightened it up a bit. Even my mom can't taste the difference.

Serves: 8
Hands-on time: 20 minutes
Cooking time: 20 minutes

- 2 pounds baby red potatoes, unpeeled
- ½ cup reduced-fat oil and vinegar salad dressing
- 2 tablespoons Dijon mustard
- ¼ cup chopped parsley or fresh cilantro, rinsed, dried, and chopped
- 1 bunch green onions, thinly sliced on the diagonal
- 2 garlic cloves, minced
- ½ cup diced celery
- ¼ cup chopped dill pickle
- salt to taste
- ½ teaspoon ground black pepper

Boil the potatoes until cooked through but not too soft, about 15 to 20 minutes. Drain and cool until just warm. Dice the potatoes to ½-inch cubes; place them in a large bowl.

Mix the oil and vinegar dressing with the mustard; sprinkle onto the warm potatoes to absorb the dressing. Add the parsley or cilantro, green onions, garlic, celery, and pickle. Toss well, taking care not to break up the potatoes or tear the skins. Season with salt and pepper, and more vinaigrette as needed. Stir gently and serve.

COOK'S TIP

Enhance the flavor by letting the salad stand at least 30 minutes before serving. This allows the flavors to infuse into the potatoes.

NUTRITION PER SERVING	
Serving size	½ cup
Calories	110 kcal
Fat	7 g
Saturated fat	1 g
Cholesterol	0 mg
Sodium	300 mg
Carbohydrates	10 g
Dietary fiber	4 g
Protein	3 g

Sautéed Herbed Wild Mushrooms

Martha Marino, M.A., R.D., C.D.

Serves: 6
Hands-on time: 10 to 15 minutes
Cooking time: 15 minutes

Each September, a friend and I head out to the damp woods in western Washington to hunt for chanterelles. It's an adult version of an Easter egg hunt: we look under logs and behind mossy rocks, and we squeal when we are lucky enough to find them. This recipe is equally good with mushrooms purchased at the supermarket.

- 2 tablespoons butter
- 2 tablespoons olive oil
- ¼ cup chopped onion
- 2 cloves garlic, minced
- 1 pound chanterelle mushrooms, thinly sliced
- 1 pound mixed crimini and button mushrooms, thinly sliced
- 2 tablespoons chopped parsley
- 2 teaspoons fresh thyme
- 1 teaspoon salt
- ¼ teaspoon pepper

Melt the butter with the olive oil in a large skillet over medium heat. Add the onion and garlic and cook for 2 or 3 minutes or until the onion is softened. Add the mushrooms; increase the heat to medium-high and cook, stirring, 5 to 6 minutes or until lightly browned around the edges. Stir in the parsley, thyme, salt, and pepper.

COOK'S TIP

To clean the mushrooms, use a clean, dry vegetable brush. Avoid getting the mushrooms too wet as they will become soggy even after cooking.

NUTRITION PER SERVING

Serving size	½ cup
Calories	130 kcal
Fat	9 g
Saturated fat	3 g
Cholesterol	10 mg
Sodium	410 mg
Carbohydrates	9 g
Dietary fiber	3 g
Protein	5 g

Tiger Fries

Kristine Napier, M.P.H., R.D.

Sliced red potatoes from Idaho tossed with sweet potato strips yield a dish that's as pretty as it is great tasting. It's also kid-pleasing!

Serves: 4
Hands-on time: 10 minutes
Cooking time: 20 minutes

vegetable oil cooking spray
1 large sweet potato (about ½ pound), peeled
2 to 3 red potatoes (about ½ pound), scrubbed with peel on
2 tablespoons extra-virgin olive oil
1 teaspoon salt
½ teaspoon black pepper

Preheat oven to 400°F. Spray a large baking sheet with the cooking spray. Slice the potatoes very thinly (use a food processor if you have one). Place the potatoes in a bowl; add the oil, salt, and pepper. Toss to coat. Transfer the potatoes to a baking sheet. Spread them out in a single layer.

Bake for 10 minutes; turn the potatoes over. Bake for an additional 5 to 10 minutes, or until the potatoes are slightly crisp and golden brown.

SUBSTITUTION

Substitute an equal weight of an Idaho or a Russet potato for the red ones; scrub well and follow the recipe.

NUTRITION NUGGET

Scrub the sweet potatoes and slice with the skin on. It's edible and adds fiber.

NUTRITION PER SERVING	
Serving size	¾ cup
Calories	160 kcal
Fat	7 g
Saturated fat	1 g
Cholesterol	0 mg
Sodium	590 mg
Carbohydrates	23 g
Dietary fiber	2 g
Protein	2 g

Mom's Baked Beans

Barbara J. Pyper, M.S., R.D., C.D., F.H.C.F.A., F.C.S.I.

Serves: 8
Hands-on time: 20 minutes
Cooking time: 10 hours

Bean pots were commonplace in Montana kitchens when I was growing up. My mom, Betty Pyper, cooked beans in her bean pot overnight. Although bean pots are long gone from most kitchens, you can still make this fiber-rich recipe in the oven.

vegetable oil cooking spray
2 cups uncooked great northern beans
1 medium-size onion, diced
¼ pound extra-lean ham
¼ cup molasses
2 tablespoons brown sugar
1 to 2 teaspoons dry mustard
¼ cup ketchup

Preheat oven to 300°F. Spray a 3-quart oven-safe dish with the cooking spray. Wash the beans and place in the prepared dish. Add 5 cups water and the onion and meat. Cover the dish tightly. Cook 5 hours.

Uncover; add the molasses, brown sugar, mustard, and ketchup. Increase the temperature to 375°F. Cook for 1 additional hour.

VARIATION

Use 4 slices center-cut bacon, chopped and uncooked, in place of the ham.

FOOD TRIVIA

Baked beans were first made because of religious reasons by the colonists who settled in the Northeast. They cooked the beans on Saturday so that they would have something to eat on Sunday when no cooking was allowed.

NUTRITION NUGGET

This recipe uses dry mustard rather than prepared mustard, which reduces the sodium level considerably. To spice it up, use a little extra dry mustard.

NUTRITION PER SERVING	
Serving size	¾ cup
Calories	230 kcal
Fat	1.5 g
Saturated fat	0 g
Cholesterol	5 mg
Sodium	310 mg
Carbohydrates	43 g
Dietary fiber	10 g
Protein	13 g

Barley Pilaf

Kristine Napier, M.P.H., R.D.

Barley, native to the Palouse region, is a great alternative to rice and pasta. Using quick-cooking barley and frozen vegetables, this dish cooks up quickly, is pleasing to the eye, and is delicious!

Serves: 4
Hands-on time: 10 minutes
Cooking time: 15 minutes
Standing time: 5 minutes

- 1 teaspoon sesame oil
- 1 medium-size onion, chopped
- 1 14-ounce can reduced-sodium chicken broth
- 1 cup quick cooking barley
- 1 10-ounce package frozen peas and carrots, thawed
- 2 tablespoons chopped fresh parsley (optional)

Heat the oil in a large heavy kettle over medium heat. Add the onion; sauté for 3 to 5 minutes or until the onion is translucent. Increase the heat; add the broth. Bring the liquid to a boil. Add the barley, cover, reduce heat, and simmer for 10 minutes.

Remove from heat. Stir in the vegetables. Cover and let stand for 5 minutes. Top with the chopped fresh parsley just before serving.

SUBSTITUTION

Substitute a 10-ounce box of chopped broccoli for the peas and carrots.

NUTRITION PER SERVING

Serving size	1 cup
Calories	190 kcal
Fat	2.5 g
Saturated fat	0 g
Cholesterol	0 mg
Sodium	60 mg
Carbohydrates	39 g
Dietary fiber	7 g
Protein	7 g

Lemon Fresh Tabbouleh

Kristine Napier, M.P.H., R.D.

Serves: 6
Hands-on time: 15 minutes
Standing time: 3 hours, 25 minutes

SUBSTITUTIONS
Substitute an equal amount of chopped fresh mint for the parsley. If you use mint, also try using an equal amount of orange juice instead of lemon juice.

Tabbouleh is a classic Middle Eastern dish. This version, inspired by the Palouse region's vast wheat fields, is considerably slimmed down from the traditional version. Enjoy it for a main course or a side-dish salad.

½ cup fresh lemon juice
2 cups (12 ounces) uncooked bulgur
1 teaspoon extra-virgin olive oil
1 teaspoon freshly ground black pepper
¼ teaspoon salt
1 cup chopped fresh parsley
1 bunch (5 or 6) green onions, chopped
2 cloves garlic, crushed
4 tomatoes, chopped

In a medium-size saucepan, bring the lemon juice and 3½ cups water to a boil; add the bulgur, oil, pepper, and salt. Remove from heat; cover, and let stand 20 to 25 minutes.

In a large bowl, combine the parsley, green onions, and garlic; toss to mix well. Add the bulgur mixture; toss again to mix well.

Transfer the bulgur mixture to a large serving bowl; refrigerate covered at least 3 hours until thoroughly chilled. Stir in the chopped tomatoes just before serving.

NUTRITION PER SERVING	
Serving size	1½ cups
Calories	200 kcal
Fat	2 g
Saturated fat	0 g
Cholesterol	0 mg
Sodium	125 mg
Carbohydrates	43 g
Dietary fiber	10 g
Protein	7 g

Lentil and Bead Soup

Martha Marino, M.A., R.D., C.D.

The rolling hills of the Palouse area in eastern Washington and western Idaho produce most of the lentils grown in the United States. The beads in this soup are tiny rounds of pasta called acini di pepe. *Some Italian-American families give their* bambini *(babies) acini di pepe pasta as one of their first foods, sometimes with a little olive oil or butter.*

Serves: 8
Hands-on time: 20 minutes
Cooking time: 45 minutes

- 2 tablespoons olive oil
- 1½ cups chopped onion
- 1 teaspoon minced garlic
- 2 cups shredded carrots
- 1 49-ounce can fat-free chicken broth or regular chicken broth
- 1½ cups dried lentils
- ⅓ cup acini de pepe pasta (or orzo)
- ¼ teaspoon salt
- ¼ teaspoon fresh ground pepper
- 1 cup shredded Italian cheese such as Parmesan, Romano, or Parmegianno Reggiano

Heat the olive oil in a large stock pot over medium-low heat. Add the onion and cook 7 to 8 minutes or until softened. Add the garlic and carrots and cook, covered, over low heat about 5 minutes or until softened. Add the broth and 2 cups water; heat to boiling. Stir in the lentils and return to a boil, stirring occasionally. Reduce heat to low, cover but leave the lid slightly ajar, and simmer until the lentils are tender, about 30 to 40 minutes.

While the lentils are cooking, bring 2 cups of salted water to a boil over high heat in a saucepan. Add the pasta, return to boil, and cook 10 to 12 minutes or until al dente. Drain.

Stir the cooked pasta into the lentil mixture. Add salt and pepper to taste. Serve with a bowl of Italian cheese at the table.

SERVING SUGGESTION

For a comforting meal on a chilly evening, add a loaf of rustic bread and a simple salad.

NUTRITION NUGGET

This hearty soup provides nourishing complete proteins with its combination of legumes and grains.

NUTRITION PER SERVING

Serving size	1 cup
Calories	270 kcal
Fat	8 g
Saturated fat	3 g
Cholesterol	10 mg
Sodium	360 mg
Carbohydrates	34 g
Dietary fiber	10 g
Protein	17 g

Pasta Fazool (Pasta e Fagioli)

Martha Marino, M.A., R.D., C.D.

Serves: 8
Hands-on time: 15 minutes
Standing time: soak beans 8 to 12 hours
Cooking time: 1 hour, 30 minutes

VARIATION

A delicious adaptation of this recipe is to add chopped pancetta or a ham hock with the onion, and proceed with the recipe. If the ham does not fall off the bone into bite-sized pieces, simply remove the bone before adding the pasta, cut the ham into pieces, and return the meat to the broth.

COOK'S TIP

If you prefer a vegetarian soup, substitute vegetable broth for the chicken stock.

NUTRITION PER SERVING

Serving size	1 cup
Calories	200 kcal
Fat	6 g
Saturated fat	1.5 g
Cholesterol	5 mg
Sodium	410 mg
Carbohydrates	28 g
Dietary fiber	9 g
Protein	11 g

Dean Martin sang about pasta fazool in the well-loved song, "That's Amore": "When the stars make you drool just like pasta fazool, that's amore!" An Italian-American favorite with as many variations as there are immigrants, the mainstays are beans and pasta. Here is our family's recipe that developed over the years in our Washington home.

- 8 ounces (1¼ cups) dried canellini beans or navy beans
- 2 tablespoons olive oil
- ¾ cup chopped onion (about 1 medium-size)
- 3 garlic cloves, minced or put through garlic press
- 1 tablespoon dried parsley
- 1 teaspoon dried oregano
- ½ teaspoon dried basil
- 1 14-ounce can Italian peeled tomatoes diced in purée, including juice
- 1 cup peeled and chopped carrots (about 2 medium-size)
- 8 cups chicken stock (or 4 14-ounce cans low-sodium chicken broth plus water to make 8 cups)
- ¾ cup ditalini or tubetini pasta, may be called salad macaroni
- 1 teaspoon salt (or to taste)
- ½ teaspoon fresh ground pepper
- grated Parmesan or Romano cheese to taste

Rinse the beans and pick them over to remove any grit. Place in a bowl, add 4 cups water, cover, and soak overnight.

Drain and discard the water the next day. Place the beans in large pot and add plenty of water. Bring the water to a boil, reduce heat, and simmer until the beans are almost tender, about 1 hour. Drain and discard the water, reserving the beans.

Heat the olive oil in large pot or Dutch oven over low heat. Add the onion and sauté, stirring, until it is very soft and translucent but not brown, about 25 minutes. Add the garlic and cook 1 to 2 minutes longer. Stir in the parsley, oregano, and basil. Add the undrained tomatoes, carrots, chicken stock, and reserved beans. Bring to a boil, then reduce heat to low and simmer uncovered for 45 minutes.

Add the pasta, salt, and pepper to the bean mixture and cook 10 to 15 minutes, depending on the pasta package directions, until the pasta is al dente. Serve in soup bowls with a bowl of grated Italian cheese at the table.

Palouse Winter Stew with Millet

Anita Crook, R.D., C.D.

This rich-tasting stew is perfect for a cold winter night. I developed it to take advantage of two of the crops grown in the Palouse region of the inland Northwest: lentils and chick-peas. The creamy texture and mild, nutty flavor of the millet is a good complement to the stew. It is a great way to incorporate whole grains into the meal and proves that millet is not just for the birds!

Serves: 6
Hands-on time: 20 minutes
Cooking time: 30 minutes

- 1 cup millet, washed with any field debris removed
- ½ teaspoon sea salt
- ½ cup lentils
- 1 tablespoon olive oil
- ¼ to ½ bunch Swiss chard to equal 2 cups of chopped chard leaves (remove stems from the leaves, chop, and set aside)
- ½ cup chopped onion
- 2 cloves garlic, minced
- ½ teaspoon cumin
- ½ teaspoon oregano
- 1 tablespoon chili powder
- 1 8-ounce can no-salt-added tomato sauce
- 1 tablespoon red wine vinegar
- 1 tablespoon molasses
- ¼ cup raisins
- ¾ cup 50% less sodium chick-peas, drained and rinsed
- ½ cup roasted, salted cashews, chopped

Bring 2 cups of water to boil in a medium-size saucepan. Add the millet and sea salt. Reduce heat to low, cover, and simmer for 20 minutes or until the millet is done. If there is water on top of the millet after cooking, stir it back into the millet.

Bring 1½ cups of water to boil in another medium-size saucepan. Add the lentils, reduce heat to medium low, cover, and simmer for 25 minutes or until the lentils are tender.

SERVING SUGGESTION

Serve with a green salad, whole-grain rolls, and baked pears topped with vanilla yogurt.

NUTRITION PER SERVING

Serving size	about ½ cup of stew mixture, ⅓ cup millet, and 1½ tablespoons cashews
Calories	370 kcal
Fat	11 g
Saturated fat	2 g
Cholesterol	0 mg
Sodium	420 mg
Carbohydrates	56 g
Dietary fiber	12 g
Protein	13 g

Palouse Winter Stew with Millet *(continued)*

COOK'S TIP

A rice cooker is a great appliance for cooking millet or other whole grains that require slow cooking at low heat and that can scorch easily if forgotten. Just put the proper measurements of grain, water, and salt into the rice cooker, turn it on, and forget about it until serving time.

Heat the olive oil in a medium-size (9½-inch) skillet over medium heat. Add the chard stems. Sauté for 2 minutes, then add the onion and garlic and sauté for another 5 to 10 minutes until golden brown. Add the cumin, oregano, chili powder, tomato sauce, red wine vinegar, molasses, raisins, and chard leaves to the skillet. Cover and simmer on low heat for 5 minutes. Add the cooked lentils and canned chick-peas. Cover and simmer for 5 more minutes.

Divide the cooked millet into 4 bowls. Top each with about ¾ cup of the stew and 2 tablespoons of the chopped cashews.

Sam's Greek Roasted Chicken

Naomi Kakiuchi, R.D., C.D.

In this Greek-inspired recipe, my dad roasts red potatoes, carrots, and parsnips alongside chicken in our Chinese home in Seattle. He always serves it with a leafy green salad topped with feta, tomatoes, and Kalamata olives.

Serves: 6
Hands-on time: 20 minutes
Cooking time: 1 hour

- vegetable oil cooking spray
- 1 whole chicken, washed
- 6 red potatoes, scrubbed (peel on)
- 2 carrots, peeled and sliced in half lengthwise
- 2 parsnips, peeled and sliced in half lengthwise
- 1 tablespoon extra-virgin olive oil
- 2 tablespoons Greek seasoning

Preheat oven to 400°F. Coat the roasting pan with the cooking spray. Place the chicken in the pan. Toss the potatoes, carrots, and parsnips with the olive oil and then place them in the roasting pan around the chicken. Sprinkle the chicken and vegetables with Greek seasoning.

Bake for 10 minutes and then lower the heat to 350°F. Continue to bake until the chicken temperature is 165°F (test with cooking thermometer near chicken thigh), approximately 45 minutes to 1 hour. Baste the chicken and vegetables at least twice with the cooking juices. Remove and discard the chicken skin. Serve hot.

COOK'S TIP
To intensify the flavor, sprinkle 1 tablespoon of Greek seasoning inside the chicken.

NUTRITION PER SERVING

Serving size	4 ounces cooked chicken plus 1¼ cups cooked potatoes and vegetables
Calories	300 kcal
Fat	6 g
Saturated fat	1 g
Cholesterol	80 mg
Sodium	115 mg
Carbohydrates	31 g
Dietary fiber	4 g
Protein	29 g

Cucumber Sunomono Salad

Naomi Kakiuchi, R.D., C.D.

Serves: 4
Hands-on time: 10 minutes
Standing time: 15 minutes

Preparing my native Japanese foods in my Seattle home is easy with the plethora of seafood and produce available. Sunomono is the Japanese word for "vinegared things," such as these salad ingredients, which are coated with a sweet-vinegar sauce. Sunomono ingredients include a wide variety of raw or cooked vegetables: broccoli, cabbage, carrots, cauliflower, celery, cucumber, daikon, lettuce, mushrooms, onions, pea pods, spinach, string beans, and seaweed.

- ¼ cup rice (or rice wine) vinegar
- 3 tablespoons sugar
- ¼ teaspoon salt
- 1 medium-size English or 2 medium-size Japanese cucumbers, skin scrubbed well and left on
- ½ pound cooked small shrimp, chilled
- 1 small head radicchio, chopped

Combine the vinegar, sugar, and salt in a container with a secure lid. Cover and shake until the sugar dissolves.

Cut the cucumbers in half lengthwise; slice thinly. Combine the cucumbers and shrimp in a medium-size bowl. Pour dressing over the top, stir well, cover, and let stand 15 minutes at room temperature to allow the cucumbers to soften and the flavors to mingle.

Serve the salad on a bed of chopped radicchio.

VARIATIONS

Use 3 cups of your favorite vegetables in place of the cucumbers. To spice it up, sprinkle ⅛ to ½ teaspoon wasabi powder for a hotter version.

NUTRITION PER SERVING

Serving size	1½ cups
Calories	120 kcal
Fat	1 g
Saturated fat	0 g
Cholesterol	85 mg
Sodium	240 mg
Carbohydrates	14 g
Dietary fiber	1 g
Protein	13 g

Baked Halibut Bristol Bay

Tami J. Cline, M.S., R.D., F.A.D.A., S.F.N.S.

Alaskan bush pilots cook a lot of halibut over campfires, including a simpler version of this recipe. While this recipe is simple, you'll love the flavor burst as red onion and celery leaves fuse with the lemon juice.

Serves: 2
Hands-on time: 10 minutes
Cooking time: 15 minutes

- 2 5- to 6-ounce halibut steaks
- 1 tablespoon extra-virgin olive oil
- 2 tablespoons lemon juice
- ¼ cup finely chopped celery leaves
- ¼ cup red onion, finely chopped
- ½ teaspoon black pepper
- ¼ teaspoon salt

Preheat oven to 400°F. Line a 9-by-13-inch baking dish with aluminum foil, allowing enough extra on each end to fold and seal into a pouch. Place the halibut steaks in the foil.

Combine the oil, lemon juice, celery leaves, onion, pepper, and salt in a small bowl; spoon evenly over the halibut. Seal the foil. Bake at 300°F or on a heated grill for approximately 15 minutes.

COOK'S TIP

The seasoning works well with other white fish.

FOOD TRIVIA

Halibut can weigh in at half a ton, but is commonly between 50 and 100 pounds. Fresh halibut is most abundant from March to September. The finest selection of halibut is the very young fish, called chicken halibut.

NUTRITION PER SERVING

Serving size	1 halibut steak plus ¼ cup sauce
Calories	160 kcal
Fat	9 g
Saturated fat	1.5 g
Cholesterol	25 mg
Sodium	350 mg
Carbohydrates	3 g
Dietary fiber	0.72 g
Protein	17 g

Northwest Cioppino

Martha Marino, M.A., R.D., C.D.

Serves: 6
Hands-on time: 20 minutes
Cooking time: 1 hour, 20 minutes

VARIATIONS

As with many soups and stews, this recipe serves as a guide. The amount of halibut (or other fin fish) can be doubled for a sturdier stew. Other shellfish, such as clams, can be substituted or added.

SERVING SUGGESTION

Serve with crusty Italian bread and a green salad (greens, tomatoes, and artichoke hearts).

COOK'S TIPS

When purchasing mussels, scallops, and clams, buy only those with tightly closed shells. After cooking thoroughly, eat only the shellfish whose shells have opened and discard those that did not open.

NUTRITION PER SERVING	
Serving size	2 generous cups
Calories	330 kcal
Fat	12 g
Saturated fat	2 g
Cholesterol	70 mg
Sodium	870 mg
Carbohydrates	18 g
Dietary fiber	2 g
Protein	30 g

The Pacific Northwest boasts an abundance of fish and shellfish. Italian immigrants to this area created this delicious tomato-based fish and shellfish stew. Adapt this version of cioppino to whatever is fresh and in season. To eat cioppino, you and your guests will dig right in with your fingers to fish out the mussels, clams, and shrimp. Set out extra napkins and empty bowls for shells.

¼ cup olive oil
1 large onion, diced (about 2 cups)
3 cloves garlic, minced
¼ cup chopped Italian flat-leaf parsley
1 teaspoon dried or 1 tablespoon fresh basil
1 teaspoon dried or 1 tablespoon fresh oregano
1 teaspoon salt
½ teaspoon fresh ground pepper
1 28-ounce can Italian crushed tomatoes in purée
1 8-ounce can tomato sauce
1 cup white wine (or water)
¾ pound halibut or firm white fish such as cod or snapper, skin removed, cut into 1½-inch cubes
½ pound mussels (about 12 to 14), shells scrubbed clean
½ pound bay scallops (about 12 to 14)
¼ pound fresh shrimp (about 12 to 14), shelled and deveined

Heat the oil over medium-low heat in a large stock pot. Add the onion and cook until the onion is softened, about 5 to 7 minutes. Add the garlic and cook for 1 to 2 minutes longer. Add the parsley, basil, oregano, salt, and pepper. Add the crushed tomatoes, tomato sauce, and wine, and bring just barely to a boil. Reduce to simmer, cover, and cook 30 minutes.

Add the fish, cover, and cook for 10 to 20 minutes longer. Add the mussels and/or clams, scallops, and shrimp, and simmer for 10 minutes or until the shells open. Serve immediately.

North Pacific Seafood Wrap

Lori A. Miller, R.D., L.D.

Can you hear the foghorns off the Seattle coast and smell the sea air? Succulent seafood sparked with a zesty wasabi sauce and delicate crispy Chinese Napa cabbage make these Northwest-inspired wraps unforgettable. If desired, serve on a lettuce leaf as a salad.

Serves: 8
Hands-on time: 15 minutes
Cooking time: 20 minutes

- 3 cups cooked and chilled seafood (scallops, shrimp, halibut), coarsely chopped
- 2 cups Chinese Napa cabbage, shredded
- ⅓ cup celery, chopped
- ⅓ cup green onion, thinly sliced
- 1 cup Red Bell Pepper Wasabi Sauce (see recipe on page 381)
- 8 10-inch flour tortillas

Combine the seafood, cabbage, celery, and onion in a large bowl. Add the Red Bell Pepper Wasabi Sauce; toss lightly.

Place ½ cup of the seafood mixture on the bottom edge of one tortilla. Fold the bottom edge of the tortilla in, fold the sides over the end, and roll forward wrapping tightly, burrito style. Tuck in the tortilla end securely by folding over about ½ inch. Wrap the tortilla diagonally in parchment paper; cut it in half. Repeat using the remaining tortillas and the filling.

SHOPPING TIP

Chinese Napa cabbage, available year-round, is thin, crisp, and delicate in flavor. The ruffled edges hold much of the sauce and still maintain its crunch.

SUBSTITUTIONS

Shredded lettuce may be used in place of Chinese Napa cabbage. For a much quicker version, blend 1 teaspoon wasabi with 1 to 2 teaspoons soy sauce for each wrap. Give it more color by substituting finely shredded red cabbage for the Napa version; around the Christmas holidays, the blend of red cabbage and green onions is delightful. If you are allergic to shellfish, substitute artificial crab meat, but read the label to ensure that the brand you choose does not have natural shellfish flavoring.

NUTRITION PER SERVING

Serving size	1 wrap
Calories	370 kcal
Fat	10.5 g
Saturated fat	3.5 g
Cholesterol	49 mg
Sodium	506 mg
Carbohydrates	47 g
Dietary fiber	3 g
Protein	19 g

All-American Ground Beef Casserole

Barbara J. Pyper, M.S., R.D., C.D., F.H.C.F.A., F.C.S.I.

Serves: 4
Hands-on time: about 30 minutes
Cooking time: 40 to 50 minutes

As we know them today, American casseroles are indeed a relatively modern invention—like this recipe. It is originally from my great aunt, Evelyn Meuli, who called it Delitzia. When we would visit her each summer, she would make this casserole—something we looked forward to! Although we've tried to trace the very ethnic-sounding "Delitzia," today we think she created the word to make it seem like fancy food.

- 3 cups uncooked wide egg noodles
- vegetable oil cooking spray
- ½ pound (8 ounces) extra-lean ground beef
- 1 large onion, diced
- 1 medium-size green pepper, diced
- 1 medium-size red pepper, diced
- 1 14¾-ounce can creamed corn
- 1 10½-ounce can condensed cream of tomato soup
- ¼ to ½ teaspoon black pepper
- 1 teaspoon garlic powder
- 1 cup (4 ounces) shredded sharp cheddar cheese

Cook the egg noodles as directed on the package. Preheat oven to 350°F. Spray a 2-quart casserole with the cooking spray; set aside.

Brown the ground beef and onion in a large nonstick skillet until the beef is cooked through. Remove from heat. Stir in the peppers, creamed corn, tomato soup, black pepper, garlic powder, and cooked noodles. Transfer the mixture to a prepared baking dish and bake uncovered for 30 minutes.

Remove the casserole from the oven. Top it evenly with the cheddar cheese. Bake 10 to 20 minutes more, or until the cheese bubbles and is golden brown.

SERVING SUGGESTION

Finish the meal with something healthy *and* sweet. Mix 1 teaspoon cinnamon with 1 tablespoon sugar. Slice one apple per person; dip the slices in the cinnamon/sugar mixture.

COOK'S TIP

This dish can also be made on the stove top. Brown the meat as directed in the recipe; stir the remaining ingredients into the skillet. Sprinkle evenly with cheese. Cover the skillet tightly and allow the cheese to melt, about 5 minutes. Serve.

FOOD TRIVIA

The word *casserole* has two meanings. For one, it means the dish or pot in which food is cooked or baked. Casserole also means "a combination of foods cooked together in a slow oven." As a cooking method, casseroles date back to the ancient practice of stewing meat slowly in earthenware containers.

NUTRITION PER SERVING

Serving size	1¾ cups
Calories	480 kcal
Fat	17 g
Saturated fat	9 g
Cholesterol	80 mg
Sodium	950 mg
Carbohydrates	58 g
Dietary fiber	4 g
Protein	27 g

German Beef Rolls (Rouladen)

Bonnie Athas, R.D.

What goes together better than beef, paprika, mushrooms, and barley? I'll walk you through rolling a dill pickle around sliced beef to create this easy version of a traditional German dish that is served often in the many German homes throughout Utah.

Serves: 4
Hands-on time: 20 minutes
Cooking time: 45 minutes

- 2 medium-size onions, chopped (divided)
- 2 turkey bacon slices, chopped
- 2 carrots, peeled and finely chopped
- 2 cloves garlic, minced
- 1 tablespoon hot Hungarian paprika, divided
- 1 tablespoon sweet Hungarian paprika, divided
- ¼ cup dry bread crumbs
- 1 pound round steak, thinly sliced and cut into 4 (4-ounce) pieces
- 2 tablespoons stone-ground mustard
- 1 large dill pickle, cut lengthwise into 4 pieces
- 2 tablespoons canola oil
- 1 14-ounce can reduced-sodium beef broth
- 2 cups sliced mushrooms
- 1 cup fat-free sour cream
- 3 cups cooked barley, hot

Combine half of the onions, bacon, carrots, and garlic and 1 teaspoon of each type of paprika in a large, heavy skillet. Cook over medium-low heat until the onions are translucent. Add the bread crumbs; stir well. Set aside to cool.

Place the beef slices between sheets of plastic wrap; pound or roll out until very thin. Spread evenly with the mustard.

Divide the vegetable mixture into four equal parts and spoon it over each piece of beef. Press the mixture onto the meat leaving a ½-inch border at each edge. Place 1 pickle piece on each beef slice. Roll the meat over the pickle, burrito style, enclosing the filling completely. Secure the roll with toothpicks.

Heat the oil over medium-high heat; add the beef rolls and the remaining half of the onions. Brown all sides of the rolls, about 8 minutes total. Reduce heat and add the broth, mushrooms, and the remaining 2 teaspoons of each type of paprika; stir gently. Bring the sauce to a boil; reduce heat, cover, and simmer until the beef is tender (about 30 minutes). Turn the rolls occasionally.

Remove the beef from the pan. Add the sour cream and simmer 5 minutes uncovered, allowing the sauce to reduce (cook off some liquid). Serve the beef rolls over hot barley.

FOOD TRIVIA

Roulade comes from the French word *rouler,* which means to roll.

SUBSTITUTION

Instead of the dill pickle, roll up green chilis or bell pepper strips.

COOK'S TIP

Pound the beef (or other meat) using a meat tenderizer or a mallet. Place the plastic-wrapped meat on a lucite or plastic cutting board (never wood, because it can hold the bacteria from raw meat) to avoid damaging your countertop. Wash the tenderizer or mallet and cutting board well with hot soapy water (or place in the dishwasher).

NUTRITION PER SERVING

Serving size	1 beef roll, ¾ cup cooked barley, ⅓ cup sauce
Calories	550 kcal
Fat	14 g
Saturated fat	3 g
Cholesterol	79 mg
Sodium	1,075 mg
Carbohydrates	65 g
Dietary fiber	10 g
Protein	40 g

Frikadeller (Danish Meatballs)

Martha Marino, M.A., R.D., C.D.

Serves: 8
Hands-on time: 30 minutes
Cooking time: 20 to 30 minutes

Both the Swedes and the Danes in my family have their own traditional versions of meatballs. Here in my Seattle home, I adapted my Grandmother Jorgensen's Danish recipe by substituting lean ground pork for pork sausage, substituting nonfat milk for whole milk, and using the leanest ground beef available. The mix is flavorful with traditional spices: nutmeg, allspice, and cloves.

1 cup dry bread crumbs
1 cup nonfat (skim) milk
2 eggs
1½ teaspoons salt
½ teaspoon nutmeg
½ teaspoon allspice
¼ teaspoon cloves
¼ cup white flour
1½ pounds extra-lean ground beef
½ pound lean ground pork
1 tablespoon butter

In the bowl of an electric mixer, combine the bread crumbs and milk. Let this mixture stand for 10 minutes.

Add the eggs, salt, nutmeg, allspice, cloves, and flour. Beat for 2 minutes on medium speed. Add the beef and pork; beat on low speed just until combined. Do not overmix.

Shape the meat mixture into meatballs about 2 inches in diameter, using about 3 tablespoons of meat mixture for each meatball. (A small ice-cream scoop may be used for consistent portions.)

Melt the butter in a heavy skillet over medium heat. Place the meatballs in the skillet and flatten slightly (frikadeller aren't perfect orbs). Cook 8 to 10 minutes until the meatballs are browned on both sides and are no longer pink in the middle. Depending on the size of the skillet, the meatballs likely will need to be prepared in batches. Place the cooked meatballs on a platter and keep them warm.

SERVING SUGGESTION

We serve frikadeller with red cabbage, boiled new potatoes or mashed potatoes, and lingonberries. Although we generally don't use gravy with our meatballs, packaged beef gravy could be served on the side.

COOK'S TIP

Leftover frikadeller can be placed in a zip-top food storage bag and frozen for a future meal.

NUTRITION PER SERVING

Serving size	3 or 4 meatballs
Calories	330 kcal
Fat	17 g
Saturated fat	7 g
Cholesterol	110 mg
Sodium	660 mg
Carbohydrates	15 g
Dietary fiber	Less than 1 g
Protein	27 g

Montana Roasted Beef Tenderloin

Barbara J. Pyper, M.S., R.D., C.D., F.H.C.F.A., F.C.S.I.

Where I grew up in Montana, we were serious about our beef. Slices of this savory entrée, wedges of roasted red onion, and creamy mashed potatoes make a decadent trio.

Serves: 8
Hands-on time: 10 minutes
Cooking time: 40 minutes

2 tablespoons prepared horseradish
2 tablespoons mustard, stone-ground or Dijon
½ teaspoon kosher salt
½ to 1 teaspoon black pepper, freshly ground
3 cloves garlic, minced
1 large shallot, minced
1 tablespoon dried thyme leaves
vegetable oil cooking spray
1 tablespoon olive oil
1 (2-pound) beef tenderloin
4 large red onions, quartered

Preheat oven to 425°F. Process the horseradish, mustard, salt, and pepper in a food processor or blender until smooth. Combine the garlic, shallot, thyme, and oil with the horseradish mixture in a small bowl to make the seasoning rub.

Place the trimmed tenderloin (small end tucked) and the quartered onions in a roasting pan sprayed with the cooking spray. Spread or pat the seasoning rub on the tenderloin. Insert a meat thermometer in the thickest part of the meat.

Cover and roast for 20 minutes. Baste with the meat juices; roast, uncovered, for another 10 to 20 minutes to desired doneness.

COOK'S TIP

Use the following guide from the National Cattlemen's Beef Association for meat temperatures: rare = 140°F; medium rare = 145°F; medium = 160°F; well done = 170°F. The meat temperature will continue to rise after removal from the oven—count on approximately 5 to 10°F.

NUTRITION NUGGET

Beef can be a healthy choice: a 3-ounce serving of tenderloin contains 180 calories and 8.6 grams of fat.

NUTRITION PER SERVING	
Serving size	3 ounces beef and ½ onion
Calories	260 kcal
Fat	13 g
Saturated fat	4.5 g
Cholesterol	70 mg
Sodium	280 mg
Carbohydrates	10 g
Dietary fiber	2 g
Protein	24 g

Korean Ribs

Barbara J. Pyper, M.S., R.D., C.D., F.H.C.F.A., F.C.S.I.

Serves: 5 to 6
Hands-on time: 15 minutes
Cooking time: 20 minutes

This is a great summer barbecue recipe. My sister first served me these savory ribs here in Seattle; the ribs are marinated in a blend of typical Korean ingredients. Now I love sharing the recipe with others. The marinade can easily be doubled or tripled if you're serving a crowd.

- 2 cups reduced-sodium soy sauce
- 2 tablespoons minced garlic, about 3 cloves
- 1 tablespoon grated ginger
- 1 cup sliced green onions, bulbs and stems
- 1 cup granulated sugar
- ⅔ cup packed brown sugar
- ¼ cup sesame seeds
- 1 teaspoon ground black pepper
- 1 teaspoon crushed red pepper
- 6 tablespoons sesame seed oil
- 1 tablespoon canola oil
- 10 pounds Korean style beef short ribs (cut across the bone, ½- to ¾-inch thick)

Mix together the soy sauce, garlic, ginger, onion, granulated sugar, brown sugar, sesame seeds, black pepper, red pepper, sesame seed oil, and canola oil until smooth. Place the ribs in a large, plastic or glass bowl; pour the marinade over the ribs. Cover the bowl and refrigerate overnight.

Preheat grill. Turn it on high 15 minutes prior to use. If using a charcoal grill, allow 20 to 30 minutes for the coals to reach the white ash stage.

Grill over hot coals for 2 to 4 minutes on each side, while continuously basting with the marinade. Discard any leftover marinade.

COOK'S TIP

Marinate the ribs and then freeze them in the marinade. When you're ready to use them, just thaw and grill. Discard any unused marinade.

NUTRITION PER SERVING

Serving size	about 2 pounds bone-in ribs
Calories	250 kcal
Fat	13 g
Saturated fat	4 g
Cholesterol	50 mg
Sodium	830 mg
Carbohydrates	15 g
Dietary fiber	less than 1 g
Protein	18 g

Pastitso (Greek Lasagna)

Bonnie Athas, R.D.

This is one of the best-known Greek entreés known outside of Greece, including here in Utah. Notably, this dish differs from Italian lasagna in that it calls for tubular pasta, a white sauce rather than a red sauce, and is flavored with cinnamon. Sometimes, feta cheese is added to the lasagna.

Serves: 8
Hands-on time: 20 minutes
Cooking time: 1 hour

vegetable oil cooking spray
1 2-ounce package tubular macaroni
¾ pound (12 ounces) extra-lean ground beef
1 cup onions, minced (2 small or 1 medium-size = 1 cup)
1 14½-ounce can diced tomatoes
1 8-ounce can no-salt-added tomato sauce
1 cup grated Romano cheese, divided
1½ teaspoons ground cinnamon, divided
1½ tablespoons butter
½ cup all-purpose flour
3 cups nonfat milk
¼ to 1 teaspoon black pepper (to taste)
¼ teaspoon salt
1 cup liquid egg substitute

Preheat oven to 350°F. Spray a 9-by-13-inch baking dish with the cooking spray. Cook the macaroni as directed on the package. Brown the beef with the onions in a large pan over medium heat, about 8 to 9 minutes. Add the diced tomatoes, tomato sauce, ¼ cup Romano cheese, and 1 teaspoon cinnamon. Remove the pan from the heat and set aside.

Béchamel Sauce

Melt the butter in a heavy saucepan. Combine the flour and milk in a bowl and whisk until smooth. Pour into the melted butter, whisking until the mixture thickens. Add the remaining ½ teaspoon cinnamon, black pepper to taste, and salt. Remove from heat.

NUTRITION NUGGET

Using just the right combination of salt-added and no-salt-added tomato products can bring the sodium level of your finished dish just where you need it to be.

NUTRITION PER SERVING	
Serving size	⅛ of pan
Calories	290 kcal
Fat	6 g
Saturated fat	3 g
Cholesterol	30 mg
Sodium	370 mg
Carbohydrates	39 g
Dietary fiber	2 g
Protein	20 g

Pastitso (Greek Lasagna) *(continued)*

To Put It All Together

Drain the cooked pasta; return it to the pot (but not on the hot burner). Add the egg substitute and ½ cup Romano cheese; stir well.

Place ½ of the macaroni mixture (3 heaping cups) on the bottom of the prepared baking dish; top with all of the meat mixture; cover with the remaining macaroni mixture (3 heaping cups). Pour the béchamel sauce over the top. Sprinkle with the remaining ¼ cup Romano.

Bake uncovered for 1 hour, or until the mixture bubbles.

Pork Roast with Gingersnap Gravy

Bonnie Athas, R.D.

I don't think there is a type of food that ginger won't enhance. If you're not from a German background, you may be surprised to learn that ginger and molasses-rich cookies flavor this savory gravy which is often served over sauerbraten or pork roast.

Serves: 8
Cooking time: 10 minutes

- vegetable oil cooking spray
- 2 pound lean pork roast, such as a boneless loin
- salt, pepper, and garlic powder to taste
- 1 14-ounce can reduced-sodium beef broth
- 12 gingersnap cookies, crushed
- 1 8-ounce container reduced-fat sour cream

Preheat oven to 375°F. Coat a roasting pan with the cooking spray. Place the roast in a roasting pan. Season to taste. Roast 45 minutes. Turn and roast an additional 45 minutes, or until internal temperature reaches 160°F.

Bring the broth to boil in a medium-heavy saucepan. Add the crushed cookies, a few at a time, whisking constantly. Reduce heat to a simmer; whisk in the sour cream. Serve while still hot.

COOK'S TIP

An 8-ounce container of sour cream measures about 1 cup.

NUTRITION NUGGET

Using reduced-fat sour cream instead of regular cuts about 20 calories per serving (and over 2 grams of total fat).

NUTRITION PER SERVING	
Serving size	3 ounces cooked roast and ⅓ cup gravy
Calories	265 kcal
Fat	12 g
Saturated fat	5 g
Cholesterol	80 mg
Sodium	135 mg
Carbohydrates	8 g
Dietary fiber	0 g
Protein	26 g

Cheesiest Lasagna

Laura Faler Thomas, M.Ed., R.D., L.D.

Serves: 12
Hands-on time: 20 minutes
Cooking time: 1 hour

What better place to bake whole wheat noodles into lasagna than in Idaho, the heart of wheat growing? The cheesy flavors meld with the whole wheat to produce a rich, yet trendy flavor. Make it even trendier with a ladle of jarred marinara sauce over the top just before serving.

vegetable oil cooking spray
2 cups (8 ounces) shredded, part-skim mozzarella cheese, divided
1 cup (4 ounces) small curd nonfat cottage cheese
1 20-ounce bag frozen chopped broccoli, thawed
1 medium-size onion, minced
2 cloves garlic, minced
1 medium-size red bell pepper, trimmed, seeded, and minced
1⅓ cups plain nonfat yogurt
9 whole wheat lasagna noodles, cooked and drained
½ cup (2 ounces) fresh shredded Parmesan cheese
jarred marinara sauce for garnish, if desired

Preheat oven to 350°F. Coat a 9-by-13-inch baking dish with the cooking spray. Mix 1 cup of the mozzarella cheese and the cottage cheese, broccoli, onion, garlic, red pepper, and yogurt in a large bowl. Place three noodles on the bottom of the baking dish. Spread half of the cheese-broccoli mixture over the noodles. Repeat. Top with the last three noodles. Sprinkle with the remaining 1 cup mozzarella cheese and all of the Parmesan cheese.

Cover with aluminum foil, creating a tent to prevent the cheese from sticking to the foil; crimp the edges to create a seal. Bake for 45 minutes. Uncover and bake for an additional 5 to 10 minutes, or until the cheese is melted and slightly browned. Let stand for 10 minutes before cutting.

Add one ladleful of jarred marinara sauce before serving each piece, if desired.

SUBSTITUTION
Substitute chopped spinach for broccoli. Or be adventurous and try any vegetables you think would be tasty.

NUTRITION PER SERVING	
Serving size	1/12 of casserole
Calories	212 kcal
Fat	6 g
Saturated fat	4 g
Cholesterol	21 mg
Sodium	330 mg
Carbohydrates	24 g
Dietary fiber	4 g
Protein	17 g

Orange-Glazed Cranberry Cake

Barbara J. Pyper, M.S., R.D., C.D., F.H.C.F.A., F.C.S.I.

This incredibly moist cake was a fall favorite in my home state of Montana where cranberries are a native crop. It's still a favorite in Seattle where I now live.

Serves: 12
Hands-on time: 15 minutes
Cooking time: 40 minutes

CAKE
2 cups all-purpose flour
1¼ teaspoons baking powder
½ teaspoon baking soda
3 tablespoons butter, softened
1 cup sugar
2 eggs
⅔ cup nonfat plain yogurt
2 cups fresh or frozen cranberries, chopped
vegetable oil cooking spray

ORANGE GLAZE
½ cup confectioner's sugar
4½ teaspoons fresh orange juice
1 teaspoon grated orange peel

Preheat oven to 350°F. Sift together the flour, baking powder, and baking soda. Cream the butter and sugar until fluffy. Add the eggs, one at a time, beating well after each addition. Beat the flour mixture into the creamed mixture alternately with the yogurt, beating well after each addition. Fold in the cranberries.

Spray a 10-inch fluted tube pan with the nonstick cooking spray. Transfer the cake batter into the pan. Bake for 40 minutes or until a toothpick inserted into the center of the cake comes out clean. Cool the cake in the pan for 10 minutes. Finish cooling it on a wire rack.

Mix together all the glaze ingredients. Drizzle the orange glaze onto the cooled cake.

NUTRITION PER SERVING	
Serving size	1/12 of cake
Calories	190 kcal
Fat	4 g
Saturated fat	2 g
Cholesterol	45 mg
Sodium	70 mg
Carbohydrates	36 g
Dietary fiber	1 g
Protein	4 g

Swedish Cream

Barbara J. Pyper, M.S., R.D., C.D., F.H.C.F.A., F.C.S.I.

Serves: 10
Hands-on time: 20 minutes
Cooking time: 20 minutes

In Montana, we served Swedish Cream with native-grown cranberries. For a real Swedish treat, look for fresh or frozen lingonberries to use instead of cranberries. These miniature berries are found in the wild throughout the Nordic region.

SHOPPING TIP
When cranberries are available fresh in the supermarket, buy extra bags and freeze them. Place the package inside a tightly sealed plastic bag and freeze up to six months.

1½ teaspoons unflavored gelatin
1 cup heavy whipping cream
⅓ cup sugar
¾ cup nonfat sour cream
¼ cup nonfat plain yogurt
2 tablespoons orange-flavored liqueur (such as Grand Marnier)
1 teaspoon pure vanilla extract

Place 2 tablespoons cold water in a cold 1-quart saucepan; sprinkle the gelatin into the water. Let it stand until softened, about 3 minutes. Add the heavy cream and sugar; cook and stir over low heat until the gelatin is dissolved. Do not boil. Remove the pan from heat; cool for 20 minutes, stirring occasionally.

Fold in the sour cream, yogurt, liqueur, and vanilla. Pour into serving dishes and refrigerate until ready to serve. If desired, serve topped with Cranberry Orange Sauce.

Cranberry Orange Sauce

1 cup (5 ounces) fresh or frozen cranberries
½ cup sugar
1 tablespoon orange-flavored liqueur
1 teaspoon grated orange peel

Combine ½ cup water and the cranberries and sugar in a medium-size saucepan; bring to a boil, stirring occasionally. Reduce heat and simmer for 10 minutes until the cranberry skins begin to pop open. Remove from heat and cool 5 minutes.

Transfer the sauce to a food processor; process using a metal blade for 1 minute, or until puréed. Stir in the liqueur and orange peel. Serve atop Swedish Cream.

NUTRITION PER SERVING

Serving size	¼ cup cranberries plus 3 tablespoons sauce
Calories	170 kcal
Fat	9 g
Saturated fat	6 g
Cholesterol	35 mg
Sodium	20 mg
Carbohydrates	20 g
Dietary fiber	0 g
Protein	1 g

Cinnamon Apple Peanut Butter Bars

Barbara J. Pyper, M.S., R.D., C.D., F.H.C.F.A., F.C.S.I.

Kids and adults alike will love these all-American wholesome bars that make great after-school treats or lunchbox fillers. You can make them all year, but we especially love them in the fall with freshly picked Washington State apples.

Serves: 24
Hands-on time: 15 minutes
Cooking time: 30 minutes

- vegetable oil cooking spray
- ¾ cup packed brown sugar
- ½ cup applesauce
- 1 cup peanut butter
- 1 cup liquid egg substitute
- 1 cup all-purpose flour
- ½ cup wheat germ
- 1 tablespoon plus 1 teaspoon cinnamon
- 1 teaspoon baking soda
- 3 cups old-fashioned oats
- ⅓ cup nonfat milk
- 1 tablespoon pure vanilla extract
- 1 cup packed raisins
- 2 medium-size apples, chopped

Preheat oven to 350°F. Coat a 9-by-13-inch baking dish with the nonstick cooking spray. Beat the brown sugar, applesauce, peanut butter, and egg substitute on the medium speed of a mixer until the mixture is smooth and creamy. Add the flour, wheat germ, cinnamon, baking soda, oats, milk, and vanilla; blend well. Stir in the raisins and apples.

Pour into the prepared baking dish and bake for 25 to 30 minutes, or until firm to the touch. Cool the bars before cutting.

SUBSTITUTION

Use 4 whole (large) eggs for the 1 cup of egg substitute.

VARIATION

Use an equal quantity of your favorite dried fruit instead of raisins.

NUTRITION PER SERVING	
Serving size	1/24 of pan
Calories	190 kcal
Fat	7 g
Saturated fat	1.5 g
Cholesterol	0 mg
Sodium	75 mg
Carbohydrates	28 g
Dietary fiber	3 g
Protein	7 g

Lemon Sauce

Barbara J. Pyper, M.S., R.D., C.D., F.H.C.F.A., F.C.S.I.

Serves: 10
Hands-on time: 10 minutes
Cooking time: 10 minutes

Tart and refreshing are words my family in Cut Bank, Montana, would use to describe their favorite dessert sauce. My preferred way to serve it is with angel food cake. I find that the tartness of the lemon makes a nice contrast to the sweetness of the cake.

- 1 cup sugar, granulated
- 2 tablespoons cornstarch
- ½ cup liquid egg substitute
- rind and juice of 1 lemon (3 to 4 tablespoons juice plus 1½ teaspoons grated rind)
- 2 tablespoons butter

Mix the sugar and cornstarch together in a saucepan. Add the egg substitute and mix well. Add 1½ cups hot water, then the lemon rind, lemon juice, and butter. Cook, stirring all the time until the mixture comes to a full rolling boil; continue to cook and stir 5 more minutes. Serve hot or cold.

COOK'S TIP

To safely store your lemon sauce, refrigerate it in a nonreactive container, such as one made of glass or plastic. Reactive containers, made of aluminum, copper, and cast iron, react with certain foods, especially acidic ones. Lemon juice, tomatoes, and vinegar are some examples of acidic foods. When acidic foods come into contact with reactive cookware, a metallic taste forms and the food can become discolored.

NUTRITION PER SERVING	
Serving size	¼ cup
Calories	115 kcal
Fat	3 g
Saturated fat	1.5 g
Cholesterol	6 mg
Sodium	50 mg
Carbohydrates	22 g
Dietary fiber	Less than 1 g
Protein	2 g

Triple Chocolate Cake

Lisa Poggas, M.S., R.D.

Cake mixes became a staple in pantries across the United States after they were developed in the 1940s. Creative bakers continue to transform a basic mix into incredible creations using good old American ingenuity. This Colorado-born recipe highlights how a few changes and additions to the mix can create a decadent dessert for any occasion (without going overboard on calories or fat). This cake is delicious by itself or dress it up by drizzling it with Wild Blueberry Sauce (page 62).

Serves: 16 or 20
Hands-on time: 20 minutes
Cooking time: 45 to 50 minutes

vegetable oil cooking spray
2 tablespoons unsweetened cocoa powder
1 18¼-ounce box devil's food cake mix
1 3⁹⁄₁₆-ounce package instant chocolate fudge pudding mix, sugar-free or regular
1 cup plain nonfat yogurt
¼ cup canola oil
¼ cup light mayonnaise
¾ cup liquid egg substitute
1 teaspoon vanilla extract
½ cup semisweet chocolate chips
3 tablespoons sifted powdered sugar

Coat a 10-inch fluted tube pan with the cooking spray. Coat the inside of the pan with the cocoa powder or flour and shake out the excess. Set aside.

In a large mixing bowl, combine the cake mix, pudding mix, yogurt, oil, ½ cup water, mayonnaise, egg substitute, and vanilla. Beat with an electric mixer on low speed until combined; beat on medium speed until smooth, about 2 to 3 minutes. Stir in the chocolate chips. Spoon the batter evenly into the prepared pan.

Bake in a 350°F oven for about 45 to 50 minutes or until a wooden toothpick inserted near the center comes out clean. Cool in the pan on a wire rack for 10 minutes. Remove from the pan and cool completely on wire rack. Sprinkle with the powdered sugar before serving.

VARIATION

Use 3 eggs or 6 egg whites in place of the ¾ cup liquid egg substitute.

NUTRITION NUGGET

We've provided nutrition for ¹⁄₁₆ and ¹⁄₂₀ of the cake so that you can decide what size piece fits into your calorie budget.

NUTRITION PER SERVING	
Serving size	¹⁄₁₆ of cake
Calories	250 kcal
Fat	9 g
Saturated fat	2.5 g
Cholesterol	0 mg
Sodium	320 mg
Carbohydrates	38 g
Dietary fiber	1 g
Protein	4 g

NUTRITION PER SERVING	
Serving size	¹⁄₂₀ of cake
Calories	200 kcal
Fat	7 g
Saturated fat	2 g
Cholesterol	0 mg
Sodium	260 mg
Carbohydrates	30 g
Dietary fiber	1 g
Protein	3 g

New-Fashioned Whole-Grain Cookies

Laura Faler Thomas, M.Ed., R.D., L.D.

Yield: 6 dozen
Hands-on time: 20 minutes
Cooking time: 9 to 10 minutes for freshly made dough

Don't let the kids know these gems are so healthy. The secret is to use a bag of whole-grain hot cereal mix from your supermarket's cereal aisle; use it dry and you've essentially baked a nutritious bowl of hot cereal into some tasty treats. It seems only logical that such a whole-grain delight would be created in Idaho, in the heart of America's grain basket.

3¼ cups flour
1½ teaspoons baking soda
½ teaspoon salt
4 cups 5-grain cereal, uncooked
½ cup butter
⅓ cup canola oil
½ cup unsweetened applesauce
⅓ cup sugar
⅓ cup packed brown sugar
1 cup liquid egg substitute
2 teaspoons vanilla
1 cup raisins
½ cup chocolate chips
1 cup sweetened dried cranberries

Preheat oven to 375°F. Combine the flour, baking soda, salt, and cereal; set aside.

In a large mixing bowl, beat together the butter, oil, applesauce, sugars, egg substitute, and vanilla until smooth. Slowly beat the flour mixture into the wet mixture. Stir in the raisins, chocolate chips, and cranberries.

Drop by rounded tablespoonfuls onto an ungreased cookie sheet. Bake for 9 to 10 minutes or until golden brown but still soft to the touch.

SHOPPING TIP

Five-grain cereal mix can be found in the cooked cereal section of most grocery stores. You can also choose 10-grain or 12-grain cereal.

COOK'S TIP

Freeze tablespoon-size dollops of cookie dough unbaked. Store in an airtight container in the freezer. To bake a tray of fresh cookies, just place pieces of the frozen dough on a baking tray and allow them to thaw for about 15 minutes. Then bake according to the recipe directions. Baking time may vary; adjust as necessary.

SERVING SUGGESTIONS

Eat them for breakfast. Or, for a tasty, nutritious after-school snack, serve these cookies with a glass of milk. Together the milk and cookies provide energy, protein, calcium, iron, B-vitamins, fiber, and other vitamins and minerals active growing kids need.

NUTRITION PER SERVING

Serving size	1 cookie
Calories	100 kcal
Fat	3.5 g
Saturated fat	1 g
Cholesterol	5 mg
Sodium	25 mg
Carbohydrates	16 g
Dietary fiber	2 g
Protein	2 g

Lemon Yogurt Cheese over Summer Fruit

Martha Marino, M.A., R.D., C.D.

Fresh, ripe fruit is key to the flavor of this simple dessert. Try a local farmers' market for luscious seasonal fruit in your area, as I do in Seattle. Many farmers will provide you with a taste of their berries, apricots, peaches, and other fruit they have grown to make sure you will be happy with your purchase.

Yogurt cheese is a delicious, lower-fat substitute for cream cheese or sour cream. When placing yogurt in a strainer, the liquid whey is drained off, leaving remaining curds as thick as a cheese-like spread.

Serves: 4

Hands-on time: 15 minutes plus time for the yogurt to drain overnight

- 2 cups reduced-fat vanilla yogurt
- ¼ cup sugar
- 1 teaspoon grated lemon zest
- 1 tablespoon fresh lemon juice
- 2 to 3 cups fresh fruit, cut into bite-sized pieces (blueberries and cantaloupe; strawberries, raspberries, and Marion berries; peaches and raspberries)

Set a strainer lined with cheesecloth over a large bowl (or use an unlined fine-mesh strainer or a strainer lined with a coffee filter). Place the yogurt in the strainer, cover it loosely with plastic wrap, and refrigerate overnight (6 to 24 hours). The yogurt will thicken and the liquid will be expelled into the bowl, leaving about 1 cup of yogurt cheese in the strainer. Reserve the yogurt cheese; discard the liquid.

Whisk together in a small bowl the yogurt cheese, sugar, lemon zest, and lemon juice. Let it stand until the sugar has dissolved, about 10 to 15 minutes.

Divide the fresh fruit among four dessert bowls or plates, top with about ¼ cup yogurt cheese, and serve.

VARIATION

Try another use for yogurt cheese—blend yogurt cheese made from plain low-fat yogurt with your favorite herbs and spices to create a vegetable dip.

COOK'S TIP

Yogurt cheese may be prepared ahead and refrigerated for up to three days.

NUTRITION PER SERVING	
Serving size	¼ cup sauce plus ¾ cup fruit
Calories	190 kcal
Fat	2 g
Saturated fat	1 g
Cholesterol	5 mg
Sodium	85 mg
Carbohydrates	39 g
Dietary fiber	3 g
Protein	7 g

Poached Pears with Caramel Sauce

Martha Marino, M.A., R.D., C.D.

Serves: 4
Hands-on time: 15 minutes
Cooking time: 15 minutes

Pears are plentiful in northwest orchards in the fall. This recipe, which combines pears with the rich taste of caramel, is a great way to enjoy them—not only in the autumn, but all year.

- 4 firm ripe medium-size pears, such as Bosc or Bartlett
- ¼ cup lemon juice
- ¼ cup prepared caramel sauce or caramel topping

Peel the pears, leaving the stems attached. Cut a thin slice from the bottom of each pear so that the pear will stand upright. Place the pears in a saucepan large enough to fit 4 pears without the fruit toppling. Add the lemon juice and 4 cups water. Bring to a boil, reduce heat to simmer, and cook for 10 to 15 minutes or until tender but not falling apart. Drain the liquid. Place the pears on a plate, cover, and chill 3 hours or overnight.

Arrange the pears on individual dessert dishes. Drizzle caramel sauce over the pears, making a small puddle of sauce on the plate.

VARIATION

Instead of using lemon juice and water, use 1 quart (4 cups) of apple juice to cook the pears. If the pears are short on flavor, this will give them a boost.

NUTRITION PER SERVING

Serving size	1 pear
Calories	100 kcal
Fat	0.5 g
Saturated fat	0 g
Cholesterol	0 mg
Sodium	20 mg
Carbohydrates	24 g
Dietary fiber	3 g
Protein	1 g

Zwetschgenkuchen (Plum Tart)

Nancy Becker, M.S., R.D., L.D.

My mother used to make this typical German Jewish tart every year for Rosh Hashanah, the Jewish New Year. Here in Oregon, Brooks plums are abundant in the fall, so I have continued the tradition. The crust is also special: a cookielike pie crust called muerbeteig.

Serves: 10
Hands-on time: 45 minutes
Cooking time: 40 minutes

- 1 cup plus 2 tablespoons unbleached white flour
- 1 tablespoon sugar
- ½ cup butter or margarine
- 1 egg yolk (optional, or equivalent egg substitute)
- dash salt
- 2 tablespoons brandy, divided
- 3 pounds Italian (Brooks) plums, washed, pitted, and quartered (about 4 cups)
- ½ cup sugar
- 1 teaspoon grated lemon peel
- ⅓ cup currant jelly

Preheat oven to 375°F. Mix the flour and sugar. Using a food processor or pastry blender, cut in the margarine until the mixture resembles coarse crumbs. Add the egg yolk, salt, and 1 tablespoon brandy to moisten the crust.

Gather the dough into a ball and turn out onto a board. Knead very briefly (unnecessary if you're using a food processor). Place the dough in the center of a 9-inch pie plate or tart pan and pat it with your fingers or the back of a wooden spoon so that it covers the bottom and about ½ inch of the sides of the pan.

Place the plums in a bowl. Add the sugar, lemon peel, and the remaining 2 tablespoons flour. Toss gently to coat all of the fruit.

Spread the currant jelly on the crust. Place the plums cut-side up in a circle on the crust so that each piece overlaps another in ever smaller circles. Sprinkle the arranged plum pieces with brandy. Bake for 40 to 50 minutes until the crust is golden brown and the plums are bubbling. Cool to room temperature or serve slightly warm.

SUBSTITUTION
When (and where) Brooks plums are not available, substitute sliced pears or tart baking apples.

VARIATION
Serve tart wedges with whipped cream or á la mode with vanilla ice cream.

NUTRITION NUGGET
Plums are rich in phytochemicals and even though the crust is quite rich, the serving size is small; you get an explosion of flavor in a small slice.

NUTRITION PER SERVING	
Serving size	1 slice
Calories	290 kcal
Fat	11 g
Saturated fat	6 g
Cholesterol	45 mg
Sodium	0 mg
Carbohydrates	46 g
Dietary fiber	2 g
Protein	3 g

9

FUSION DEFINED

The Cuisines of California and Hawaii

Kristine Napier, M.P.H., R.D.

California is often called the culinary crossroads of America. The same can be said for its neighbor to the west, Hawaii. Both cuisines are melting pots of foods and recipe traditions from cultures that have spanned centuries. True, many of the cultures left culinary threads in both places. The distinctive food fabrics that were eventually woven, though, are as different as plaid from polka dots.

Under the warm California sun and in the trade winds cooling the Hawaiian Islands, very distinctive cuisines evolved. Their recipes begin with an abundance of fresh ingredients grown in native rich soils—and in farmers' dream climates. Both stake their culinary personalities on freshness and innovative ways to use just-plucked produce. Seas hugging their coasts boast another culinary (and nutritional) asset: treasure chests of fish.

The earliest chefs in both Hawaii and California cooked with a tremendous variety of foods—from which they learned an enviable range of culinary skills. Borrowing from the diverse cultures in their own backyards, these cooks also learned a skill that has become so trendy today: fusion cooking.

Hot sauces sweetened with coconut speak of the Thai and Filipino influences in both Hawaii and California. Chinese food, with its delectable sauces and wealth of cooked-to-perfection vegetables, brings much to Californian and Hawaiian tables. Hot peppers boldly imprint the personalities of Mexico and South America on many characteristic California recipes.

Common Global Influences

Despite so many similar influences, the cuisines of each state simmered differently over time. Let's look at the global influences that affected the cuisines of both Hawaii and California. From there, we'll take a glimpse at cultures and factors that apparently touched one but not the other.

Chinese

The Chinese have enviable culinary goals: a desire and the ability to extract from every ingredient its distinctive and most pleasurable quality. Note the care taken to create a stir-fry of many colors, textures, and flavors. Indeed, the Chinese plate is really a palette of pleasing-to-the eye foods. Vegetables are a perennial focal point of Chinese cuisine. Mushrooms, bamboo shoots, water chestnuts, and bean sprouts are ever present, but are certainly not the only ones in these nutritionally wealthy dishes.

The tenets of classic Chinese cuisine dovetail well with today's nutritional goals. For one, we know that enjoying small portions of several different foods quells the appetite sooner than eating a larger quantity of one food. Also, we taste first with our eyes—one of the reasons that a visually pleasing plate quiets hunger before the first bite. Certainly, enjoying a range of multicolored vegetables is an excellent strategy to control weight and reduce risk of disease.

Soy-derived foods play a key role in Chinese cuisine, including tofu (also called bean curd) as a protein source. In China, soybeans were once known as the poor man's cow, as they can be made into products that resemble milk and cheese. Versatile soy can also be made into many different seasonings, including soy sauce; hoisin sauce, a thicker, brownish-red, sweet-sour version of soy sauce (Hoisin Chicken Spinach Salad, page 452); and Chinese black beans, which are really fermented soybeans preserved with salt and ginger. Chinese black beans, in fact, often take the place of salt as a seasoning in Chinese recipes. Rice is a mainstay in most meals.

Stir-fry cooking is attributed to the Chinese. Today, we celebrate this culinary style as one that retains not only brilliant color and crisp texture, but also life-giving nutrients.

Japanese

Similar, but deliciously distinctive, are the Japanese imprints on Californian and Hawaiian cuisines. For example, painstaking presentation is central to almost all Japanese meals. While rice is a Japanese staple, soba noodles are also frequent fare. Fish is a common protein food, but may be served as sashimi (raw fish) or as tempura (deep fried) in addition to conventional seafood cooking methods. While food historians believe that the Japanese introduced tempura (for cooking fish, vegetables, and fruits) to Hawaii, it was the Portuguese traders who taught the Japanese.

Thai

Thai cuisine may be one of the world's oldest fusions. During the earliest years of the first millennium, Chinese and Indian culinary styles blended in Thailand to emerge as its own food style. Nam prik, a spicy-hot condiment, is used in a plethora of ways to create many different flavors (Thai Green Beans in Coconut Milk, page 332). Thin stews, reminiscent of India's liquid curries, are commonly mixed with rice. Coconut is a central ingredient.

Filipino

The Filipino culinary handprint is found, for one, in the use of fermented fish paste and sauce (bagoong and patis, respectively). Gastronomic experts say the single most characteristic taste of Filipino food is a sour-salty taste (Tangy Braised Beef with Beans and Peppers, page 469). Coconut in its many forms has always been a key ingredient in Filipino cooking, as it is in many other Southeast Asian cuisines.

Delicious Inspirations of California Kitchens

In the world of cuisine firsts, California claims credit for the Caesar (Hola Caesar, page 446) and the Cobb Salads—and the doggie bag, which originated with Lawry's Prime Rib House in 1938 (what a great contribution to portion control!). Let's time-travel to a place in history centuries ago to catch a glimpse of the foods and recipes that have been left behind for present-day Californians to enjoy and share with the rest of the country.

California's Native American Food Influences

California had a thriving Native American population long before Spanish explorers walked the land. Traveling from north to south, most tribes made their homes along the coast, taking advantage of the abundance of the sea. The Tilpai-Ipai, deep in southern California and Northern Baja, also ate of the abundant cacti and prickly pear, as well as indigenous cherries, berries, acorns, and clover. Southwest of the San Bernardino Mountains, the climate and soil were ideal for the Cahuilla tribe to plant the three sisters—corn, beans, and squash—that their ancient ancestors established as a viable (and incidentally, nutritionally complete) crop group.

From central to northern California, the food supply diversified. In addition to the acorns, seeds, nuts, and berries, the Miwok, Yuki, Wintun, Karok, Hupa, Achomawi, and Pomo tribes enjoyed a wide range of small and large game, as well as fresh- and saltwater fish.

The Spanish Influence on California

Spanish influence on cuisine wound its way to California from Spain through at least two hundred years of interaction with the native people of South and Central America. Food historians argue that the Hispanic influence was so significant on Californian cuisine because of the state's proximity to Mexico and Central and South America. Undoubtedly, large numbers of Hispanic people immigrated to California from these lands.

Religion, too, played a pivotal role in California's early agricultural history. Spanish missionaries introduced wheat to California in the eighteenth century. Trying very hard to turn wheat into a golden crop, they grew it only during the winter, when coastal California receives most of its rainfall. Corn and barley were at most secondary crops in the Spanish missions, even though these latter crops (especially corn) fared much better in the climate and terrain. Ultimately, wheat would fail in California but would become a key American crop in the Mississippi Valley and the Palouse (see chapter 8). Corn, too, moved east and barley went both north and east.

Spanish missionaries first produced wine in California from indigenous Mission grapes, but it wasn't until after the 1849 California gold rush that the wine industry burgeoned. Franciscan monks planted the first orange grove of any size at San Gabriel mission, east of Los Angeles, in the early 1800s. Today, orange groves are a common sight—as well as a significant industry—from San Diego to Sacramento. Cuisine, too, reflects the citrus appeal.

Mexican Fare Travels North

By the time it reached California, Mexican food was already a fusion of the food ways of its indigenous tribes and Spanish influences. The fundamental ingredients of Aztec cooking before the Spanish arrived included beans, corn, chili peppers, and tomatoes. The Spanish complemented these foods with cinnamon, garlic, onions, rice, sugar cane, wheat, and hogs from Europe.

Together, the fusion created what we know as classic Mexican food and flavors, including:

- Corn tortillas filled with pork
- Tomato, chili, and onion sauces, which we know as salsa (see Tomatillo-Chipotle Salsa, page 435; Fresh Salsa, page 328)
- Refried beans (frijoles refritos), made possible by the availability of pork fat (Tom 'n' Henry's Refried Beans, page 334—a slimmed-down version of traditional recipes).

The Gold Rush Demands Further Innovation in Food

Another wave of innovation hit California cuisine in the nineteenth century: the gold rush. People arrived in California by horse and wagon or by ship from the East Coast. Other vessels descended on California from Europe and the Orient, bringing even further diversity to the culinary scene. Starting in 1860 (and continuing for a century) California's population doubled on average of once every two decades.

The first American settlers that headed west were midwestern farmers of Anglo-Saxon descent. Their movement west, say food historians, brought the emergence of American regional cuisine. Written for the benefit of western housewives, *The Great Western Cookbook* illustrates how ingredients and cooking methods were adapted as settlers migrated west and needed simplicity in cooking. It includes recipes for "California Soup," "Corn-Meal Batter Cakes," and "Veal—Western Fashion."

Sourdough bread arose during the gold rush era as a way to make bread in the great outdoors. Contrary to popular belief, it wasn't until the Alaskan Klondike gold strike in 1897 that miners became known as "sourdoughs." Still today, sourdough remains San Francisco's favorite bread. Purportedly, it is leavened with a sourdough starter dating back so long ago that no one remembers anymore. Stories abound that a crock of San Francisco sourdough starter, once removed from its native city, loses its power to produce top-quality bread.

The gold rush produced many interesting recipes, including Hang Town Fry. This omelet of oysters and eggs was concocted at Hang Town (modern Placerville, California) during the gold rush, when miners who struck it rich in the gold fields asked for the most expensive dinner money could buy.

Twentieth-Century Influences on California Cuisine

From Hollywood to the White House, the contemporary influences on California cuisine are notable. A closer look, though, reveals that they repeat themes established centuries earlier. The Coconut Grove opened in 1921 serving distinctive dishes made with fresh, local ingredients. Its food was a favorite among Hollywood greats including Charlie Chaplin and Judy Garland. Chasen's created an ever-so-popular chili using ingredients founded in Mexican cuisine. Elizabeth Taylor sent for Chasen's chili while on the set of Cleopatra in Rome, and President Richard Nixon served it to world dignitaries.

The use of fresh, native ingredients resurfaced as an important theme again in the 1970s when Alice Waters opened Chez Panisse in 1971. Waters, in fact, coined the term *California cuisine* with the use of tender baby vegetables and varietal tomatoes grown by local farmers. Food became a form of art in the influential Asian tradition. A decade later the chef Wolfgang Puck reiterated a light, fresh bill of fare. Designer pizzas are said to have originated at his original Hollywood restaurant Spago's (try out some designer pizzas for yourself, such as Sacramento Delta Pear Pizza, page 473 and Smoked Salmon Pizza, page 379).

Does Caesar Salad sound Italian? The classic blend of romaine lettuce, garlic, olive oil, croutons, Parmesan cheese, Worcestershire sauce, egg yolks, lemon, and anchovies was first created about 1920 by Caesar Cardini in Mexico. Purportedly, it was first introduced to a U.S. restaurant in San Diego (Hola Caesar, page 446).

Agriculture and the Sea Dominate California Cuisine

No matter how you slice it, California's food is defined first by the land, the sea, and the climate, and *then* by the people and cultures that crafted it.

California Agriculture

California is this country's leading agricultural producer; for some crops it is the nation's sole domestic source. Innovation emerges again as an important factor in defining California cuisine, especially in the form of irrigation, which played a significant role in California's becoming a key agricultural state. Important farm products produced in California include:

- Almonds
- Broccoli

- Dates
- Figs
- Lemons (Lemon-Dijon Asparagus, page 438)
- Lettuce (sometimes called California's green gold, the most important vegetable grown in California; over two-thirds of lettuce grown in the United States is produced there)
- Peaches
- Prunes
- Strawberries (Fresh Strawberry Glacé Pie, page 475)
- Sugar beets
- Tomatoes (Grilled Tuna with Warm Cherry Tomato Salsa, page 460)
- Walnuts (Turkey, Walnuts, Blue Cheese Salad, page 458)
- Turkey
- Rice (Turkey, Sun-Dried Tomato, and Basil Rice, page 456)

LETTUCE IN ANCIENT EGYPTIAN TOMBS?

Lettuce was first domesticated and grown as a food crop in ancient Egypt. Paintings and carvings inside ancient Egyptian tombs depict lettuce plants associated with Min, the god of vegetation and procreation. In ancient times the leaf was eaten as today, but lettuce seeds also were used. Lettuce seeds were pressed to extract oil, or crushed and prepared as bread.

California's Fishing Industry

Fishing, too, remains a financially important industry to California. In 2002, California fishermen caught approximately 5 million pounds of salmon, 10 million pounds of anchovies, and 160 million pounds of squid. Other fish that are key financial catches include flounder and tuna.

The Hawaiian Melting Pot

Captain Cook wrote of Hawaii's distinctive culinary style during his first visit over two hundred years ago. The people and circumstances that had already peppered the Hawaiian culinary personality spanned more than one thousand years. Then, as today, Hawaii's cuisine was characterized as elegantly simple, built around wholesome local food that unites cultures from Asia and Europe. Today, those influences have grown to include the mainland of the United States.

Hawaii's First Inhabitants

Historians believe that Polynesian voyagers arrived in Hawaii during the fifth century, with a second wave in the ninth and tenth centuries. They carried with them their dietary mainstays:

- Taro: a root vegetable with an edible green top.
- Breadfruit: a starchy vegetable similar to the potato (also called ulu—Spicy Breadfruit, page 187; Ulu Home Fries, page 442). From green to ripe, Hawaiians cook breadfruit in many ways: boiling, frying, simmering in coconut milk, and baking.
- Pigs (Hawaiian Pork and Peas, page 470; Maui Pineapple Pork Roast, page 471).
- Bananas: the first bananas, called plantains, were ones that had to be cooked. Sweet bananas would come to the islands much later with the Brazilians and the Chinese.
- Coconuts: they used the meat, the milk (for drinking and cooking), the shells, and the leaves.
- Sweet potatoes and yams: in addition to enjoying the potatoes, Hawaiians ate the leaves of the sweet potato plant.

Hawaii's earliest inhabitants are thought to have eaten a diet rich in fish. Some 1,500 years later, we know that eating fish regularly can be an important tool in reducing heart disease risk. Some fish is high in omega-3 fats, a special fat with heart benefits (see page 572). Overall, fish has less saturated and total fat than most meat.

Hawaii as a Stepping Stone for Explorers

Captain Cook is believed to be the first European to stop in Hawaii. He was the first of many European and American explorers, trappers, and whalers who used the Hawaiian Islands as stepping-stones for fresh supplies. Together, these explorers' influence on island life—including its cuisine—was profound.

An unfortunate series of events drastically changed Hawaii's cultural mix. When Cook arrived in 1778, the Hawaiian population numbered about 300,000. Diseases brought by global visitors, however, reduced the population to about 70,000 over the next one hundred years. The population decrease coincided with a thriving sugar cane industry. Desperate, the Hawaiian islanders sought labor to keep their chief industry alive. Workers arrived from Asia, Europe, the United States, and the tropics. These different peoples settled there and wove their cultural threads into the Hawaiian fabric.

The Chinese brought more vegetables, noodles, ginger, and stir-fry cooking. The Japanese introduced tempura, and the Portuguese left their culinary influence by way of spicy pork dishes, especially stews like Hawaiian Pork and Peas (page 470). The Koreans brought garlic and spicy peppers (Korean Ribs, page 406), and people from the Philippines reintroduced the Spanish and Malaysian flair of their homelands.

Not only did these people stir different foods into the Hawaiian cooking pot, but they also diversified the agricultural output. While sugar cane would remain the most important crop, pineapple, squash, peppers, tomatoes, and lettuce emerged as important cash crops—and, of course, significant fresh ingredients in local recipes.

Religious Influences in Hawaii

Religion, too, played a part in the formation of Hawaiian cuisine. Traveling from the east coast of the United States to Hawaii in the early 1800s, missionaries carried everyday mainland staples: potatoes, apples, salt cod, corned beef, cheese, and butter. These foods, too, would make their way into Hawaiian cuisine.

Hawaii's Agricultural and Marine Influences

Let's take a look at some of the other ingredients that are so central to Hawaiian cuisine:

- Macadamia nut: known for its crunchy, buttery rich flavor, the Macadamia nut originally hails from Australia (Ono Mango Macadamia Nut Bread, page 432).
- Mahimahi: you'll find this slightly sweet fish on most Hawaiian menus, cooked in a plethora of wonderful ways.
- Maui Onion: rivaling Georgia's sweet Vidalia and Oregon's Walla Walla, the Maui onion grows on the slopes of Mount Haleakala where temperatures are cool and the soil is fertile (Maui Pineapple Pork Roast, page 471).

Oatmeal à la Canela

Elsa Ramirez Brisson, M.P.H., R.D.

Serves: 1
Hands-on time: 5 minutes
Cooking time: 10 minutes

Inspired by my Mexican heritage and our generous use of cinnamon, this oatmeal will warm your soul and provide yet another opportunity to enjoy a hearty, nutritious breakfast. While we simmer old-fashioned oats with a cinnamon stick, you can make it much quicker with ground cinnamon.

½ cup rolled oats
1 cup nonfat milk
2 tablespoons raisins
¼ teaspoon cinnamon
1 teaspoon molasses

Combine all the ingredients in a heavy saucepan and stir. Simmer over low heat, stirring occasionally, for 10 minutes, or until creamy.

COOK'S TIP

Use the microwave: combine all of the ingredients with ¼ cup water in a microwave-safe container; cook for 2 minutes at 50 percent power. Stir and cook on high for 1 more minute; stir and cook 1 minute on high.

VARIATIONS

- Stir in 2 tablespoons flaxseed and cook as directed.
- Substitute 1 teaspoon honey, brown sugar, or maple syrup for the molasses.
- Top the oatmeal with 2 tablespoons walnuts, almonds, peanuts, or soy nuts.
- Substitute 1 apple (chopped with peel) for the raisins.
- Substitute 2 tablespoons of your favorite dried fruit for the raisins.
- Double the amount of raisins (or other dried fruit) and omit the molasses (or other sweetener).
- Stir in 1 teaspoon vanilla extract (or other favorite extract) after cooking.
- Omit the raisins and cook as directed. Top with ½ cup sliced fresh strawberries or other fresh fruit.

NUTRITION PER SERVING	
Serving size	1¼ cups
Calories	330 kcal
Fat	2.5 g
Saturated fat	0 g
Cholesterol	5 mg
Sodium	140 mg
Carbohydrates	61 g
Dietary fiber	6 g
Protein	16 g

Coconut Banana Muffins

Beverlee Kell, R.D.

This fusion of all-American banana bread with an Asian flair—so common in California cuisine—provided by coconut and wheat germ to provide a touch of health is a wonderfully unique version of an all-time favorite.

Serves: 24
Hands-on time: 15 minutes
Baking time: 25 to 30 minutes

- vegetable oil cooking spray
- 2 cups all-purpose flour
- ½ cup toasted wheat germ
- 2 teaspoons baking soda
- ½ teaspoon cardamom
- ½ cup canola oil
- ½ cup applesauce
- 1½ cups sugar
- 5 very ripe bananas
- ½ cup chopped hazelnuts
- ½ cup shredded sweetened coconut

Preheat oven to 350°F. Coat 24 regular muffin tins with the cooking spray.

Mix the flour, wheat germ, baking soda, and cardamom in a small bowl; set aside. Combine the oil, applesauce, sugar, bananas, nuts, and coconut in a medium-size bowl. Fold the flour mixture into the wet ingredients, stirring until just blended.

Fill the muffin cups ¾ full. Bake for 25 to 30 minutes, or until a toothpick inserted in the middle comes out clean.

SUBSTITUTION
Substitute chopped walnuts for the hazelnuts.

NUTRITION PER SERVING

Serving size	1 muffin
Calories	190 kcal
Fat	7 g
Saturated fat	1 g
Cholesterol	0 mg
Sodium	110 mg
Carbohydrates	30 g
Dietary fiber	2 g
Protein	2 g

Ono Mango Macadamia Nut Bread

Paula Williams, R.D., C.E.C.

Serves: 16
Hands-on time: 20 minutes
Baking time: 1 hour

To say "delicious" in Hawaiian, you say "ono." And this is a very ono bread, which showcases local ingredients. My neighbor at Kula has dozens of macadamia nut trees in her backyard, and was generous in letting me gather as many of the fallen crop as I wanted. No one warned me that these ono nuts are nearly impossible to crack. They have an extremely hard shell. I resorted to wedging one in a crack of my concrete sidewalk, smacked it with a small hammer, and sent it right through my window! This only made me crave the ono nutmeats more, so I finally perfected a method using a small c-clamp and a larger hammer. I strongly recommend the purchase of already-shelled macadamia nuts.

vegetable oil cooking spray
½ cup chopped macadamia nuts
1¼ cups sugar
2 teaspoons ground cinnamon
1¼ cups all-purpose flour
¾ cup toasted wheat germ
2 teaspoons baking soda
3 eggs
¼ cup canola oil
½ cup applesauce
2 teaspoons vanilla extract
2 cups cubed ripe mangoes (about 2 medium-size mangoes—reserve extra for Cucumber and Mango Salad on page 244)

Preheat oven to 350°F. Coat a 9-by-5-by-3-inch loaf pan with the cooking spray. Combine all the dry ingredients in a large bowl; mix well.

Whisk the eggs in a separate bowl; add the oil, applesauce, and vanilla and beat vigorously for 1 to 2 minutes. Pour the wet ingredients into the dry; stir just until the mixture is blended. Fold in the mangoes; some will break up, which is okay. Pour the mixture into the pan. Bake it for 1 hour.

SUBSTITUTIONS

Substitute equal amounts of papaya for the mango and almonds for the macadamia nuts.

NUTRITION NUGGET

Reduce the sugar and calories by using ¾ cup sugar and ½ cup spoonable sugar replacement.

NUTRITION PER SERVING

Serving size	1/16 of loaf
Calories	220 kcal
Fat	8 g
Saturated fat	1 g
Cholesterol	40 mg
Sodium	170 mg
Carbohydrates	33 g
Dietary fiber	2 g
Protein	4 g

Tropical Breeze Smoothie

Catherine Hoffmann, M.S., R.D.

Blend this smoothie and sip it with your eyes closed. You'll think you're in Hawaii or Tahiti!

Serves: 2

1 cup nonfat milk
½ cup crushed pineapple (in juice)
1 medium-size banana
1 medium-size papaya, peeled and cubed
4 to 6 ice cubes

Combine all the ingredients in a blender on high until smooth. Serve at once.

COOK'S TIP
Slice and freeze the banana to make the smoothie extra thick.

NUTRITION PER SERVING	
Serving size	1¼ cups
Calories	190 kcal
Fat	1 g
Saturated fat	0 g
Cholesterol	0 mg
Sodium	70 mg
Carbohydrates	44 g
Dietary fiber	5 g
Protein	6 g

All-Year Christmas Salsa

Dona Richwine, M.S., R.D.

Serves: 8
Hands-on time: 30 minutes

SUBSTITUTION

Use jarred grapefruit sections, available in the dairy or refrigerated produce section of the supermarket.

VARIATION

If tangerines aren't available, add an extra orange.

COOK'S TIP

To avoid staining your hands when seeding the pomegranate, seed it in a bowl of ice cold water.

NUTRITION NUGGET

Pomegranates are an excellent source of potassium; on average, each one has about 400 mg potassium.

NUTRITION PER SERVING	
Serving size	½ cup salsa with 1½ ounces chips
Calories	270 kcal
Fat	12 g
Saturated fat	2.5 g
Cholesterol	0 mg
Sodium	320 mg
Carbohydrates	40 g
Dietary fiber	5 g
Protein	4 g

This salsa looks like a shimmering bowl of jewels. Ruby red pomegranates are in season during the winter holidays, as are grapefruits here in California. When you can't get pomegranates, simply omit for a refreshing citrus salsa any time of year.

- 2 medium-size navel oranges
- 2 medium-size tangerines
- 1 medium-size ruby red grapefruit
- 1 medium-size red bell pepper
- 2 jalapeño peppers (to taste)
- ½ medium-size red onion, diced
- seeds of 1 pomegranate
- ½ bunch cilantro, chopped
- ½ cup lime juice
- ¼ teaspoon salt
- 1 13-ounce bag baked tortilla chips

Peel the oranges and tangerines with a sharp knife to remove the rinds; cut them into small ¼-inch pieces, remove any seeds. Peel the grapefruit with a sharp knife to remove the rind; cut out each section so that no membrane remains. Cut the sections into small ¼-inch pieces, remove any seeds. Seed the red pepper and jalapeños; mince both. For a hotter salsa, use some of the jalapeño seeds. Combine with the onion and fruit in a large bowl. Add the cilantro, lime juice, and salt. Transfer the salsa to a serving bowl and serve with the baked tortilla chips.

Tomatillo-Chipotle Salsa

Elsa Ramirez Brisson, M.P.H., R.D.

Spicy chipotles with refreshing salsa create this traditional Mexican dish.

Serves: 8
Hands-on time: 15 minutes
Cooking time: 5 minutes
Standing time: 30 minutes

- 2 medium-size onions, chopped and divided
- 1½ cups tomatillos
- 2 to 3 cloves garlic, minced
- 3 canned chipotle peppers, chopped
- 1 cup chopped fresh cilantro

Combine ¼ cup onion, the tomatillos, and ½ cup water in a small saucepan; bring to a boil and cook for 5 minutes. Drain and coarsely chop the mixture.

Stir together the cooked tomatillo mixture, the remaining onion, and the garlic, peppers, and cilantro in a large bowl; let stand 30 minutes before serving.

COOK'S TIP

Store leftover salsa in the refrigerator for up to 2 weeks in a tightly sealed container.

NUTRITION PER SERVING	
Serving size	⅓ cup
Calories	35 kcal
Fat	0 g
Saturated fat	0 g
Cholesterol	0 mg
Sodium	5 mg
Carbohydrates	7 g
Dietary fiber	2 g
Protein	1 g

Korean Beef and Pineapple Kabobs

Judy Lee-Norris, M.P.H., R.D.

Serves: 8
Hands-on time: 15 minutes
Standing time: 6 hours
Cooking time: 5 minutes

The signature blend of soy sauce, dark sesame oil, sherry, garlic, and cayenne make this Korean-seasoned appetizer a favorite. The pineapple sweetens it just a bit, and also makes it the perfect party kabob.

3 tablespoons soy sauce, low sodium
1 teaspoon brown sugar
2 tablespoons sesame oil, divided
1 teaspoon sherry
4 cloves garlic, minced
¼ teaspoon cayenne pepper
2 slices ginger root (about ½-inch-thick slices), minced
1 pound very lean beef, cut into cubes
1 20-ounce can pineapple chunks in juice, drained

Combine the soy sauce, sugars, 1 tablespoon oil, sherry, garlic, cayenne, and ginger in a flat glass or plastic dish. Add the beef and pineapple chunks.

Cover and marinate at least 6 hours; overnight is fine.

Heat the remaining tablespoon of oil in a large nonstick skillet over high to medium-high heat; add the beef cubes and sauté until cooked through. Add the pineapple chunks and remove the pan from heat.

Skewer the beef and pineapple on party toothpicks.

NUTRITION PER SERVING

Serving size	3 to 4 kabobs
Calories	130 kcal
Fat	6 g
Saturated fat	2 g
Cholesterol	25 mg
Sodium	230 mg
Carbohydrates	9 g
Dietary fiber	0 g
Protein	10 g

Mediterranean Quesadillas

Laura Faler Thomas, M.Ed., R.D., L.D.

Fuse fresh vegetables with Mediterranean flavors and spices and you have a fabulous quesadilla that's great for appetizers or a main course.

Serves: 12 as an appetizer or 6 as a main course
Hands-on time: 15 minutes

1 unpeeled cucumber, chopped
1 medium-size tomato, chopped
½ cup nonfat plain yogurt
1 cup prepared hummus (for recipe, see page 230)
6 10-inch garlic- or tomato basil-flavored tortillas
1 cup tomato-basil feta cheese crumbles (or plain feta cheese crumbles) (4 ounces)
vegetable oil cooking spray

Combine the cucumber, tomato, and yogurt in a medium-size bowl; set aside.

Spread ⅓ cup hummus evenly over each of three tortillas. Sprinkle each with ⅓ cup cheese. Top each with another tortilla.

Coat a large nonstick skillet with the cooking spray and cook each quesadilla 1 minute per side or until the cheese is melted. Cut each into 4 wedges; serve with the vegetable mixture.

COOK'S TIP

Freeze leftover tortillas in a tightly sealed plastic bag; thaw at room temperature for 30 minutes or in the microwave for 30 to 60 seconds.

NUTRITION PER SERVING	
Serving size	4 wedges, main course
Calories	360 kcal
Fat	12 g
Saturated fat	3 g
Cholesterol	10 mg
Sodium	360 mg
Carbohydrates	50 g
Dietary fiber	6 g
Protein	14 g

NUTRITION PER SERVING	
Serving size	2 wedges, appetizer
Calories	180 kcal
Fat	6 g
Saturated fat	1.5 g
Cholesterol	5 mg
Sodium	180 mg
Carbohydrates	25 g
Dietary fiber	3 g
Protein	7 g

Lemon-Dijon Asparagus

Sanna James Delmonico, M.S., R.D.

Serves: 4 to 8
Hands-on time: 10 minutes
Cooking time: 3 minutes

Spring is the time for asparagus in California: steamed asparagus, grilled asparagus, cream of asparagus soup, asparagus frittata, and this easy salad.

- 1½ pounds fresh asparagus, ends trimmed
- 2 tablespoons extra-virgin olive oil
- 2 tablespoons lemon juice
- 1 tablespoon Dijon mustard
- 2 teaspoons minced lemon zest
- ¼ teaspoon ground pepper
- 1 teaspoon sugar
- 1 tablespoon minced fresh parsley
- 1 tablespoon minced fresh chives

Blanch the asparagus in boiling water for 3 minutes. Plunge it into a bowl of ice water to stop the cooking and preserve the bright green color. Drain well. Whisk together the remaining ingredients in a small bowl. Pour over the asparagus and serve at room temperature.

SHOPPING TIP

Look for asparagus with freshly cut ends, tight tips, and no signs of decay or sliminess.

VARIATION

Use any combination of fresh herbs; try basil, tarragon, thyme, and oregano.

NUTRITION PER SERVING	
Serving size	1 cup
Calories	110 kcal
Fat	8 g
Saturated fat	1 g
Cholesterol	0 mg
Sodium	95 mg
Carbohydrates	9 g
Dietary fiber	2 g
Protein	6 g

Asian-Style Slaw

Libby Mills, M.S., R.D., L.D.

Stressing simple elegance using wholesome foods—so characteristic of Hawaiian cooking—this recipe uses just green cabbage. It is highlighted with vinegar, soy sauce, and red pepper, giving it two of the three typical tastes coleslaw can have (spicy and tangy; sweet is the third). Enjoy it for a few days; it gets better over time!

Serves: 4
Hands-on time: 20 minutes
Cooking time: 5 minutes

¼ cup sugar
4 cups (10 ounces) cleaned and thinly sliced green cabbage
¼ teaspoon red pepper flakes
1 teaspoon white rice wine vinegar
1 tablespoon light soy sauce
2 teaspoons toasted sesame seed oil
½ cup chopped fresh cilantro

In a small saucepan, combine ⅓ cup water and the sugar; bring to a boil over medium-high heat, stirring until all the sugar dissolves, approximately 5 minutes. Remove from heat.

In a large mixing bowl, combine the cabbage, red pepper flakes, vinegar, soy sauce, and sesame seed oil. Stir in the water-sugar mixture. Stir in the chopped cilantro.

Serve at once or refrigerate for at least 1 hour before serving.

SHOPPING TIP
1 head of cabbage (about 12 ounces) will yield 4 cups of shredded cabbage.

COOK'S TIP
This dish may be refrigerated for up to 4 days.

FOOD TRIVIA
The term coleslaw comes from the Dutch koolsla, meaning "cool cabbage."

NUTRITION PER SERVING

Serving size	¾ cup
Calories	90 kcal
Fat	2.5 g
Saturated fat	0 g
Cholesterol	0 mg
Sodium	150 mg
Carbohydrates	17 g
Dietary fiber	2 g
Protein	1 g

Sesame Orange Snow Peas

Libby Mills, M.S., R.D., L.D.

Serves: 4
Hands-on time: 5 minutes
Cooking time: 10 minutes

Forget Chinese take-out when you can make this flavor-packed vegetable dish in just minutes. Asian flavors of toasted sesame, fresh ginger, orange, and soy—commonly found in California and Hawaii—create a zesty sauce for crisp-tender snow peas anywhere in the United States.

4 cups fresh snow peas
5 cloves garlic, minced
1 tablespoon minced ginger
2 tablespoons light soy sauce
⅓ cup orange marmalade
2 tablespoons sesame seeds

Clean the snow peas by breaking off the stem ends and removing the fibrous strings running the length of the pod; wash well.

In a medium-size nonstick skillet, combine the peas, garlic, ginger, soy sauce, and marmalade. Cover and cook over medium heat for 7 to 10 minutes or until the peas are bright green and still crisp.

Meanwhile, in another medium-size skillet, toast the sesame seeds over medium-high heat, stirring several times, until golden—about 5 to 6 minutes.

Transfer the peas to a serving bowl; top with sesame seeds.

VARIATION

Enjoy another texture in this recipe by choosing a chunky orange marmalade that contains pieces of orange peel.

COOK'S TIP

To clean snow peas, hold in your nondominant hand with the tip of the "string" end up and the entire string side toward your dominant hand. Pinch the end with your thumb and forefinger and pull the string away from the pod; discard.

NUTRITION PER SERVING	
Serving size	½ cup
Calories	110 kcal
Fat	2 g
Saturated fat	0 g
Cholesterol	0 mg
Sodium	320 mg
Carbohydrates	21 g
Dietary fiber	0 g
Protein	2 g

Flash-Fried Romaine

Stacy Haumea, R.D.

Hawaii is the only place I've ever had cooked romaine lettuce. The symphony of peanut oil, romaine, and bacon is fabulous, as is the texture. Remember, this recipe calls for just a "flash in the pan"!

Serves: 4 to 8
Hands-on time: 5 minutes
Cooking time: 5 minutes

- 4 slices bacon
- 2 bunches romaine lettuce, rinsed and spun dry (about 16 cups)
- ½ teaspoon salt
- ½ teaspoon ground black pepper
- 1 tablespoon peanut oil

Fry the bacon in a wok or a very large frying pan over medium-high heat; remove from heat. Clean the pan. Drain the bacon on paper towels; cool and chop it into ½-inch pieces.

Shred the romaine; season it with salt and pepper.

Heat the oil in a wok; add the lettuce. Flash-fry just 1 to 3 minutes, turning constantly.

Garnish with the bacon pieces. Serve hot.

NUTRITION PER SERVING	
Serving size	1¼ cups
Calories	100 kcal
Fat	7 g
Saturated fat	1.5 g
Cholesterol	5 mg
Sodium	450 mg
Carbohydrates	6 g
Dietary fiber	4 g
Protein	6 g

Ulu Home Fries

Stacy Haumea, R.D.

Serves: 6
Hands-on time: 10 minutes
Cooking time: 1 hour, 35 minutes

Native to the Pacific, breadfruit is a favorite in Hawaii. Try this recipe and you'll quickly understand why we love it.

1 medium-size ulu (breadfruit)
1 teaspoon salt, divided
¼ cup canola oil
2 tablespoons butter

COOK'S TIP
Ulu skin is not edible; remove before or after cooking.

Preheat oven to 325°F. Clean the outer ulu skin with a damp cloth. Bake the whole breadfruit until a skewer pokes through the skin easily (similar to a baked potato), for approximately 1 hour, 15 minutes. Remove the ulu and let it cool completely (about 1½ to 2 hours).

Cut the ulu into quarters and remove all the skin. Cut out the center rib and the seeds. Slice the quarters into ¼-inch thick slices.

Heat a large skillet over medium-high heat; add the oil and butter. Place the ulu slices in the pan; lightly sprinkle with salt. Sauté until golden brown (about 10 minutes) then turn to brown the other side (about 7 to 8 minutes).

Remove from the pan and place on a paper towel to remove the excess oil.

NUTRITION PER SERVING	
Serving size	1 cup
Calories	180 kcal
Fat	13 g
Saturated fat	3 g
Cholesterol	10 mg
Sodium	290 mg
Carbohydrates	17 g
Dietary fiber	3 g
Protein	1 g

Minted Corn, Cucumber, and Tomato Salad

Sanna James Delmonico, M.S., R.D.

This recipe will transport you to a summer day at a farmers' market in California's Napa Valley—my own inspiration for this salad. Yes, fresh raw corn from the cob is excellent!

Serves: 4

Hands-on time: 10 to 12 minutes

- 1 cup fresh corn kernels (about 2 ears), or 1 cup frozen
- ½ English cucumber, diced (peel on)
- 1 cup cherry tomatoes, cut in halves
- 2 tablespoons fresh chopped mint
- pinch of salt
- pinch freshly ground pepper
- 1 tablespoon lime juice
- ½ teaspoon sugar
- 2 teaspoons extra-virgin olive oil

Combine the corn, cucumber, and tomatoes in a medium-size bowl; set aside. In a separate small bowl, whisk together the mint, salt, pepper, lime juice, sugar, and oil. Pour the sauce over the vegetables; toss. Let the salad sit for at least 30 minutes in the refrigerator before serving so that the flavors blend.

SHOPPING TIPS

When you bring a bunch of fresh mint home, cut the ends and store the bunch upright in a glass of water, just as you would a bunch of flowers. This will help it stay fresh longer.

COOK'S TIP

A pinch is equivalent to 1⁄16 of a teaspoon.

SERVING SUGGESTION

Serve this salad on a hot summer night alongside grilled salmon or trout.

NUTRITION PER SERVING	
Serving size	1 cup
Calories	70 kcal
Fat	3 g
Saturated fat	0 g
Cholesterol	0 mg
Sodium	45 mg
Carbohydrates	11 g
Dietary fiber	2 g
Protein	2 g

Rosemary Roasted Vegetable Medley

Lisa Turner, R.D.

Serves: 6
Hands-on time: 15 minutes
Cooking time: 40 minutes

Californians love anything fresh and also multiple layers of taste. This is just what is accomplished when rosemary and vinegar are blended together. You may even get your family to beg for more vegetables when you serve this!

vegetable oil cooking spray
1 pound red skin potatoes, cut into bite-size chunks
2 cups (12-ounce bag) very tiny baby carrots
1 small head cauliflower, trimmed and separated into bite-size florets
3 tablespoons extra-virgin olive oil
1 teaspoon balsamic vinegar
2 tablespoons minced fresh rosemary (or 2 teaspoons dried)
1 teaspoon salt
½ teaspoon black pepper

Preheat oven to 450°F and spray a 13-by-9-inch baking pan with the cooking spray. Combine the potatoes, carrots, and cauliflower in the baking pan. Stir together the oil, balsamic vinegar, rosemary, salt, and pepper in a small bowl; pour over the vegetables and toss.

Cover tightly and bake for 20 minutes. Uncover, stir, and bake for an additional 10 to 20 minutes, or until the potatoes are fork-tender.

SUBSTITUTIONS

Substitute 2 teaspoons dried oregano and 1 teaspoon garlic powder for the rosemary.

COOK'S TIP

Cook the vegetables on the grill instead of in the oven. Combine all the ingredients in a large bowl; cover and let stand 30 minutes at room temperature. Place in a grilling basket (suited for small items) and grill over a medium-hot flame for 10 to 20 minutes, turning frequently. Grill until potatoes are fork-tender.

NUTRITION PER SERVING	
Serving size	1½ cups
Calories	130 kcal
Fat	7 g
Saturated fat	1 g
Cholesterol	0 mg
Sodium	440 mg
Carbohydrates	14 g
Dietary fiber	5 g
Protein	4 g

Hawaiian Salad with Sesame Dressing

Lisa C. Peterson, M.S., R.D., C.D.N.

This is a favorite at the annual New England–style Hawaii we host every summer. It's just different enough for those n with genuine island cuisine. It's also great for entertaining ing and the vegetables can be prepped the day before and just before serving.

Serves: 4 as a main cours
or 12 as a side dish.
Hands-on time: 20
Cooking time: 10

SUBS
Cri

SALAD

1 6-ounce can sliced water chestnuts, drained
1 medium-size red bell pepper, thinly sliced and slices halved
¼ cup scallions, sliced
1 cup celery, thinly sliced on diagonal
2 cups fresh mung bean sprouts, blanched until just wilted (½ pound)
1 cup bok choy, thinly sliced on diagonal
½ cup sliced almonds, toasted

DRESSING

½ cup toasted sesame oil
¼ cup reduced-sodium soy sauce
½ teaspoon sugar
1 tablespoon fresh lemon juice
½ teaspoon freshly ground black pepper

Make the salad by combining the water chestnuts, peppers, scallions, celery, sprouts and bok choy in a salad bowl (can be refrigerated overnight).

Make the dressing by combining the sesame oil, soy sauce, sugar, lemon juice, and pepper; whisk to blend.

To serve, toss the vegetables with the dressing. Sprinkle with the almonds; serve immediately.

COOK'S TIP

Blanch sprouts by bringing 2 quarts of water to a boil in a 3-quart kettle. Add the sprouts, stir, and remove and drain immediately.

NUTRITION PER SERVING	
Serving size	2 cups
Calories	190 kcal
Fat	17 g
Saturated fat	2.5 g
Cholesterol	0 mg
Sodium	290 mg
Carbohydrates	8 g
Dietary fiber	3 g
Protein	3 g

Hola Caesar!

Susan Kell Peletta, R.D.

This recipe introduces some interesting San Francisco twists to the famous salad, which, contrary to popular belief that it comes from Europe, actually hails from Tijuana, Mexico.

e

inutes
minutes

ITUTIONS
mbled feta or shred-
ded Parmesan can be substituted for cotija cheese. Sunflower seeds can be substituted for pumpkin seeds.

COOK'S TIP
Dress it up by slicing a ripe avocado into thin strips and garnishing the salad bowl or each plate.

NUTRITION PER SERVING	
Serving size	2 cups, main course
Calories	270 kcal
Fat	18 g
Saturated fat	3 g
Cholesterol	5 mg
Sodium	450 mg
Carbohydrates	17 g
Dietary fiber	4 g
Protein	12 g

NUTRITION PER SERVING	
Serving size	¾ cup, side dish
Calories	90 kcal
Fat	6 g
Saturated fat	1 g
Cholesterol	0 mg
Sodium	150 mg
Carbohydrates	6 g
Dietary fiber	1 g
Protein	4 g

- vegetable oil ooking spray, butter flavored
- 3 6-inch corn tòrtillas cut into thin strips
- 1 bunch fresh cilantro leaves (about 1½ cups)
- 2 cloves garlic, peeled
- 3 tablespoons lime juice
- 3 tablespoons canola oil
- ½ cup liquid egg substitute
- ¼ teaspoon Worcestershire sauce
- ¼ teaspoon salt
- (additional) lime juice to taste
- coarse ground pepper to taste
- 1 10-ounce bag cut romaine lettuce
- 1 medium-size red bell pepper, quartered and cut into thin strips
- ½ cup cotija cheese, crumbled
- ¼ cup roasted pumpkin seeds

Preheat oven to 400°F. Spray a baking pan with the cooking spray. Cut the tortillas in half, then into thin strips. Spread them out evenly on the baking pan. Spray the tortilla strips evenly with the cooking spray.

Bake the tortilla strips for about 10 minutes, until crisp and golden brown, shaking the pan and separating the strips with tongs halfway through the cooking time. Remove from the oven and set aside to cool.

Combine the cilantro, garlic, lime juice, oil, egg substitute, Worcestershire, and salt in the blender. Whip for 1 minute. Scrape the sides of the blender down with a rubber spatula. Repeat, whipping for a total of 2 minutes. The dressing will be thin but silky. Add more lime juice and pepper to taste.

Toss the romaine, tortilla strips, bell pepper, cheese, and pumpkin seeds with the dressing. Serve immediately.

VARIATIONS
To add some protein, toss in grilled chicken breast strips or cooked shrimp; for vegetarian style, add black beans.

Sopa de Elote (Mexican Corn Soup)

Linda Ferber, M.S., R.D.

Satisfying and delicious, this soup is filled with the authentic flavors of regional Mexican cooking so prevalent in San Diego. It's also economical!

Serves: 6
Hands-on time: 30 to 40 minutes
Cooking time: 35 minutes

- 5 cups corn kernels, fresh or frozen
- 6 cups reduced-salt chicken broth
- vegetable oil cooking spray
- 2 teaspoons olive oil, divided
- 1 small onion, chopped
- 1 medium-size clove garlic, chopped
- 1 cup celery, chopped (2 ribs)
- 1 large ripe tomato or 3 ripe roma tomatoes, chopped
- 2 medium-size, fresh poblano chilis, seeded and cut into 2-by-¼-inch strips
- ¼ cup chopped cilantro, divided
- ½ teaspoon salt
- ¼ teaspoon black pepper
- ⅓ cup light sour cream

Place the fresh or frozen corn in a 4-quart pot with the chicken broth. Bring to a boil over medium heat; reduce to a simmer and cook for 10 minutes. Remove 1 cup of the corn from the broth and reserve.

Coat a nonstick skillet with the cooking spray and place over medium heat; add 1 teaspoon olive oil and sauté the onion, garlic, and celery for 5 minutes until softened.

Purée the onion mixture, broth, corn, and tomatoes in a blender until smooth. Add the purée to the pot and cook for 5 minutes.

Using the same nonstick skillet, sauté the chilis in the remaining teaspoon of oil for 5 minutes. Add to the pot along with the reserved corn. (The peppers will blacken and become soft.) Add 2 tablespoons of cilantro and the salt and pepper to the soup; cook for 5 minutes.

Remove from heat. Add ⅓ cup of light sour cream and blend well. Garnish each serving with 1 teaspoon of chopped cilantro and serve hot.

VARIATION

Substitute plain low-fat or nonfat yogurt for the light sour cream. Or make a nondairy version with your favorite vegetarian sour cream or yogurt.

COOK'S TIP

Two pounds of frozen corn kernels or about 10 ears of corn will yield 5 cups.

NUTRITION PER SERVING

Serving size	1 cup
Calories	200 kcal
Fat	6 g
Saturated fat	2 g
Cholesterol	10 mg
Sodium	330 mg
Carbohydrates	33 g
Dietary fiber	4 g
Protein	8 g

Hawaiian Star Soup (Hoku Soup)

Paula Williams, R.D., C.E.C.

Serves: 6
Hands-on time: 20 minutes
Cooking time: 40 minutes

Food is a way of sharing yourself and your heritage, especially when you live on Maui. Every event is a potluck, with each participant bringing something special to share for the meal—and there is always a meal associated with every event. Hoku is Hawaiian for star, and because so many events are held outside in the evenings, with the stars seeming closer and brighter than possible, I wanted to create a simple yet tasty soup to complement the vast variety of other foods shared.

- 3 tablespoons cornstarch
- 4 14-ounce cans reduced-sodium chicken broth
- 2 ribs celery, thinly sliced
- 3 medium-size carrots, peeled and thinly sliced
- 2 tablespoons grated fresh ginger root
- ¼ cup reduced-sodium soy sauce
- 1 teaspoon cayenne pepper, ground
- ½ teaspoon chili paste
- ¼ cup chopped fresh parsley
- 1 pound cooked chicken, diced
- ½ cup uncooked star pasta
- 2 green onions, sliced thinly
- black pepper, optional, to taste

Dissolve the cornstarch in ½ cup cold water in a large stock pot. Add the broth, celery, carrots, ginger, soy sauce, cayenne, chili paste, and 2 cups water. Simmer 30 minutes. Add the parsley, chicken, and pasta; bring the soup to a boil. Cook the pasta as directed on the package and add it to the soup.

Garnish the soup with the green onions. Adjust the spiciness with black pepper or more cayenne, if desired.

NUTRITION NUGGET

I've reduced the sodium by using reduced-sodium chicken broth and light soy sauce. The other seasonings carry the flavor beautifully.

NUTRITION PER SERVING

Serving size	1½ cups
Calories	220 kcal
Fat	4 g
Saturated fat	1.5 g
Cholesterol	65 mg
Sodium	520 mg
Carbohydrates	18 g
Dietary fiber	3 g
Protein	28 g

Tropical Chicken with Mango Salsa and Coconut Rice

Christina Blais, M.Sc., P.Dt.

Pacific Rim flavors are right at home in Montreal, Canada, where I live. Let the fresh flavors of ginger, lime, cilantro, and coconuts take you on a culinary adventure to Hawaii. Montreal, our home, has become a multicultural city. Our markets carry foods from around the world, making cooking an even more satisfying experience. The fresh and tangy flavors of Hawaiian and Thai cooking fuse together beautifully in this easy meal. Serve leftovers cold over lettuce the next day.

Serves: 4
Hands-on time: 20 minutes
Cooking time: 20 minutes

- 1 pound boneless, skinless chicken breast halves
- ¼ cup reduced-sodium soy sauce
- 1 tablespoon minced ginger
- 1 cup coconut milk
- 1 teaspoon salt
- 1 cup basmati rice

Slice the chicken in half horizontally and trim the fat. Combine the soy sauce and ginger in a large bowl. Add the chicken and marinate for at least 30 minutes or up to 2 hours in the refrigerator, turning occasionally.

Drain the chicken and discard the marinade. Cook on a greased grill over medium-high heat, turning once until nicely browned and no longer pink inside, about 8 to 10 minutes.

Bring the coconut milk, 1 cup water, and the salt to a boil in a medium-size saucepan. Add the rice; reduce heat and simmer, covered, for 15 minutes or until tender. Remove from heat and let stand 5 minutes. Fluff with a fork just before serving.

COOK'S TIP

How to peel and slice a mango: Cut off the stem of the mango. Cup the fruit in the palm of your nondominant hand, holding it upright. Use a potato or vegetable peeler or a paring knife with your dominant hand to remove the peel; follow the curves of the fruit. Lay the fruit on its flat end and slice it lengthwise (working around the flat seed in the middle). Carve away the remaining flesh by turning the mango as you cut.

NUTRITION PER SERVING

Serving size	½ chicken breast, ⅔ cup cooked rice, ¼ cup salsa
Calories	350 kcal
Fat	3.5 g
Saturated fat	1 g
Cholesterol	65 mg
Sodium	790 mg
Carbohydrates	49 g
Dietary fiber	3 g
Protein	31 g

Tropical Chicken with Mango Salsa and Coconut Rice *(continued)*

SHOPPING TIP
To pick a ripe mango, choose one that "gives" ever so slightly with a gentle squeeze.

COOK'S TIP
Lime, lemon, and orange rind are called zest.

Mango Salsa

- 1 medium-size ripe mango, peeled, diced into ½-inch cubes
- ¼ cup chopped fresh mint leaves
- ¼ cup cilantro and/or chives
- 1 tablespoon fresh lime juice
- 1 teaspoon minced fresh ginger
- 1 teaspoon Thai fish sauce (optional)
- ½ teaspoon grated lime rind
- dash salt

Combine the mango, herbs, lime juice, ginger, fish sauce, and lime rind in a medium-size bowl. Add salt to taste. Chill until ready to serve.

Serve the marinated chicken topped with the mango salsa over the coconut rice.

Korean Style Chicken with Green Beans

Judy Lee-Norris, M.P.H., R.D.

The signature blend of soy sauce, dark sesame oil, sherry, garlic, and cayenne make this Korean-seasoned meal one to remember. You'll find it easy to prepare when time is short.

Serves: 4
Hands-on time: 15 minutes
Standing time: 2 hours
Cooking time: 15 minutes

- 3 tablespoons reduced-sodium soy sauce
- 2 tablespoons dark sesame oil, divided
- 1 tablespoon sherry
- 1 tablespoon packed brown sugar
- 4 cloves garlic, minced
- ¼ to ½ teaspoon cayenne pepper (or Thai red chili paste to taste)
- ¼ to ½ teaspoon black pepper
- 1 pound boneless, skinless chicken thighs, cut into strips
- 2 medium-size onions, quartered and sliced thinly
- 1 pound fresh green beans, sliced into 1½-inch slivers

Mix the soy sauce, 1 tablespoon of the oil, the sherry, sugar, garlic, and peppers. Add the chicken and marinate for at least 2 hours; overnight is fine.

Heat the remaining tablespoon oil in a frying pan on medium-high heat; add the onions and green beans. Sauté 5 to 7 minutes, stirring constantly, until the onions are wilted. Remove the vegetables from the pan and keep warm.

Add the chicken to the same pan. Stir-fry 5 to 7 minutes, stirring constantly, until the meat is cooked through. Add the green bean mixture and reheat briefly.

SHOPPING TIP
Sesame oil is available dark (also called toasted) or light; choose the dark for this recipe.

SUBSTITUTION
Save time by substituting 1 pound frozen, French-style green beans for the fresh. Thaw them first before using in this recipe.

NUTRITION PER SERVING

Serving size	2 cups
Calories	230 kcal
Fat	9 g
Saturated fat	1.5 g
Cholesterol	80 mg
Sodium	410 mg
Carbohydrates	15 g
Dietary fiber	2 g
Protein	24 g

Hoisin Chicken Spinach Salad

Lori Martinez-Hassett, R.D.

Serves: 4
Hands-on time: 30 minutes
Cooking time: 8 minutes

Asian inspired as so many recipes are in San Francisco, this flavor-packed salad entrée is also appealing and colorful. You may have to purchase the hoisin sauce and pickled ginger in the Asian section of your grocery store if you don't already have them on hand. But you'll find these ingredients popping up in other recipes you'll want to try too.

- 2 tablespoons peanut oil
- ¼ cup rice vinegar
- 3 tablespoons hoisin sauce
- 1 small shallot, finely minced
- ½ pound boneless, skinless chicken breasts or thighs
- 1 10-ounce bag baby spinach leaves
- ¼ cup roasted cashew nuts
- 2 tablespoons chopped pickled ginger (sushi ginger)
- 1 medium-size orange, peeled and sectioned

Preheat grill or broiler. Whisk together the oil, vinegar, hoisin, 1 tablespoon water, and the shallot (or pulse briefly with a food processor or immersion blender). Divide the dressing into 2 containers (⅓ cup each). Use ⅓ cup of the dressing for basting the chicken breasts. Use the remainder as dressing for the salad.

Broil or grill the chicken while basting continuously with the dressing. Cook until thoroughly done, about 3 to 4 minutes per side. Remove the skin and slice into ½-inch strips.

Place 2 cups of spinach on each of 4 plates. Top evenly with sliced chicken.

Add 1 tablespoon cashew nuts to each salad. Top with ginger and orange segments. Drizzle the salads with the dressing.

SHOPPING TIP

Many grocery stores and almost all Asian markets carry hoisin sauce and pickled ginger.

SUBSTITUTIONS

If you don't have shallots, substitute ¼ small onion (minced). Instead of rice wine vinegar, use an equal amount of white wine vinegar.

COOK'S TIP

For food safety, use only the reserved dressing for the salad; discard the portion you used to marinate the chicken.

NUTRITION PER SERVING

Serving size	3 cups
Calories	240 kcal
Fat	12 g
Saturated fat	2 g
Cholesterol	35 mg
Sodium	460 mg
Carbohydrates	17 g
Dietary fiber	4 g
Protein	17 g

Chinese Chicken Salad

Stacy Haumea, R.D.

In our Hawaiian home, we enjoy this salad with and without the chicken. Spice up the dressing with more cayenne if you like.

Serves: 4 as a main course or 8 as a side dish
Hands-on time: 20 minutes
Cooking time: 15 minutes

1 pound boneless, skinless chicken breasts
1 14-ounce can reduced-sodium chicken broth
3 tablespoons white or apple cider vinegar
3 tablespoons sugar
3 tablespoons sesame oil
⅛ to ¼ teaspoon cayenne pepper, ground
2 cups shredded red cabbage
1 bunch watercress, coarsely chopped (optional)
½ cup chopped cilantro leaves
4 cups shredded romaine lettuce
2 medium-size carrots, shredded
1 medium-size cucumber, thinly sliced (peel on)
2 medium-size ripe tomatoes, chopped
½ cup chow mein noodles

Combine the chicken and the broth in a skillet; cover and simmer until the chicken is cooked through, about 15 minutes. Cool the chicken and chop into ½-inch pieces.

Meanwhile, boil the vinegar and sugar in a saucepan until clear, about 2 minutes. Let the liquid cool. Whisk in the sesame oil and the cayenne; set the dressing aside.

Combine the cabbage, watercress, cilantro, lettuce, carrots, cucumber, and tomatoes in a large salad bowl. Divide the salad mixture among 4 plates.

Chop the cooked chicken; coat the chicken in the dressing and stir well. Pour the chicken and dressing over the salads. Top with the chow mein noodles.

SUBSTITUTION
Substitute one additional cup red cabbage for the watercress.

NUTRITION PER SERVING	
Serving size	3 cups, main course
Calories	350 kcal
Fat	15 g
Saturated fat	2.5 g
Cholesterol	70 mg
Sodium	190 mg
Carbohydrates	26 g
Dietary fiber	4 g
Protein	32 g

Asian Chicken Salad

Maria Vargas, M.S., R.D.

Serves: 6
Hands-on time: 20 minutes
Cooking time: 20 minutes

My kids love sweets and are not vegetable eaters, but this recipe solved that problem. The sweet and sour dressing is a fusion of flavors. The salad combines a variety of raw vegetables that they love to eat on hot summer days. This salad is best served cold. Please note that you can use the dressing on any combination of vegetables—as a main meal or a great side dish.

½ cup rice wine vinegar
¼ cup reduced-sodium soy sauce
3 tablespoons packed brown sugar
1 tablespoon dark sesame oil
1 medium-size head (1¼ pound) Napa cabbage, cored and shredded
½ cup shredded red cabbage
½ cup julienne-cut carrots
1 medium-size red bell pepper, trimmed, seeded, and diced
2 chopped green onions, using both bulb and stems
1 cup cooked soba noodles, cooled
1 pound cooked boneless, skinless chicken breast halves, sliced into strips
2 tablespoons sesame seeds

Whisk together the vinegar, soy sauce, brown sugar, and oil; set aside.

Toss lightly the cabbage, carrots, red pepper, and onions in a large salad bowl. Drizzle the vegetables with dressing; toss them to coat. Add the cooked noodles; toss and top with the chicken strips. Sprinkle with the sesame seeds and serve.

COOK'S TIP

To save time, you can use bagged shredded cabbage and matchstick-cut carrots, which are sold in the produce section of the supermarket.

NUTRITION PER SERVING	
Serving size	2 cups
Calories	230 kcal
Fat	7 g
Saturated fat	1.5 g
Cholesterol	65 mg
Sodium	490 mg
Carbohydrates	17 g
Dietary fiber	3 g
Protein	27 g

California Chicken Wrap

Elizabeth Arvidson, R.D.

Wraps have revived the somewhat weary sandwich, and with good reason. They can be filled with flavorful veggies, meat, and condiments and are ready to go at a moment's notice. This wrap also does double duty as an appetizer when it is cut into small slices.

Serves: 16 as an appetizer or 8 as a main course
Hands-on time: 15 minutes
Cooking time: 15 minutes

- 1 pound boneless, skinless chicken breast halves
- 2 teaspoons dried rosemary or Italian seasoning or other favorite herbs
- 1 14-ounce can reduced-sodium chicken broth
- 1 7¼-ounce jar roasted red bell pepper, water packed, divided
- 1 medium-size green bell pepper, trimmed, seeded, and minced
- 4 ounces light cream cheese, softened
- ½ teaspoon garlic powder
- ¼ teaspoon ground cumin
- ¼ teaspoon cayenne pepper
- 4 10-inch flour tortillas
- 2 cups (about 4 ounces) shredded romaine

Place the chicken, rosemary (or other seasoning) and broth in skillet; cover. Simmer for 15 minutes or until the chicken is cooked through. Cool slightly and slice into thin strips.

Mince half of the roasted peppers; set aside the other half. Combine the minced red and green bell peppers, cream cheese, garlic powder, cumin, and cayenne. Spread the mixture evenly over each tortilla. Place the chicken evenly among the 4 tortillas. Top with the remaining roasted peppers and romaine.

To assemble the wrap: Place the filling across the lower third of the wrap (or tortilla). Fold the bottom edge of the tortilla over the filling. Fold both the right and left sides inward. Continue rolling up tightly, tucking the ends in, and enclosing the filling. Place seam-side down on parchment wrap or foil, and then wrap it up. Cut in half diagonally. Slice each roll into 4 pieces just before serving. Secure with a toothpick if necessary.

COOK'S TIP

For faster assembly, substitute precooked chicken, available in the meat case.

NUTRITION PER SERVING

Serving size	1 wrap
Calories	510 kcal
Fat	17 g
Saturated fat	5 g
Cholesterol	75 mg
Sodium	820 mg
Carbohydrates	49 g
Dietary fiber	4 g
Protein	37 g

Turkey, Sun-Dried Tomato, and Basil Rice

Lori Martinez-Hassett, R.D.

Serves: 6
Hands-on time: 20 minutes
Cooking time: 45 minutes

Although it's a bit more labor-intensive than cooking other types of rice, making risotto from arborio rice is well worth the effort. The result is a creamy rice like none other you've tried. Here in San Francisco, we like to blend in lots of other ingredients, such as this Italian combination of sun-dried tomatoes, basil, and saffron.

- 1 49-ounce can reduced-sodium chicken broth, divided use
- ½ teaspoon saffron threads, crushed
- 2 tablespoons extra-virgin olive oil
- 1 medium-size onion, chopped
- 4 cloves garlic, chopped
- ½ pound (8 ounces) boneless, skinless turkey breasts, cubed
- 2 cups arborio rice
- ¼ cup sun-dried tomatoes
- ½ pound mushrooms, sliced (suggested crimini or brown mushrooms)
- ¼ teaspoon white pepper
- 3 tablespoons chopped fresh basil (or 1 tablespoon dry)
- 1 tablespoon chopped fresh thyme (or 1 teaspoon dry)
- ½ cup white wine
- 4 tablespoons freshly shredded Parmesan cheese

Combine all of the broth and crushed saffron in a small saucepan. Simmer until the saffron is evenly dispersed, about 3 to 4 minutes. Remove from heat.

Heat the oil in a large 3-quart kettle. Add the onion and garlic and sauté for 3 to 5 minutes, or until the onion is soft. Add the turkey to the sautéed onion and garlic; cook for 4 to 6 minutes, or until the turkey is cooked through. Add ½ cup of the saffron-infused broth to the turkey mixture; stir and loosen the brown bits from the bottom of the pan (which will help to flavor the food). Add the rice, sun-dried tomatoes, mushrooms, and white pepper. If you are using dry herbs, add those.

SUBSTITUTION

Substitute an equal amount of chicken for the turkey.

NUTRITION PER SERVING

Serving size	1 cup plus 1 tablespoon Parmesan
Calories	440 kcal
Fat	10 g
Saturated fat	3 g
Cholesterol	30 mg
Sodium	200 mg
Carbohydrates	69 g
Dietary fiber	3 g
Protein	22 g

Over medium heat, stir the rice until it is well coated and starts turning opaque, about 2 to 3 minutes. Add the white wine and cook until the liquid has evaporated. Add 1 additional cup of saffron-infused broth. Stir the rice and cook over medium heat until the liquid is absorbed. Add more saffron-infused broth, 1 cup at a time, stirring occasionally until all the liquid is again absorbed. Repeat this process until the risotto is cooked al dente (20 to 25 minutes). You will use all of the 7 cups of broth.

Note: Do not cover the rice while it is absorbing the chicken broth.

Add fresh herbs to the risotto. Top with freshly grated Parmesan cheese just before serving.

Turkey, Walnuts, and Blue Cheese Salad

Tami J. Cline, M.S., R.D., F.A.D.A., S.F.N.S.

Serves: 4 servings
Hands-on time: 15 minutes

Here's a salad that combines a lot of great tastes and textures. The dressing is "fire and nice" from Tabasco and honey. The salad greens team up with smoked turkey, fresh veggies, tangy blue cheese, and crunchy walnuts for a sensational main dish. Both walnuts and turkey are important agricultural commodities in my home state of California.

- 2 tablespoons extra-virgin olive oil
- 1 small onion, chopped
- 2 tablespoons red wine vinegar
- 2 tablespoons honey
- 1 to 2 teaspoons Tabasco sauce
- 8 cups assorted greens
- 8 ounces smoked turkey white meat, diced
- 1 large tomato or 2 small plum tomatoes, chopped
- ⅓ cup crumbled, reduced-fat blue cheese
- ½ cup frozen sweet corn, thawed and drained
- ¼ cup finely chopped walnuts, toasted

Combine the oil, onion, vinegar, honey, and Tabasco sauce in a blender and purée. (The dressing can be made ahead of time, but bring it to room temperature before serving.)

Combine the assorted greens in a large bowl. Toss with the dressing. Add the remaining ingredients, except for the walnuts. Toss gently, then top with the walnuts.

SUBSTITUTION

Substitute an equal amount of your favorite nut for the walnuts. Pecans, like walnuts, team up with the other ingredients to create a flavor explosion.

NUTRITION PER SERVING

Serving size	3 cups
Calories	290 kcal
Fat	17 g
Saturated fat	4 g
Cholesterol	35 mg
Sodium	740 mg
Carbohydrates	22 g
Dietary fiber	4 g
Protein	17 g

Fish Stock

Lori Martinez-Hassett, R.D.

Some recipes seem intimidating just by their name. Fish stock, though, is incredibly easy to make anywhere in the United States. Make a large batch and freeze it for later use in all your recipes that call for fish stock.

Serves: 4
Hands-on time: 20 minutes
Cooking time: 30 minutes

1 tablespoon olive oil
½ cup onions, chopped
1 stalk celery, thinly sliced
1 medium-size carrot, thinly sliced
peels from ½ pound shrimp
4 sprigs parsley, chopped
½ teaspoon salt
½ teaspoon pepper

Heat the olive oil in a large saucepan. Toss in the onions, celery, and carrot; sauté over medium heat until the onions are soft. Add 2 cups water and the shrimp peels, parsley, salt, and pepper. Simmer over medium heat until the liquid is reduced to approximately half, about 30 minutes. Strain the liquid, discarding the solids.

COOK'S TIP

If you don't have time to make fish stock now, make it later. Freeze the shells in a tightly sealed plastic container. Toss them in frozen and add the remaining ingredients. (Cook an additional 15 minutes if the shells are frozen.)

NUTRITION PER SERVING	
Serving size	1 cup
Calories	50 kcal
Fat	3.5 g
Saturated fat	0.5 g
Cholesterol	0 mg
Sodium	310 mg
Carbohydrates	4 g
Dietary fiber	1 g
Protein	1 g

Grilled Tuna with Warm Cherry Tomato Salsa

Sanna James Delmonico, M.S., R.D.

Serves: 4
Hands-on time: 20 minutes
Cooking time: 8 to 16 minutes

Fusing the freshness of Napa, the seafood of California, and the Tuscan way of spicing food resulted in this easy tuna recipe. If you can't find fresh tuna, use any firm fish, such as halibut or salmon.

4 small tuna steaks (about 4 to 6 ounces each, with bone)
1 tablespoon plus 2 teaspoons extra-virgin olive oil, divided
1 tablespoon lemon juice
vegetable oil cooking spray
½ teaspoon salt
¼ cup finely diced red onion (½ onion)
2 cloves garlic, minced
2 cups cherry or pear tomatoes, cut in halves
2 tablespoons chopped fresh flat-leaf parsley
1 tablespoon capers, optional
freshly ground black pepper, to taste

Rinse the fish and pat it dry with paper towels. Place it in a glass pie plate and drizzle with olive oil and lemon juice. Let the fish marinate in the refrigerator for at least 15 minutes and up to 4 hours.

Preheat grill. Place the tuna on a double-thick sheet of aluminum foil that has been sprayed with the cooking spray; place it on the grill. Grill the fish, turning it once, until it flakes and is not quite opaque in the center. This takes between 4 and 8 minutes per side, depending on the thickness of the fish.

Preheat oven to 400°F. Combine the remaining 2 teaspoons of olive oil, the chopped onion, and the garlic in a glass, oven-safe pie plate. Bake for 7 to 8 minutes, stirring halfway through. Mix the salt into the tomatoes; stir the tomatoes into the onion mixture and continue to roast for 4 or 5 minutes, until the tomatoes are warmed and the onion is starting to brown. Remove from the oven, stir in the chopped parsley and capers, if using. Spoon the mixture evenly over the grilled tuna steaks. Add the desired amount of black pepper.

COOK'S TIP

As an alternative cooking method, roast the tuna steaks for 10 to 15 minutes, depending on the thickness of the fish, in the oven at 400°F in a pan coated with vegetable oil cooking spray. Turn the tuna once for even cooking. Italian, or flat-leaf, parsley is more flavorful than curly parsley. Curly parsley is more commonly used as a garnish rather than to flavor food.

NUTRITION PER SERVING

Serving size	1 tuna steak plus ¼ cup sauce
Calories	230 kcal
Fat	8 g
Saturated fat	1 g
Cholesterol	64 mg
Sodium	355 mg
Carbohydrates	7 g
Dietary fiber	1 g
Protein	34 g

Shrimp with Lobster Sauce

Lisa Turner, R.D.

You're not alone if you think lobster is missing from the ingredient list of this recipe. There is no lobster in the lobster sauce! Asian kitchens, such as mine in California, commonly produce recipes with a name that doesn't match the ingredient list. Fermented black beans impart a characteristic flavor to this mouth-watering entrée. The black beans are actually soybeans that turn black during fermentation; they're available in the international section of many supermarkets or in Asian markets. They're quite salty, so use sparingly.

Serves: 4
Hands-on time: 20 minutes
Cooking time: 10 minutes

- 1 tablespoon cornstarch
- ¼ teaspoon salt
- 2 tablespoons rice wine or dry sherry
- 1 egg white
- 1 pound shelled and deveined shrimp
- 1 tablespoon minced fresh ginger
- 4 cloves garlic, minced
- 2 scallions, thinly sliced (reserve some for garnish)
- 2 tablespoons fermented black beans, rinsed and drained
- 1 large egg
- 1 tablespoon dark sesame oil
- ¼ pound lean ground pork
- 1 tablespoon rice wine or dry sherry
- 1 14-ounce can reduced-sodium chicken broth
- ½ teaspoon sugar
- 1 teaspoon cornstarch plus 1 tablespoon cold water
- 2 scallions, sliced thinly

Whisk together the cornstarch, salt, wine (or sherry), and egg white until smooth. Add the shrimp; toss to coat and marinate in the refrigerator for 15 minutes (or, alternatively, overnight).

Combine the ginger, garlic, scallions, and black beans in a small bowl; cover until ready to use.

Beat the egg in a small bowl; set aside.

Place the sesame oil in a wok or heavy pan and place over medium-high heat. Add the shrimp and stir-fry for 20 seconds (the shrimp will *not* be pink or done); remove the shrimp and set it aside. Add the ginger mixture and stir, but do not brown. Add the pork, breaking it into small pieces. Brown thoroughly. Add the shrimp and stir-fry for about 1 minute. Add the wine or sherry, chicken broth, and sugar. Drizzle the

SUBSTITUTION

If you have shellfish allergies, use artificial lobster or crabmeat, but read the label to make sure the product you choose is free of natural shellfish flavors.

COOK'S TIP

Spice it up by sprinkling in cayenne pepper to taste.

NUTRITION PER SERVING

Serving size	1½ cups
Calories	320 kcal
Fat	14 g
Saturated fat	4 g
Cholesterol	250 mg
Sodium	420 mg
Carbohydrates	10 g
Dietary fiber	0 g
Protein	34 g

Shrimp with Lobster Sauce *(continued)*

beaten egg slowly into the hot mixture, whisking constantly to prevent the egg from clumping. Dissolve the cornstarch in cold water; stir it into the shrimp mixture. Stir until the sauce is thickened; remove from heat.

Serve over hot rice. Garnish with the scallions.

Grilled Halibut with Gremolata

Sanna James Delmonico, M.S., R.D.

Gremolata is a mixture of chopped lemon zest, parsley, and garlic. In t[...] spirit of Californians' desire for freshness, gremolata gives a fresh touch to rich foods. Sprinkle it on grilled fish, chicken, and meat, as well as into stews, cooked rice, or risotto just before serving.

2 tablespoons extra-virgin olive oil
2 tablespoons lemon juice
½ teaspoon salt
1 teaspoon black pepper
2 pounds halibut steaks (purchase 4 pieces totaling 2 pounds)

GREMOLATA

zest of one lemon (remove only the yellow of the lemon skin with a vegetable peeler, zester, or grater)
½ cup chopped fresh Italian flat-leaf parsley leaves (no stems)
1 to 3 cloves garlic, finely chopped
pinch salt

Combine the oil, lemon juice, salt, and pepper in a 9-by-13-inch baking dish. Add the halibut; turn to coat the other side; cover and set aside. Marinate at room temperature for no more than 30 minutes. You can make the marinade ahead of time and marinate the fish for up to 4 hours in the refrigerator.

Preheat grill or broiler. Chop the lemon zest; combine it in a bowl with the parsley, garlic, and salt. Mix well and set aside.

Grill the fish, turning it once, until it flakes and is not quite opaque in the center. This takes between 4 and 8 minutes per side, depending on the thickness of the fish. Transfer the fish to a serving platter and spoon the gremolata evenly over the top.

S[...]
Inst[...]
tute s[...]
steaks.

FOOD TRIVIA
A pinch is about [...] teaspoon, a dash about 1/16 teaspoon, and a smidgen 1/32 teaspoon. Some specialty kitchen stores sell these tiny measuring spoons.

NUTRITION NUGGET
Control your calorie intake. Enjoy dessert on a night when you have a lighter entrée, such as this one.

NUTRITION PER SERVING	
Serving size	1 halibut steak and ¼ cup gremolata
Calories	320 kcal
Fat	12 g
Saturated fat	1.5 g
Cholesterol	75 mg
Sodium	490 mg
Carbohydrates	2 g
Dietary fiber	Less than 1 g
Protein	48 g

h, Chinese Style

lawaiian culinary ease creates this fabu-
ıp a fish and forget about it while you
e garnish: a sizzling black bean–cilantro
de which is better—the taste or the

Serves: 4
Hands-on time: 15 minutes
Cooking time: 8 to 16 minutes

e fish (deheaded)

sed, drained, and coarsely chopped

SUBSTITUTION
ead of halibut, substi-
lmon or tuna

...as
...gh smoke
point. That means that
it can be heated to
high temperatures
without burning.

... rim the green onion tops and slice ... onions. Reserve the remains. Cut enough heavy-... aluminum foil to wrap the fish lengthwise. Line the foil with the remaining stems of the green onions. Place the fish over the greens and along the center of the foil. Bring up the sides of the foil and fold over the fish to form a tent. Double-fold the edges for a tight seal and secure the ends. Place the wrapped fish on a large baking sheet.

Bake the fish until it is opaque and beginning to flake, about 40 to 50 minutes. Do not overcook. Remove the skin from the fish and then place the fish on a serving platter; keep warm.

Heat the peanut oil in a large skillet over high heat. Add the beans, soy sauce, onions, and cilantro. Stir and cook just until hot.

Sprinkle the hot salsa mixture over the fish at tableside for a beautiful presentation.

NUTRITION PER SERVING	
Serving size	5 ounces cooked fish plus ¼ cup bean sauce
Calories	360 kcal
Fat	97 g
Saturated fat	2 g
Cholesterol	129 mg
Sodium	563 mg
Carbohydrates	9 g
Dietary fiber	3 g
Protein	54 g

Monterey Bay Salmon Salad

Caroline Margolis, R.D.

This easy herb-crusted salmon, a few veggies, and a drizzle of honey-mustard dressing liven up an ordinary mixed green salad to make it the star of the meal.

Serves: 4
Hands-on time: 10 minutes
Cooking time: 10 to 12 minutes

Salad

- 8 cups or 1 10-ounce package mixed greens
- 2 cups cherry or grape tomatoes, halved (1 pint)
- 2 cups frozen whole kernel corn, thawed
- ½ cup low-fat or fat-free honey mustard dressing

Lightly toss the greens, tomatoes, corn, and dressing. Divide among 4 dinner plates.

Salmon

- vegetable oil cooking spray
- 1 tablespoon dried basil
- 2 teaspoons dried oregano
- 1 teaspoon lemon-flavored pepper
- ¼ teaspoon crushed red pepper
- 1 teaspoon garlic powder
- ½ teaspoon salt
- 1 tablespoon lemon juice
- 2 teaspoons extra-virgin olive oil
- 1 pound salmon fillet (add an extra 2 to 3 ounces if fillet has skin)
- 1 red onion, thinly sliced, separated into rings

Preheat oven to 450°F. Line a baking pan with foil and coat the foil with the cooking spray.

Combine the basil, oregano, lemon pepper, crushed red pepper, garlic powder, and salt. Add the lemon juice and oil; stir well. Place the salmon skin-side down on the prepared baking pan. Spread the herb mixture evenly over the fish.

Bake for 10 to 12 minutes; let cool slightly. Slice the salmon into thin strips and place on top of the salad. Garnish with the red onion slices.

SUBSTITUTION

Make this salad in a hurry using canned salmon. Dress it with oregano, lemon pepper, crushed red pepper, garlic powder, salt, lemon juice, and oil.

NUTRITION NUGGET

When you choose canned salmon, select one that still has the bones. Remove any skin you see, but leave the bones in (break them up a bit). Salmon bones boost calcium intake.

NUTRITION PER SERVING

Serving size	2 cups salad and 3 ounces cooked salmon
Calories	380 kcal
Fat	13 g
Saturated fat	2 g
Cholesterol	80 mg
Sodium	790 mg
Carbohydrates	34 g
Dietary fiber	7 g
Protein	35 g

Napa Valley Glazed Salmon

Mary Abbott Hess, L.H.D., M.S., R.D., F.A.D.A.

Serves: 4
Hands-on time: 10 minutes
Baking time: 20 minutes

Elegant and gourmet-delicious, this salmon recipe is ready in less than thirty minutes. I like to serve it with grilled leeks over white beans seasoned with vinegar, honey, and fresh thyme, or atop gently steamed baby spinach, both Napa Valley trendy.

2 tablespoons honey
1 teaspoon dried thyme
2 teaspoons Dijon mustard
1 teaspoon finely grated lemon zest
1 teaspoon white pepper
1¼ pounds salmon, cut into 4 pieces

Preheat oven to 350°F.

Combine the honey, thyme, mustard, lemon zest, and pepper in a small bowl. Arrange the salmon in a shallow roasting pan lined with cooking foil. Using the back of a spoon, spread the honey mixture to coat the top of each fillet.

Bake, uncovered, for 20 minutes, or until the salmon flakes with a fork.

VARIATION

Substitute your favorite dried or fresh herb for the thyme—or combine several.

COOK'S TIP

To store fresh fish a day or two after purchase, rinse and place in a bag with ice. Pour off melted ice and replace with more ice chunks.

SERVING SUGGESTION

Slice leftover salmon and place on top of a bed of mixed greens and chopped tomatoes for an easy lunch or dinner.

NUTRITION NUGGET

The white droplets accumulating on the top of salmon are rich in omega-3s. So is the gray-colored meat right next to the skin. Enjoy both to reap the most omega-3s.

NUTRITION PER SERVING

Serving size	3 ounces roasted salmon
Calories	270 kcal
Fat	11 g
Saturated fat	1.5 g
Cholesterol	90 mg
Sodium	135 mg
Carbohydrates	10 g
Dietary fiber	0 g
Protein	32 g

Spicy Indian Salmon

Madhu Gadia, M.S., R.D., C.D.E.

For spicy salmon with a flavorful twist, try it with a blend of Indian spices, which I continue to make in my Iowa home much as we did in India. Grill or bake for a quick dish. If desired, marinate the salmon overnight in the refrigerator.

Serves: 4
Hands-on time: 10 minutes
Marinating time: 20 minutes
Cooking time: 20 minutes

- vegetable oil cooking spray
- 1 pound salmon (without skin; add ⅓ pound if skin)
- 2 cloves garlic, minced
- 1 teaspoon finely grated fresh ginger
- ¼ teaspoon salt
- ¼ teaspoon turmeric
- ½ teaspoon ground cumin
- ½ teaspoon black pepper
- ½ teaspoon cayenne pepper, optional
- ½ teaspoon garam masala (recipe follows)
- 1 tablespoon fresh lime juice

Coat a baking dish with the cooking spray. Arrange salmon in the baking dish. Combine the garlic, ginger, and spices, and rub into the salmon. Prick the salmon with a fork a few times. Cover and marinate for 20 minutes at room temperature or up to 24 hours in the refrigerator.

Preheat oven to 400°F.

Bake the salmon, uncovered, for 15 to 20 minutes. Or grill the salmon, wrapped in foil with a tent for venting, for 10 to 15 minutes. The salmon is done when it easily flakes with a fork.

Sprinkle with the lime juice before serving.

Garam Masala

- ¼ cup cumin seeds
- 3 tablespoons whole black peppercorns
- 3 tablespoons whole cardamom pods
- 1 teaspoon cloves
- 2 teaspoons dry ginger powder
- 2 cinnamon sticks

Lightly dry-roast the cumin seeds in a skillet over medium heat. Roast until the seeds turn color, about 7 to 10 minutes. Cool to room temperature. Combine all the spices and grind to a fine powder in a coffee grinder or blender. Sift to eliminate any chunks. Store in an airtight container. Makes about ½ cup.

FOOD TRIVIA

Garam masala, a blend of several spices, is frequently used in Indian recipes. Buy it in markets or make your own.

NUTRITION PER SERVING	
Serving size	3 ounces cooked salmon
Calories	170 kcal
Fat	7 g
Saturated fat	1 g
Cholesterol	60 mg
Sodium	200 mg
Carbohydrates	1 g
Dietary fiber	0 g
Protein	23 g

Barbecued Tri Tip

Rita Storey Grandgenett, M.S., R.D.

Serves: 8
Hands-on time: 15 minutes
Standing time: 4 days
Cooking time: 45 minutes

My son-in-law, Chuck Edmunds, developed this fabulous recipe for barbecued beef. While he uses a tri-tip cut of beef, use any lean beef. Tri-tip comes from the hip section and is more commonly used in California than in the Midwest.

2 pounds tri-tip beef (angular cut from the hip)

MARINADE

1 12-ounce can beer (recommended: ale type)
¼ cup teriyaki sauce
1 tablespoon Worchestershire sauce
5 cloves garlic, minced
1 medium-size onion, minced
1 teaspoon black pepper
¼ teaspoon cayenne
¼ teaspoon chili powder
1 tablespoon dried parsley (or ¼ cup chopped fresh parsley)

Combine all the marinade ingredients in a container large enough to hold the meat. Immerse the meat in the marinade, cover, and refrigerate 4 days. (Be sure that the meat is fully covered with the marinade.) Turn the meat once per day.

Preheat grill to medium-low heat. (When it's hot, you should still be able to hold your hand over the flame for just a second.) Grill the meat slowly, marinating for the first 20 minutes. Discard the remaining marinade and continue to grill until the meat is cooked through—30 minutes to 60 minutes, depending on the thickness.

Slice or shred the meat and serve it on whole-grain buns with a side of teriyaki or barbecue sauce.

VARIATION

Instead of grilling the meat, prepare it in the oven. Marinate the beef as directed. Preheat oven to 350°F. Transfer the beef to a roasting pan; pour the marinade in the pan until it reaches one inch up the side of the pan. (Discard the remaining marinade.) Roast the meat for one hour, marinating occasionally.

COOK'S TIPS

Use two forks to shred the beef rather than slicing it with a knife. An alternative marinating technique is to place the marinade ingredients into a tightly sealed, heavy-duty plastic bag.

NUTRITION PER SERVING	
Serving size	¾ cup shredded beef with sauce
Calories	250 kcal
Fat	12 g
Saturated fat	5 g
Cholesterol	60 mg
Sodium	440 mg
Carbohydrates	6 g
Dietary fiber	1 g
Protein	25 g

Tangy Braised Beef with Beans and Peppers

Elsa Ramirez Brisson, M.P.H., R.D.

Inspired by Philippine spices and cooking, this delightfully different stir-fry can be spicy or mild; just dial up or down the chili powder and/or fish sauce as I do in my southern California home.

Serves: 6
Hands-on time: 20 to 25 minutes
Cooking time: 40 minutes

- 1 tablespoon vegetable oil
- 1 pound lean beef cut into chunks
- 1 small sweet onion, sliced
- 1 28-ounce can crushed tomatoes
- 2 tablespoons peeled, grated fresh ginger
- 1 clove garlic, finely chopped
- 1 teaspoon chili powder
- ½ teaspoon turmeric
- 1 pound green beans, diagonally trimmed, 1-inch lengths
- 1 medium-size green bell pepper, sliced
- 1 medium-size red bell pepper, sliced
- 2 tablespoons chopped cilantro
- 2 teaspoons fish sauce or soy sauce, if desired

Heat the oil in a large nonstick skillet or wok. Add the meat and onion. Cook, stirring often, until the meat is browned. Add the tomatoes, ginger, garlic, chili powder, and turmeric. Stir well. Cover, reduce heat, and simmer slowly for 15 minutes. Add the green beans, and the red and green bell peppers. Cover and simmer for another 10 minutes. Add the cilantro and, if desired, the fish sauce or soy sauce; simmer 5 minutes more, until the beans are tender-crisp.

FOOD TRIVIA
Fish sauce is one of the signature ingredients of Philippine cooking.

COOK'S TIP
Take a short cut—use 1 pound frozen cut green beans (thawed) instead of fresh.

NUTRITION PER SERVING

Serving size	1½ cups
Calories	220 kcal
Fat	9 g
Saturated fat	3 g
Cholesterol	40 mg
Sodium	400 mg
Carbohydrates	20 g
Dietary fiber	5 g
Protein	20 g

Hawaiian Pork and Peas

Stacy Haumea, R.D.

Serves: 6
Hands-on time: 10 minutes
Cooking time: 35 minutes

Pork and peas are a favorite combination in Hawaii, as is the unique blend of seasonings in this almost complete meal. Just cook some rice and your meal is done.

- 2 teaspoons canola oil
- 1 pound lean pork, cut into chunks
- 2 cloves garlic, chopped
- 2 tablespoons reduced-sodium soy sauce
- 1 14½-ounce can spicy stewed tomatoes
- 1 7-ounce jar roasted red peppers in brine, drained and chopped
- 1 4-ounce jar chopped pimientos with juice
- ⅛ teaspoon ground cinnamon (or 1 cinnamon stick)
- ⅛ teaspoon ground black pepper
- 1 bay leaf
- 1 10-ounce package frozen petite peas
- 3 cups cooked white or brown rice

Heat the oil in a large nonstick skillet. Sauté the pork and garlic for 10 minutes. Drizzle the soy sauce over the pork. Stir in the tomatoes, red peppers, pimientos, cinnamon (or cinnamon stick), black pepper, and bay leaf. Bring to a boil; reduce heat, cover, and simmer for another 20 minutes. Meanwhile, cook the rice as directed on the package. Add the peas to the pork mixture. Return to a simmer. Cover and simmer for 5 more minutes. Remove the bay leaf.

Serve the meat over rice.

COOK'S TIP

This dish may be made 1 to 2 days ahead of time and reheated; the longer the meat and vegetables marinate, the more intense the flavors.

NUTRITION PER SERVING

Serving size	¾ cup meat mixture plus ½ cup rice
Calories	300 kcal
Fat	7 g
Saturated fat	2 g
Cholesterol	45 mg
Sodium	500 mg
Carbohydrates	36 g
Dietary fiber	4 g
Protein	22 g

Maui Pineapple Pork Roast

Paula Williams, R.D., C.E.C.

Pork is the meat of choice in Hawaii. It is served at most celebrations, whether prepared underground in an "imu" or roasted on a spit over a keawe wood fire. For those of us who have returned to the mainland, we have to resort to the use of an oven.

Serves: 8
Hands-on time: 10 minutes
Cooking time: 1 hour, 10 minutes

- 2 pounds fat-trimmed, rolled pork roast
- vegetable oil cooking spray
- 1 8-ounce can crushed pineapple, juice-packed, undrained
- 1 medium-size sweet onion, chopped
- 2 cloves garlic, minced
- 2 tablespoons apple cider vinegar
- 3 tablespoons light soy sauce
- 1 teaspoon ground ginger (or 1 tablespoon fresh grated ginger)
- 1 tablespoon brown sugar
- 1 tablespoon cornstarch
- 2 medium-size green bell peppers, thinly sliced
- 1 20-ounce can pineapple rings (juice-packed), juice and rings separated

Preheat oven to 325°F. Place the pork roast in a roasting pan sprayed with the cooking spray. Mix the crushed pineapple, pineapple juice, onion, garlic, vinegar, soy sauce, ginger, and brown sugar. Spoon the mixture over the pork.

Bake, covered, about 40 minutes. Uncover, turn the roast, and bake uncovered for 20 to 30 more minutes, or until the internal temperature reaches 150°F, basting frequently with the pineapple mixture. Remove to a heated platter; keep warm.

Transfer the cooking juice to large skillet. Skim the fat. Heat to boiling.

Mix the cornstarch into 3 tablespoons cold water until smooth; stir into the pan juices. Whisk until the sauce thickens. Add the green pepper slices, cover, and steam for 5 minutes, just until they are crisp-tender but still brilliant green.

Arrange the pineapple rings around the roast; top the rings with the green pepper slices. Pour the sauce over all.

COOK'S TIP

If you are looking for some traditional Hawaiian accompaniments to this dish, try baked sweet potatoes, cut in 1-inch wheels; spinach cooked in coconut milk; steamed sticky rice; and a medley of tropical fruit for a refreshing dessert.

NUTRITION NUGGET

Because regular soy sauce is high in sodium, this recipe uses light soy sauce, which is a reduced-sodium variety.

NUTRITION PER SERVING	
Serving size	3 ounces cooked pork plus ½ cup vegetables/fruit/sauce
Calories	300 kcal
Fat	15 g
Saturated fat	5 g
Cholesterol	75 mg
Sodium	300 mg
Carbohydrates	19 g
Dietary fiber	2 g
Protein	24 g

Portabella Mushroom Wraps

Elizabeth Arvidson, R.D.

Serves: 4
Hands-on time: 15 minutes
Cooking time: 15 minutes
Standing time: 5 minutes

À la California style, this wrap is filled with layers of flavor that fuse together well. If you haven't tried quinoa, this is a great recipe to start with. Quinoa is an ancient grain from South America. It was a staple for the Incas.

- 1 tablespoon extra-virgin olive oil
- ⅓ cup soy sauce
- ⅓ cup Merlot or any red wine
- ⅓ cup balsamic vinegar
- 1 tablespoon garlic powder
- 1 teaspoon crushed red pepper
- 2 medium-size portabella mushrooms, sliced
- ½ cup uncooked quinoa
- 8 ounces reduced-fat cream cheese, room temperature
- 1 7-ounce jar sun-dried tomatoes, drained
- 4 10-inch whole-wheat tortillas (or other designer flavor, such as garlic-herb)
- 2 cups fresh baby spinach, washed and dried

Combine the oil and the soy sauce, wine, vinegar, garlic powder, and red pepper; add the portabella mushrooms. Cover and marinate overnight in the refrigerator.

Combine the marinated mushrooms and ½ cup water in a medium-heavy saucepan. Bring to a boil; add the quinoa; reduce heat, cover, and simmer 15 minutes. Remove from heat; stir, cover, and let stand 5 minutes.

Meanwhile, blend the cream cheese and tomatoes in a food processor on medium speed until smooth. (Alternatively, finely chop the tomatoes and stir them into the softened cream cheese.)

To prepare the wraps: spread the cream cheese mixture evenly over the tortillas. Top with ¼ cup of the cooked mushroom-quinoa mixture and ½ cup of the spinach leaves. Tuck in the upper and lower edges of the tortilla and roll it into a cylinder. Serve warm.

SUBSTITUTION

Substitute brown rice for the quinoa; increase the simmer time to 35 minutes.

VARIATION

Add drained, chopped artichoke hearts to the filling mixture.

NUTRITION PER SERVING

Serving size	1 wrap
Calories	420 kcal
Fat	13 g
Saturated fat	2 g
Cholesterol	5 mg
Sodium	1,360 mg
Carbohydrates	62 g
Dietary fiber	8 g
Protein	20 g

Sacramento Delta Pear Pizza

Paula Benedict, M.P.H., R.D.

The Sacramento Delta region produces a bounty crop of Bartlett pears, supplying much of America's canned pear needs. After attending the annual Pear Festival in the quiet little river town of Courtland near Sacramento last July, I came home with ten pounds of fresh pears and a real need to find new ways to eat them. I've always enjoyed the flavor trio of Gorgonzola cheese, walnuts, and fresh pears in spinach salads, and this pizza improves on those flavors by melting Gorgonzola and browning pears and walnuts atop a traditional pizza.

Serves: 6
Hands-on time: 15 minutes
Cooking time: 15 minutes

1 cup pizza or marinara sauce
1 pizza crust (10 to 12 ounces), ready-made
1¼ cups part-skim mozzarella cheese, coarsely grated
2 ripe pears, (preferably Bartlett)
⅓ cup Gorgonzola blue cheese, crumbled
⅓ cup walnut pieces

Preheat oven to 425°F. Spread the pizza sauce evenly over the pizza crust. Sprinkle with the mozzarella cheese. Wash, quarter, and core the pears. Slice each pear quarter lengthwise into three thin slices. Place the pear slices on top of the mozzarella, fanning the pears outward from the center of the crust and placing 3 to 4 slices in the center. Sprinkle the Gorgonzola cheese on top of the pear slices. Top with the walnut pieces.

Place the pizza on a baking sheet and bake for 12 to 15 minutes, or until the cheeses have melted and the walnut pieces are browned. Remove from the oven; cool slightly, and cut into 6 wedges. Serve warm.

SUBSTITUTION
Substitute ⅓ cup of goat or feta cheese for the Gorgonzola, or devise your own blend of cheeses.

NUTRITION PER SERVING	
Serving size	⅙ of pie
Calories	310 kcal
Fat	12 g
Saturated fat	4.5 g
Cholesterol	20 mg
Sodium	760 mg
Carbohydrates	37 g
Dietary fiber	3 g
Protein	14 g

Ham Sandwich with Grandma Baker's Homemade Mustard

Marilyn Baker Jouini, M.S., R.D., A.R.M.

Serves: 4 (with leftovers of mustard)
Hands-on time: 15 minutes

Easter in our California home would not be Easter in our family without this mustard on our ham. While my grandmother added "a lump of butter the size of an egg," the recipe is absolutely scrumptious with much less.

1 tablespoon flour
2 tablespoons sugar
2 tablespoons dry mustard
1 large egg
¾ cup cider vinegar
2 tablespoons butter
6 ounces deli-sliced lean ham
8 slices rye bread
1 large tomato, sliced thinly
2 to 3 leaves of lettuce

In a medium-heavy saucepan, whisk together the flour, sugar, dry mustard, and large egg until smooth. Stir in the vinegar. Cook over medium heat until the mixture is smooth and thick. The mixture should thicken near the boiling point. Remove from heat and stir in the butter. Serve hot or cold.

Build 4 sandwiches on rye bread.

SERVING SUGGESTIONS

Use this mustard on baked ham, broiled chicken or fish, or as a salad dressing.

COOK'S TIP

Store leftover mustard in a tightly sealed container up to 2 weeks.

NUTRITION PER SERVING

Serving size	1 tablespoon mustard + 2 slices rye + 1½ ounces ham + 2 tomato slices
Calories	380 kcal
Fat	15 g
Saturated fat	7 g
Cholesterol	100 mg
Sodium	770 mg
Carbohydrates	47 g
Dietary fiber	5 g
Protein	17 g

Fresh Strawberry Glacé Pie

Carol Mergen, M.S., R.D.

Across California and across the country, gardeners gather strawberries at their peak of perfection. And there is no better way to showcase nature's bounty than in a strawberry pie. If you don't have your own strawberry patch, check out a u-pick patch or a farmers' market for the most flavorful berries.

Serves: 8
Hands-on time: 25 minutes
Chill time: 2 hours

- 1 (9-inch) baked pie crust
- 5 cups whole strawberries, washed and hulled (reserve 1 cup for glaze)
- ⅔ cup sugar
- 3 tablespoons cornstarch
- 1 teaspoon lemon juice
- 1 cup nonfat whipped topping

Line the baked pie crust with select strawberries placed large end down. For the glaze, crush the remaining 1 cup of strawberries with a fork or in a food processor or blender. Combine the strawberries and sugar in a 2-quart saucepan. Slowly bring the mixture to a boil over medium heat; simmer 1 minute. Mix ¾ cup cold water and the cornstarch until smooth; gradually add to the hot strawberry mixture. Bring to a boil; reduce heat and cook, stirring constantly, until the mixture thickens. Boil and stir for 1 minute. Remove from heat. Stir in the lemon juice; cool slightly.

Spoon the glaze over berries. Gently shake the pan to evenly distribute the glaze. Refrigerate for 2 hours. Top each serving with whipped topping. Serve chilled.

COOK'S TIPS

You will need about 20 to 25 medium-size strawberries to place in the pan. Hull the strawberries (remove the green leaves and stem) just before using to keep them at their freshest.

NUTRITION PER SERVING	
Serving size	⅛ of pie
Calories	200 kcal
Fat	6 g
Saturated fat	1.5 g
Cholesterol	0 mg
Sodium	110 mg
Carbohydrates	36 g
Dietary fiber	2 g
Protein	1 g

Gingered Mango-Pineapple Crisp in a Crunchy Wonton

Roberta L. Duyff, M.S., R.D., F.A.D.A., C.F.C.S.

Serves: 12
Hands-on time: 15 minutes
Cooking time: 20 to 25 minutes

This Hawaiian-inspired dessert brings together many tropical and Asian ingredients that I've enjoyed on the islands: pineapple, mango, macadamia nuts, ginger, and wonton wrappers. Wonton wrappers make a quick, convenient pastry dough for this individually portioned, crisp dessert.

SHOPPING TIP

Look for crystallized ginger in the baking aisle of your supermarket. If it's not available, substitute grated fresh ginger or dried, chopped apricots for a flavor burst.

vegetable oil cooking spray
24 (3½-inch square) wonton wrappers
2 medium-size fresh, ripe mangoes
1 15-ounce can pineapple tidbits, drained
½ cup macadamia nuts, chopped and toasted
⅓ cup flour
¼ cup crystallized ginger, chopped
¼ cup sugar
¼ teaspoon salt
¼ cup (4 tablespoons) butter or margarine
edible flowers, for garnish (optional)

NUTRITION NUGGET

Although high in fat, macadamia nuts contain mostly monounsaturated fat, the heart-healthy type that tends to lower total and LDL ("bad") blood cholesterol levels. They're also a rich source of vitamin E, an antioxidant. Go easy, though; macadamia nuts have 200 calories per ounce.

Preheat oven to 375°F. Spray a 12-muffin tin with the cooking spray. Press 2 wonton wrappers into each cup in the muffin tin.

Peel and remove the seeds from the mangoes. Cut them into ½-inch pieces. Fill each wonton cup with mango and pineapple, to ¾ full.

Combine the nuts, flour, ginger, sugar, and salt in a mixing bowl. Add the butter or margarine to the nut-flour mixture; cut it into the dry ingredients using a pastry cutter (or use two knives, cutting through the mixture at cross angles) to make a coarse crumb. Top the fruit with the nut-flour-butter mixture.

Bake for about 25 minutes until golden brown, or just bubbling. Serve warm. Garnish with the edible flowers, if desired.

NUTRITION PER SERVING

Serving size	1 muffin
Calories	190 kcal
Fat	8 g
Saturated fat	3 g
Cholesterol	10 mg
Sodium	140 mg
Carbohydrates	29 g
Dietary fiber	2 g
Protein	3 g

FOOD TRIVIA

Macadamia nuts are native to the subtropical east coast Australian rainforest. The indigenous people there have eaten them for thousands of years. In the early 1900s they were taken to Hawaii where they were developed for commercial production.

PART 2

Eating Healthy for Life

10

NUTRITION BASICS

The Reasons for Our Luscious Food

Kristine Napier, M.P.H., R.D.

After strolling through pages of luscious recipes—and enjoying many of them—we hope you arrived at our critical message: food created with your health in mind tastes fabulous.

We've purposefully presented *first* a diversity of gourmet-tasting (but oh-so-easy-to-prepare) recipes to entice you to learn what we dietitians usually teach first. Instead of weighing you down with facts and numbers, we wanted you to taste the rich goodness of food that nourishes your body well. In this section, we'll use the recipes to impart nutrition basics in a more general sense so that you can feed yourself and your family well at each meal, every day.

Food: Always the First Choice

In teaching you about nutrition through the enjoyment of food and cooking, we emphasize a critical point: the best nutrition is found wrapped in Mother Nature's intricate packages—*food*—not in nutrient-supplement tablets. We think that Mother Nature does nutrition better, for many reasons:

- Even with the most advanced nutritional science, we have not yet determined what, in addition to nutrients, Mother Nature provides in that complex package we call food. For example, we are just beginning to realize the potential importance of phytochemicals in food. (Phytochemicals are the nonnutrient substances in foods thought to help fight chronic disease, including cancer and heart disease.) No doubt there are other substances in food that are critical to health that scientists have yet to discover. Eating a wide variety of foods, especially fruits, vegetables, and whole grains, ensures not only that we get essential nutrients but also these nonnutrient substances. (Find more about boosting phytochemical intake later in this chapter.)
- Real foods interacting with one another do the most good in making our bodies strong and disease resistant. In fact, studies regarding specific nutrients and their ability to prevent cancer, for example, have been strikingly disappointing. On the other hand, thousands of studies corroborate one consistent result: people who eat lots of fruits, vegetables, whole-grain foods, and legumes are much less likely to suffer from cancer, heart disease, and high blood pressure.

All Foods Fit—Portion Size Makes It Happen

You may have pondered the recipe for Chocolate-Mandarin Ganache Layered Cake (page 316) or Triple Chocolate Cake (page 415), wondering, "Why in the world would a dietitian develop recipes—for my good health—for chocolate cake and other decadent desserts?" There are three reasons for including such a wide variety of foods in this cookbook:

- People who eat varied diets—that is, many different types of foods—are the healthiest. Our recipes bring you dietary diversity—and that means enjoying delicious desserts.
- It is normal and healthy to take pleasure in good-tasting food, every day. Food is meant to be a celebration of life—after all, food *is* life sustaining. We cannot work hard enough to dispel "old-fashioned dietitian adages" such as "good-for-you food has to taste bad."
- Desserts (as well as beef and foods created with a touch of butter or sour cream), when balanced with other nutrient-dense foods and an active lifestyle, can add interest and enjoyment to your daily life without compromising good health.

Although we believe in eating a wide variety of food, we also feel very strongly that appropriate portioning of all food is a golden rule of good health. Just as measuring carefully the ingredients for the Sweet Potato Scones in this book is key to baking up a delightful breakfast treat, serving a suitable portion of Triple Chocolate Cake or Roasted Beef Tenderloin is key to achieving health goals.

Dietary Diversity and Your Health Goals

Dietary diversity, or eating a wide variety of foods, is also called the "whole-diet approach." Researchers reported in the prestigious *Journal of the American Medical Association* about their fifteen-year study of more than forty-two thousand women (average age sixty-one) and how dietary diversity affected their health. In this study:

- From a list of sixty-two foods, participants circled those foods eaten in the past year.
- For each woman, researchers selected twenty-three of the sixty-two foods that met dietary guidelines, and then counted how many of these twenty-three foods each woman ate at least once each week.
- Using these numbers, researchers calculated a "food diversity" score—the higher the number, the more different types of foods eaten each week.

Researchers found a very strong affect of dietary diversity on overall health. Women with the highest food diversity scores had 30 percent lower risk of dying of any cause than those with the lowest scores; specifically, those with highest scores were:

- 40 percent less likely to die of cancer
- 33 percent less likely to die of heart disease
- 42 percent less likely to die of stroke

Take note of the critical message from this study: *eating a diverse diet that meets dietary guidelines can improve health and longevity*. This is, indeed, an important message, especially when juxtaposed to how Americans are eating. The National Health and Nutrition Examination Survey, an ongoing study of American's eating habits, reveals disconcerting details about American dietary diversity:

- One-quarter (25 percent) of Americans eat foods from three or even fewer food groups.
- A paltry one-third (33 percent) of Americans eat foods from all five food groups.

- Fruit is the most common food group missing from American diets—nearly half (46 percent) of Americans do not eat fruit.
- On average, women eat 1.9 servings of vegetables daily, and men eat 2.5. Note that these figures include french fries as a vegetable, so the true number of vegetable servings is lower than these figures.

An Adventure in Achieving Dietary Diversity

You're about to embark on a delightful adventure in food shopping and eating, one that helps you expand the types and varieties of food you eat and increases your body's ability to ward off disease. We're sensitive to family preferences as well as the time it takes to prepare different foods, which is why we offer an array of strategies for including lots of fabulously assorted foods.

Here is the easiest way to achieve dietary diversity: eat ten to fifteen different foods every day. While that may not seem like a lot, note that most Americans eat the same four to seven foods every day. To diversify your dietary selections:

- Choose at least three different vegetables daily, and try to select three different colors (e.g., green peas, creamy cauliflower, red bell peppers).
- Enjoy at least three different fruits, going after three distinct colors (an orange tangerine, purple grapes, a green apple).
- Diversify starches, including three different whole grains daily (hearty whole-grain bread for lunch, an oatmeal cookie as a snack, and barley pilaf for dinner). How about including whole wheat pasta, brown rice, bulgur, barley, rye, quinoa, and amaranth on other days?
- Try three different protein foods each day—peanut butter (on toast for breakfast), lentils (in soup for lunch), and grilled beef tenderloin for dinner. Then there are tofu, chicken, pork, black beans, lamb, and game to include on other days.
- Pour, spoon, or slice into dairy—nonfat milk, low-fat yogurt, and cheese—to round out your day.

What's in Food?

To keep it simple, think of food as containing three essential elements:

- Macronutrients: carbohydrates, protein, fat, and water
- Micronutrients: vitamins and minerals
- Nonnutritive substances: phytochemicals and fiber

Fueling Up on Macronutrients

Asleep or awake, the body demands fuel—alias, calories—every single microsecond, to walk, talk, sleep, breathe, and make the chemicals that keep bodies functioning optimally. We get calories from three substances in food: carbohydrates, protein, and fat. There is a fourth, alcohol, but we don't consider that a macronutrient needed for good health.

While we often think of fruit as carbohydrate or meat as protein, it is rare for calories in food to come from just one macronutrient. While we don't want to bog you down with unnecessary numbers, here are a few examples of where calories come from in certain common foods:

- Skim milk: about six parts carbohydrate calories, three parts protein calories and one part fat calories
- Oatmeal: about seven parts carbohydrate calories, two parts protein calories and one part fat calories
- Walnuts: less than one part carbohydrate calories, slightly more than one part protein calories and eight parts fat calories
- Salmon: no carbohydrate calories, a little over half protein calories, a little under half fat calories

More about Carbohydrates

When it comes to nutrition, one day we hear that we should eat carbs and no fat. The next day we hear that we must avoid all carbs and eat a high-protein diet. Yet another day we hear that we should eat only low-glycemic carbs. Sadly, if you are trying to avoid carbohydrate-containing foods because of some recent fad, you will miss out on nature's bounty of fruits, vegetables, legumes, and whole-grain foods.

You might also hear the word "sugar" or "starch" when people speak of carbohydrates. Sugar, or glucose, is the simplest building block of the carbohydrates. Carbohydrate foods are made from just one or as many as thousands of glucose-building blocks hooked together. Starch foods (although a term now out of vogue) have thousands of glucose units joined together.

Food Sources of Carbohydrates

Remember, we're keeping this simple, so let's cut right to the chase: listed below are five groups of food that are excellent sources of carbohydrate. For optimal health and disease prevention we recommend eating some of each of these foods every day. Each food is listed with its nutrient bonuses:

- Fruits. Rich in fiber, vitamin A, vitamin C, folate, potassium, and sometimes vitamin E.

- Vegetables. In addition to the nutrients and fiber in fruit, vegetables have a wider variety of minerals than fruit and also contain some protein.
- Legumes, such as black beans, lentils, and kidney beans. Excellent source of protein, fiber, folate, potassium, iron, and several minerals.
- Whole grains and whole-grain foods, such as bread, oatmeal, rice, barley, and whole-grain bread and pasta. Very rich in minerals, rich in fiber, protein, and B vitamins.
- Dairy foods, with an emphasis on low-fat and fat-free varieties, such as skim milk, nonfat yogurt, and low-fat yogurt. Excellent sources of protein, calcium, phosphorus, and sometimes vitamin D. In many cases, reduced-fat varieties have more calcium than the regular fat versions.

You can tell by the nutrient bonuses we listed with each type of carbohydrate that having more of one—say, whole grains—cannot substitute for skipping another (such as vegetables). Remember, diversity is key to achieving health goals.

Empty-Calorie Carbohydrates

There is a sixth group of carbohydrates (in our keep-it-simple scheme): empty-calorie carbohydrates. These foods are void, or empty, of nutrients—although many have lots of calories. This category causes most of the confusion about eating carbohydrate-containing foods; as a result, many people shun the five types of nutrient-rich carbohydrate groups listed previously. Put another way, empty-calorie carbohydrates give even good carbohydrate-containing foods a bad reputation. Some examples of empty-calorie carbohydrates include:

- Soda pop. 12-ounce can: 141 calories, with no nutrients
- Snack items, such as cookies and chips. Twenty-five cheese-flavored, tiny crackers: 64 calories, 37 percent of which are fat calories, 10 percent of which are artery-clogging saturated fat, 88 grams of cholesterol (while not the maximum for the day, a lot for 64 calories), and some thiamin (in the fortified white flour used to make them)

Are we telling you that these foods should never touch your lips? No. But eating too many empty-calorie foods does the following:

- It fills you up on calorically dense foods that contribute a large amount of calories in a small amount of food (e.g., soda pop).
- It offers little appetite-holding power, because these foods generally have neither fiber nor protein, they do not keep the appetite at bay. As a result, you end up hungry soon after eating or drinking them.

- It contributes nothing to your nutritional profile except calories. This means you have fewer calories left for foods that supply the nutrients your body needs for good health.

More about Protein

Like carbohydrates, protein is a macronutrient or calorie-supplying nutrient. Unlike carbohydrates, protein has an even more important job than just supplying calories to the body. Let's take a look at the vital roles protein plays in our health:

- Protein is the most important nutrient-supporting growth and tissue repair substance at work in every cell of the body.
- Protein-rich substances drive the body's never-ending chemical reactions that make us breathe, keep our heart beating, and simulate every other action vital to life.
- Without protein, our hormones, antibodies (essential to fighting infections), and genes (the body's code for making any tissue or cell) could not function.
- Protein substances also maintain the most optimal chemical mix in the blood for awesome health.

It is no wonder, then, that the term protein comes from the Greek *proteios*, which means "holding first place."

Protein is constructed of building blocks called amino acids, of which there are two categories: essential and nonessential. These categories have nothing to do with whether they are important in the functioning of the human body. Rather, they distinguish between amino acids the body can make on its own from those it cannot. Of the twenty-two amino acids needed by the human body, nine are dietary *essentials*, or must be eaten in foods. The remaining thirteen are *nonessential* dietary components because the body can make them from scraps of leftover carbohydrates, fats, and other amino acids. If you lack a single essential amino acid for any period of time—no matter what quantity of other amino acids you eat—your body will break down your own muscle tissue to harvest that essential amino acid it needs.

Foods of animal origin (e.g., meats, fish, milk, cheese, and yogurt) contain all the essential amino acids, which is why we call them complete proteins. Nearly all plant foods—except soybeans and foods made from them—are missing at least one of the essential amino acids and are hence incomplete proteins. But they are still great sources of protein when paired with other proteins, both complete and incomplete, the problem is solved. We call this "complementing" proteins, and you can solve the problem of incomplete proteins by pairing up the following foods:

QUICK RULE: GRAIN FOODS + LEGUMES GENERALLY = COMPLETE PROTEIN

- Lentils and corn (such as lentil soup and corn bread)
- Rice and kidney beans
- Tofu (or other forms of soy) and rice
- Peanut butter and whole wheat bread
- Corn tortilla and pinto beans
- Meatless chili with beans and whole wheat bread
- Navy beans and rye bread
- Rice cakes and peanut butter
- Chick-peas and corn bread
- Black-eyed peas and corn bread

The good news is that you only have to have a complement of incomplete proteins over the course of a day, rather than in the same meal. This makes it much easier to sometimes make vegetable-protein meals. For many years, nutrition experts thought that incomplete proteins had to be complemented within the same meal to ensure their use as protein instead of as fuel. That's what happens to scraps of essential amino acids: they get sent to the junk heap to be recycled as fuel, and not even the best type of fuel for the human body (see the following section). Now we know that having a very small quantity of a complete protein food during the course of the day—say, a bit of cheese or a glass of milk—also ensures that the protein in the incomplete protein food will hook up with the other essential amino acids in the bloodstream they need to make a complete protein.

What Do Plant Proteins Have to Do with Me, a Meat Lover?

We know you are not alone if you are wondering why we're telling you about plant sources of protein—alias, vegetarian eating. No matter how we try to sugarcoat it, to many, meatless eating is still vegetarian eating. You may be thinking that vegetarian main courses will never touch your lips. At least start thinking about including some meals that do not include meat, poultry, or fish at least once or twice each week for dinner. Including more plant sources of protein can have the following huge payoffs to your health:

- They reduce the risk of artery-clogging heart disease (atherosclerosis).
- They reduce total fat and calorie intake.

- They increase fiber, mineral, and phytochemical intake.
- They increase antioxidant intake.
- If nothing else, they reduce the amount you spend on food.

Eating more plant sources of protein is a great way to eat for far less money. Don't worry: the recipes in this book will get you started on fabulous meals that just don't happen to contain any meat.

Why Protein Isn't the Body's Primary Energy Source

We use an analogy to make this important point. Many people heat their homes with natural gas. While there are some by-products in the process of burning natural gas, they are relatively few, especially compared to the seemingly outrageous alternative of producing heat by burning your grandmother's varnished mahogany dining room table. Yes, burning the table would produce heat, but at great cost—not only the financial loss of a family antique but also the not-so-pleasant by-products released when the stain and the varnish burn.

As outrageous as this example seems, it is somewhat akin to relying on protein as your main source of calories, by going on a high-protein diet. The unwanted by-products of burning protein for energy, ketones among them, must pass through the kidneys for excretion through the urine. While many people can handle the process of getting rid of all of these unwanted by-products, others cannot. In addition, by relying exclusively on protein-rich foods like meat, poultry, or eggs as your main source of calories, you can get more fat and cholesterol than your body needs. Just as seriously, you are missing out on nutrients, fiber, and phytochemicals.

Many people ask if eating more protein can help them build more muscle or lean body tissue. There is no evidence to indicate that you can increase muscle mass, or bulk up, by eating more protein. In fact, exercise experts have shown in repeated studies that people who work out may need *less* protein than those who do not, because exercising regularly helps the body retain nitrogen, one of the building blocks of protein. The best—and only—way to build more muscle tissue is to use your muscles. Yes, that tired old adage "use it or lose it" is still true. Use your muscle tissue every single day, as much as you can, and you will not only retain it but also build more.

Diversifying Protein—It Really Does Matter

Just as diversifying carbohydrates help you obtain a wider variety of essential nutrients and fiber, so does mixing up protein foods. In addition, eating a wide variety of protein throughout the day can help significantly in reducing intake of dietary cholesterol and saturated fat. Getting some protein from plant foods also increases the intake of fiber and phytochemicals—neither of which you can get from animal protein sources. Try these easy ways to diversify protein at each meal during the day:

Breakfast protein. Choose from the following sources of protein at breakfast:

- Eggs
- Egg whites
- Liquid egg substitute
- Tofu (you'll find some great recipes for smoothies and tofu scrambles)
- Skim milk or reduced-fat, fortified soy milk
- Nonfat or reduced-fat cottage cheese
- Bacon or sausage (on occasion, and in appropriate portion sizes)
- Bacon or sausage made from soy products
- Cheese, soy cheese, reduced-fat cheese

Lunch protein. A long-term goal should be to enjoy a vegetable source of protein at nearly every lunch, such as a black bean salad, lentil soup, or a garbanzo bean pocket. For most people, this is a new way of eating, so start with:

- A vegetable protein one day each week
- Another new recipe from our book that uses vegetable protein until you have achieved five, six, or seven days of this type of eating.
- On one or two days of the week, enjoy a leftover meat loaf or a grilled cheese sandwich, or a favorite lunch meat.

Dinner protein. Think of your dinner protein in seven-day cycles. In each cycle, try to plan:

- At least two fish meals; more is better. Canned fish is okay; see chapter 16 for more information.
- At least one vegetable source of protein; more is better.
- For the other four days, choose either:

  Two poultry meals and two red-meat meals (red meat is beef, pork, veal, lamb, and red game meat). Of course, you don't have to have these meals; it's perfectly okay—and even better—to substitute more fish or more vegetable sources of protein.

  Three poultry meals and one red-meat meal.

Take a look at the following monthly protein plan, using recipes from our book as one way to diversify dinner protein:

Monday	Tuesday	Wednesday	Thursday	Friday	Saturday	Sunday
Korean-Style Chicken with Green Beans	Twenty-Minute Stove-Top Goulash (beef)	Garden Fresh Tomato-Basil Pasta	Anna's Salmon Patties	Easy Chicken Wraps	Grilled Herbed Pork Chops	Bristol Bay Halibut
Minnesota Chicken and Wild Rice Casserole	All-American Chili (beef, pork, or vegetarian)	Inside-Out "Fried" Chicken	Pacific Northwest Tuna Salad	Confetti Sloppy Joes	Dijon Honey-Glazed Roasted Salmon	Sam's Greek-Roasted Chicken
West Texas Chipotle Chicken Salad	Oven-Roasted Peppers and Parmesan Pasta	Cajun Style Lemon Chicken Breasts	Citrus-Roasted Salmon	Philly Cheesesteak Packets (beef)	Paul Bunyan Wild Rice Soup (pork)	Pan-Seared Grouper with Warm Tomato Jam
No-Nonsense Clam Chowder	Grandma's Famous Mexican Casserole (beef)	Asian Chicken Salad	Turkey Pot Pie	The Best Meat Loaf We Could Find	Tuna Rotini Casserole	Maui Pineapple Pork Roast

It is the rare American who consumes too little protein. One of the main reasons for this overconsumption of protein is that our protein portions are too large. In the best of all worlds we would use a food scale and weigh our protein portions, but this isn't always possible. Here are some visuals, along with appropriate portion sizes:

- Meat, poultry, and fish: 3 ounces. To get an idea of portion size, visualize:

  The size of a deck of playing cards in height, width, and thickness.

  A 1-pound package of lean ground sirloin. A package this size should serve four people.

  Two chicken thighs. This would be an optimal portion size (sans skin).

  Three index fingers. The average index finger is one ounce.

- Legumes and dried beans, such as black beans and lentils: 1 cup cooked. To get an idea of portion size, visualize:

  The size of a baseball.

  The portion must fit into an average woman's hand.

- Tofu: 6 ounces. Tofu comes water-packed or in a shelf-stable brick (such as in a cardboard box). To get an idea of portion size, visualize:

  Half of a container.

  A tennis ball.
- Cheese: 1 ounce or ¼ cup, if shredded. To get an idea of portion size, visualize:

  Four dice (if the cheese is not shredded).

  One slice of presliced cheese.

  One-fourth of a tennis ball.

More about Fat

As with carbohydrates and protein, when it comes to fat, portion control remains a golden rule of good health. Instead of diversifying your fat intake, as was discussed for carbohydrates and proteins, our goal here is helping you choose better fats.

Without fat, the body's millions of cells cannot form properly, as fat is an essential ingredient in every cell. Nor can cells control the traffic of nutrients, hormones, and chemicals essential for life (yes, fat-containing substances stand guard at the entry and exit of many cells). Hormones couldn't form or function without fat, nor could the body absorb certain nutrients and phytochemicals.

You're not alone if you're asking, "If I need fat in every cell in my body, then why is fat in my food such a problem?" We summarize Americans' dietary fat concerns as follows:

- Fat calories sneak up on many of us, hidden in fast food and prepackaged items, as well as in food labels that go unread.
- Portion sizes of fats and fat-containing foods are often too large and not measured (including cooking fat portion sizes).
- Foods you wouldn't suspect contain significant amounts of fat in fact do.
- We don't replace high-fat foods with low-fat foods on a lifelong basis.
- We often think cholesterol-free foods are fat-free foods—a dangerous misconception.
- Choosing better fats is much too confusing.

We'll suggest solutions to these problems, but first, a quick guide to understanding the different types of dietary fat.

Dietary Fat and Cholesterol Facts

Dietary fats are made of building blocks called triglycerides. In turn, each triglyceride is constructed of one glycerol molecule connected to three fatty acids. The fatty-acid portion is the key ingredient: it distinguishes one type of triglyceride or dietary fat from the other, both in terms of flavor and the fat's effect within the human body. There are three main types of naturally occurring fatty acids (trans fatty acids are another group, but they are made in the food manufacturing industry):

1. Saturated
2. Monounsaturated
3. Polyunsaturated

Trans fatty acids also occur naturally, but the overwhelming majority is made during food manufacturing.

Every food that naturally contains fat has all three types of fatty acids, but one type predominates. For example:

- Olive oil

  Mono: 77 percent

  Poly: 9 percent

  Saturated: 14 percent
- Canola oil

  Mono: 59 percent

  Poly: 30 percent

  Saturated: 7 percent
- Peanuts

  Mono: 36 percent

  Poly: 23 percent

  Saturated: 10 percent
- Walnuts

  Mono: 14 percent

  Poly: 56 percent

  Saturated: 7 percent
- Almonds (sliced)

  Mono: 47 percent

  Poly: 18 percent

  Saturated: 6 percent
- Butter

  Mono: 29 percent

  Poly: 4 percent

  Saturated: 62 percent

Fats that are predominantly poly- and monounsaturated fatty acids are liquid at room temperature. Fats with mostly saturated fatty acids are solid. Picture a bottle of liquid olive oil (predominately monos) versus a stick of butter (mostly saturated fats) at room temperature.

Fats from plant foods, such as vegetable oils, are almost entirely poly and mono (the two exceptions are coconut and palm, which are predominantly saturated fat). Animal fats—those in dairy foods, beef, pork, and chicken—are predominantly saturated.

Cholesterol Is Not a Dietary Fat

Cholesterol does not have calories, either. Rather than being a fat, cholesterol is a waxy substance found in every cell of the human body, as well as the cells of every animal. The most important facts about cholesterol include:

- The majority of cholesterol in the human body does not come from the food we eat—it is made right inside the liver.
- Only foods that come from animals (e.g., meat, poultry, fish, dairy products, and eggs) can have cholesterol; even plant foods that are all fat—such as olive oil and canola oil—cannot have cholesterol.
- Cholesterol in the food we eat does not automatically become cholesterol in the bloodstream; rather, dietary cholesterol is just one factor that determines blood cholesterol levels (see sidebar about types of cholesterol in the blood).
- Cholesterol is important to good health; however, trouble brews when blood cholesterol levels rise too high.

Trans Fats: A Man-Made Dietary Fat

Trans fatty acids, also known as trans fats, are found naturally in small quantities in some foods, including beef, pork, lamb, butter, and milk. But most trans fatty acids in the diet come from hydrogenated foods. Oils are hydrogenated to give food a more desirable taste quality, or to make foods last longer. Hydrogenation enables some types of peanut butter to have a creamier consistency and is used to make stick margarine from vegetable oil. To create a visual, picture first a bottle of canola oil (which is liquid at room temperature), and then a stick of canola-oil margarine (which is solid at room temperature). Hydrogenation converts the first (the liquid) to the second (the solid).

But margarine is not the most significant source of trans fatty acids. Convenience foods, such as packaged cakes, cookies, and snack foods, as well as fast foods all contain significant amounts of trans fatty acids.

Although they are created from heart-friendlier vegetable oils, trans fatty acids undergo more than a physical transformation when they are hydrogenated; the way they affect the body also changes dramatically. Once hydrogenated or partially hydrogenated, these fats act more like detrimental saturated fats and may even be worse. Trans fatty acids:

- Increase total blood cholesterol levels
- Increase low-density lipoprotein (LDL) cholesterol levels
- Decrease high-density lipoprotein (HDL) cholesterol

You can reduce your intake of trans fatty acids by:

- Choosing crackers, cookies, and other convenience products carefully by reading labels. Just because a product says "no saturated fat" or "no cholesterol," it may still contain trans fats. Check the ingredients label; if you see an ingredient beginning with "partially hydrogenated" or "hydrogenated" you'll know it contains trans fatty acids.
- Using liquid oils instead of solid shortenings and margarines as much as possible. If you use margarine, choose one that claims to be "trans fat free."
- Reducing the frequency of eating fast food. If you do choose a fast-food burger or other sandwich, add a salad on the side (with low-fat dressing).

Fat, Cholesterol, and the Heart

Saturated fat is the heart's greatest food enemy. It is the most significant dietary culprit in raising blood cholesterol levels, especially LDL cholesterol, the type of cholesterol that builds up on arterial walls and narrows them. For every 1 percent increase in dietary saturated fat intake, serum cholesterol increases 2.4 mg/dl.

Overall, saturated fats contribute about 11 to 12 percent of calories to the American diet. Because of their potent hypercholesterolemic nature, the American Heart Association recommends limiting them to 8 to 10 percent of total calories, and to less than 7 percent of calories in people who have high cholesterol levels or have atherosclerotic heart disease.

One of the ways saturated fat is thought to raise LDL cholesterol levels is by impairing the liver's cholesterol-removal machinery. LDL receptors stand ready as if they were large grappling hooks on the ends of liver cells, ready to snag LDL cholesterol as it flows by. The LDL particles are then packaged for removal from the body via the intestinal tract.

CHOLESTEROL IN THE BLOOD

There are several types of cholesterol in the bloodstream. According to the National Cholesterol Education Project at the National Heart, Lung, and Blood Institute, three types are key to predicting a person's risk of heart disease (there are several other types, but they aren't as key in predicting heart disease risk):

- Total cholesterol: the sum of all types of cholesterol in the blood

  <200 = desirable

  200–239 = borderline high

  ≥ 240 = high

- LDL cholesterol, or bad cholesterol, because it increases heart disease risk. Lower levels are better:

  <100 = optimal

  100–129 = near optimal/above optimal

  130–159 = borderline high

  160–189 = high

  ≥ 190 = very high

- HDL cholesterol, or good cholesterol, because it reduces heart disease risk. Higher levels are better:

  <40 = low

  ≥ 60 = high

OTHER LIFESTYLE CHOICES THAT CAN REDUCE HEART DISEASE RISK

In addition to making smart food choices consistently, you can reduce heart disease risk by:

- Stepping up activity. Walk, cycle, dance, garden, put laundry away, clean the house—try to clock sixty minutes of active time daily.
- Achieving and maintaining a recommended body weight.
- Not smoking—not even a little bit.
- Enjoying a stress-free time—even just five minutes—every single day.

Saturated fat, however, prevents these grappling hooks from working properly. In a simplistic sense, saturated fat gums up the works by reducing the number of LDL receptors and impairing their efficiency. This is one big reason saturated fat is such a major culprit in keeping LDL cholesterol, or bad cholesterol, too high.

As substitutes for saturated fat, polyunsaturated and monounsaturated fats can help reduce heart disease risk. One type of polyunsaturated fat, omega-3, may also reduce this risk. It is found in some types of fish: salmon, tuna, halibut, anchovies, and sardines, for example. Choosing omega-3 foods is definitely a way to get better fats.

Solutions for Using Fat Wisely

We don't expect you to get out the calculator every day to find nutrition solutions for you and your family. To simplify matters, let's take a look at the common American dietary fat woes with an eye toward everyday solutions.

Why do fat calories sneak up on us? Fat is much more calorically dense than the other macronutrients (protein and carbohydrates). While each gram of protein and carbohydrate has four calories, one gram of fat has nine calories—making fat two-and-one-quarter times more calorically dense. This explains why a small piece of chocolate or cheesecake racks up hundreds of calories, but a large bowl of salad has significantly less. Use your knowledge about density in choosing fats wisely and portioning them carefully.

How do we measure healthier added fat portion sizes, fat for cooking, and foods containing fat?

- Learn portion sizes for added fats such as margarine, butter, salad dressing, and mayonnaise (see the table later in this chapter).
- Use measuring teaspoons and tablespoons when adding margarine, butter, and oil to cooking pans and pots.
- Make your portioning tools readily available. Place a pretty coffee mug or small flowerpot on your kitchen counter with two or three

sets of measuring spoons so you'll never look for your only set in the sink or dishwasher.

- Order salad dressings and other added fats on the side when eating out and add sparingly.
- Learn and use low-fat cooking methods regularly (see our suggestions later in this chapter).
- Portion foods with fat, especially meats, cheeses, and desserts.

Unsuspecting foods contain significant amounts of fat. Did you know, for example, that restaurant hamburgers often contain butter, margarine, or oil on the bun? (No wonder we like them so much.) Broiled fish in some restaurants—probably many—often contains oil or butter on the top (yes, that's why it's so moist); even broiled steaks are topped with melted butter. Crackers, snack bars, cereals, and boxed rice and pasta dishes can contain significant amounts of fat. Some whole-grain cereals have up to 5 grams of fat per serving; crackers can have double that amount, and packaged rice and pasta dishes can contain 15 to 20 grams per serving.

- Take control of food you order when eating out. Make a point of asking for a bun without butter or oil; ditto for fish, steak, and pasta.
- Read labels carefully.
- Choose cereals, crackers, and snack bars with less than 5 grams of fat per serving.
- Choose packaged rice and pasta dishes with 7 grams of fat per serving or less; check for instructions on how to prepare the dishes with less added fat.
- Diversify protein sources.

We don't always think about finding replacements for some high-fat foods on a lifelong basis. Tell yourself that today is tomorrow and start today with the following solutions:

- Dial down the fat in your milk one notch today, and another notch in two weeks. Do you drink whole milk? Switch to 2 percent today, 1 percent in two weeks, ½ percent in another two weeks, and then to nonfat.
- Try reduced-fat sour cream, cream cheese, and yogurt.
- Focus on herbs, spices, and high-flavor vegetables to increase flavor rather than using fat. Accent reduced-fat sour cream with minced basil, chives, garlic, or other favorite herbs and spices. Sauté fresh herbs and minced onions, shallots, and garlic in 1 measured teaspoon of butter for your potato, fish, or vegetables—making 1 teaspoon seem like 2 or 3.

- Learn about low-fat baking methods and use them consistently. Try some of the recipes in our book and prove to yourself that reduced-fat baked goods can taste even better than traditional versions. For example, in the Gooey Double Fudge Brownies, we've replaced some of the butter with puréed black beans (a must-try recipe!); in the Sweet Potato Scones, the sweet potato is actually the replacement for some of the butter.
- Find alternative thickeners for soups, stews, and sauces. Cooked and puréed rice, boiled potatoes, green peas, and cornstarch blended into nonfat milk or broth, water, or fruit juice will thicken kitchen creations with fewer calories and fat grams, and no sacrifice in flavor.
- Don't be afraid to try one of these new methods, but be sure to follow one of our tried-and-true recipes.

We often think cholesterol-free foods are fat-free foods—a dangerous misconception. We've come by this misconception quite honestly, given that many foods are advertised as being "cholesterol-free." However, we have learned that cholesterol is not a type of fat and is found only in foods of animal origin. Vegetable foods can be exceptionally high in fat and have absolutely no cholesterol. Read labels carefully, especially those with the claim, "cholesterol-free."

The concept of choosing better fats is confusing. On the one hand, it is great news that some dietary fats are not as atherogenic as others, meaning they are less likely to increase the risk of artery-clogging heart disease. On the other hand, confusion arises over how to include foods with these good fats into our everyday eating plans. For example, because olive and canola oils contain better fat, can we be less careful about amounts when cooking with them than when we cook with artery-clogging butter? The same goes for peanuts, almonds, walnuts, and other nuts that contain better fats: you're not alone if you've heard that you should try to eat more because they're "good for you." Here are some concepts we've put together to reduce all the confusion:

- Understand the four types of fat in food.
- Use less fat whenever possible, no matter what the type.
- Choose better fats when you must use fat, and among them choose monounsaturated fats over polyunsaturated fats.
- Plan carefully when you want to include foods with saturated fat (the most atherogenic), and portion such foods fastidiously.
- Avoid foods with trans fats as much as possible.
- Remember the bottom line about fat: a little dab will do ya.

How to Portion Added Fat

Whether you use them in cooking or on food, measure added fats carefully. One fat serving of the following foods is generally:

- Salad dressings (reduced fat): 2 tablespoons
- Salad dressings (regular fat): 1 tablespoon
- Mayonnaise (reduced fat): 2 tablespoons
- Mayonnaise (regular): 1 tablespoon
- Butter or margarine: 1 teaspoon
- Oil: 1 teaspoon
- Sour cream (reduced fat): 2 tablespoons
- Sour cream (regular): 1 tablespoon
- Cream cheese (reduced fat): 2 tablespoons
- Cream cheese (regular): 1 tablespoon

Low-Fat Cooking Methods

- Stir-sizzle: this is the low-fat way to stir-fry. You have two options: Avoid the use of oil altogether by first spraying a nonstick pan with vegetable oil spray. Add vegetable, chicken, or beef broth as the moisture needed to stir-fry. Alternatively, start with a teaspoon or two of canola or olive oil, and then add broth as needed for moisture.
- Baking: convert cookie, cake, and quick-bread recipes that call for oil, butter, or shortening into low-fat versions. In most cases, you can substitute applesauce or puréed prunes for up to half of the fat. Also, use one of the better fats, such as olive or canola oil. If you do not like the taste of olive oil, use the light version for less of an olive flavor. Be aware, however, that it has the same number of calories as other olive oils.

Micronutrients: Vitamins and Minerals

The body needs dozens of vitamins and minerals to do the following:

- Digest, absorb, and metabolize food
- Grow
- Heal injuries
- Fight disease
- Drive the thousands of chemical reactions taking place in the body every microsecond

It's the rare nutrient that works alone to accomplish a task; most work in concert with one another. For example, calcium, vitamin A, phosphorus, fluoride, copper, and manganese are all necessary to form bone tissue. Red blood cells need at least iron, vitamin C, copper, B_6, B_{12}, and riboflavin for their good health. This takes us back to critical points presented earlier in this chapter: choosing foods with diversity in mind helps us harvest the plethora of vitamins, minerals, and other healthful substances in food.

Using the guidelines for achieving diversity in carbohydrates, protein, and fat mentioned earlier, as well as those for boosting phytochemical intake, you will more than likely harvest the vitamins and minerals your body needs. Many people want to know more details about individual vitamins and minerals. The following chart provides information about their function, source, and guidelines for use.

Vitamins

Nutrient	Why We Need It	Problems with Getting Too Much	Foods Rich in This Nutrient
Vitamin A (retinol)	• Essential for vision • Enhances immunity • Builds and maintains bone	• Headache • Vomiting • Blurred vision • Liver damage • Birth defects	• Orange fruits • Leafy green vegetables
Vitamin B_1 (thiamin)	• Releases energy from carbohydrates, protein, and fat • Essential for nerve function	• Not toxic if taken orally	• Yeast • Legumes • Seeds • Nuts • Unrefined cereal
Vitamin B_2 (riboflavin)	• Releases energy from carbohydrates, fat, and protein • An ingredient in hormones • Prevents anemia • May prevent migraine headache at higher doses	• Not toxic	• Skim milk • Leafy green vegetables • Whole-grain bread • Skim milk or low-fat yogurt • Skim or 1% fat cottage cheese • Meat
Vitamin B_3 (niacin)	• Releases energy from carbohydrates, fats, and proteins • Helps prevent anemia	• Upper limit of safe intake: 35 mg • Flushing • Liver problems • Aggravates asthma • Ulcers • Glucose intolerance associated with type II diabetes	• Legumes • Nuts • Whole-grain bread • Fish • Meats

Nutrient	Why We Need It	Problems with Getting Too Much	Foods Rich in This Nutrient
Vitamin B_6 (pyridoxine)	• Helps break down protein • Essential for healthy nerve function • New evidence suggests may prevent high blood cholesterol and heart disease; may prevent depression; may ensure clear thinking later in life	• Prolonged use of more than 250 mg per day can cause sensitivity to light and irreversible neurological symptoms	• Bananas • Many vegetables, including peas, potatoes, sweet potatoes • Chicken (without the skin) • Fish • Lean pork
Biotin	• Necessary for energy reactions • Makes fatty acids • Breaks down amino acids, the building blocks of protein	• Not toxic at doses up to 10 mg	• Soybeans and soy products • Yeast
Folate (folic acid, folacin)	• Helps make new cells • Prevents anemia • Prevents some birth defects • May prevent high blood cholesterol and heart disease, cancer, and depression • May ensure clear thinking in later life	• Upper limit: 1,000 mcg • At levels >1 mg • Masks the symptoms of B_{12} deficiency • Pernicious anemia	• Yeast • Leafy green vegetables, such as spinach, romaine lettuce, mustard greens, and many others • Fruits, such as oranges, bananas, and papayas • Legumes, such as lentils, black beans, and many more
Vitamin B_{12} (cobalamin)	• Helps make new cells • Maintains healthy nerve fibers • May prevent high cholesterol and heart disease • May prevent depression	• No toxicity up to 100 mcg	• Clams • Oysters • Skim milk • Seafood • Egg whites • Fortified soy milk • Fish and lean meat
Pantothenic acid	• Necessary to make fatty acids	• None known	• Whole grains • Legumes • Mushrooms • Avocado • Broccoli • Yeast
Vitamin C (ascorbic acid)	• Acts as extra cellular antioxidant • Helps form essential hormones • Recycles vitamin E; as an antioxidant	• Nausea and diarrhea • May decrease copper levels • Reduces serum levels of B_{12} • Inhibits utilization of beta-carotene	• Citrus fruits • Berries • Nearly all vegetables, higher in green vegetables, peppers, tomatoes, and potatoes

(continued)

VITAMINS *(continued)*

Nutrient	Why We Need It	Problems with Getting Too Much	Foods Rich in This Nutrient
Vitamin C (ascorbic acid) (continued)	• May prevent atherosclerotic heart disease when obtained through food, but not in high-dose supplements	• May increase risk of atherosclerosis when taken in high-dose supplements	
Vitamin D	• Helps absorb calcium • An essential component of hormones	• Leaches calcium from bones and teeth • Kidney damage • Artery hardening • Death	• Sunlight, if you do not wear sunscreen, if you do not have dark skin, and if you are under the age of sixty • Fattier fish, such as salmon and mackerel (the type your body needs) • Skim milk • Fortified soy milk
Vitamin E (tocopherol)	• Prevents anemia and neurological abnormalities; as an antioxidant • Helps protect cells from the damage caused by oxygen-free radicals	• Gastrointestinal discomfort • Impaired immune function • Flulike symptoms	• Vegetable oils • Wheat germ • Nuts • Green leafy vegetables • Many fruits and vegetables
Vitamin K	• Necessary for normal blood clotting • New research suggests it's needed for building bone	• No evidence of toxicity	• Green leafy vegetables • Milk • Cabbage • Soybean oil

Minerals

Nutrient	Why We Need It	Problems with Getting Too Much	Foods Rich in This Nutrient
Arsenic	• Growth • Optimal iron use	• Very quickly toxic at doses over the recommended	• Fish • Grain • Cereal products
Boron	• Healthy cell membranes • Hormone function	• Vomiting • Diarrhea • Fatigue • Encourages loss of riboflavin through the urine	• Leafy vegetables • Nuts • Legumes • Noncitrus fruits

Nutrient	Why We Need It	Problems with Getting Too Much	Foods Rich in This Nutrient
Calcium	• Forming bones • May lower blood pressure • May prevent colon cancer	• Upper limit: adults >age nineteen: 2,500 mg • Inhibits absorption of other minerals, especially iron and magnesium (take calcium, iron, and magnesium supplements at different times of the day) • Increases vitamin C metabolism (therefore causing loss of vitamin C) • Causes: Kidney stones Fatigue Muscle weakness Depression Anorexia Nausea	• Nonfat milk and dairy products • Green leafy vegetables • Sardines • Salmon, especially pink salmon canned with bones • Low-fat tofu • Fortified soy milk
Chloride	• Necessary for fluid balance • Essential ingredient in stomach acid	• Elevated blood pressure	• Dietary salt and salt substitutes containing chloride, such as potassium chloride
Chromium	• Helps metabolize carbohydrates and fats • Needed for insulin to work properly	• Decreases zinc absorption	• Mushrooms • Prunes • Nuts • Asparagus • Some lean meats • Whole grains • Cheese
Cobalt	• Important ingredient of vitamin B_{12}	• May interfere with iron absorption	• Foods rich in B_{12}, such as meat and milk
Copper	• Essential ingredient in a wide variety of enzymes needed for using iron, making connective tissue, and forming energy	• Decreases zinc and iron absorption • Increases metabolism of riboflavin and B_6, which means these nutrients are lost from the body	• Legumes • Seafood and shellfish • Whole grains • Nuts • Seeds • Vegetables
Fluoride	• Increases hardness of bones and teeth	• Fluorosis, or mottling of teeth	• Fluoridated water
Iodine	• Needed for making thyroid hormones	• Intakes up to 2 mg apparently not dangerous	• Iodized salt • Dairy products

(continued)

MINERALS *(continued)*

Nutrient	Why We Need It	Problems with Getting Too Much	Foods Rich in This Nutrient

Iron	• Prevents anemia	• Iron overload can
		  • Damage the pancreas, liver, and heart
		  • Reduce copper levels
		  • Interfere with zinc and calcium absorption (take iron, zinc, and calcium supplements at different times of the day)
		  • Increase metabolism of B_{12}, riboflavin, niacin, and folate
			• Lean meats
			• Fish
			• Poultry
			• Organ meats
			• Legumes
			• Nuts and seeds
			• Whole grains
			• Dark molasses
			• Green leafy vegetables

Magnesium	• Necessary for absorbing and using calcium • May help control blood pressure	• Increases metabolism of thiamin, vitamin C, and B_6, which means these nutrients are lost from the body	• Unprocessed whole grains (note that 80 percent of magnesium is lost during processing of whole grains into refined products) • Legumes • Nuts and seeds • Chocolate • Dark green vegetables • Bananas
Manganese	• Used to make many enzymes • Needed for energy reactions	• Toxicity from dietary intake is rare • Affects the brain when it does occur • Decreases magnesium absorption • Increases metabolism of riboflavin, niacin, and thiamin, which means these nutrients are lost from the body	• Whole-grain cereal products • Many fruits and vegetables • Many legumes • Tea
Molybdenum	• Needed in producing energy	• Not known	• Milk • Beans • Breads • Cereals • Widely distributed in food supply; deficiency unlikely
Nickel	• Not entirely understood; but probably an ingredient of a number of enzymes	• Gastrointestinal irritation	• Chocolate • Nuts • Dried beans and peas • Grains

Nutrient	Why We Need It	Problems with Getting Too Much	Foods Rich in This Nutrient
Phosphorus	• Necessary for: • Forming cells essential to metabolism of carbohydrates, protein, and fat • Transporting fat in bloodstream • Moving nutrients into and out of cells	• Causes bone loss • Interferes with calcium absorption	• Many fruits and vegetables • Cereal grains • Skim milk • Low-fat milk products • Lean meat
Potassium	• Essential for proper muscle function • Regulates heart beat	• Causes irregular heart beat, cardiac arrest	• Fruits • Vegetables • Legumes • Meat
Selenium	• Functions as antioxidant	• Damages nervous system • Causes skin lesions, thicker but more fragile nails • Loss of hair and nails • Nausea • Abdominal pain • Diarrhea • Fatigue • Irritability • Interferes with antioxidant balance of cell, which is not good • Increases copper metabolism, which causes copper to be lost from the body	• Brazil nuts (one Brazil nut gives you all the selenium you need for the day) • Seafood • Lean meat • Egg whites • Whole grains • Legumes
Silicon	• Helps form connective tissue; necessary for making strong bones	• No known toxic effects	• Unrefined grains with high fiber content • Root vegetables, such as potatoes, carrots, parsnips, and more
Sodium	• Regulates fluid balance in body; helps in metabolism of carbohydrates and protein	• Fluid retention • In some people, hypertension • Pulls calcium from bones	• Processed foods
Vanadium	• Thought to regulate enzyme and hormone functions	• May cause gastrointestinal problems, such as cramps and diarrhea	• Shellfish • Mushrooms • Parsley • Black pepper

(continued)

Nutrient	Why We Need It	Problems with Getting Too Much	Foods Rich in This Nutrient
Zinc	• Necessary for: • Growth • Immune function • Blood clotting • Wound healing	• Lowers: • Good HDL cholesterol • Levels of copper • Shrink's red blood cells, which decreases the amount of oxygen they can carry • Impairs immunity • Increases metabolism of: • Niacin • B_6 • Vitamin E • Vitamin A • Causes these nutrients to be lost from the body	• Lean meat • Eggs • Seafood • Nuts • Whole grains

Aluminum, tin, cadmium, lead, germanium, lithium, and rubidium have all been studied, but there is insufficient evidence that they are essential to human health.

Nonnutrient Substances in Food: Fiber and Phytochemicals

Plant foods have fiber and phytochemicals. We call these nonnutritive substances because they don't contribute calories and are not required to live.

Fiber: Essential Threads of Good Health

The four categories of foods in which we find fiber are:

- Fruits
- Vegetables
- Whole-grain foods
- Legumes

Indeed, fiber is found only in plant foods—another reason why these fabulously versatile and diverse foods are so important to great health.

What Is Fiber?

The fiber in plants is somewhat akin to the fibers or threads that form your clothing. Just as threads give cloth structure, fiber lends structure and strength to plants. Partly owing to this strength, fibers in fruits and vegetables are indigestible, which means our bodies cannot break them down. From a health perspective this is great news. Fiber adds weight to intestinal waste—the reason fiber-containing foods are called bulky foods—and helps them pass more quickly through the body.

Just as there is more than one type of thread in cloth, there are many types of fiber found in plants, and they're divided into two main types: insoluble and soluble.

- Insoluble fiber soaks up water—much like a sponge—to make stools softer and easier to eliminate. Wheat bran, many vegetables, and other whole grains are good sources of insoluble fiber.
- Soluble fiber dissolves in the watery contents of the gastrointestinal tract to form a gel, which traps substances in the intestinal tract that the body could eventually turn into fat and cholesterol; the gel is then passed from the body as part of the body's intestinal wastes. This process works exceptionally well when the intake of insoluble fiber is also high, because the stools are heavier and pass through the intestinal tract much faster. Oats, barley, some fruits, dried beans, and dried peas are excellent sources of soluble fiber.

Health Benefits of Fiber

We've worked hard to bump up the fiber in our recipes, but you probably haven't noticed anything but the great taste. Here's a quick summary of why we've made such an effort (and we hope you will, too). Fiber does the following:

- It normalizes intestinal function to prevent constipation. More than an issue of comfort, preventing constipation can help prevent health problems down the road, such as diverticulosis (a condition by which pockets form in the intestinal wall after repeated straining to pass the stool).
- It reduces heart disease risk by helping to corral and eliminate fatty substances from the intestinal tract.
- It assists with weight control. High-fiber foods fill you up on far fewer calories, making weight control naturally easier.
- For people with type 2 diabetes it slows the rise of blood glucose after a meal, which helps reduce the number of peaks, or too high of an increase in blood sugars. Over the long term, fiber may help reduce complications associated with diabetes.
- Decreases the risk of colon cancer.

How Much Fiber?

The National Academy of Sciences recommends:

- 38 grams fiber for men and 25 for women up to age fifty
- 30 and 21 grams, respectively, after age fifty

Everyday solutions for increasing fiber include:

- Pour it into your cereal bowl. Choose a breakfast cereal with at least 5 grams of fiber per serving.

  Make a transition to a high-fiber cereal by mixing your current cereal with a high-fiber one—gradually phasing out the former.

  Bump up the fiber a notch with fresh or dried fruit on your cereal (and count them as one of your fruit and vegetable servings, too).

- Blend it into a smoothie. Add ¼ cup oats to your favorite smoothie and/or 2 to 4 tablespoons milled/ground flaxseed. Count an additional 2 to 8 grams of fiber (4 in 2 tablespoons of flaxseed and 2 for ¼ cup of oats).
- Do you love toast and peanut butter in the morning? Top it with sliced strawberries, bananas, raisins, or other fresh or dried fruit. Slice up another bowl of fruit on the side, or grab a piece of fruit for the car. Start your day with 2 to 6 grams of fiber just by adding fruit; use whole-grain bread and proudly claim another 2 to 5 grams.
- Enjoy the crunch of a lunch vegetable. At home, work, school, or a restaurant, include one vegetable daily with lunch, and you'll be 2 to 4 grams closer to your fiber goal. Check out our list that follows for ideas for easy lunch vegetables no matter where you are.
- Plan two for dinner—that's two vegetables of two different colors. Having a serving of two different kinds of vegetables makes it easier to enjoy the amount that your body needs for good health.
- Diversify your grains at lunch and dinner; always think a rainbow of colors and textures. A rainbow of colors in grains—aren't they all some shade of brown or yellow? Yes, but what a rainbow range of shades! Try the following:

  Trade one rice meal each week for a barley pilaf.

  Ladle hot soup over barley rather than over rice or noodles.

  Toss whole wheat pasta with white pasta—a great way to make the step toward using more whole-grain pasta.

  Stir up a bulgur salad for lunch one day. Try the recipes in this book or buy a boxed product.

Try cornmeal muffins rather than crackers with chili. Check the index for our delicious and easy recipes using cornmeal.

- Stir whole grains into baking as a matter of kitchen policy.

  Most recipes work fine with half whole wheat flour; you may have to bump up the baking powder by ½ to 1 teaspoon to assist with rising.

  Add ½ to 1 cup ground or milled flaxseed to most bread and muffin recipes (do not reduce the flour).

- Experiment with more dried beans and peas, such as black beans, lentils, and split peas.

  Toss black beans or garbanzo beans with chopped vegetables and reduced-fat mayonnaise; stuff this mixture into a whole-grain pita pocket for an easy and high-fiber lunch.

  Serve up beef-and-bean burritos at dinner. Use half the usual ground beef and stir in a can of (fat-free) refried beans.

  Simmer a pot of bean soup once a month and freeze in four batches—one for each week. Not only will you save cooking time but also you'll bump up the fiber. Try our French Market Soup.

- Last, but certainly not least, drink plenty of water to help the fiber work for you. Increasing fiber intake without drinking enough water can make stools hard and very difficult to pass (constipation).

Vegetables On the Go

If you find it hard to chop and cook vegetables from scratch, try some of these ideas to work more vegetables into your eating plan—in a flash:

- Visit the salad bar when shopping for groceries and package three salads (without dressing so it holds longer) or purchase premixed salad-in-a-bag.
- Buy cut-up vegetables, including those marked for stir-fry, to have on hand for lunches, snacks, and even as meal solutions.
- Choose a variety of frozen vegetables each time you shop, planning two colors for each meal of the week. Toss a handful on lunchtime salads, or pack some into a sealable container for an easy lunchtime or snack vegetable.

FIBER CHART

Food Item	Amount	Grams of Total Fiber
Fruits		
Avocados	½ each	8.5
Bananas, medium	1 each	3.1
Banana chips	½ cup	3.2
Dried apple rings	8 each	4.5
Dried apricots	½ cup	4.7
Dried cranberries	½ cup	4.6
Dried figs	5 each	4.1
Dried peaches	½ cup	6.6
Dried prunes	½ cup	6.0
Kiwi, large, without skin	1 each	2.7
Pear, medium	1 each	5.1
Raspberries	½ cup	4.0
Strawberries, sliced	½ cup	1.7
Vegetables		
Asparagus, medium	10 each	3.4
Broccoli, chopped, raw	1 cup	2.3
Carrots	2 large	4.0
Spinach, cooked	2 cups	8.6
Corn, cooked	½ cup	2.3
Sun-dried tomatoes	½ cup	3.3
Winter squash (acorn), cooked	½ cup	3.2
Grains		
Bagel, oat bran, 4-inch	1 each	3.2
Bagel, plain, 4-inch	1 each	2.0
Barley, cooked	½ cup	3.0
Bran flakes cereal	1 cup	6.2
Bulgur wheat, cooked	½ cup	4.1
Flaxseed	1 tablespoon	3.3
Grape nuts cereal	½ cup	5.0
Pumpernickel bread	1 piece	1.7
Raisin bran	1 cup	7.7
Rye bread	1 piece	1.9
Rye crisps	8 each	2.6
Rye melba toast	8 each	3.2
Rye wafers/crackers	8 each	20.1
Shredded wheat and bran cereal	1 cup	6.3
Toasted wheat germ	¼ cup	4.3
Whole wheat pita pocket	1 each	4.7
Legumes		
Black beans, cooked	½ cup	7.5
Black-eyed peas, cooked	½ cup	5.6
Chick-peas, cooked	½ cup	6.2

Food Item	Amount	Grams of Total Fiber
Lentils, cooked	½ cup	7.8
Lima beans, cooked	½ cup	6.6
Mung beans, cooked	½ cup	7.7
Navy beans, cooked	½ cup	6.7
Pinto beans, cooked	½ cup	7.0
Red kidney beans, cooked	½ cup	8.2
Roasted soybeans	½ cup	7.0
Split peas, cooked	½ cup	8.1
Nuts and Seeds		
Blanched almonds	½ cup	7.5
Dry-roasted pecans	4 ounces	10.7
Dry-roasted pistachios	½ cup	6.3
Dry-roasted sunflower seeds	½ cup	7.1
Spanish peanuts	½ cup	7.0
Snack Foods		
Air-popped popcorn	3 cups	3.6

WHAT ARE ANTIOXIDANTS AND HOW DO THEY WORK?

Antioxidants protect the health of every cell in the body. Oxygen, an essential element for life, can create damaging by-products during normal cellular metabolism. Antioxidants counteract these cellular by-products, called free radicals, and bind with them before they can cause damage. If left unchecked, free radicals may cause heart damage, cancer, cataracts, and a weak immune system.

- Antioxidants work by binding to the free radicals, transforming them into nondamaging compounds, or by repairing cellular damage. Antioxidants come in a variety of forms that include vitamin C, vitamin E, the carotenoids, and selenium.
- Good sources of antioxidants include fruits and vegetables. The highest concentrations are found in fruits and vegetables with the deepest or brightest colors (spinach, carrots, red bell peppers, tomatoes, cantaloupe, berries).

Everyday Solutions for Boosting Phytochemical Intake

Phytochemicals generally travel in colors. Eating three to five different colors of fruits and vegetables daily helps ensure a wider array of phytochemicals as well as vitamins, minerals, and more fiber. Try these solutions for diversifying the colors of fruits and vegetables you enjoy daily:

- Red apples, orange tangerines, green beans, red bell peppers, deep green spinach, purple grapes

- Red grapes, creamy white bananas, orange peaches, green pears, green peas, yellow corn
- Orange acorn squash, yellow papaya, red radishes, deep green romaine lettuce, purple onions, red tomatoes
- Green onions, red radicchio, orange apricots, green Granny Smith apples, purple eggplant, creamy white/brown mushrooms

11

PORTION SAVVY

Less Is More!

Susan Kell Peletta, R.D., and Kristine Napier, M.P.H., R.D.

Benjamin Franklin warned of being penny wise and pound foolish. His advice is applicable to Americans who are too often captured by the lure of "super-sized" meals and food products. From the fast-food restaurant to the movie concessions counter, we are continually bombarded with offers such as "For just a few pennies more, you can upsize your beverage, fries, or burger." But the offer is no bargain to your health. An additional 50 cents, for example, buys a 670-calorie instead of a 300-calorie pastry at a popular food chain.

Larger portion sizes have become a fact of life in grocery stores, too. In the 1950s an average soda pop was served in a 6½-ounce bottle and had just 80 calories. Today, however, the typical size is 20 ounces, a change that adds 160 calories, for a sum of 240. When the bagel was introduced to the United States from Poland, it weighed 1½ ounces and contained 116 calories. Today's U.S. bagel has nearly tripled in size and calories. It weighs from 4 to 4½ ounces and may contain over 300 calories.

Researchers Lisa R. Young, Ph.D., and Marion Nestle, Ph.D., of New York University published their survey of portion sizes in the *American Journal of Public Health* (February 2002). Compared to standard portion sizes recommended by the U.S. Department of Agriculture's (USDA) Food Guide Pyramid, they found that:

- Cookies were as much as seven times standard portion sizes.
- Servings of cooked pasta were often nearly five times standard portion sizes.
- Muffins weighed in at over three times standard portion sizes.

Overall, Young and Nestle found that marketplace food portions are consistently larger now than in the past. For example, their research discovered that a popular fast-food chain offered only one portion size of french fries in the mid-1950s. Today, across the industry, that size is now labeled "small" and is one-third the weight of the largest portion size available.

Do We Eat These Larger Portions?

Unfortunately, the majority of us eat most of the food set before us. The American Institute for Cancer Research found in a 2001 survey that 67 percent of Americans usually eat everything or almost everything on their plates. According to the Pennsylvania State University nutrition researcher Barbara Rolls, Ph.D., even lean young men who typically are careful about regulating food intake are tempted out of control when large portions are put before them. In one study, they ate 10 ounces of a 16-ounce portion of macaroni. When offered 25 ounces, however, they ate 15 ounces, a 50 percent increase!

Do Larger Portions Really Add Up?

At home or dining out, portion size may be the single worst culprit causing weight gain. For example, what if you meant to have:

- 12 ounces of fat-free milk for breakfast, but instead poured 16 ounces?

  Calorie increase: 40
- 1 tablespoon of peanut butter on your bagel in the morning, but instead had 4 teaspoons?

  Calorie increase: 30
- A healthy-sized 3-ounce bagel, but instead had a large one at 5 ounces?

  Calorie increase: 150

- 6 whole wheat crackers with your salad, but instead grabbed 3 extra for a total of 9?

  Calorie increase: 50
- 1 teaspoon of extra-virgin olive oil (with balsamic vinegar and herbs) on your salad, but instead had 2 teaspoons?

  Calorie increase: 40
- 3 ounces of chicken on your lunchtime salad, but instead had 4?

  Calorie increase: 43
- 3 ounces of grilled, poached, or baked salmon, but instead had 5 ounces?

  Calorie increase: 100
- 1 cup of wild rice at dinner, but instead had 1¼ cups?

  Calorie increase: 54

Maybe you've already done the math in your head, but if you haven't, you will be surprised to learn that seemingly small increases in portion size of these wholesome foods add up to a whopping 500-calorie difference for the day. Day after day, this can mean the difference between successfully or unsuccessfully maintaining a healthy weight, or losing weight slowly and keeping it off. Here's another interesting fact that will help put this weight into perspective: to lose 1 pound of body weight, you must have a deficit of 3,500 calories.

Five Options for Managing Portion Size

With such large portions available, no wonder we need help with serving ourselves and family members portion sizes that enhance health. We suggest five strategies:

- Purchase portion-controlled foods.
- Serve foods with measuring spoons and cups instead of serving spoons and ladles.
- Select bowls, glasses, cups, and plates that hold specific portion sizes.
- Learn and use visual serving-size cues.
- Measure and weigh foods.

The following details will help you determine which options work best for you.

Purchase Portion-Controlled Foods

At the supermarket, select foods that take the chore and the guesswork out of portioning at home. For example:

- Purchase the amount of meat, poultry, or fish needed for a meal; if you do not see the size package you need, ask someone in the meat or seafood department to package the amount you need. (There generally is no extra charge for this.)

  Purchase 4 ounces uncooked (boneless and skinless) meat or poultry for each family member.

  Purchase 5 ounces uncooked fish for each family member.
- At the bakery, ask the clerk to package just the number of cookies or pieces of cake, for example, that you need to serve your family for dessert.
- Purchase dried raisins and other snack foods in individual-serve boxes and packages.

Serve with Measuring Spoons or Cups

Enjoy serving savvy at every meal with this very easy strategy. Instead of serving pasta, rice, and mashed potatoes with a serving spoon, use a long-handled measuring cup. Purchase two or three one-half and one-cup measures with long handles. (Having several on hand helps ensure there is always a clean one.) Similarly, serve yourself butter, margarine, oil, and salad dressings with measuring spoons.

Set out a pretty mug or small ceramic flowerpot in an accessible spot in your kitchen and fill it with two or three sets of measuring spoons, separated, so that you don't dirty an entire set at once. Stack measuring cups next to the spoons, or choose a larger container and store all the items together. Making these tools for healthy living readily accessible helps you make them a regular good habit.

Select Bowls and Glasses with Your Portion in Mind

Enjoy a treasure hunt in your own kitchen by searching for dishes that help you serve optimal portions. You'll need measuring cups in your search for some of these valuables.

- Find a drinking glass that holds 8 ounces. Using your measuring cup as a guide, select the glass you think is closest to this amount. Then put your eye to the test and measure how much your choice holds. If you cannot find a glass in your cabinet that holds 8 ounces, mark 8 ounces with an indelible marker by pouring a measured 8 ounces into the glass.
- Find a bowl that holds 1 cup (plus a little extra room to prevent spillage), or at least has a pattern on the inside that provides a mark

for 1 cup. Use this bowl for cereal, rice, pasta, mashed potatoes, and other foods for which you generally enjoy a 1-cup portion. (Remember, though, that 1 cup of rice or potatoes counts for two servings of your daily total, and 1 cup of pasta counts for three servings.

- Locate a bowl that holds ½ or ¾ cup. Verify the capacity with measuring cups. Use this petite treasure for ice cream, pudding, and other treats.

Learn and Use Visual Cues

Common items serve as excellent visual cues for "eyeballing" serving sizes—especially in restaurants, at picnics, or at parties. Take advantage of these common visual cues:

- Computer mouse = 1 medium potato
- Hockey puck = 3-ounce bagel
- Audiocassette tape = 3 ounces cooked meat or poultry
- Deck of playing cards = 3 ounces cooked meat or poultry
- Household checkbook = 3 ounces grilled fish
- Four dice = 1 ounce cheese
- Three dice = 1 tablespoon peanut butter
- One die = 1 teaspoon peanut butter
- Baseball = 1 cup salad greens
- Cardboard box from Chinese carryout = 2 cups

Your hand also provides excellent visual cues when portioning food. For example:

- Index finger = 1 ounce meat or poultry
- Woman's closed fist = 1 cup
- Man's closed fist = 1½ cups

Weigh and Measure Foods

Even though we listed this strategy last, we believe that weighing and measuring food is the gold standard for achieving portion control. Buy yourself a good food scale, a gift that speaks of both commitment and health. You don't have to measure meat, poultry, and fish portions daily. Rather, measure as much as you need to when you get started—probably for two or three days. Then choose one day of the week and check how well you are doing eyeballing portion sizes.

Do the same with measuring cups. Use them for portioning everything from vegetables to fruits to pastas and rice. This is a great way to train your eye to portion without measuring devices.

SERVING-SIZE HELP

Breads, Cereals, Rice, and Pasta

Food	Serving Size
Bread	1 slice
Pasta	½ cup (cooked)
Rice	½ cup (cooked)
Hot cereal	½ cup (cooked)
English muffin	½ each
Bagel (2 ounces whole)	½ each
Cold cereal	1 ounce (about ¾ cup)
Crackers	4 small
Tortilla (corn or flour)	1 (6-inch)

Fruits and Vegetables

Food	Serving Size
Raw vegetables	1 cup
Cooked vegetables	1 cup
Vegetable juice	¾ cup
Whole fruit	1 medium piece
Berries	¾ cup
Cooked or canned fruit	½ cup
Dried fruit (such as raisins)	¼ cup
Fruit juice	½ to ¾ cup

Dairy Foods

Food	Serving Size
Milk	1 cup (8 ounces)
Yogurt	1 cup (8 ounces)
Cheese	1 ounce

Meat, Poultry, Fish, Dried Beans, Eggs, and Nuts

Food	Serving Size
Meat, fish, poultry (lean)	2 to 3 ounces (cooked)
Dried beans/peas (such as black beans or lentils)	1 cup (cooked)
Nuts (such as peanuts or almonds)	⅔ cup
Nut butters (such as peanut butter)	2 to 3 tablespoons
Cottage cheese	1 cup (choose reduced fat)
Tofu	6 ounces
Egg	2 whole or 4 egg whites

12

CREATING THE KITCHEN DEDICATED TO FLAVOR AND GOOD HEALTH

Kristine Napier, M.P.H., R.D.

Enjoying great-tasting food that meets your health goals is much easier when your kitchen is stocked with the equipment and food that make it easy to prepare a meal—especially at the last minute—and in record time. We've pooled ideas from our 1,500 culinary-focused dietitians to create this handy list of utensils, pots, pans, and other equipment. Most important, we've tried to keep kitchen tools to a bare minimum for people on limited budgets. There are two lists: "Definitely Good to Have" includes a short list of equipment that helps you prepare food with greater ease. "Nice Extras" includes additional equipment that can make food preparation even easier, if your budget allows for them. The well-stocked kitchen should be accessible to everyone.

Utensils

Definitely Good to Have

- Grater (choose different sizes for grating cheese; lemon, orange, or lime zest; fresh ginger)

- Vegetable peeler
- 6-inch paring knife
- 8-inch chef's knife
- Spatulas (one narrow and one wide, long-handled, and heat resistant)
- Wooden cooking spoons
- Rubber or plastic utensils for nonstick pans
- Tongs
- Whisks (small and large)
- Colanders, plastic or metal (variety of sizes)
- Cutting boards, two if possible (choose ones that fit into and are safe for the dishwasher)
- Ladles (small and large)
- Strainers (medium and small if possible)

Nice Extras

- Potato masher
- Steamer basket
- Baster and baster brush
- Funnels
- Jar opener

Electric Appliances

Definitely Good to Have

- Electric mixer (if finances permit, a heavy-duty mixer on a stand, with a dough hook for making bread, eliminating the need for a bread maker)
- Blender

Nice Extras

- Food processor (large and, if possible, a mini version)
- Toaster oven or toaster
- Coffee grinder for grinding seeds, nuts, and grains
- Rice cooker (doubles as a vegetable steamer)

Pots and Pans

Definitely Good to Have

- Nonstick skillets with glass lids (medium and extra large, if possible)

- Heavy saucepans with lids (small and medium, if possible; medium, if not)
- Large pasta or stock pot (if possible, with colander insert)

Nice Extras

- Wok or stir-fry pan with glass lid
- Slow cooker (optional, depending on your projected use)

Measuring Equipment

Definitely Good to Have

- Liquid and dry measuring cups
- Measuring spoons

Nice Extras

- 1-cup heat-tempered glass measuring cup
- 1- and 2-quart heat-tempered glass bowls and mixing cups (with lids, if possible)
- Unconventional measuring cup sizes, such as ⅔ cup and ¾ cup
- An extra set of measuring cups and measuring spoons

Baking Bowls and Pans

Definitely Good to Have

- Metal and tempered-glass baking pans (9-inch square pan, 9-by-13-inch pan)
- Large glass, plastic, or metal mixing bowl
- 2- and 3-quart tempered-glass baking dish
- Nonstick loaf pans (regular and mini)
- Nonstick muffin tins (regular and mini)

Nice Extras

- Stacking metal mixing bowls

Other Kitchen Utensils

Definitely Good to Have

- Food scale
- Meat or instant-read food thermometer

Nice Extras

- Freezer-to-microwave containers

- Kitchen shears
- Digital timer
- Freezer-to-oven containers
- Gravy separator and pitcher

What's in the Pantry, the Refrigerator, and the Freezer?

You'll be much closer to achieving your health goals if you have on hand the tools you need to cook the food your body needs. This includes food in your pantry, refrigerator, and freezer. With the staples you keep on hand, you should be able to cook at least one full meal.

Pantry Suggestions

Stocking your shelves with ingredients that you use often can make cooking easier and more enjoyable. As with the equipment lists, we've distinguished the "nice extras" in some of the lists. As always, purchase what you are most likely to use.

- Baking ingredients:

  Cornstarch

  Baking soda

  Baking powder

  Nonstick cooking spray

  Nonfat dried buttermilk or nonfat dried milk powder

  Sugar (white and dark brown)

  Flour (all-purpose unbleached white, whole wheat)
- Canned ingredients, definitely good to have:

  Beans

  Chicken and beef broth (reduced sodium)

  Fat-free evaporated milk

  Fat-free sweetened condensed milk

  Fruit, canned in juice (mandarin oranges, peaches, pears, fruit cocktail, pineapple)

  Salmon

  Soups (regular and reduced sodium)

  Tomato products (puréed, diced, crushed, stewed, paste, sauce)

  Tuna (albacore, canned in water)

  Vegetables (water chestnuts, pumpkin, corn)

- Canned ingredients, nice extras:

  Light coconut milk

  Roasted red peppers
- Dressings, sauces, and condiments—definitely good to have (read labels to determine which are to be refrigerated after opening):

  Salsa

  Marinara or pasta sauce

  Soy sauce (reduced sodium)

  Vinegars (white, apple cider, and balsamic)

  Favorite reduced-fat salad dressing

  Jelly, jam, or preserves

  Ketchup and barbecue sauce

  Maple syrup

  Mustard (brown, yellow and Dijon)

  Horseradish

  Honey

  Hot sauce
- Dressings, sauces, and oils—nice extras:

  Rice-wine and red-wine vinegar

  Hoisin and oyster sauces if you prepare Asian food
- Dried fruit (raisins, apricots, sweetened cranberries, other favorites)
- Grains and grain foods:

  Bread crumbs (seasoned and plain)

  Bulgur

  Cold and hot cereals (high-fiber choices)

  Crackers, whole grain (reduced sodium and reduced fat)

  Barley (medium and quick cooking)

  Oats (old-fashioned for baking)

  Pasta (regular and whole wheat in assorted shapes)

  Pretzels and rice cakes

  Rice (brown and white)

  Couscous (regular, whole wheat)
- Microwave popcorn (reduced fat)
- Nuts (your favorite almonds, peanuts, pecans, soy nuts, walnuts)
- Pastas (your favorite shapes)

- Peanut butter
- Produce (garlic, onions, potatoes, and sweet potatoes, kept in a cool place)
- Oils, definitely good to have:

  Canola

  Extra-virgin olive
- Oils, nice extras:

  Dark sesame and/or peanut, if you prepare Asian recipes
- Tea (herbal, green, black, oolong)
- Wraps for sandwiches:

  Corn tortillas

  Whole wheat flour tortillas

What's in the seasoning rack?

- Salt and pepper (whole peppercorns to grind)
- Dried herbs

  Essential

  Basil
  Cayenne pepper
  Chili powder
  Chives
  Cilantro
  Curry powder
  Dill
  Ground cinnamon
  Ground ginger
  Mustard powder
  Nutmeg
  Onion powder
  Oregano
  Parsley
  Rosemary
  Sage
  Thyme

  Nice to have

  Allspice
  Black pepper
  Caraway seeds
  Cardamom
  Celery seed
  Chipotle chili
  Cloves
  Filé powder
  Old Bay seasoning
  Tarragon
  Turmeric
  White pepper
- Extracts

  Essential: Vanilla

  Nice to have: White vanilla and almond

What's in the refrigerator?

- Juices (calcium-fortified, if possible)
- Fresh herbs (including ginger root, cilantro, and parsley)
- Produce
- Tofu
- Eggs and egg substitute
- Dairy products:

  Milk (nonfat and fat-free)

  Sour cream (reduced-fat)

  Cream cheese (reduced-fat)

  Cottage cheese (calcium-fortified and reduced-fat or fat-free)

  Butter or alternative spread

  Yogurt (reduced-fat or nonfat)

  Parmesan (block or freshly grated)

  Cheese (block and shredded, of favorite varieties)

What's in the freezer?

- Frozen fruit and berries:

  Strawberries, blueberries, raspberries, mixed berries (no sugar added)

  Peaches (no sugar added)
- Frozen juice concentrate (orange, grapefruit, apple, cranberry)
- Frozen vegetables:

  Broccoli

  Brussels sprouts

  Corn

  Green beans

  Peas

  Edamame, shelled (green soybeans)

  Spinach (chopped)

  Winter squash
- Garden (soy) burgers
- Finfish: steaks (mahimahi or tuna), salmon, shrimp
- Poultry: one roasting chicken plus individually wrapped boneless, skinless breasts and thighs; one turkey breast
- Beef: two 1-pound packages extra-lean ground; one sirloin tip roast

(buy 4 ounces for each family member); one pot roast (5 ounces for each family member)

- Pork: one tenderloin (4 ounces for each family member); center-cut sirloin chops (one for each family member)
- Bread dough (multiloaf package of 1-pound loaves)

Food Safety in the Kitchen

Unwashed fruits and vegetables are responsible for about the same number of reported cases of food-borne illness (often called food poisoning) as are beef, chicken, fish, and eggs, combined.

Good food is great medicine. Making sure food is safe is just as important as enjoying the foods you need for optimal health. Indeed, the final step in preparing and serving health-enhancing food is to keep it safe from food-borne illnesses caused by bacteria and other pathogens (microscopic organisms—what we frequently call germs). We've compiled the most commonly asked questions and provided the following answers:

What are the most important steps to take in the kitchen to prevent food-borne illness?

- Wash your hands when you enter the kitchen, and wash often during meal preparation.
- Keep raw meat, poultry, and fish separate from ready-to-eat foods—in the grocery cart, in grocery bags, and in the refrigerator.
- Cook foods to proper and safe internal temperatures.
- Refrigerate all foods promptly to below 40°F.

How often should hands be washed when preparing meals?

- After handling raw meat, poultry, or seafood
- When switching tasks, such as handling meat and then cutting vegetables
- After taking out garbage
- After sneezing or using a tissue
- Touching a dog, a cat, or another pet

How—and for how long—do I need to wash my hands in order to remove germs?

- Sing two choruses of "Happy Birthday" while you lather with soap, which is the same as washing for about 20 seconds.
- Wash hands front and back and up to your wrists, between fingers, and under fingernails.
- Dry with a clean hand towel or disposable paper towels.

What type of soap should I use for washing hands?

- Washing hands for twenty seconds with any type of soap in warm water is effective in reducing bacteria. There is no scientific evidence that using anti-bacterial soap versus ordinary soap reduces the incidence of any disease.

Are sponges safe to use?

- Sponges are safe only when cleaned properly. Bacteria live and grow in damp conditions.
- Wash dishcloths, sponges, and towels often in the hot cycle of the washing machine, then dry completely in the clothes dryer.
- Replace worn sponges frequently.

Can sponges be washed in the dishwasher or microwave?

- The preferred method is to wash them in the hot cycle of your washing machine.

Which kind of cutting board is best to use, plastic or wood?

- It is acceptable to use plastic, wood, marble, or acrylic. More important than the type is how you use it:

  Have one cutting board for meat, poultry, and seafood, and another for ready-to-eat foods like breads, fruits, and vegetables.

  Wash cutting boards thoroughly in hot, soapy water after each use.

  Discard cutting boards that are worn with cracks, crevices, or excessive knife scars.

How do I prevent cross-contamination of foods?

- Use two cutting boards (see previous list).
- Use separate and clean plates, containers, and utensils for raw and cooked foods.
- Wash hands properly (see previous list).
- Place raw meat, poultry, and seafood on the bottom shelf of the refrigerator so their juices don't drip onto other foods.
- Place washed produce into clean storage containers, not back into their original ones.
- Use two separate clean towels or cloths in the kitchen, one for kitchen surfaces and the other for drying hands.
- Use separate utensils for tasting food and stirring or mixing food. Each time you taste, use a clean utensil.
- Use clean scissors or knife blades to open bags of food; keep a pair of kitchen-only scissors that you wash thoroughly with hot, soapy water (or in the dishwasher) after each use.

- Wear latex gloves if you have a cut or sore on your hand.

How do I know when meat, poultry, fish, eggs, and leftovers are cooked to the proper temperatures?

- Harmful bacteria are destroyed when food is cooked to proper internal temperatures (see the following table).
- Just because the outside of the food looks good doesn't mean the inside temperature is high enough to kill bacteria. A meat or instant-read thermometer used to check internal temperatures is the only reliable way to ensure that foods are cooked thoroughly and are safe to eat.
- An added benefit: cooking foods to the right temperature gives a better taste.

SAFE COOKING TEMPERATURES

Food	Safe Internal Cooked Temperature
Beef, Lamb, Veal	
Ground products	
Hamburger (prepared as patties, meatballs, etc.)	160°F
Nonground products	
Roasts and steaks	
Medium-rare	145°F
Medium	160°F
Well-done	170°F
Poultry	
Ground chicken or turkey	165°F
Whole chicken or turkey	180°F
Boneless turkey roasts	170°F
Poultry breast and roasts (white meat)	170°F
Poultry thighs, wings, and drumsticks (dark meat)	180°F
Duck, goose	180°F
Stuffing (cooked alone or in a bird)	165°F
Pork	
All cuts including ground products	
Medium	160°F
Well-done	170°F
Fresh, raw ham	160°F
Fully cooked ham, to reheat	140°F
Egg dishes, casseroles	160°F
Leftovers, reheated	165°F

Adapted from and consistent with guidelines from the U.S. Department of Agriculture and the U.S. Food and Drug Administration.

How do I use a meat or instant-read thermometer properly?

- Red meats, roasts, steaks, chops, and poultry pieces: insert in the center of the thickest part, away from bone, fat, and gristle.
- Poultry (whole bird): insert in the inner thigh area, near the breast, but not touching the bone.
- Ground meat and poultry: place in the thickest area of the meat loaf or patty; with thin patties, insert sideways, reaching the very center with the stem of the thermometer.
- Egg dishes and casseroles: insert in the center or thickest area of the dish.
- Fish: insert sideways, reaching the very center with the stem of the thermometer.

Always remember to wash the thermometer stem thoroughly in hot, soapy water after each use.

How cold should the refrigerator be?

- Keep the temperature between 33°F and 40°F.
- Note that the internal temperature of your refrigerator is based on many variables, including the quantity of food inside, how often the door is opened, and the kitchen temperature.
- Monitor the refrigerator temperature with a refrigerator thermometer, and lower the temperature setting if needed.

How long can food be left out of the refrigerator?

- After two hours food reaches temperatures at which harmful bacteria multiply rapidly.
- In hot weather (above 90°F) do not leave food out longer than one hour.

Is it okay to defrost meat or other food on the kitchen counter?

- No, nor should you defrost food in warm water.
- Most food-borne pathogens thrive at room temperature.
- Two safe methods of defrosting food are in the refrigerator or in the microwave oven.
- In the refrigerator, place it on the bottom shelf, with a container underneath so that juices don't drip onto other foods.
- When using the microwave oven to thaw food, remember that it must be cooked immediately after defrosting.

HOW LONG ARE LEFTOVERS SAFE TO EAT?

Leftovers	Keeps Refrigerated Up To
Cooked fresh vegetables	3 to 4 days
Cooked pasta	3 to 5 days
Cooked rice	1 week
Deli-counter meats	5 days
Greens	1 to 2 days
Meat:	
Ham, cooked and sliced	3 to 4 days
Hot dogs, opened	1 week
Lunch meats, prepackaged, opened	3 to 5 days
Cooked beef, pork, poultry, fish, and meat casseroles	3 to 4 days
Cooked patties and nuggets, gravy and broth	1 to 2 days
Seafood, cooked	2 days
Soups and stews	3 to 4 days
Stuffing	1 to 2 days

13

EVERYDAY SOLUTIONS FOR ENJOYING MORE VEGETABLES AND FRUITS

Kristine Napier, M.P.H., R.D., Linda Marmer, M.S., R.D., L.D.;
Dorothy Chen-Maynard, Ph.D., R.D.; Barbara J. Pyper, M.S., R.D., C.D., F.H.C.F.A., F.C.S.I.;
Barbara LaVella, M.B.A., R.D., L.D., Peggy Eastmond, R.D.

Looking for more information on how to slice, chop, and stir more vegetables and fruit into your eating plan? We've got some great answers that supply loads of options and equip you with the information that helps you turn the science of nutrition into delicious food on your plate.

Fresh, Frozen, or Canned?

If you're like most families, you probably need all three in your kitchen. Produce experts say that using canned or frozen vegetables may be the answer to eating more vegetables, especially when:

- Fresh produce is out of season.
- Fresh produce is in poor quality at the time you shop.
- Frequent shopping is not an option.
- Convenience is important.

Certainly there is no science in how to choose fruits and vegetables. But there are some strategies for determining an approximate mix of fresh, frozen, and canned produce for you and your family. When collating your grocery list for the week:

- Plan mostly fresh produce for meals and snacks during the first four days of the week.
- Pencil in frozen or canned varieties to cover the last three days of the week.
- If your budget allows, toss in an extra container or two of frozen and canned vegetables and fruit for busier moments and emergency backup menu partners.
- Check your supply of potatoes, onions, carrots, apples, and other produce that hold up well (properly stored) for a week or more; plan on buying more as needed for the following week.

FRUIT AND VEGETABLE BUYING AND STORAGE TIPS

Type of Produce	Buying Tips	Storage Tips
Fresh	• Choose produce with a good complexion—without bruises, cuts, or other damages. • Buy the amount you can use in three to five days. • Buy mature fruit whenever possible. Some fruit, such as a cantaloupe that was picked too green, will never become sweet and juicy, although it will soften and appear ripe. Also, some fruits, such as pineapple, don't ripen after picking. • Buy cut produce only when it is refrigerated or on ice. • Place produce in plastic bags and close tightly before placing in the shopping cart. • Do not place raw meats, poultry, or fish on top of produce (to avoid contamination).	• Refrigerate produce that needs refrigerating (see the buying, storage, and cooking table that follows) • Use the crisper drawer of your refrigerator, as it has a higher humidity than the rest of the refrigerator. • Refrigerate all cut produce (even those that can be stored at room temperature) in a tightly covered clean container or plastic bag for up to two days. • Transport vegetables—whole or cut—to a picnic or potluck meal by first packing in a clean, airtight container or plastic bag. Then, place in a cooler with ice or ice packs. Upon arriving, discard the ice used in the cooler.
Frozen	• Packages should be firm and solidly frozen. • Packages should not be limp, wet, or sweating. (These are signs that the vegetables have defrosted or are in the process of defrosting.) • Pass by those packages with stains or that are coated with ice. (This signals that the package thawed at some point.)	• Check your freezer temperature, and make sure it is at 32°F or lower. • Once the whole package thaws, store leftovers in the refrigerator (tightly sealed) and use within three days. • If you remove just what you want to use and return the rest to the freezer promptly (sealed tightly), the rest will keep for eight to twelve months.

Type of Produce	Buying Tips	Storage Tips
Frozen *(continued)*	• On a regular basis, choose vegetables that are just vegetables. Save frozen vegetables in sauces for special treats, and plan ahead for their extra calories, fat, and sodium.	
Canned	• Choose perfect cans, without bulges, swells, leaks, or dents. • Ensure that the lid of vegetables in glass jars is not loose.	• Store canned vegetables at no more than 75°F, and use within two years of purchase for peak quality. Once opened, transfer the unused portion to a plastic or a glass container with a tightly fitting lid and refrigerate.

How long can I store cooked fruits and vegetables?

Most cooked vegetables keep up to three or four days in the refrigerator, provided they are refrigerated within two hours after cooking. Place in a plastic or a glass container with a tightly fitting lid.

Are canned and frozen fruits and vegetables as nutritious as fresh?

Yes. Canned or frozen, they are harvested and preserved at the peak of freshness and are comparable in nutrition to most fresh vegetables and fruit.

What about the sodium in canned vegetables?

Of all the choices—fresh, frozen, and canned—canned is the only variety with added sodium. (Frozen vegetables can have added sodium if they contain sauces or flavorings.) Sodium, one part of table salt, is added to many canned foods. One way to reduce the sodium is to drain and rinse canned vegetables, which can cut the sodium by about 40 percent. If you are on a sodium-restricted diet, look for no-salt-added or reduced-sodium varieties.

What should I know about choosing frozen fruit?

Many types of berries, peaches, and an increasing variety of other fruits are available frozen. These are an excellent way to enjoy fruits out of season, or simply to have fruits on hand for eating, cooking, or baking. But choosing carefully is key, given that frozen fruits can be packaged with some or a lot of added sugar. Let's take a look at how frozen fruit with and without added sugar stacks up:

- ½ cup frozen strawberries, no added sugar: 40 calories, 10 grams carbohydrate
- ½ cup frozen strawberries, with added sugar: 125 calories, 33 grams carbohydrate

You can enjoy fruit from the freezer case without the added sugar by reading labels carefully. On the front of the label, look for "No Sugar Added." To be sure, though, check the ingredients list. The only ingredient should be the type of fruit you wish to purchase.

How do I select canned fruit?

Canned fruit is fabulous for packing into lunches (especially those sold in individual-serve, pop-top cans), or for enjoying when a fruit variety is out of season. As with frozen, though, you have to read labels if you choose to avoid added sugar. In general, the best choice is fruit canned in its own juice. Look for "Canned in Juice" on the front label; on the ingredients list, you should find just fruit and fruit juice.

Let's take a look at how the different types of canned fruit stack up:

- Peaches canned in juice, 1 cup: 110 calories, 29 grams carbohydrate
- Peaches canned in light syrup, 1 cup: 160 calories, 40 grams carbohydrate
- Peaches canned in heavy syrup, 1 cup: 250 calories, 68 grams carbohydrate

Buying More for Your Money

If you shop at one store consistently, read the weekly advertisement (in the newspaper, online, or in the store) and plan menus around produce on sale. When it comes to frozen and canned vegetables, save by choosing cut, sliced, or diced versions—if they work in your recipe. Whole vegetables generally cost more than cut styles because they are specially selected for appearance and uniformity of size, shape, and color.

Safety in the Kitchen: Cleaning Fresh Vegetables and Fruit

Properly cleaning vegetables and fruit before eating can effectively wash away dirt, bacteria, and water-soluble pesticides, says the U.S. Food and Drug Administration. Don't forget to wash produce you peel (such as bananas and apples), tripled-washed bagged salad, and baby carrots.

The Best Time to Clean Vegetables

Wash vegetables just before use, not when you bring them home. Cleanse just the amount you will use for the next meal, leaving the others in their original storage containers.

How to Clean Vegetables

Shower, don't bathe, your fruits and vegetables. Here's how:

- Use constantly running cool, drinkable tap water.

- Wash even those vegetables you plan on peeling or cutting (such as melons) as bacteria on the surface can be transferred onto the knife.
- Scrub firm produce, such as cucumbers, melons, potatoes, and root vegetables, with a clean produce brush, even if you plan to peel them.
- Rinse berries and other fragile fruits and vegetables in a colander with copious amounts of water.
- Cut away damaged or bruised areas immediately because bacteria thrive in them (such as a bruise on an apple).
- Remove and discard the outer leaves of leafy vegetables (e.g., cabbages, romaine lettuce) before washing. Shower for five full minutes in clear, cold running water.

Water alone is effective in washing fruits and vegetables, say food safety experts. Be cautious with dish detergents, bleach, or special produce washes. Produce is porous, which means it can absorb detergents and bleaches; subsequently, you could consume them.

To Peel or Not to Peel?

Keep peels on whenever you can and enjoy not only the texture and taste but also the health benefits of extra fiber, minerals, and vitamins. Try our mashed potatoes, a recipe that includes the potato peel. Most vegetable skins and many fruit skins are edible. Refer to the following guide for specific information on each type of fruit and vegetable.

If you do elect to peel fruits and vegetables, try to peel them just before using to retain nutrients and flavor as well as to avoid browning (such as in apples and potatoes). If you need to peel them ahead, stop browning by sprinkling them with lemon juice (if you prefer, rinse off the juice just before cooking).

The Ultimate Vegetable Buying, Storage, and Cooking Chart

How many pounds of green beans should you buy to serve eight people for Sunday dinner? How long should you steam broccoli, and how? What should asparagus look like when you buy it?

We've collected the best information on how to buy, store, and cook vegetables. We've also ferreted out some culinary advice to make cooking more fun and creative, including spices that can enhance vegetables or give them a whole new taste for your family. Refer to the following pages for general guidelines on microwaving, steaming, sautéing, grilling, and roasting vegetables.

THE ULTIMATE VEGETABLE BUYING, STORAGE, AND COOKING CHART

Vegetable and Equivalent Measures	How to Buy Fresh: Qualities to Look For	How to Store Fresh	How to Microwave Fresh	How to Steam Fresh	Ideas for Enjoying More and Seasoning Suggestions
Alfalfa sprouts 1 pound = 6 cups	• Crisp buds still attached	Refrigerate	• Not recommended	• Not recommended	• Add crunch to cold or hot sandwiches • Mix with greens as a salad base • Use as salad topper
Artichokes 1 pound = 2 medium	• Tight, compact heads that feel heavy for their size • Surface brown spots okay	Refrigerate	• Not recommended	• 35 to 40 minutes	• Use bottled or canned in salads, pita pockets, wraps, stir-fry dishes, dips • Seasonings: marjoram, paprika, parsley, savory
Arugula 1 pound = 8 cups	• Deep green leaves • Crispness	Refrigerate	• Rinse well; leave slightly wet; chop coarsely; cover • 2 minutes per cup • 7 to 10 minutes per 1¼ pound	• Rinse; remove stems; tear into bite-size pieces • 1 to 5 minutes	• Raw in salads or sandwiches • Steamed and tossed with pasta
Asparagus 1 pound = 16 to 20 stalks, or 2½ cups cooked pieces	• Firm, bright green almost entire length (or pale ivory for white variety) • Tightly closed, dry tips	Refrigerate	• Point tips toward center; add 2 tablespoons water; cover • 2 to 3 minutes per cup	• Remove tough lower portion • 3 to 5 minutes for ½-inch-diameter spears • 5 to 10 minutes for spears greater than ½ inch in diameter	• Raw as snack or appetizer; in salads and pita pockets • Hot: steamed whole; sliced in stir-fry dishes and casseroles • Cooked and puréed with nonfat milk for soup • Seasonings: basil, chives, dill, fennel, lemon juice/zest, marjoram, mint, parsley, saffron, savory, tarragon
Beans, green 1 pound = 3 cups (1-inch pieces)	• Slender • Crisp • Bright green • Blemish-free • Avoid beans with with large seeds and swollen pods	Refrigerate	• Whole: add 2 to 3 tablespoons water; cover • 3 to 4 minutes per ½ pound • Cut or sliced into 1-inch pieces: add ¼ cup water and cover • 3 minutes per cup cut • 7 to 12 minutes per pound, cut or whole	• 15 to 18 minutes per pound; stir after 10 minutes	• Raw: whole for snack or appetizer; chopped for salad or pita pockets • Cold: cooked fresh, frozen, or canned; in salads and pita pocket sandwiches • Hot: in stir-fry dishes, soups, casseroles, stews • Seasonings: basil, cayenne, chives, cilantro, cumin, dill, fennel, garlic, mint, parsley

Vegetable and Equivalent Measures	How to Buy Fresh: Qualities to Look For	How to Store Fresh	How to Microwave Fresh	How to Steam Fresh	Ideas for Enjoying More and Seasoning Suggestions
Beans, wax 1 pound = 4 cups (1-inch pieces)	• Pale yellow	Refrigerate	• Whole: add 2 to 3 tablespoons water; cover • 3 to 4 minutes per ½ pound • Cut or sliced; add 2 tablespoons water and cover • 2 to 3 minutes per cup	• 15 to 18 minutes per pound; stir after 10 minutes	• Steam or microwave raw in the pod • Roast in the pod for a snack • Cooked fresh, canned, or frozen in salads, pita pockets, soups, stews • Seasonings (see Beans, green)
Bean sprouts 1 pound = 8 cups	• Crisp buds still attached • Firm • Not overly moist or slimy	Refrigerate	• Add 1 tablespoon water; cover • 1 to 2 minutes per cup	• 1 to 4 minutes	• Raw in sandwiches and salads • Hot in stir-fry dishes, soups, stand-alone side dish • Seasonings: chili powder or chilis, cilantro, curry powder, garlic, ginger, soy sauce
Beets 1 pound (without greens) = 2 cups sliced 1 pound = 3 to 4 beets Skin is edible, but scrub well	• Firm, smooth-skinned • Small to medium • If attached, leaves should be deep green and crisp	Refrigerate	• Slice; add 3 to 4 tablespoons water; cover • 5 to 6 minutes per cup	• 30 to 40 minutes	• Raw slices plain or dipped in horseradish • Roast with rosemary, thyme, or dill • Grill thin slices brushed with extra-virgin olive oil and sprinkled with cloves and cinnamon • Additional seasonings: anise seed, caraway seed, chives, coriander, fennel, ginger, mustard, parsley, savory
Bok choy or Chinese cabbage 1 pound = 12 to 16 cups, sliced	• Several white, bunched stems with thick green leaves • Stems don't form a head	Refrigerate	• Slice or chop; add 2 tablespoons water; cover • 2 to 3 minutes per cup	• Slice or chop; 5 to 8 minutes	• Chop raw stems and leaves for salads, coleslaw • Stir-fry in Asian dishes • Cooked in soups • Seasonings: cayenne, sesame seeds and/or oil, soy sauce
Breadfruit 1 fruit = 2 to 5 pounds Peel is not edible (peel raw or after cooking)	• Resembles green bumpy melon before ripe; brown when ripe • Creamy white inside	Refrigerate	• Not recommended	• Not recommended	• Ripe: enjoy raw • Unripe: slice and bake, boil, or panfry

(continued)

THE ULTIMATE VEGETABLE BUYING, STORAGE, AND COOKING CHART *(continued)*

Vegetable and Equivalent Measures	How to Buy Fresh: Qualities to Look For	How to Store Fresh	How to Microwave Fresh	How to Steam Fresh	Ideas for Enjoying More and Seasoning Suggestions
Broccoli 1 pound = 4 cups pieces; = 2 cups florets; = 3 cups spears	• Tight, closed buds • Brilliant dark green and/or purplish blue-green • Leaves should be crisp • Avoid leaves with yellowish or brownish tint and thick woody stems	Refrigerate	• Point florets toward center; add 2 tablespoons water; cover • 2 to 3 minutes per cup	• 13 to 15 minutes per pound for spears • 5 to 8 minutes per pound for florets • 4 to 6 minutes for 1 pound of pieces	• Raw or frozen (thawed) as snack or appetizer • Frozen works well in nearly all cooked dishes and in pita pockets • Seasonings: garlic, lemon juice/zest, mace, nutmeg, pepper (black/red), Parmesan
Brussels sprouts 1 pound = 4 cups	• Small, bright green sprouts that are tightly closed • Feel firm and heavy for their size	Refrigerate unwashed in an airtight plastic bag	• Peel away wilted or brown outer leaves; add 2 tablespoons water; cover • 3 to 4 minutes per cup • 8 to 10 minutes per pound	• Cut "X" into stems • 15 to 20 minutes per pound	• Steam or microwave lightly; overcooking tends to bring out bitter flavor • Seasonings: basil, chives, garlic, horseradish, mustard, sweet-and-sour sauce, thyme
Cabbage, red or green 1 pound = 4 cups shredded	• Firm heads that feel heavy • Outer leaves have good color and are free of blemishes	Refrigerate	• Remove outer leaves; cut into chunks; add 2 tablespoons water; cover • 4 to 6 minutes per average cabbage	• Trim outer leaves; cut into quarters or shred • 20 to 23 minutes per average cabbage in quarters • 8 to 12 minutes per average cabbage shredded	• Great raw or cooked • Seasonings: basil, caraway, cumin, dill, garlic, ginger, mustard, pepper (black or red), savory, vinegar, sesame seeds
Cactus pads	• Look like cactus leaves	Refrigerate	• Not recommended	• Remove thorns; slice • 8 to 10 minutes per pound	• Simmer on stove top or steam in microwave
Carrots 1 pound = 2½ cups shredded or 2½ cups diced Skin is edible	• Firm, well-shaped with bright orange-gold color • If tops are attached, should be crisp • Avoid carrots that are withered or soft	Refrigerate	• Slice; add 2 tablespoons water; cover • 3 to 4 minutes per cup	• Cut into ¼-inch slices or leave whole • 16 to 19 minutes per pound if sliced; stir once after 10 minutes • 21 to 24 minutes whole; stir once after 10 minutes	• Raw or frozen (thawed) as snacks, in sandwiches • Boil, steam, sauté in stir-fry dishes, cooked and mashed • Seasonings: caraway, cinnamon, cloves, dill, mace, nutmeg, tarragon

Vegetable and Equivalent Measures	How to Buy Fresh: Qualities to Look For	How to Store Fresh	How to Microwave Fresh	How to Steam Fresh	Ideas for Enjoying More and Seasoning Suggestions
Cassava (also yucca) 1 pound = 2 cups cooked Skin is edible, but not when it is waxed for longer keeping	• Thick brown peel • Inside, white or yellow like a potato • Two varieties: sweet (crisp white flesh) and bitter (toxic until cooked)	Refrigerate	• Not recommended	• Not recommended	• Cooked in dishes similar to potatoes (boiled, mashed) • Needs moist-heat cooking, such as boiling or in soups; dries out when baked • Seasonings: allspice, basil, curry powder, nutmeg, paprika
Cauliflower 1 small = 1½ pounds (4 cups florets)	• Firm compact creamy-white heads (without brown spots) • Florets pressed tightly together • Leaves crisp and bright green • Avoid yellow tinge and spreading florets, which indicate over-maturity	Refrigerate	• Separate into florets; add 2 tablespoons water; cover • 3 to 4 minutes per 2 cups • 8 to 10 minutes per pound	• Remove core; cut into 2-inch-diameter florets • 20 to 25 minutes per average cauliflower; stir once after 15 minutes	• Roast with dill, beets, extra-virgin olive oil • Purée cooked or frozen (thawed) with nonfat milk for soup • Seasonings: basil, cumin, dill, ginger, lemon juice/zest, mace, marjoram, mustard, nutmeg, savory, tarragon, thyme
Celeriac (member of celery family) 1 pound = 2½ cups grated = 1 cup cooked, puréed Skin and leaves are not edible	• Fibrous brown bumpy peel		• Not recommended	• Peel, slice root only • 8 to 12 minutes per cup	• Enjoy root but not leaves • Peel and enjoy raw as a snack or in salads • Peel and boil or steam; top with favorite seasonings • Use in place of celery in soups or stews • Seasonings: basil, fennel, marjoram, tarragon
Celery 1 rib = ½ cup sliced	• Crisp rigid green ribs surrounding a tender heart, topped with leaves, forming a stalk • Fresh-looking leaves • Avoid limp stalks, wilted and/or brown leaves	Refrigerate	• Slice or chop; add 2 table-spoons water; cover • 2 to 3 minutes per cup	• Slice • 8 to 12 minutes per cup	• Raw as a snack or an appetizer, plain or filled with peanut butter and raisins or other diced fruit; dipped in salsa • Seasonings: anise seed, basil, caraway seed, celery seed, fennel, mace, marjoram, parsley, tarragon, turmeric

(continued)

THE ULTIMATE VEGETABLE BUYING, STORAGE, AND COOKING CHART *(continued)*

Vegetable and Equivalent Measures	How to Buy Fresh: Qualities to Look For	How to Store Fresh	How to Microwave Fresh	How to Steam Fresh	Ideas for Enjoying More and Seasoning Suggestions
Chard (also Swiss chard) 1 pound = 1⅓ to 2 cups cooked	• Greens on creamy white or red stalks • Large, crinkled dark green leaves	Refrigerate	• Rinse well; leave slightly wet; chop coarsely; cover • 2 minutes per cup • 7 to 10 minutes per 1¼ pound	• Rinse; remove stems; tear into bite-sized pieces • 1 to 5 minutes	• Use cooked or frozen (thawed) like spinach and collards; sautéed, soup, stir-fry dishes • Seasonings: basil, cardamom, cayenne, chervil, nutmeg, sesame seed
Chayote 1 pound = 3 cups sliced = 1 cup cooked and mashed	• Pale green, pear-shaped, gourdlike fruit used like a vegetable • Creamy white flesh	Refrigerate	• Not recommended	• Scrub well; cut in half • 30 to 35 minutes per medium	• Use as you would squash; bake, broil, braise, stuff, and bake • Choose assertive seasonings to enhance its mild flavor: cayenne, chives, dill, ginger, oregano, tarragon
Chilis 1 pound = 2½ cups chopped; = 3 cups sliced Skin and seeds are edible, but they add more "heat"	• Deep, vivid colors • Smaller chilis much hotter than larger ones	Refrigerate; can be dried and stored in a tightly sealed container at room temperature	• Not recommended	• Slice or chop, using gloves	• Use latex gloves when chopping chilis, as the capsaicin they contain can get into cuts and be transferred to eyes, resulting in painful burning
Corn 2 medium ears = 1 cup kernels	• Green husks • Moist stems • Silk ends free of decay or worm injury • When pierced with a thumbnail, kernels should give a squirt of juice • Avoid tough skins, which indicate overmaturity	Refrigerate	• Wrap each ear of corn in plastic wrap; microwave 10 to 13 minutes on high	• Husk and remove silk • 20 minutes	• Seasonings: chili powder, chives, cilantro, coriander, cumin, dill, oregano, sage, tarragon
Cucumbers 1 pound = 50 to 60 slices. Skin is edible	• Firm, dark green and slender • Avoid soft or yellow	Refrigerate	• Not recommended	• Not recommended	• Seasonings: dill, mint, oregano, parsley
Daikon (also Asian radish) 1 medium = 1½ cups chopped or sliced	• Looks like smooth thick white parsnip • Should be very white with a minimum of cracking; should not look dry • Has sweet flavor and juicy white crisp flesh	Refrigerate	• Slice; add 2 tablespoons water; cover • 3 to 4 minutes per cup	• Slice • 8 to 12 minutes per cup	• Raw in salads and sushi • Shredded raw as a garnish • Chop and sauté in stir-fry dishes • Seasonings: cayenne, garlic, parsley, sesame seed

Vegetable and Equivalent Measures	How to Buy Fresh: Qualities to Look For	How to Store Fresh	How to Microwave Fresh	How to Steam Fresh	Ideas for Enjoying More and Seasoning Suggestions
Dasheen (also called yautia) 1 pound = 2½ cups cubed Skin is edible, but is often removed	• Large round root vegetable with a coarse brown peel (looks much like taro)	Refrigerate	• Slice; add 2 tablespoons water; cover • 3 to 4 minutes per cup	• Slice • 8 to 12 minutes per cup	• Raw (but very strong flavor) • Baked • Boiled, alone or in soup • Leaves used as greens • Seasonings: basil, chives, garlic, nutmeg
Eggplant 1 pound = 8 1-inch slices or 4 cups diced Peel is edible and adds fiber and nutrients	• Firm, heavy for size, with taut glassy deeply colored skin • Stems bright green	Refrigerate	• Slice thinly; 4 minutes on high	• Slice into ½-inch slices • 15 to 20 minutes per pound	• Boil, grill, bake, stuff and bake • Seasonings: basil, garlic, oregano, sage, thyme
Fennel 1 pound = 3 cups chopped = 2½ cups grated = 2 cups cooked	• Looks like a squat bunch of celery with feathery leaves • Licorice aroma	Refrigerate	• Slice; add 2 tablespoons water; cover • 3 to 4 minutes per cup	• Slice • 8 to 12 minutes per cup	• Bulb or stalks also braised, sautéed, roasted, used in soups • Leaves used in salads, as an herb for flavoring other foods • Seasonings: basil, cardamom, garlic, lemon, lemon pepper, mace, oregano
Jerusalem artichoke 1 pound = 3 cups chopped or sliced	• Knobby and irregular shape • Light brown or purplish red peel • No relation to globe artichokes	Refrigerate	• Slice; add 2 tablespoons water; cover • 3 to 4 minutes per cup	• Slice • 8 to 12 minutes per cup	• Enjoy raw • Often cooked in its peel; a little lemon juice in the cooking water keeps peeled Jerusalem artichokes from browning • Cook and use in dishes calling for potatoes • Seasonings: basil, chives, mustard, nutmeg, thyme
Jicama 1 pound = 2 cups chopped = 2½ cups sliced Skin not edible; peel and discard prior to use	• Firm, well-formed tubers free of blemishes • Thin brown outer skin • Size does not affect flavor, but larger roots tend to have a coarse texture • White, crisp flesh that is sweet, nutty and refreshing	Refrigerate for optimum quality up to 3 weeks before cutting; after cutting, wrap tightly and refrigerate up to 1 week	• Slice; add 2 tablespoons water; cover • 3 to 4 minutes per cup	• Slice • 10 to 15 minutes per cup	• Raw: peel and slice into thin strips and dip into salsa; use in place of water chestnuts; season with lime juice, cayenne, and garlic for an interesting salad • Cook in stir-fry dishes or boil and mash (as you would potatoes)

(continued)

THE ULTIMATE VEGETABLE BUYING, STORAGE, AND COOKING CHART *(continued)*

Vegetable and Equivalent Measures	How to Buy Fresh: Qualities to Look For	How to Store Fresh	How to Microwave Fresh	How to Steam Fresh	Ideas for Enjoying More and Seasoning Suggestions
Kelp	• Brown seaweed that is harvested, sun-dried, and formed into sheets	Refrigerate	• Not recommended	• Not recommended	• Used in Japanese cooking • Raw, wrapped around sushi • Pickled, used as a condiment
Kale 1 pound = 1⅓ to 2 cups cooked	• Doesn't form a head • Richly colored, deep grayish-green leaves with no signs of wilting or yellowing	Refrigerate	• Rinse well; leave slightly wet; chop coarsely; cover • 2 minutes per cup • 7 to 10 minutes per 1¼ pound	• Rinse; remove stems; tear into bite-sized pieces • 1 to 5 minutes	• Use in salads raw, mixed with milder flavored greens, such as romaine or red-leaf lettuce • Cook and use as you would spinach • Sauté with a dash of extra-virgin olive oil, lemon juice, and fresh ginger as side dish • Add to soups, such as Lentil-black bean soup with a Tex-Mex flair and wild rice soup
Kohlrabi 1 pound = 2½ cups cubed or chopped Skin is edible	• Looks like a turnip • Can be light green, white, or purple • Should have young tender bulbs with fresh green leaves; the smaller the bulb, the more delicate the flavor and texture • Avoid those with scars and blemishes	Refrigerate	• Slice; add 2 tablespoons water; cover • 3 to 4 minutes per cup	• Slice • 10 to 15 minutes per cup	• Trim away woody, tough skin of larger varieties • Enjoy raw slices as snacks and on appetizer trays, or in salads with shredded carrots, water chestnuts, sesame seeds, green onions, and vinaigrette dressing • Slice and use in stir-fry dishes • Steam and season with favorite herbs and spices
Lettuce, endive 1 head = 1¼ pounds = 6 cups bite-sized pieces = 10 cups shredded; 1 pound = 25 to 30 leaves	• Fresh crisp tender leaves free of blemishes or yellow color • Look for deeply colored leaves • Avoid bunches with thick, coarse-veined leaves	Refrigerate	• Not recommended	• Not recommended	• Raw in salads, enhanced by walnuts and pears • Braised as side dish

Vegetable and Equivalent Measures	How to Buy Fresh: Qualities to Look For	How to Store Fresh	How to Microwave Fresh	How to Steam Fresh	Ideas for Enjoying More and Seasoning Suggestions
Lettuce, iceberg 1 head = 1¼ pounds = 6 cups bite-sized pieces = 10 cups shredded; 1 pound = 25 to 30 leaves	• Tight heads, medium green in color • Avoid heads with yellow discoloration or brown leaves	Refrigerate; does not freeze well	• Not recommended	• Not recommended	• Remove outer leaves before using • Raw in salads or sandwiches
Lettuce, romaine 1 pound = 6 cups leaves	• Dark green, broad crisp leaves • Avoid those with yellowed, browned or shriveled leaves	Refrigerate; does not freeze well	• Generally not recommended	• Not recommended	• Raw in salads and sandwiches • Flash-fried Hawaiian style (recipe page 441)
Lettuce, chicory or curly endive 1 pound = 6 cups leaves	• Frizzy green leaf in a loose head	Refrigerate; does not freeze well	• Not recommended	• Not recommended	• Adds a nice touch to mixed-green salads (can be bitter, so use in small amounts)
Lettuce, escarole 1 pound = 6 cups leaves	• Green leaves have a reddish tinge • Leaves form a loose head	Refrigerate; does not freeze well	• Rinse well; leave slightly wet; chop coarsely; cover • 2 minutes per cup • 7 to 10 minutes per 1¼ pound	• Not recommended	• Raw in salads • Cooked in soups and as side dish
Lettuce, radicchio 1 pound = 6 cups leaves	• Small, purplish head of leaves with white ribs	Refrigerate; does not freeze well	• Rinse well; leave slightly wet; chop coarsely; cover • 2 minutes per cup • 7 to 10 minutes per 1¼ pound	• Rinse; remove stems; tear into bite-sized pieces • 1 to 5 minutes	• Raw, adds nice touch to salads • Steamed or stir-fried, great addition to pasta or stir-fry dishes
Lotus root 1 pound = 2¼ cups diced Skin is edible, but scrub well Root, stem, leaves, and seeds all edible	• Root of the water lily • Outside, root is smooth and green • Inside, several large air pockets run length of root (which makes it buoyant in water)	Refrigerate; does not freeze well	• Slice; add 2 tablespoons water; cover • 3 to 4 minutes per cup	• Slice • 10 to 15 minutes per cup	• Often eaten peeled • Stir-fried, steamed, or braised with mixed Chinese dishes • Seasonings: chili powder, coriander, curry powder, ginger, paprika, turmeric

(continued)

THE ULTIMATE VEGETABLE BUYING, STORAGE, AND COOKING CHART *(continued)*

Vegetable and Equivalent Measures	How to Buy Fresh: Qualities to Look For	How to Store Fresh	How to Microwave Fresh	How to Steam Fresh	Ideas for Enjoying More and Seasoning Suggestions
Mushrooms 1 pound = 6 cups sliced, or 4 cups diced	• Blemish-free, without slimy spots or signs of decay • Tightly closed caps	Refrigerate	• Slice; add 2 tablespoons water; cover • 3 to 4 minutes per cup	• Slice • 8 to 12 minutes per cup	• Raw in salads, sandwiches, appetizer tray • Cooked sliced in stir-fry dishes, soups, casseroles • Side dish (with garlic and onions) • Seasonings: garlic, oregano, rosemary, tarragon, thyme
Okra 1 pound = 2 cups chopped	• Small to medium in size • Deep green and free of blemishes • Pods should snap or puncture easily with slight pressure	Refrigerate	• Slice; add 2 tablespoons water; cover • 5 to 6 minutes per cup	• Slice • 15 to 20 minutes per cup	• Cooked in gumbos, soups, stews • Seasonings: basil, Cajun and Creole, garlic, oregano
Onions, white, red, or yellow 1 pound = 3 large 1 large = 1 cup chopped	• Heavy for size • Avoid onions with soft spots or with sprouting green shoots	Store whole at room temperature in cool dry place; refrigerate cut	• Chop; add 2 tablespoons water; cover • 3 minutes per cup	• Slice • 8 to 12 minutes per cup	• Raw or cooked • Seasonings: cinnamon, garlic, nutmeg, savory • Tip: Have a hard time cutting raw onion because your eyes water? Try putting the onion in the freezer for 20 minutes to 1 hour before peeling and chopping—and cry no more
Onions, green (also called scallion) 1 bunch (6 to 8) = 4 ounces = ⅓ cup chopped = 1 cup sliced	• Crisp, bright green tops and clean white bottoms • Evenly colored green stems that are wilt-free • Firm, dry, with brittle outer skin	Refrigerate	• Chop; add 2 tablespoons water; cover • 3 minutes per cup	• Slice • 8 to 12 minutes per cup	• Raw, use tops and bulbs, one or both, depending on recipe and color interests • Cooked, slice thinly and use in a wide variety of soups, casseroles, stir-fry dishes, vegetable sides
Onions, leeks	• Looks like a bigger, sturdier, flat-leaved version of green onions • Clean white bottoms and crisp fresh-looking green tops	Refrigerate	• Slice or chop; add 2 tablespoons water; cover • 3 minutes per cup	• Slice • 10 to 15 minutes per cup	• Prior to cooking, clean well to remove soil that gets between the leaves (slit in half lengthwise to better wash out dirt) • Milder in flavor than onions add great flavor to cooked and raw dishes • Bulbs often sliced and used in soups or baked in casseroles • Leaves used raw in salads

Vegetable and Equivalent Measures	How to Buy Fresh: Qualities to Look For	How to Store Fresh	How to Microwave Fresh	How to Steam Fresh	Ideas for Enjoying More and Seasoning Suggestions
Parsnips 1 pound = 4 medium Skin is edible	• Small to medium, smooth, firm, well shaped, and creamy white in color • Avoid large roots because they may have a woody core	Store at room temperature in cool dry place	• Slice; add 2 tablespoons water; cover • 3 to 5 minutes per cup	• Scrub well; slice into 1-inch slices • 16 to 19 minutes per pound	• Blend well with many flavors • Slice and use in beef stew, with roasted pork tenderloin, roasted with carrots, or cooked and mashed with reduced-fat cream cheese, nonfat milk, salt, and pepper • Seasonings: allspice, basil, curry powder, nutmeg, paprika
Peas 1 pound (green, in pod) = 1 cup shelled	• Small plump, bright green pods that are firm, crisp, and well-filled	Refrigerate	• Add 2 to 3 tablespoons water; cover • 3 to 4 minutes per cup		• Steamed, microwaved, or boiled fresh or frozen and thawed, use cold in salads, pita pockets, or heated in casseroles, soups, stir-fry dishes • Seasonings: chervil, horseradish, mint, pepper
Peppers, bell 1 large = 6 ounces =1 cup diced 1 pound = 2 to 3 medium	• Bright, glossy, firm, and well-shaped • Avoid those with soft spots or gashes	Refrigerate	• Slice or chop; add 1 to 2 tablespoons water; cover • 1 to 2 minutes per cup	• Slice or chop • 5 to 8 minutes per cup	• Cold, sliced or chopped: in salads, stuffed into pita pocket sandwiches, folded into wraps, or for snack or appetizer • Hot, sliced, or chopped: in stir-fry dishes, casseroles, soups • Hot, whole: stuffed with rice, meat, chicken, seafood, and/or other vegetables, and baked • Seasonings: basil, garlic, oregano
Potatoes, red, white, and baking Red 1 pound = 4 medium White 1 pound = 3 medium = 2¼ cups diced or sliced = 1¾ cups mashed Baking 1 pound = 1 large Skin is edible	• Firm, smooth, with no wrinkles, sprouts, cracks, bruises, decay, or bitter green areas	Store at room temperature in cool dry place	• Scrub skin well with brush and water; pierce 5 to 6 times with a fork; place on paper towel • 4 to 5 minutes per one medium potato • Add 2 to 3 minutes per each additional potato cooked at same time	• Scrub well with brush and water; cut in half • 30 to 35 minutes per medium potato	• Boil or bake • Seasonings: caraway, dill, garlic, mint, pepper, rosemary, thyme

(continued)

THE ULTIMATE VEGETABLE BUYING, STORAGE, AND COOKING CHART *(continued)*

Vegetable and Equivalent Measures	How to Buy Fresh: Qualities to Look For	How to Store Fresh	How to Microwave Fresh	How to Steam Fresh	Ideas for Enjoying More and Seasoning Suggestions
Potatoes, sweet 1 pound = 3 medium Skin is edible	• Firm, well shaped with bright, uniformly burnt orange skin	Store at room temperature in cool dry place	• Scrub skin well with brush and water; pierce 5 to 6 times with a fork; place on paper towel • 4 to 5 minutes per 1 medium potato • Add 2 to 3 minutes per each additional potato cooked at same time	• Scrub well with brush and water; cut in half • 30 to 35 minutes per medium potato	• Bake, boil, or use in stir-fry dishes • Seasonings: cardamom, cinnamon, cloves, nutmeg
Pumpkins 1 medium = about 5 pounds; 1 pound = 4 cups (pared, cubed), or 1 cup (cooked, mashed) Skin is very tough, but is edible when boiled (scrub well)	• Choose evenly orange/burnt orange pumpkin without soft spots	Store at room temperature in cool dry place	• Scrub skin well with brush and water; cut into serving-sized pieces; remove seeds and fiber; place in dish (cut side up); sprinkle surface with ¼ cup water or fruit juice; cover • 10 to 13 minutes per small	• Scrub well; cut in half • 30 to 35 minutes per medium	• Bake whole, seasoned with brown sugar, cinnamon, and cloves • Peel, cube, boil, and mash with reduced-fat cream cheese and nonfat milk • Peel, cube, boil, and purée for pies • Seasonings: cardamom, cinnamon, cloves, nutmeg
Radishes 1 pound = 45 to 50 each	• Firm when gently squeezed • Attached leaves should be green and crisp	Refrigerate	• Not recommended	• Not recommended	• Enjoy raw, whole, or sliced • Flavor varies from mild to peppery • For added crispness, soak radishes in ice water for a couple of hours • Radishes can also be cooked
Rutabagas 1 pound = 2½ cups cubed; while skin is edible, most people peel before using (scrub well if eating peel)	• Root vegetable with a turniplike appearance • Thin, pale yellow skin and a slightly sweet, firm flesh of the same color • Choose rutabagas that are small to medium, smooth, firm, and heavy for their size	Store at room temperature in cool dry place	• Slice; add 2 tablespoons water; cover • 4 to 6 minutes per cup	• Scrub well; slice into 1-inch slices • 16 to 19 minutes per pound	• Use in any recipe that calls for turnips, such as soups, stews, and casseroles; can also be boiled and mashed

Vegetable and Equivalent Measures	How to Buy Fresh: Qualities to Look For	How to Store Fresh	How to Microwave Fresh	How to Steam Fresh	Ideas for Enjoying More and Seasoning Suggestions
Seaweed (also kelp, nori)	• Purchase dried	Refrigerate or store at room temperature in cool, dry place	• Not recommended	• Not recommended	• Used most often in Asian dishes and some Irish, Welsh, and Scottish dishes • Use in soups, sushi, as tea
Shallots 1 large = 1 tablespoon minced	• Firm, papery-covered bulbs that are pale brown, pale gray or rose	Store at room temperature in cool dry place	• Chop; add 2 tablespoons water; cover • 3 minutes per cup	• Not recommended	• Use raw or cooked when you want a mild, gentle onion flavor
Spinach 1 pound = 10 cups leaves = 1½ cups cooked	• Small leaves with deep green color and a crisp, springy texture • Sweet-smelling leaves with fairly thin stems • Avoid wilted, crushed or bruised leaves	Refrigerate	• Rinse well; leave slightly wet; chop coarsely; cover • 2 minutes per cup • 7 to 10 minutes per 1¼ pound	• Rinse; remove stems; tear into bite-sized pieces • 1 to 5 minutes	• Raw in salads, sandwiches • Cooked as vegetable side (steamed, wilted, sautéed, stir-fried) • In soup, pasta, and stir-fry dishes • Frozen spinach works well in many recipes • Seasonings: garlic, lemon juice/zest, nutmeg, pepper
Squash, summer (also zucchini) 1 pound = 3 cups sliced = 2½ cups chopped Skin is edible, but scrub well	• Yellow squash and zucchini of medium size with firm, smooth, glossy, tender skin • Heavy for its size	Refrigerate	• Slice; add 2 tablespoons water; cover • 3 minutes per cup	• Cut into ¼-inch slices • 15 minutes per pound; stir once after 9 minutes	• Raw: slice, chop, or grate for appetizer • Seasonings: allspice, chives, dill, ginger marjoram, paprika, tarragon
Squash, winter 1 pound = 1 cup mashed Skin is very tough, but is edible (scrub well)	• Hard, thick skins and seeds • Many colors; choose one that is deep-colored and free of blemishes or moldy spots	Store at room temperature in cool dry place	• Scrub skin well with brush and water; cut into serving-sized pieces; remove seeds and fiber; place in dish (cut side up); sprinkle surface with ¼ cup water or fruit juice; cover • 10 to 13 minutes per 1½ to 2 pounds cut into chunks; 4 to 5 minutes per cup	• Scrub well; cut in half • 45 to 60 minutes for 1½ to 2 pound squash	• Remove seeds and bake, simmer, soufflé, steam • Roast the seeds for a crunchy snack • Seasonings: caraway, cardamom, cayenne, cinammon, cloves, nutmeg

(continued)

THE ULTIMATE VEGETABLE BUYING, STORAGE, AND COOKING CHART *(continued)*

Vegetable and Equivalent Measures	How to Buy Fresh: Qualities to Look For	How to Store Fresh	How to Microwave Fresh	How to Steam Fresh	Ideas for Enjoying More and Seasoning Suggestions
Taro 1 pound = 2½ cups diced, chopped, or sliced Skin is *not* edible Taro *must* be cooked as its sap may irritate the throat; cooking eliminates it	• Rough, brown or purplish tuber that looks much like a yam, although some varieties do not	Refrigerate	• Chop; add 2 tablespoons water; cover • 4 to 6 minutes per cup	• Scrub well; slice into ¼-inch slices • 16 to 19 minutes per pound	• Leaves are edible and generally cooked in soup • Taro is peeled and usually boiled, baked, or fried, much like potatoes • Used to make Hawaiian "poi"
Tomatillos 1 pound = 16 medium Skin is edible, but scrub well	• Paperlike husk • Under husk, looks like small green tomato	Refrigerate	• Not recommended	• Not recommended	• Often used in food like a green tomato, especially in Southwest and Mexican dishes • Dice for use in salads • Dice and boil with jalapeño peppers for salsa • Dice and combine with onions for an omelet • Seasonings: cilantro, coriander, cumin
Tomatoes, cherry or grape 1 pint = about 25 tomatoes	• Smooth, well formed, firm; not hard • Avoid those with puckers or soft spots	• Store ripe tomatoes at room temperature and use within a few days • Refrigeration can make flesh pulpy and greatly lessens flavor • Unripe tomato can be ripened by placing in in pierced paper bag with an apple for several days at room temperature • Do not set in sun	• Not recommended	• Not recommended	• Cooked or raw • Seasonings: allspice, basil, celery seed, chives, cilantro, dill, garlic, oregano, parsley, sage, tarragon

Vegetable and Equivalent Measures	How to Buy Fresh: Qualities to Look For	How to Store Fresh	How to Microwave Fresh	How to Steam Fresh	Ideas for Enjoying More and Seasoning Suggestions
Tomatoes, all large varieties 1 pound = 4 small, 3 medium or 2 large; 1 medium = 1 cup chopped; 1 pound (peeled and seeded) = 1½ cups pulp, or 12 slices	• Firm, well-shaped, richly colored for their variety • Free from blemishes, heavy for size • Should give slightly to palm pressure	• Store ripe tomatoes at room temperature and use within a few days • Refrigeration can make flesh pulpy and greatly lessens flavor • Unripe tomato can be ripened by placing in pierced paper bag with an apple for several days at room temperature • Do not refrigerate or set in sun	• Not recommended	• Not recommended	• Raw or fresh in a multitude of ways • Seasonings: allspice, basil, celery seed, chives, cilantro, dill, garlic, oregano, parsley, sage, tarragon
Turnips 1 pound = 3 medium = 2 cups cooked Skin is edible, but many people remove	• Firm, smooth, small to medium size; heavy for their size • Greens fresh, without yellowing or wilting	Store at room temperature in cool dry place	• Slice; add 2 tablespoons water; cover • 4 to 6 minutes per cup	• Scrub well; slice into ¼-inch slices • 16 to 19 minutes per pound	• Boil, bake, or roast • Greens are edible—as well as tasty and highly nutritious • Steam or sauté gently • Seasonings: allspice, anise seed, curry powder, rosemary, savory
Yams Skin is edible, but scrub well	• Firm, well shaped with uniformly colored skin • Not related to sweet potato, yams are mellow yellow in color • Sweeter flavor than sweet potato	Store at room temperature in cool dry place	• Scrub skin well with brush and water; pierce 5 to 6 times with a fork; place on paper towel • 4 to 5 minutes per 1 medium potato • Add 2 to 3 minutes per each additional potato cooked at same time	• Scrub well with brush and water; cut in half • 30 to 35 minutes per medium potato	• Bake, boil for use in stir-fry dishes • Add chopped raw pieces to soups and stews • Mash • Seasonings: cardamom, cinnamon, cloves, nutmeg
Yucca (see Cassava)					
Zucchini (see Squash, summer)					

Microwaving

Microwaving vegetables is an excellent cooking technique for preserving nutrients, bright color, and fresh taste. A wonderful bonus is that you can serve the vegetables in the cooking dish, so cleanup is a snap. Follow these guidelines for optimal results:

- Use microwave-safe containers.
- Cut vegetables into same-sized pieces for even cooking.
- Stir halfway through the cooking time. (Refer to the preceding vegetable table and follow package directions for cooking frozen vegetables.)
- Cover food loosely so that steam escapes. (Use waxed paper, a reusable microwave cover, or leave the lid of the cooking container slightly ajar to allow for steam release.)
- Pierce whole, unpeeled vegetables to speed cooking time and to prevent them from bursting during cooking.
- Remove vegetables from the microwave oven when barely tender, as they continue to cook. Stir upon removing, and let stand three to five minutes covered.

Steaming

Steaming is another excellent way to help retain vegetable flavor and nutrients. An additional advantage is that you can cook vegetables without adding fat. Place steamed vegetables in a steaming basket over, never in, the cooking water. Instead, steam encircles the food to cook it. To steam vegetables:

- Choose a pot deep enough to accommodate the steaming basket (so that it remains above the water).
- Pour 1 to 2 inches of water in the pot.
- Put the steaming basket into the pot; it should sit about ½ to 2 inches above the water.

Cut the vegetables into small pieces; place them in the basket.

Cover the pot with a lid.

Heat the water to boiling; cover.

Check the water occasionally; add additional water to the bottom of the pot as needed.

Add lime juice, lemon juice, fresh herbs, and/or wine to the cooking water to infuse interesting flavors into the vegetables.

Sautéing

Sauté vegetables alone or as part of a stir-fry dish with poultry, meat, fish, or tofu. While traditional recipes often call for oil or butter in fairly large amounts, note that very little fat is needed to create fabulous sautéed or stir-fried dishes. To sauté vegetables easily and with less fat:

- Choose a nonstick pan; spray it with nonstick cooking spray.
- Use 1 teaspoon to 2 tablespoons vegetable oil, such as extra-virgin olive, canola, sesame, peanut, or walnut.
- Enhance the flavor by adding herbs, minced garlic, minced fresh ginger, or minced onions to the oil. Add any combination of these flavor enhancers and sauté over low heat for three to five minutes, allowing the flavors to fully release into the oil.
- Clean and slice or chop the vegetables into bite-sized pieces. That helps the flavor-enhancing ingredients contact more of the vegetable, thereby yielding a tastier product.
- Extend the oil (if needed) with chicken, beef, or vegetable broth, or fish stock, depending on the mix of ingredients.

Grilling

Grilling provides a different way to enjoy vegetables. In addition, if you are grilling your main course, all of your cooking efforts are centralized in one place, making cooking easier and more efficient. To grill:

- Blanch vegetables that require more cooking time, such as potatoes, to shorten the grilling time.
- Marinate vegetables thirty minutes at room temperature or a minimum of two hours if refrigerated. Use reduced-fat salad dressings, or create your own marinade with herbs, juices, vinegars, and measured amounts of oils. Marinating not only makes vegetables more flavorful but also helps them cook faster.
- Scrub the grill grates with a metal brush before and after cooking.
- Lubricate the grill by dipping a soft cloth in vegetable oil and lightly coating the grates before turning on the grill to avoid getting burned.
- Heat the grill to medium-high:

  Place the vegetables on the grill grates and sear the skins. Turn every one to two minutes with tongs.

  Alternatively, place the vegetables in a grilling basket, which allows you to turn vegetables less often with a large spoon or a spatula.

Pierce the vegetables with a fork to determine doneness. Vegetables are done when they are fork-tender.

Roasting

Roasting intensifies flavors, and it too can be a wonderful adventure in enjoying vegetables. Roasting caramelizes the natural sugars in vegetables and brings out many complex taste sensations. During roasting, vegetables cook in their own natural juices.

To roast, you'll need just a heavy roasting pan or a clay roaster with a tightly fitting cover. If lacking a lid, use heavy foil. Then:

1. Preheat the oven to 400°F.
2. Scrub the vegetables with a brush and water.
3. Cut or chop the vegetables into uniform-sized pieces.
4. Toss with a measured amount of extra-virgin olive oil, herbs, and/or minced garlic.
5. Seal the pan tightly to decrease the roasting time and enhance the flavors.
6. To brown further, uncover the vegetables during the last ten to fifteen minutes of roasting time.

Fruit Buying, Storage, and Use Guide

Fresh fruit can be difficult to buy; storing can be even more of a mystery. Use our guide to help you enjoy your favorite fruits—and some new ones, too. Note that we have included varietal information for some fruits and not others, based on what you need to know to purchase and use the fruit.

IS DRIED FRUIT A HEALTHY ALTERNATIVE?

In addition to being perennially available, dried fruit is an excellent way to enjoy fruit on the road, in baking, and on salads. In addition, tropical fruits not available fresh or frozen might be sold in dried form. Dried fruit is calorically dense, so watching portion size can help you keep an eye on your calorie goals.

Dried fruits may be preserved with sulfite, which can trigger allergic reactions in some people. If you or someone you prepare food for is sulfite-sensitive, read the labels to find out if sulfites are present.

HOW TO BUY, STORE, AND USE FRUIT

Fruit	Subtype of Fruit; Color and Taste	Preparation Methods and Tips	Buying Tips	How to Store
Applesauce 1-pound jar = 2 cups	Cortland • Red with white flesh • Pleasant tartness	• Breaks down with cooking, best for applesauce	• Firm fruit • Avoid bruises, broken skin, or brown spots • Choose fruit with a pleasant smell • Skin coloration depends on the variety	• Apples continue to ripen at room temperature ten times faster than when refrigerated • Store less than 7 days at room temperature. If storing more than 7 days (up to 3 weeks), place in back of refrigerator in plastic bag
Apples Dried 1 cup = 2⅔ cups cooked 6-ounce package = 1 cup Fresh 1 medium = 1 cup sliced 1 pound = 3 cups sliced	Empire • Red or green • Tart-sweet • Cross between Red Delicious and McIntosh	• Eaten raw or applesauce		
	Fuji • Yellowish green • Sweet/spicy • Japanese origin	• Eaten raw		
	Gala • Golden/rosy • Sweet/crisp • New Zealand origin	• Raw, sautéeing, or slow baking		
	Golden Delicious • Yellowish • Sweet/juicy • Flesh does not darken as readily	• Raw, frying, pies • Holds shape during cooking		
	Granny Smith • Bright green • Sweet/tart • Australia origin	• Raw, sautéeing, baking		
	Honeycrisp • Large with streaks of red and green • Mellow/juicy/crisp	• Raw or cooked		
	Jonathan • Golden with red stripes • Juicy yellow flesh	• Raw, baking or cooking		
	McIntosh • Red skin • Crisp/juicy • Available in fall	• Flesh softens with cooking, applesauce		

(continued)

HOW TO BUY, STORE, AND USE FRUIT *(continued)*

Fruit	Subtype of Fruit; Color and Taste	Preparation Methods and Tips	Buying Tips	How to Store
Apples *(continued)*	Red Delicious • Dark red/red • Sweet/juicy • Available all year but best in summer • Buy during peak season for best quality	• Raw or applesauce, not for baking or frying		
	Rome Beauty • Large red • Sweet-tart	• Baking whole/stuffed		
Apricots Dried 1 cup = 2 cups cooked 1 6-ounce package = 1 cup Fresh 1 pound = 2 cups sliced 1 pound = 8 to 12 medium 2 medium = ½ cup sliced	• Range from orange with deep yellow flesh to golden yellow with red blush • Fragrant, juicy, rich flavor	• Eaten raw, dried, cooked	• Best when ripened on tree since they don't improve in flavor after they are picked • Choose uniform gold-orange plump fruit • Choose fragrant fruit that yield slightly when gently squeezed • Avoid hard fruit or pale, greenish, soft/mushy ones	Refrigerate unwrapped up to 2 days once ripe • Wash just before using
Avocados 1 pound = 1½ cups pulp 1 pound = 2 medium	• Several varieties • Green to black • Buttery/rich when ripe	• Best eaten uncooked • Slice for salad or sandwiches • Mash for spreads and dips	• Ripe fruit gives slightly to the touch	• If unripe, ripen at room temperature • To speed ripening, place in a paper bag with an apple, banana, or tomato • Store ripe fruit up to 1 week in refrigerator • Store cut avocado in sealed container or plastic bag

Fruit	Subtype of Fruit; Color and Taste	Preparation Methods and Tips	Buying Tips	How to Store
Bananas 1 medium = 1 cup sliced 1 pound = 1¾ cups mashed 1 pound = 3 medium	Cavendish • Yellow when ripe • Sweetness increases with ripeness • Available all year	• Fresh for eating • Fresh or frozen in smoothies or in baked goods	• Look for bright firm yellow fruit • Bananas are fully ripe when brown spots appear	• Store only at room temperature • Ripen well off the tree
	Plantain • Large, green with tapered ends • Starchy • Available all year	• Must be cooked • Boil and mash • Slice and fry (especially when ripe)	• Skin blackens as fruit ripens	• Store at room temperature
Blueberries Fresh 1 pound = 3½ cups 1 pint = 2 to 3 cups Dried: 1 pound = 2½ cups	• Wild and cultivated varieties • Dark blue with powdery white bloom • Availability: late spring to summer • Small, wild berries more flavorful than larger cultivated ones	• Eaten raw or cooked as sauces, preserves, baked goods	• Berries are too old if the white bloom is absent	• Can be refrigerated up to 1 week
Cantaloupe 1 6-inch melon = 3 pounds 3 pounds = 25 balls (⅞ inch) 3 pounds = 4 to 4½ cups cubed	Aromatic orange flesh, with raised netting on skin	• Slice and eat • Cube and use in smoothies • Cube and freeze to make sorbet, ice cream	• Smell the fruit for strong aroma • Ripe melons have flatter side with paler color compared to the rest of the melon • Ripe melons give to gentle pressure on blossom end • Look for moist stem but not moldy	• Store only at room temperature • Refrigerate cut melons in airtight container up to 2 days
Cherries Canned, tart 16 ounces pitted = 1½ cups drained Dried, tart 3 ounces = ½ cup	Bing • Large heart-shaped, red to black color • Firm sweet flesh • Excellent for eating fresh	• For eating	• Look for brightly colored fruit that is plump, clean, glossy, without broken skin, mold, or soft spots • Stems should be pliable, green, and still attached	• Ripe fruit will keep up to 3 days in refrigerator in tightly closed container, as cherries are prone to absorbing strong flavors from other foods such as leeks, onions, and peppers

(continued)

HOW TO BUY, STORE, AND USE FRUIT *(continued)*

Fruit	Subtype of Fruit; Color and Taste	Preparation Methods and Tips	Buying Tips	How to Store
Cherries *(continued)* Fresh 1 pound = 1¾ cups pitted Frozen, tart, pitted 1 pound = 2 cups	Royal Anne • Golden/white with red cheek • Crisp, sweet • Excellent for eating fresh	• For eating • For baking	• Available late spring to summer	• Wash just before using
	Black Tartarian • Deep red			
	Lambert • Deep red, smaller than Bing • Sweet	• Excellent for eating raw		
	Rainier • Golden with a pink blush • Sweet	• Excellent for eating raw		
	Morellos • Dark, short stem • Sour, juicy	Acidic, best cooked in jams or pies		
Coconut Flaked 7-ounce package = 2½ cups 3½-ounce can = 1¼ cups Fresh 1 pound = 1 medium 1 pound = 3 cups grated	• The green husk may be removed, exposing the hard shell with thick flesh • Sweet crunchy white flesh with thin white liquid in the center	• To split a coconut in the shell, pierce the eyes with a screwdriver and drain clear liquid, which is sweet • Using a hammer, give the center of the shell a sharp blow and the nut should split into two halves • Flesh is good raw, or can be toasted in 400-degree oven for 15 minutes	• Choose heavy "nut" for juicy flesh • Look for eyes that are not dried out	• Store at room temperature for a few weeks • Refrigerate for longer shelf life

Fruit	Subtype of Fruit; Color and Taste	Preparation Methods and Tips	Buying Tips	How to Store
Cranberries Dried 6-ounce package = 1⅓ cups Fresh 1 pound = 4 cups	• Red round fruit sold in bags • Tart	• Fresh in relish uncooked • Cook fresh for sauces, chutneys, fritters, jellies, compotes, relishes, or pies with sugar or sweetener • Dried cranberries for eating or using in baked goods or on salads	• Look for bright dry plump and unshriveled fruits • Most available fall through mid-winter	• Keep unwashed up to 2 weeks in refrigerator • Freeze in tightly sealed container • Wash just before use
Currants 1-pound package = 3 cups	• Red, white, or black • White less acidic than red/black • Tart	• Fresh raw (note that many are tart) • Fresh cooked in jams, preserves, syrup • Dried for eating or in baked goods	• Look for small, firm berries, free of mold • Fresh most available mid-to-late summer	• Refrigerate up to 2 days • Wash just before use
Dates Dried, diced, sugared 1 pound = 2⅔ cups Dried, pitted 8 ounces = 1¼ cups Dried, unpitted 1 pound = 2½ cups pitted Fresh 1 pound = 3½ cups pitted	• Fresh have smooth brown skin with soft yielding flesh and a mild sweet rich flavor • Dried have increased sugar content and sweetness	• Fresh for eating raw • Dried for eating or baking	• Soft dates have high moisture with low sugar • Look for whole, shiny, and plump dates Avoid fruit with mold at stem, cuts, or bruises • Dried may be wrinkled	• Dried can be stored at room temperature in airtight container • Dried may keep for weeks in tightly sealed container in refrigerator • Store fresh dates tightly wrapped in the refrigerator up to 2 weeks
Figs Dried 1 pound = 4 cups cooked 1 pound = 40 medium 1 pound = 3 cups chopped Fresh 1 pound = 2½ cups chopped 1 pound = 9 medium	Mission • Purple black delicate skin • Pink to dark pink flesh	• Eat fresh • Remove tough stem • Can be dried in dehydrator for 12 hours or in warm dry sunny spot for a few days	• Ripe figs yield gently to pressure and may have small cracks in the skin • Avoid those with mold	• Once picked they are extremely perishable • If firm, may be allowed to ripen at room temperature • Rinse with water just before eating
	Brown Turkey • Copper and brown mixed with purple			

(continued)

HOW TO BUY, STORE, AND USE FRUIT *(continued)*

Fruit	Subtype of Fruit; Color and Taste	Preparation Methods and Tips	Buying Tips	How to Store
Figs *(continued)*	Adriatic figs • Thin green skin with red flesh • Raspberry flavor		• Too fragile for shipping so mostly available dried	
	Calimyrna • Flavor accentuated by nutty quality of seeds		• Mostly available as dried whole fruit	
Grapes Fresh 1 pound = 2½ cups seedless 1 pound = 2 cups seeded Most grapes are available with seeds or seedless	Concord • Round with purple black skin Niagara/White Concord • Pale green skin Thompson • Greenish yellow Flame • Reddish purple • Sweet Muscat • Golden/green • Rich, spicy, and musky	• Cut into smaller clusters with scissors or kitchen shears	• Look for plump, highly colored fruit for their variety • Ripe fruit has an amber glow • When ripe, some may detach from stem • Stems should be pliable • Avoid bunches that have soft, moldy, or discolored grapes	• Store in refrigerator for up to 2 weeks, although flavor may diminish • May pick up odor from other food, so store in tightly sealed container • Wash just before use
Grapefruit Fresh 1 pound = 1 medium 1 pound = ⅔ to ¾ cup juice 1 pound = 10 to 12 sections	Exterior ranges from yellow to yellow with red tinge • Interior pale beige to pink • Very juicy	• Can be halved and served with a grapefruit spoon, or peeled and segmented	• Choose fruits with smooth glossy skin that are heavy for their size • Avoid fruits that are puffy or rough as they may be dry inside	• Will keep for about a week at room temperature and several weeks in refrigerator in an open plastic bag • Wrap tightly after cutting, as they may produce odors that can be picked up by other food
Guavas	• Many varieties • Light green/yellow to pink, size varies with variety • Sweet mild flavor with multiple hard seeds through the flesh	• Cut and enjoy (do not need to peel)	• Choose soft green fruit with a fragrant aroma that intensifies with ripeness • Avoid fruit with bruises, cuts, soft spots	• Store at room temperature until ripe • Once ripe, store in refrigerator for a few days

Fruit	Subtype of Fruit; Color and Taste	Preparation Methods and Tips	Buying Tips	How to Store
Honeydew melon 1 4-pound melon = 35 balls 1 4-pound melon = 4 cups diced	• Smooth, creamy rind with green or orange flesh • Aromatic sweet firm flesh with multiple seeds in the center	• Slice and eat • Cube for use in smoothies • Cube and freeze for making sorbet or ice cream	• Ripe fruit give to gentle pressure on the blossom end	• Ripen melon at room temperature • Refrigerate only after fully ripened • Refrigerate in tightly sealed container after cutting
Kiwifruit or Chinese gooseberries 1 medium = ½ cup sliced	• Green/brown fuzzy skin with emerald green flesh • Aromatic and complex flavor, slightly tart, edible seeds	• Skin is edible, but many people remove it	• Choose plump unwrinkled fruit with unbroken skin and no dark area (bruises) • Ripe fruit will give to gentle pressure	• Usually picked unripe and stored for months • Ripens more quickly at room temperature in a loosely closed paper bag • Refrigerate 1 to 2 weeks once ripened
Kumquats	• Small, oblong orange-colored fruit • Sweet skin and tart flesh	• Eat whole or sliced for use in salads • Cooked for marmalade and preserves	• Choose plump fruit that are firm and shiny with good color	• Can be stored at room temperature for a week • Store for several weeks loosely covered in refrigerator
Lemons Lemon peel, dried 1 teaspoon = grated peel of 1 medium lemon 1 teaspoon = ½ teaspoon lemon extract 1 teaspoon = 1 to 2 teaspoons grated fresh lemon Fresh 1 pound = 4 to 6 medium 1 medium = 2 to 3 tablespoons juice 1 medium = 2 to 3 teaspoons grated peel	• Golden yellow to orange, tender skin • Grown for acidic juice and for the oil in their yellow peel that is used for flavoring	• Squeeze juice for cooking or use in lemon or limeade • For best yield, bring to room temperature, roll the fruit firmly on counter or table to soften slightly, cut in half, and squeeze • For zest, remove only the thin oily pigmented outer layer of the skin, using a zester, grater, or a swivel-bladed vegetable peeler	• Choose fruit heavy for their size, with well-colored smooth thin rinds, which indicate juicy fruit	• Avoid green, as they aren't as juicy • Avoid shriveled, hard-skinned, soft, or spongy lemons • Store at room temperature for a week • Store in refrigerator for several weeks in opened plastic bag

(continued)

HOW TO BUY, STORE, AND USE FRUIT *(continued)*

Fruit	Subtype of Fruit; Color and Taste	Preparation Methods and Tips	Buying Tips	How to Store
Limes Fresh 1 pound = ½ to 1 cup juice 1 pound = 6 to 8 medium 1 medium = 1 to 2 teaspoons grated peel 1 medium = ½ to 2 tablespoons juice	Persian lime • Shiny dark green skin, usually seedless, with juicy pale green flesh Key lime • Skin can be yellow when ripe, when some acidity is lost ripens to a yellowish green • 40% of weight is juice • More acidic than Persian		• Choose fruit heavy for size, with glossy, well-colored, smooth, thin rinds	• Refrigerate uncut limes in a plastic bag for up to 10 days. Cut limes can be stored in the same way.
Lychees	• Encased in brown papery shell with a delicate pink lining • Translucent colorless flesh enclosing a single brown glossy seed • Perfumed flavor	• Remove peel and pit • Flesh can be eaten as it is or added to sauces	• Available fresh, frozen, or canned • Fresh: look for plump heavy fruit with pleasant aroma	• Fresh fruit should be refrigerated up to a few days • Flesh will discolor and lose flavor if not fresh
Mandarins and tangerines 1 pound = 4 average 1 pound = 2 cups sections	Clementine/Algerian (common tangerines) • Small smooth bright red-orange skin • Juicy, sweet-tart flavor, may contain seeds Satsuma • Loose puffy skin, seedless • Easy to peel, sweet-tart flavor Tangelo/Minneola (hybrid) • Larger, thin skin with "neck" on stem end, red-orange skin • Easy to peel, very juicy • Cross between tangerine and grapefruit	• Enjoy fruit for snack • Split into segments and add to salads • Freeze segments for making sorbet	• Choose fruit that is heavy for its size, avoid soft spots or watery areas • Sugar level depends on climate and maturity at harvest	• Due to thin skin and tender flesh, mandarins don't keep as well as other citrus

Fruit	Subtype of Fruit; Color and Taste	Preparation Methods and Tips	Buying Tips	How to Store
Mangoes Fresh 1 medium = ¾ cup 12 ounces = 1 medium	Tommy Atkins • Medium size, oval, with bright yellow flesh and thick yellow-orange skin blushed with red • Sweet juicy smooth meat around a large seed	• Wash fruit in warm water before handling • Ripe fruit: cut flesh away from large flat seed, slicing the "cheeks" of flesh on either side of pit • Score meat inside, peel, cut away chunks of flesh • Green mangoes can be added to curry, salads, chutney	• Usually picked green since the ripe fruit is fragile • Use smell and feel to determine ripeness • Mild fruity aroma, especially at the stem end, indicates ripeness • Ripe fruit yields to gentle pressure • Avoid mangoes that are very soft or bruised • Color is not reliable guide for ripeness • Choose larger fruit for higher yield	• Ripen at room temperature until soft • Hasten ripening by placing in paper bag with an apple or banana • Fully ripe fruit will keep up to a week in the refrigerator • Bring fruit to room temperature before using for fullest flavor
	Keitt (variety from California) • Skin remains yellow to green even when ripe • Large (1 pound) oval fruit with yellow-orange low-fiber flesh • Seed is smaller than T. Atkins • Meatier, juicier flesh			
	Hayden • Yellow skin with orange and red skin, medium size			
	Kent • Green skin with dark red blush • Small seed, little fiber, rich flavor			
Nectarines 1 pound = 3 to 4 medium = 2 cups chopped = 2½ cups sliced = 1½ cups puréed	• Smooth skin, firm and fine texture • White or yellow flesh • Low acid sweet-tart rich in flavor; sweeter than a peach	• For eating	• Choose fruit that is not too hard and that is free of green spots	• Best stored at room temperature • Extras can be stored in the refrigerator, but should be brought to room temperature before eating

(continued)

Fruit	Subtype of Fruit; Color and Taste	Preparation Methods and Tips	Buying Tips	How to Store
Oranges Peel, dried 2 teaspoons = 1 teaspoon orange extract 1 tablespoon = grated peel of one medium orange Fresh 1 pound = 1 cup juice 1 medium = ⅓ to ½ cup juice 1 pound = 3 medium 1 pound = 4 to 5 tablespoons grated peel 1 medium = 5 teaspoons to 2 tablespoons grated peel 1 pound = 1 to 1½ cups sections 1 medium = ⅓ to ½ cup sections	Blood orange • Medium size with orange skin with some red streaks • Flesh streaked with purple, crimson, orange, and yellow	• For eating	• Color and sweetness depends on variety, growing area, and degree of maturity • Some purple flesh can have unpleasant musky flavor	• Best stored at room temperature • Refrigerator for prolonged storage (up to several weeks) • Bring to room temperature before eating for fullest flavor • One moldy fruit will spoil the lot quickly, so check often
	Navel • Has small secondary fruit in the blossom end of the primary fruit • Sweet crisp juicy seedless segments, easy to peel	• For zest, remove only the thin oily pigmented outer layer of the skin using a zester, a grater, or a swivel-bladed vegetable peeler • Best eaten fresh	• Orange color develops in warm days and cool nights (Calif. and Arizona) • Florida oranges may have green skin; russeting (superficial blemishing) has no effect on flavor and may indicate thinner skin and superior juiciness	
Oranges for juice	Valencia • Smooth greenish skin • Large juicy fruit with some seeds • Available February through September			
	Hamlin • Sweet and juicy, not as flavorful • Available October to December			
	Pineapple • Rich, flavorful, juicy with lots of seeds • Available January and February			

Fruit	Subtype of Fruit; Color and Taste	Preparation Methods and Tips	Buying Tips	How to Store
Oranges *(continued)* Sour oranges	• Seville • Red, orange fruits • Sour and bitter	• Used in marmalades and cooking • Not good for eating	• Not readily available in U.S. markets	
Papayas Fresh 1 pound = 1 medium 1 pound = 2 cups sliced/cubed	• Mexican (large) or Hawaiian (smaller) • Green thin skin with yellow streaks • Thick sweet juicy flesh with strong musky scent, yellow to salmon-pink flesh	• Slices of ripe papaya can be seasoned with lemon or lime juice • Green papayas are used as vegetable (shredded/sliced thinly) • Do not use in gelatin, as papaya contains enzymes that prevent jelling	• Green papayas have dark green skin • Ripe fruit have yellow/orange skin, firm but will yield to gentle pressure • Avoid fruit with cuts, soft spots, mold, or bruises • Green papayas do not ripen well off the tree, so pick fruits that are mostly yellow with some green streaks	• Store firm fruit at room temperature to soften • Can refrigerate after ripe, but bring to room temperature before eating to enjoy full flavor • Refrigerate cut papaya up to 1 week
Passion fruit 1 tablespoon of seedless pulp = 1 medium	• Purple or yellow skin • Purple sweeter richer, juicier than yellow • Golden yellow, juicy pulp with multiple edible seeds • Purple fruit has black seeds and yellow fruit has brown seeds • Yellow fruit bigger and easier to handle, used commercially • Multiple edible brown seeds	• Scoop out pulp and seeds with a spoon • If seedless pulp is needed, put through a fine-mesh strainer with rubber spatula or wooden spoon	• Unripe fruits have smooth skin • Ripe fruits have dimpled and wrinkled skin • Choose fruits that are heavy for their size	• Store unripe fruits at room temperature until ripe • Store ripe fruit in the refrigerator for about a week • Can be frozen for later use
Peaches 1 medium = ½ cup sliced fruit 1 pound = ~4 medium fruit 16-ounce can sliced peaches = 2 cups	• Sweet juicy fruit • Many varieties	• Good for eating • Use in smoothies • Cook into pies and other desserts	• Ripe peaches have deep peach aroma • Ripe peach firm but yields to gentle pressure on its shoulder • Avoid bruises, cuts, or fruits that are soft all over • Avoid green peaches, as they don't ripen well (may soften but will not sweeten)	• Store in refrigerator • Bring to room temperature before eating to enjoy full flavor • Sliced fruit browns rapidly, so slice just before eating • Lemon juice can stop browning

(continued)

HOW TO BUY, STORE, AND USE FRUIT *(continued)*

Fruit	Subtype of Fruit; Color and Taste	Preparation Methods and Tips	Buying Tips	How to Store
Pears 1 medium = ½ cup sliced fruit 1 pound = ~4 medium fruit 16-ounce can sliced pears = 2½ cups	• Depending on variety, have varying degree of sweetness	• For eating • Slice into salads • Slice and add to appetizer tray with yogurt dip • Use in baking and cooking	• Best to buy fruit that is not fully ripened and allow it to ripen at home (avoids bruising) • Test for ripeness using gentle pressure at the neck of the fruit	• Store at room temperature until ripe • Refrigerate once ripe for a few days
Persimmons 1 medium = ~4 ounces edible fruit	• Bright orange acorn-shaped fruit with thin, satiny, translucent orange-red skin • Astringent if eaten unripe	• When fully ripe, scoop out the pulp with a spoon	• Ripe fruits are very fragile • Choose fruits without cracks or bruises	• Refrigerate up to 10 days • Unripe fruit can be ripened at room temperature
Pineapples 1 medium = 3 cups cubed 1 medium = ~2 pounds 8-ounce can = 4 slices 20-ounce can = 10 slices	• Sweet, juicy	• With a sharp knife, cut the crown leaves and some of the skin on the stem end • With the fruit upright, remove the peel • To remove the eyes, use potato peeler or cut V-shaped grooves that follow the spiral patterning of the eyes • Cut the peeled fruit into wedges and trim out the fibrous core	• Must be picked fully ripe for maximum sugar content • Firm pineapple may ripen at room temperature but will not increase in sweetness • Larger fruit have higher yield • Color of the skin is not an indicator of ripeness • Should yield a bit with gentle pressure • Deep green leaves are a good sign of freshness • Avoid fruit with dried or brown leaves, fermented or sour odor, watery spots or dark patches on the skin, mold on stem end	• Store at room temperature before cutting • Refrigerate cut fruit in tightly sealed container and use in 2 to 3 days

Fruit	Subtype of Fruit; Color and Taste	Preparation Methods and Tips	Buying Tips	How to Store
Pomegranates 1 medium fruit = ½ cup pulp and seeds	• Red juicy seeds in bunches separated by ivory membranes	• Quarter fruit with sharp knife and separate the clusters of seeds by bending the skin outward • Enjoy seeds alone or in/on salad • Blenderize seeds for juice • Use fruits with split skin as soon as possible	• Skin color not a good indicator of ripeness • Choose fruit that is heavy for its size • Skin should not be dry	• Store at room temperature • Once cut, store in tightly sealed container in refrigerator
Quinces 1 pound = 3 to 4 fruits	• Aromatic with complex tropical fruit flavor	• Inedible raw due to hard gravelly texture • Cook until fork-tender, high pectin content for jelly, jam, or preserves	• Choose fruit with firm, fragrant, bright yellow or golden skin • Avoid bruises or discoloration • Ripe fruit less fuzzy than green	• Store at room temperature to ripen • Store ripe fruit in refrigerator for 1 to 2 weeks
Raspberries 1 pint = 1¾ cups	• Aromatic and flavorful when ripe	• Great for eating • Use fresh or frozen in smoothies • Use in pies, pastries, jams, or jellies	• Very fragile and perishable • Look for velvety and plump fruit • Avoid containers stained with juice of crushed berries • Avoid fruit with mold in stem cavity	• Store in refrigerator; use as soon as possible • Freezes well; freeze in single layer and then place in tightly sealed container
Strawberries 1 pint sliced = 1¾ cups 1 pint whole berries = 2½ cups 1 pint = 24 medium 1 pound frozen whole berries = 4 cups	• Aromatic and flavorful when ripe	• Great for eating • Use fresh or frozen in smoothies • Use in pies, pastries, jams, or jellies	• Very fragile and perishable • Look for shiny and plump fruit with bright leaves on top; dark berries are ripest	• Store in refrigerator; use as soon as possible • Freezes well; freeze in single layer and then place in tightly sealed container

(continued)

HOW TO BUY, STORE, AND USE FRUIT *(continued)*

Fruit	Subtype of Fruit; Color and Taste	Preparation Methods and Tips	Buying Tips	How to Store
Watermelon 20-pound melon with rind = ~20 cups cubes	• Many varieties and flesh colors	• Enjoy fresh • Freeze for use in smoothies, sorbet	• Unripened fruit will not ripen off the vine, so choose ripe • Ripe melon has yellow patch on bottom where it rests on the ground • Look for skin that has a waxy bloom; dull rather than shiny • Look for symmetrically shaped fruit	• Store uncut melon at room temperature • Store cut melon in refrigerator for a few days in airtight container

14

WHOLE GRAINS

Catching the Golden Wave of Flavor and Nutrition

Kristine Napier, M.P.H., R.D.

The mounting evidence for whole grains' ability to prevent cancer is one of the reasons that the American Dietetic Association, the American Cancer Society, and the *USDA Dietary Guidelines for Americans 2000* recommend that Americans return to the dietary habits of an earlier era, when the staff of life was more likely to be brown than white.

WHOLE-GRAIN BASICS

Nature constructs all grains alike, building each particle in three layers:

- The *outer* bran layer contains nearly all the fiber.
- The *middle* germ layer is the smallest but the most nutrient-dense. If planted, it is this nutrient-rich germ layer that would develop into a new plant; that's why it's also called the embryo.
- The *innermost* endosperm is the largest but least nutrient-dense layer; it consists mostly of starch. After milling, the endosperm is the only remaining layer.

A Faster-Paced Lifestyle Demands Faster Food, Including Faster Grain Foods

Until the mid-nineteenth century, grain-milling techniques were not as harsh as they are today. When wheat was ground into flour, for example, just the bran layer was scraped away and the germ layer was pulverized with the endosperm, dispersing the wealth of nutrients throughout the final product. But because the germ layer is high in oil, releasing it into the flour shortens the shelf life, because any oil or fat left at room temperature quickly goes rancid. To meet the demand for sliced bread readily available on supermarket shelves, food technologists developed techniques to isolate the *least* nutrient-rich endosperm and grind only it into flour. Thus, we became a society that consumed white bread and white pasta, leaving behind the golden grains—golden in both color and high nutritional value. This advance in technology was the first giant step backward in good nutrition.

Creating a white bread that stays fresh longer on grocery store shelves wasn't the only step in helping us keep up with busy schedules. We cook less whole wheat varieties such as bulgur and cracked wheat; less wild and brown rice; less barley, millet, oats, and buckwheat. Instead, we cook more white rice and white pasta and eat more low-in-fiber cereals simply as a matter of habit.

As a result, surveys indicate that the average American eats less than one serving of a whole-grain food daily. In stark contrast, the *USDA Dietary Guidelines for Americans 2000* encourages us to eat at least three of our grain servings—six to eleven, depending on age and gender—as the nutrient-, fiber-, and phytochemical-rich version. Research reveals that people who eat more whole grains:

- Take in higher amounts of vitamins and minerals than do people who do not eat whole-grain foods.
- Eat more fruit and dairy foods daily.
- Consume less total fat, less saturated fat, and fewer added sugars.

Refer to the section titled "Everyday Solutions for Using More Whole Grains" later in this chapter. Also, you'll find the everyday kitchen solutions for cooking whole grains very helpful—making whole grains far less intimidating. We're going to help you reap the golden whole-grain goodness of the past with the best of the time-saving advances we enjoy today.

Reasons for Returning to Golden Whole Grains

Preventing Cancer

Population-based studies provide good reasons for eating more whole grains. Nutrition researchers at the University of Minnesota found that eleven out of twelve studies that examined the whole-grain cancer connection confirmed that whole grains do reduce the risk of colorectal and stomach cancers. Other research makes a strong case for whole-grain protection against breast and endometrial cancers.

Reducing Heart Disease Risk

Sidestepping cancer isn't the only reason to shift to eating a wide variety of whole-grain foods. People who consistently consume whole grains have a lower risk of developing coronary artery disease or clogged arteries. The high consumption of oats and buckwheat among the Yi people of China, for example, is thought to play a key role in their notably lower total of LDL or "bad" cholesterol readings, and their desirably high HDL or "good" cholesterol levels.

Controlling Blood Glucose Levels in Diabetes

Whole-grain foods also seem to help people with diabetes avoid steep rises in blood glucose that can lead to complications. Because they're a more complex food than their refined counterparts, whole grains take longer to digest. That means the glucose units to which food is broken down are "fed" more slowly into the blood stream.

The Reasons for Whole-Grain Health Benefits

Until recently, we gave almost exclusive credit to fiber for the health benefits related to whole-grain consumption. All grains are high in insoluble fiber, which seems to cut cancer risk by ushering out carcinogens that form in or find their way into the intestinal tract. Oats and barley are also high in soluble fiber, which plays a role in lowering total and LDL cholesterol while leaving alone HDL cholesterol.

FIBER: SOLUBLE AND INSOLUBLE

Whole-grain foods, fruits, vegetables, and legumes (such as split peas, black beans, and so forth) contain two types of fiber—and we need both for better health:

- Insoluble fiber soaks up water, much like a sponge, to make stools softer and easier to eliminate. Wheat bran, many vegetables, and other whole grains are good sources of insoluble fiber.
- Soluble fiber dissolves in the watery contents of the gastrointestinal tract to form a gel, which traps substances in the intestinal tract that the body could eventually turn into fat and cholesterol; the gel is then passed from the body as part of the body's intestinal wastes. This process works exceptionally well when the intake of insoluble fiber is also high, as the stools are heavier and pass through the intestinal tract much faster. Oats, barley, some fruits, dried beans, and dried peas are excellent sources of soluble fiber.

Today, though, we focus on a multitude of factors besides fiber in the value of whole grains, looking at them in a holistic sense. Research studies indicate that their "mix" of nutrients and phytochemicals also plays a critical role in cancer and heart disease prevention, as well as helping to reduce birth defects. Let's take a look at some of the healthful-promoting and disease-fighting ingredients that Mother Nature wraps into whole-grain goodness.

B vitamins

B vitamins include the following:

- Folate, or folic acid:
  - Helps reduce the risk of birth defects, especially spina bifida and other neural tube and spinal cord defects
  - Aids in reducing heart-disease risk
  - May reduce colon-cancer risk
- Thiamin:
  - Assists the body in burning carbohydrates as fuel to keep us moving and thinking
  - Helps keep brain, nerve, and heart cells healthy
- B_6 (also called pyroxidine):
  - Helps the body use dietary protein more efficiently
  - Keeps red blood cells healthy
  - Aids in fighting infection by helping to make antibodies
  - Assists in blood-sugar control by serving as an essential ingredient in insulin
- Niacin (also called B_3):
  - Unlocks the energy in dietary carbohydrates
  - Helps keep skin, nerve, and digestive systems healthy

Minerals

Whole-grain foods (only the outer bran and middle germ portions) are one of the best dietary sources of minerals. Minerals you need include:

- Magnesium:
  - Plays an essential role in keeping hearts beating normally
  - Helps muscles to contract and nerves to function
  - Strengthens bones
- Zinc:
  - Plays an essential role in replicating DNA, the genetic material that guides the formation and function of every living cell (making it critical during pregnancy, when babies make new tissues rapidly)

Helps wounds heal
Fights infections
Bolsters the immune system
Assists in forming healthy taste buds—which helps us have the appetite that plays a role in eating healthfully

- Selenium:

Serves as an antioxidant warrior to help fight cancer, heart disease, and the effects of aging
Helps the immune system and heart muscle to function normally

- Manganese:

Strengthens bones
Helps with normal reproduction
Plays a critical role in keeping nervous-system tissues healthy

- Copper:

Bolsters bone strength
Must be present for the body to make new skin
Helps form neurotransmitters—nerve cells that communicate with each other so that we can think, walk, and perform every other action of daily living
Aids in blood clotting
Serves as an essential ingredient in red blood cells
Regulates body temperature

Phytonutrients

Phytonutrients serve as antioxidants and are thought to play a role in reducing cancer and heart disease risk, as well as the risk of other chronic health conditions.

Everyday Solutions for Using More Whole Grains

One of the best and most enjoyable strategies for using more whole grains is to look beyond those you commonly eat. Reach for grains you have never tried—and we'll help you fit them into your weekly menus.

There are at least twelve edible grains, which are also called cereal grasses:

Amaranth	Rice
Barley	Rye
Corn	Sorghum
Millet	Triticale
Oats	Wheat
Quinoa	Wild rice

Buckwheat, really an herb related to rhubarb, is often thought to be a grain because it's used like one. Neither is flaxseed a grain (it's the seed of the linen plant) but it, too, is used like one. Let's take a look at each grain to discover some of the many ways you can use it in your menus more often.

Amaranth

This ancient South American grain was once a staple of the Aztecs. It's no wonder, as it's loaded with high-quality protein, fiber, and iron. (Its leaves are also edible and highly nutritious, loaded with potassium and vitamin A.) You can find slightly sweet and delicately crunchy amaranth in whole-food markets and food co-ops, as well as in some Asian and Caribbean food markets.

Everyday solutions for using more amaranth include:

- The grain in place of rice in pilafs and casseroles
- The flour in baked bread recipes

Barley

Greek athletes ate this ancient grain to improve athletic prowess. Unfortunately, the most common use of barley in this country is in making animal food and beer and whiskey. If you haven't tasted it, you're missing a whole world of hearty whole-grain taste—especially if you've never tasted this form, which is called hulled barley. In addition to hulled barley, look for scotch or pearled barley.

Everyday solutions for using more barley with its nutty, robust, interesting flavor and chewy texture:

- In dishes traditionally calling for rice, such as:
  Spanish rice (try our recipe for Barley Pilaf on page 391)
  Stuffed peppers
- At breakfast simmered with milk, raisins, and cinnamon
- Simmered with chopped onions, carrots, garlic, and favorite herbs as the base for a pilaf; stir in peas, corn, broccoli, or any other favorite vegetables, too

Buckwheat

This distinctively flavored food isn't really a grain at all. Rather, it's an herb of the genus *Fagopyrum*, related more to rhubarb and sorrel than to wheat and other grains. Because it's not a grain, buckwheat is free of gluten, the sticky protein found in wheat and other grains that causes intestinal problems in some people. That's why buckwheat is an excellent food for people who have celiac disease, an intestinal problem, the symptoms of which can be improved by avoiding gluten.

Use buckwheat products in the following forms:

- Buckwheat groats, hulled, crushed kernels, cook up wonderfully as a side dish. Use them in place of rice once or twice per month.
- Kasha, roasted buckwheat groats, have a toastier, nutty flavor. It makes a great stuffing for winter squash or poultry.
- Stir buckwheat flour into buckwheat pancakes, one of Mark Twain's favorites, or into muffins.

Corn

Although it's really a grain, look for information on corn in chapter 13, since many people use it that way. Do note, though, that cornmeal is a fabulously delicious and richly nutritious grain. Try our recipes using cornmeal.

Flaxseed

Flaxseed is a small reddish-brown seed from the linen plant. While you may find the whole seeds in breads or other baked goods, the body is not very good at "cracking into" their outer shell. As a result, the great majority of flaxseed passes through the body unabsorbed. To harvest the goodness of flaxseed, purchase the ground or milled version. Alternatively, buy the seed whole and grind it in a coffee grinder. In addition, flaxseed is made into flour or processed for its oil. Research studies have linked flaxseed to several health benefits, including cholesterol reduction, cancer protection, and colon health.

In addition to its excellent fiber content, flaxseed is rich in omega-3 fatty acids (in a version similar to that found in some kinds of fish) and phytochemicals. One phytochemical in flaxseed is a plant estrogen. While this compound may lower the risk of breast cancer, women who already have breast cancer (or a family history of certain types of cancer) may need to moderate how much they eat. To play it safe, check with your physician before adding flaxseed to your food.

Use milled or ground flaxseed in several different ways:

- Bake milled or ground flaxseed into muffins, quick breads, and yeast breads, or stir into pancakes. Not only does it lend a delicate nutty flavor, it also adds moisture and a hearty texture. In general, mix ⅓ to ½ cup of flaxseed per 2 cups of flour into quick breads, muffins, and yeast breads. Note that the flaxseed doesn't take the place of any ingredient—it is simply an addition.
- Stir milled or ground flaxseed into yogurt along with dried fruit and nuts, creating an easy, nutrition-packed lunch.

HEALTH BENEFITS OF OMEGA-3 FATTY ACIDS

You may recognize omega-3 fatty acids as the "better" fat in salmon and other fatty fish. Omega-3s are thought to cut heart disease risk. Some grains and oil seeds (such as flaxseed) have their own version of omega-3 fatty acids. They're thought to function in a similar fashion in the human body.

Omega-3s are thought to fight inflammation, probably by keeping the body's immune system from working overtime. Specifically, omega-3 fatty acids slow down the body's production of certain components in the immune system, including prostaglandins, leukotrienes, and thromboxanes. Although the body needs a certain amount of these chemicals to function normally, too-high concentrations can lead to inflammation associated with several conditions, including arthritis and asthma.

Although just the right amount of omega-3 causes the blood vessels to contract and relax appropriately in the control of blood pressure, too much can really put the squeeze on blood vessels and cause high blood pressure. Too-high concentrations can also encourage platelets to clump in excess. While we do indeed depend on platelets to literally stick together to stop excess bleeding, too much togetherness can cause these tiny clots to clog up arteries, a condition known as atherosclerosis.

- Top your salad with 1 to 2 tablespoons of milled or ground flaxseed.
- Crush 1 cup of cornflake cereal and blend with ¼ cup ground or milled flaxseed as a topping for casseroles.
- Blend milled or ground flaxseed into smoothies, such as the Chocolate Banana Peanut Butter one on page 18.

Millet

This exceptionally interesting high-protein grain is a staple for many people in Asia and Africa. Americans, however, generally use it as animal feed and birdseed—simply because they have not been introduced to this crunchy-textured grain. Whole-food markets, health food stores, and some grocery stores carry millet grain and millet flour. You can also order these products from some bakers' catalogs.

Everyday solutions for using more millet include:

- Cooking millet in place of rice in pilaf and casserole recipes
- Boiled millet with dried fruits as a hearty breakfast cereal
- Stirring the cooked grain into yeast breads
- Blending flour into any type of baked goods. In general, you can replace up to one-half of the all-purpose flour in bakery recipes with other grains. You may have to add gluten to help these breads rise sufficiently. Find gluten in whole-food markets and some grocery stores.

Oats

This wonderful hearty grain has a rich complement of phytochemicals, fiber (including soluble), B vitamins, and minerals. It is the only grain always eaten whole. Even the quick and the instant versions are still the whole grain—they've just been cooked to varying degrees. Beyond its traditional breakfast use, you can stir oats into your diet in many other ways.

Everyday solutions for incorporating more oats in your diet include:

- Stirring them into meat loaf, replacing breadcrumbs
- Replacing part of the flour in cookies, quick breads, and yeast breads with oats. Use any version except the quick one in baked goods because instant oats are made by precooking and drying the whole oat. This process softens the oats and can turn baked goods gooey.
- Blending oats with toasted wheat germ, brown sugar, and cinnamon as a crunchy topping for fruit desserts and muffins
- Adding 2 to 4 tablespoons to smoothies
- Cooking them in adventurous ways as breakfast cereals.

Quinoa

Adding quinoa (pronounced keen'-wah) to your diet gives a fabulous new dimension to eating. Although used as grain, quinoa seeds come from a fruit. Quinoa's physical characteristics, nutritional profile, method of cultivation, and end uses, however, are much closer in similarity to the grain family. Because it's not a grain, it is low in gluten. Like buckwheat, quinoa provides another menu alternative for people who need to eat a gluten-restricted diet.

Quinoa is rich in the class of phytochemicals called saponins—so rich in them that this phytochemical tends to lend a strong taste to quinoa. The Incas, for whom this ancient seed was considered a staple grain, found the taste of quinoa so strong that they washed it in the river in an attempt to get rid of the saponins. Similarly, many recipes today recommend that quinoa be thoroughly rinsed before cooking. Doing so, however, tends to wash away the valuable saponins. Instead, try combining it with other strong flavors. You'll find the result delightfully delicious.

In addition to its rich phytochemical content (which makes it a great warrior in fighting cancer, heart disease, and possibly infections) there are a lot of other benefits to eating quinoa. It's an exceptionally great protein source, more than any other grain. In addition, quinoa contains all eight essential amino acids, unusual for a plant food, and it is high in the minerals calcium, iron, and phosphorous.

This interesting grainlike food cooks up like rice, but in half the time. Once cooked, it expands considerably and looks transparent.

Try ivory-colored, delicately flavored quinoa in:

- Soups. Cook quinoa separately and add to soups (so it doesn't soak up all the broth).
- Salads. Add orange, raspberry, or lemon tea bags to the cooking water to lend an interesting flavor and new dimension to salads.
- Stews. As with soups, cook quinoa separately and add to stews (or serve stew on top of quinoa).
- Side dishes in place of rice. Cook with onions, garlic, chopped carrots, and favorite herbs to create pilafs.
- Stuffing (for poultry or vegetables)
- Hot breakfast cereal blends
- Puddings

Rice

Americans are fond of rice. To reap the maximum nutrition from rice, don't rinse before using, as this washes out some of the precious nutrients. Similarly, don't use a large pot with extra water as this, too, washes out the nutrients. Give brown rice a try more often. It is mild, pleasant tasting, with a chewy texture and excellent nutlike flavor. Use it whenever you might use white rice, but allow a little extra cooking time.

What about rice packaged with spices and sauces? In most cases, look for an alternative to rice prepackaged with spices and sauces. Although their names and the pictures on the boxes may tickle your taste buds, packaged rice mixes are often quite high in fat and salt. Instead, try our recipes for flavoring rice while keeping it low in fat but deliciously high in flavor with some incredibly easy tricks. In general, bump up the flavor of rice by:

- Tossing an herbal tea bag into rice cooking water—lemon zinger and mandarin orange spice are especially good
- Adding minced garlic, chopped onions, and favorite herbs to the cooking water

Did you know that you can cook rice in the oven? It's a great energy-saver if that's where the rest of your dinner is cooking. Just stir rice into boiling liquid, cover tightly, and bake at 350°F for 25 to 30 minutes (30 to 40 for parboiled; 60 minutes for brown rice). As with all rice, fluff with a fork before serving.

There are many terms associated with rice. Use our guide to rice to help you understand what they mean:

- *White rice* has been stripped, or milled, from the husk, germ, and bran layers; just the kernel or "heart" remains.
- *Parboiled rice,* also called *converted rice,* is made with the whole rice kernel, which is soaked, pressure-steamed, and dried before milling. This infuses some (not all) of the nutrients from the germ and bran layers into the kernel; it also results in a fluffier rice.
- *Instant* or *precooked rice* is milled white rice that has been completely cooked and dehydrated.
- The terms *long, medium,* or *short* on the rice package refer to the length of the kernel, which determines how the rice cooks up. Long-grain rice produces light, dry grains that separate easily. The short grains produce moister kernels that stick together. Called arborio, it is used to make creamy risottos. Medium-grain rice falls somewhere in between in length, dryness, and moistness.
- *Wild rice* really isn't rice but rather a long-grain marsh grass native to the northern Great Lakes area. It has a distinctively unmatched, rich nutty flavor and unsurpassed chewy texture. Because it is pricey, many people mix it with brown or white rice to extend it. This works well, as the texture and flavor of the brown rice are deliciously strong.
- *Brown rice* is whole-grain rice with only the inedible outer husk removed. Brown rice really isn't brown at all but creamy-tan. Similar to its richer color, brown rice is richer in flavor than white. It is much easier to cook than most people think, so be sure and give it a try.

Try these everyday solutions for using more brown rice:

- Cook brown rice ahead for a month or two, which makes the extra cooking time do double, triple, or even quadruple duty. On a weekend day or evening when you plan to be at home, cook up a large pot of brown rice and then freeze in measured, family-sized portions.
- Add brown rice to soups, with extra cooking liquid to accommodate what the rice will soak up. Adding the rice while the soup simmers ensures that the rice will soak up the many wonderful flavors of the broth.
- Serve stews over brown rice.
- Use leftover brown rice as a breakfast food, stirring cinnamon, brown sugar, and raisins into it and heating it on the stove top or in the microwave.
- Blend chopped vegetables, nuts, and herbs to create your own signature pilaf.

Rye

This hearty grain is ground into four varieties of flour: light, medium, dark, and pumpernickel. The most common is medium; the darkest and coarsest is pumpernickel. If you're going to substitute some rye flour for some white flour in your favorite recipe, don't forget to add a little extra gluten, the protein part of flour that helps bread rise. Even with gluten, rye bread is generally heavier and darker than breads made from most other flours.

If you're a baker, try stirring rye flour into your next batch of bread. Not a baker? Don't worry! Enjoy rye bagels or rye rolls on occasion.

Whole Wheat

There's whole wheat—and then there's whole wheat. Your taste buds will be delighted by the wide variety of whole wheat products you can work into your eating plan, including:

- Bulgur (also spelled bulghur or bulgar). Along with wheat germ, bulgar is one of the easiest forms of wheat to work into your diet, even if you don't have much time to enjoy in the kitchen. It's made from the wheat berry after removing only the inedible hull. First the berry is steamed, then dried and crushed. Because it is already partially cooked when you buy it, you don't have to cook it very long. Try it in the classic Middle Eastern tabbouleh, or in a wonderful new breakfast sensation that blends leftover cooked bulgar with dried fruit and nuts. Try these additional kitchen tricks to using more bulgur:

  For maximum chewiness, stir in boiling water, cover tightly, and let it stand until all the water is absorbed, about thirty minutes. Another advantage of this method: you won't steam up the kitchen on a hot summer day.

  Cook it like rice: simmer for about fifteen minutes, then let it sit covered for an additional five minutes. Note that in some recipes you may have to use the simmering method.

  Cook bulgar in the microwave: cook on high for twelve minutes, turning the container every two minutes. Let stand an additional five minutes before serving.

- Whole wheat flour. Stirring whole wheat flour into your next batch of muffins, bread, quick bread, or cookies will lend a wonderful richness to your final product. In general, you can replace up to half the white flour with the whole wheat. In some cases you will have to add gluten (to help yeast bread rise) or extra baking powder.

- Wheat germ. Buy toasted wheat germ and try:

  Mixing 2 tablespoons into breakfast yogurt, along with fresh or dried fruit

Sprinkling 2 tablespoons in hot or cold cereal
Stirring some into your next baking project
Blending it into oven-fried chicken recipes
Whipping 2 or 3 tablespoons into your breakfast smoothie

- Cracked wheat. This form of wheat is exactly what its name implies; it is made by cracking the whole wheat berry when raw. Unlike bulgur, cracked wheat is not cooked at all. In terms of cooking time, cracked wheat falls between bulgur and whole wheat berries. Cook cracked wheat into pilaf. Toss cracked wheat into yeast bread, and even into quick breads, using a bit more liquid. Also serve it as breakfast food by stirring nuts, milk, and fruit into leftover cooked cracked wheat.

  Whole wheat berries. A popular food in ancient Egypt and Palestine, wheat berries are ripened kernels harvested from a head of wheat. These delicious, nutlike berries make an excellent addition to soups, stews, casseroles, breads, and muffins. Wheat berries also make a great bed for vegetables and meat. Don't be intimidated by their long cooking time. Use the guidelines that follow for cooking up extra and freezing for later use.

Easy, Everyday Solutions for Cooking and Storing Whole-Grain Foods

Like most Americans, you probably haven't grown up with this wide variety of whole-grain foods. That means you also haven't had the opportunity to learn how to weave them into your daily eating plan. Don't be intimidated. Even if you're not a cook, you'll find it incredibly easy to get more whole grains into your diet.

Ideally, we should try to have at least one different grain each day, for example, barley on Monday, brown rice on Tuesday, quinoa on Wednesday, oats on Thursday, millet on Friday, flaxseed on Saturday, and buckwheat on Sunday.

We understand that most people don't have the time to cook up whole grains at each meal, but there's an easy way around that problem because cooked grains store well in the refrigerator and in the freezer. The trick is in using moisture-tight and vapor-proof containers to prevent them from drying out and to retain maximum freshness and flavor. Make multiple batches ahead of time and freeze them. If you cook quinoa for one meal, for example, cook four times the amount you need. Store each of the other three portions in separate freezer containers, then pull one out the night before or the morning of the day you want to serve it.

Refer to the chart that follows for how to cook these whole grains. How much to cook? If you plan on storing cooked grains, follow these simple steps to determine amounts needed for one month:

1. Cook enough to yield 1 cup of cooked grain per family member for a single meal.
2. Multiply by 2, 3, or 4 (or more)—based on how many times you plan to use the grain within two months.
3. For example, if you plan on using brown rice once each week this month, and you have 4 people in your family:

   4 people × 1 cup cooked grain per week = 4 cups per week

   4 cups per week × 4 weeks = 16 cups

   Using the following chart, you find that 1 cup of raw rice yields three times that amount when cooked. Or, figuring backwards, divide the amount of cooked rice you need by 3, so:

   16 cups cooked rice divided by 3 = 5⅓ cups uncooked rice

   To determine the amount of water you'll need, multiply the amount needed to cook 1 cup by the amount of raw rice you are using. For example:

   5⅓ cups raw rice × 2 = 10⅔ cups water.

WHOLE-GRAIN COOKING CHART

Grain	Amount of Water per Cup of Raw Grain	Cooking Time	Yield
Amaranth	4 cups	15 to 20 minutes	2 cups
Barley, whole	3 cups	1 hour, 15 minutes	3½ cups
Barley, pearled	4 cups	45 minutes	3½ cups
Barley, quick-cooking	(See package label, as brands vary)		
Buckwheat	2 cups	15 minutes	2½ cups
Millet	3 cups	45 minutes	3½ cups
Quinoa	2 cups	15 minutes	2½ cups
Rice, brown	2 cups	50 minutes to 1 hour	3 cups
Rice, white	(See package label, as types and brands vary)		
Rice, wild	3 cups	50 to 65 minutes	4 cups
Wheat, bulgar (also bulgur, bulghur)	2 cups	15 to 20 minutes	2½ cups
Wheat, cracked	2 cups	25 minutes	2⅓ cups
Wheat, whole berries	3 cups	2 hours	2⅔ cups

15

LUSCIOUS LEGUMES

Beans, Peas, and Lentils

Jill Nussinow, M.S., R.D., and Kristine Napier, M.P.H., R.D.

Legumes are versatile meat alternatives, offering loads of protein and fiber without much fat.

People have eaten legumes for at least twelve thousand years, say anthropologists and historians, in almost every culture and region in the world. In the United States, their status has been elevated in the past decade from an inexpensive, affordable protein to the rank of cuisine by high-profile chefs enamored with their varied colors, textures, and flavors.

In addition to protein, beans have good amounts of B vitamins, calcium, iron, phosphorous, potassium, and zinc. They are naturally low in sodium, generally low in fat and, of course, have no cholesterol (only foods of animal origin can contain cholesterol). Legumes are a terrific source of fiber, providing 4 to 6 grams per ½ cup (cooked). Unlike meat, poultry, and fish sources of protein, legumes contain phytonutrients.

Their versatility, ease of use, and inexpensive cost make beans, peas, and lentils an excellent choice for many menu solutions, including:

- Cold, in salads and on top of salads
- Cold, blended with spices, herbs, and a sauce for a dip
- Cold, stuffed into a pita pocket with other sandwich fixings
- Hot, mashed, and rolled up with tomatoes, onions, and rice to make a burrito
- Hot, in tacos instead of meat
- Hot, in soups, casseroles, stews

While most often legumes are only available dried, occasionally you may find fresh beans in the pod, also known as "shelly beans" (named thus because they must be shelled). Shelly beans require more preparatory work, but their superior taste more than makes up for the extra time. If you are lucky enough to find black-eyed peas, Borlotti (cranberry beans), flageolet (green French kidney beans), scarlet runner, fava, or other fresh beans, do give them a try. One pound of fresh shelly beans yields one cup or so of delicious beans. These beans cook in a fraction of the time (usually ten to twenty minutes) of their dried counterparts. Some grocery stores now carry already shelled fresh legumes in the produce section—they're worth the search!

When fresh beans are unavailable, check out the vast variety of dried, canned, and even frozen beans. Most supermarkets carry the more common beans such as kidney, pinto, black, navy, Great Northern, yellow soy, and garbanzo or chick-peas. Standard brown or green lentils are usually available, as are green and yellow split peas. More unusual bean varieties, such as cannellini (Italian white kidney beans), Borlotti, flageolet, black soy, and others may be found at gourmet or natural-food stores or at various Web sites. These same sources may also carry red, black or French green lentils.

Like the recipes into which they are stirred, the names of beans are regional. Called the Jacob's cattle bean in one part of the country, this little legume is known as the trout bean elsewhere. The Anasazi bean of New Mexico is also known as the Appaloosa bean in other parts of the country. Bean regionality is also reflected by the popularity of different varieties in different areas.

Beans, Inside and Out

We've taken the guesswork out of how to use beans, starting with a glimpse into each variety's flavor and nutritional profile:

CHOOSING THE BEST BEAN FOR THE JOB

Bean	What It Looks Like	Flavor Information	Other Interesting Facts
Black beans (turtle beans)	• Black on the outside, cream colored inside	• Slightly sweet	• Combine well with rice for a great-tasting meal
Black-eyed peas (cowpeas)	• Small • White with a small black spot at the inside curve	• Gentle flavor	• One of the more easily digested beans • Two-tone, contrasting colors make them a great addition to soups
Garbanzo beans (chickpeas)	• Round • Creamy beige • Firm texture	• Mildly nutty flavor	• Good hot or cold • Great way to add protein to a salad • Frequently used mashed as a base for Middle Eastern hummus
Great Northern beans	• White, elongated	• Delicate and mild, so they accommodate a wide range of seasonings	• Often used in soup • Puréed, they make an excellent low-fat, high-in-nutrition thickener for cream sauces and soups
Kidney beans	• Firm, full-bodied slightly sweet flavor	• Red on the outside with a light-colored flesh	• Be aware that kidney beans are one of the more gas-producing beans

The Best Bean for the Job

Cooked from scratch or poured from a can, certain beans are best for certain types of foods and recipes. Here are some suggestions to get you started. Use your own kitchen creativity to find even more combinations!

- Salads: Garbanzo beans enhance texture and add a fresh nutty taste.
- Rice: Black beans add a sweet earthy flavor to plain rice or rice-based recipes like risotto or pilaf.
- Pasta: Light and dark red kidney beans give a burst of color and flavor to plain pasta; season with garlic, herbs, and/or lemon.
- Chili: Kidney and chili beans are staples in many traditional chili recipes; for new flavors, try black or Great Northern beans.
- Tacos or fajitas: Refried pinto beans and kidney beans are nutritious, convenient alternatives to pork or ground beef in a variety of Southwestern dishes.

- Mild-flavored fish: Pinto or navy beans add a savory boost of flavor when served as a side with mild fish.
- Shellfish or salmon: Great Northern beans paired with highly flavorful seafood lend a mild, clean taste to the entrée.
- Chicken: Garbanzo or black beans mixed with spinach as a bed for chicken breasts create a delicious, protein-packed meal.
- Red meat: Kidney beans mashed with chipotles and garlic complement robust flavors in filet mignon, steaks, and burgers.
- Pork: Black-eyed peas or navy beans go well as a side dish to pork chops or as an ingredient in many ham-based soups.

How to Cook Freshly Shelled or Dry Beans

Even when freshly shelled, legumes must be cooked. The amount of cooking time required for beans and lentils depends upon their age:

- Fresh-shelled beans cook the quickest.
- Recently harvested dried beans are the next fastest, especially heirloom beans. They are often of a recent harvest, and may cook up faster than their nonheirloom counterparts.
- Beans that have been on the shelf, in the store, or in your pantry take the longest to cook. Some may be so old that they never fully cook through.

  Unfortunately, you may not know the age of store-bought beans.

  At home, mark them with the purchase date and use within six months.

  Beans that are more than a couple of years old may not be worth cooking. There's only one way to tell—cook them, but don't count on them for your dinner.

Get beans ready for cooking by sorting and washing. Discard stones, dirt, and other debris; remove cracked and broken beans; rinse under running water and drain.

To Soak or Not to Soak?

There are some advantages to soaking beans:

- Cooking time can be doubled, or more, if you do not soak.
- Soaking may help reduce the intestinal gas experienced by some people after eating beans, especially those who do not eat beans often.

To presoak, choose the quick or the traditional method:

- Quick soak
  1. Cover beans with water by at least 3 inches.
  2. Bring the water to a boil and boil one minute.
  3. Remove from heat, cover the pan, and let the beans stand one hour.
  4. Drain the water.
- Traditional method
  1. Use 3 cups of water for each cup of beans.
  2. Soak for eight hours overnight or from morning until evening in the refrigerator.
  3. Drain the soaking water the from beans.

The type of bean determines cooking time (see the chart that follows for bean cooking time). Here are a couple of helpful cooking hints:

- Hard water and higher altitudes will also increase bean cooking time.
- Salt and acidic ingredients such as tomatoes, citrus juice, and vinegar inhibit the absorption of liquid and stop the softening process during cooking—resulting in tough beans. Add these ingredients after the beans are thoroughly cooked.

MORE GAS-REDUCING STRATEGIES

In addition to soaking, two other strategies may reduce some intestinal gas caused by eating beans:

- Take dietary supplements containing a food enzyme that helps the body break down the complex carbohydrates in beans and other foods that tend to cause intestinal gas. Beano is one example.
- Add the Mexican herb epazote (which has a very strong aroma).
- Add a 2-inch piece of kombu seaweed (which also helps keep the beans firm).

You Choose the Cooking Method

Beans are flexible! You can choose from a variety of cooking methods that match your style and kitchen equipment. Choose from stove-top cooking, slow cookery, and pressure cooking.

For stove-top cooking:

1. In a large saucepan combine the soaked beans and 3 cups of water for each cup of beans.
2. Bring the beans to a boil, reduce the heat to a simmer, and cover.
3. Check the beans while cooking and add more water if needed, ensuring that they stay covered with water.
4. Test the beans for doneness toward the end of the cooking time recommended in the following table (beans should be very tender when done).
5. Drain and use.

For slow cookery:

1. Presoak the beans; drain.
2. Combine the beans and 6 cups of water per pound of beans in a cooker.
3. Cover and cook on low twelve hours.

For pressure cooking:

1. Place the beans in a pressure cooker.
2. Add at least 1 cup water, or the minimum recommended by the pressure cooker manufacturer.
3. Do not fill the cooker more than half full, to allow room for expansion.
4. As with conventional cooking, pressure cooking takes about twice as long when beans are not soaked.
5. Release pressure slowly, letting it come down naturally. (This prevents beans from breaking up.)
6. Be aware of escaping steam and also very hot beans.
7. Newer cookers do not require oil, except for cooking split peas and black soybeans.

The following chart provides cooking times for beans that have already been soaked, except where indicated.

COOKING TIMES FOR SOAKED BEANS

Type of Bean	Stove-Top Cooking	Pressure Cooking
Aduzki	45 minutes to 1¼ hours	2 to 3 minutes
Anasazi	1 to 1½ hours	2 to 3 minutes
Black	1 to 1½ hours	3 to 6 minutes
Black-eyed peas	45 minutes to 1¼ hours	No presoak, 10 to 11 minutes
Cannellini	1 to 1½ hours	5 to 8 minutes
Chick-peas (garbanzo beans)	1½ to 2 hours	14 minutes
Cranberry (Borlotti)	1 to 1½ hours	5 to 8 minutes
Great Northern	1 to 2 hours	4 to 8 minutes
Kidney	1 to 2 hours	5 to 8 minutes
Lentils, brown	30 to 45 minutes	No presoak, 8 to 10 minutes
Lentils, French green	25 to 40 minutes	No presoak, 6 to 8 minutes
Lentils, red	15 to 25 minutes	No presoak, 4 to 6 minutes
Lima, baby	45 minutes to 1¼ hours	2 to 3 minutes
Lima, large	1 to 1½ hours	Add ½ teaspoon salt, 2 to 3 minutes
Mung	30 minutes to 1 hour	No presoak, 10 to 12 minutes
Navy, small white	1 to 1½ hours	3 to 4 minutes
Peas, Split	45 minutes to 1 hour	No presoak, 6 to 10 minutes
Pinto	1 to 1½ hours	2 to 3 minutes
Soybeans	2 to 2½ hours	6 to 8 minutes

Store cooked beans in the refrigerator or freezer:

- Cooked beans can be stored in the refrigerator for up to five days. Beans that are no longer edible have a sour smell and a slimy feel.
- To freeze cooked beans:
  1. Lay the beans on a cookie sheet in a single layer and place in the freezer.
  2. Once frozen, transfer the beans to airtight storage bags or containers in the amounts you commonly use.
  3. Freeze up to six months.

Canned Beans: A Fabulous Fast Food!

If you don't have time, need convenience, or just aren't inclined to cook your own beans, buy canned. The only disadvantage is their higher sodium content, but you can lower it by:

- Choosing a no-salt-added or reduced-sodium variety
- Draining and rinsing beans for one full minute under running water, which washes away up to 40 percent of the sodium.

The possibilities are endless for turning a can of beans into a quick nutrient-packed meal. Find the type of bean you like best from the following list and, after draining and rinsing, try some of the ideas listed. Or mix and match the ideas.

- Black beans: Mash with a fork, add seasoning (cumin, cayenne, garlic powder) and spread on a whole wheat flour tortilla. Add chopped tomatoes, onions, and chopped romaine, roll for an easy lunch or dinner.
- Garbanzo (also available in cans with a flip-top ring):

  Sprinkle on a bowl of salad (use prebagged salad to make it really fast; shower your salad first—under running water).

  Pop open a can for a high-protein, satisfying snack at home, work, or while out running errands.
- Great Northern: Stir into broth (chicken, beef, or vegetarian), chopped celery, chopped onion, oregano, and paprika.
- Kidney beans: Combine with chopped onion, chopped celery, chili seasoning, and fresh or frozen chopped green peppers; simmer 10 minutes.

GREAT BEAN FACTS

- 1 pound of dried beans = 2 to 2½ cups
- 2 cups dry beans = 5 to 6 cups cooked
- 1 pound of dried beans can serve 6 to 8 people

Soy Savvy: The Ultimate Soy Food Guide

It is with good reason that soy frequently makes health headlines. Solid evidence confirms that soy protein has strikingly positive health benefits, including:

- Protecting against heart disease. Soy protein can help lower "bad" blood fat levels (LDL cholesterol and triglycerides) without altering "good" or protective blood fat levels (HDL cholesterol). In 1999, the FDA determined that consuming about 25 grams of soy protein daily can reduce LDL cholesterol levels by as much as 10 percent. For example, an LDL cholesterol of 130 mg/dl could be decreased by 13 points, resulting in a reading of 117. Subsequently, the FDA approved a claim allowing food manufacturers to include the heart health benefits of soy-based foods on package labels.

  The FDA soy-protein claim, however, includes a critical caveat: to realize the heart-health benefit, a person must also reduce saturated fat and cholesterol intake (we would now add reducing trans-fat intake, too).
- Bolstering bones, reducing fracture risk. Soy protein may offer protection against osteoporosis or bone thinning, by helping bones "hang on" to calcium (the key mineral in determining bone strength).
- Protecting cells from oxidant damage. Soy protein, due to its isoflavone content (a type of phytochemical), has a strong antioxidant effect, which may help reduce the risk of cancer, heart disease, arthritis, and other conditions.
- Helping people with diabetes control blood sugar levels. The soluble fiber in soy foods helps slow absorption of glucose into the bloodstream, preventing steep rises in blood sugar. Overall, this can help reduce complications associated with diabetes. Soy's potential heart benefits are especially important to people with diabetes, who have a two- to-fourfold increase in heart disease risk.

Although evidence is not conclusive, soy isoflavones are thought to help relieve common menopausal symptoms in some women. Preliminary evidence indicates soy protein also may benefit prostate health.

Including soy foods in your meals is an excellent way to achieve protein diversity because it:

- Boasts a complete protein complement: Unlike most other vegetable proteins, soy protein contains all the essential amino acids. (Quinoa, a grain, is another.)

- Contains omega-3 fatty acids, a special type of fat that may reduce heart disease risk.
- Brims with an excellent mineral profile (including iron, zinc, and if fortified, calcium), as well as good amounts of several B vitamins (thiamin, folate and B_6).
- Adds fiber to your diet: like other vegetable proteins (but not animal), soy foods contribute valuable fiber.
- Boasts a healthier fat profile: Soy foods and soybean oil are low in saturated fat and rich in essential fatty acids. Like all vegetables, soy does not have any cholesterol. With the exception of some soy cheeses, soy foods do not have trans fats (read labels to find one that does not).

  Let's use a kitchen example to illustrate the fat point. Substituting one pound of soy crumbles for one pound of ground beef in tacos saves:

  272 calories (if serving 4 people, that's 68 calories each)

  41 fat grams (10 grams per person)

  21 saturated fat grams (5 per person)

  321 milligrams cholesterol (80 per person)

Folding Soy Foods into Your Weekly Meal Plan

Choosing soy protein for at least one meal each week can be a fun adventure. We've included some fabulous breakfast, lunch, and snack smoothies, and easy and extremely fast-in-the-kitchen strategies to include soy. We've also cooked up some great hot soy meals, which we hope you will, too!

In general, use the following guide to become acquainted with the many types of soy foods and how to use them.

ALL ABOUT SOY FOODS

Soy Food	Description	Easy Ways to Use	Grams of Soy Protein per Serving
Cereals containing soy	• Cold: flakes or granola, sometimes mixed with other grains • Hot: soy protein-fortified oatmeal	• Serve with vanilla soy milk for a rich flavor and a boost in soy content • Blend cold varieties into a trail mix of nuts (including soy nuts!) and dried fruit	• Variable; read label

(continued)

Soy Food	Description	Easy Ways to Use	Grams of Soy Protein per Serving
Edamame	• Fresh green soybeans in the pod or frozen in the pod or already shelled	• Shell edamame and discard pods, which are not edible • Enjoy cooked edamame cold or hot as: An easy snack A vegetable side In soups, salads, stews, casseroles, and entrées	• 11 grams per ½ cup (cooked)
Meat alternatives	• A textured soy protein sold frozen as burgers, crumbles, nuggets, and sausages	• Heat foods as directed and enjoy in any dish where ground beef or pork is traditionally used, such as spaghetti, sloppy joes, tacos, and casseroles • To get started, mix soy crumbles or sausages 50-50 with their meat counterpart	• 6 grams per 1 soy "sausage" link • 10 to 12 grams per 1 soy "burger"
Soybeans	• Yellow, brown, or black soybeans found dried (need cooking) or canned (already cooked)	• Toss on a salad, in soup, in casseroles—as you would use any other bean	• 15 grams per ½ cup (cooked)
Soy cheese	• Made from tofu, soy protein, and soybean oil, soy cheeses are found in most dairy cheese flavors (cheddar, mozzarella, etc.) • Reduced-fat varieties are available in some flavors	• Enjoy as you would other cheese • Try mixing soy cheese with dairy cheese to get started	• Variable; read label
Tofu	• A custardlike product made from cooked and puréed soybeans. Tofu is ideal in that it has a neutral taste—it simply absorbs flavors from other foods, spices, and herbs	• Choose the best type of tofu for your use/recipe: Soft: great for smoothies, creamy soups, and salad dressings Medium: mash or purée for dishes requiring a firm yet smooth consistency, such as some soups, dips, and desserts	• 13 grams per 4 ounces (⅓ of average tofu brick in a cardboard carton)

Soy Food	Description	Easy Ways to Use	Grams of Soy Protein per Serving
Tofu *(continued)*		Firm, extra-firm, and super-firm: ideal for slicing or cubing to use as a meat substitute. Can be marinated and grilled. Its meaty texture also makes it a good choice for crumbling into dishes such as lasagna, chili, or meatloaf	
Yogurt	Two basic versions: • Dairy yogurt with soy protein concentrate added • Cultured soy yogurt	• Use like dairy yogurt • Eat for breakfast, lunch, or a snack • Stir into muffins and other baked goods in place of water or milk • Create a dip or salad dressing	• 13 grams per cup
Soy milk	• Soybeans are soaked, ground finely, and strained to produce a fluid called soymilk. • Available: plain, vanilla, chocolate, or specialty flavors • Fortified and unfortified. Choose a variety fortified with calcium, vitamin D and B_{12}	• Use as you would dairy milk • Because soy milk does not have lactose, or milk sugar, it is often an excellent alternative for people who have lactose intolerance	• 10 grams per cup (8 ounces)
Soy nuts	• Made from soybeans soaked in water and then baked until brown • Can be found in a variety of flavors	• Salad toppers • Nutritious snacks • An addition to baked goods (chop first) • Casserole topping • Vegetable garnish	• 19 grams per ¼ cup

Bean Resources

http://www.americanbean.org—lots of recipes and other information.

http://www.michiganbean.org—great bean photos if you need help identifying different types of beans.

http://www.indianharvest.com—they carry a huge selection of heirloom beans.

http://beanbag.net/heirloom.html—another great source for heirloom beans with photos and alternate names.

http://www.phippscountry.com—a California company that grows and sells heirloom beans.

American Soybean Association
12125 Woodcrest Executive Drive
Suite 100
St. Louis, MO 63141
1-800-688-7692
http://www.amsoy.org

Soyfoods Association of North America
1723 U St. N.W.
Washington, DC 20009
(202) 986-5600

United Soybean Board
424 Second Ave. W.
Seattle, WA 98119
1-800-TALK-SOY (1-800-825-5769)
http://www.talksoy.com
http://www.soyfoods.com

16

FISH

A Guide to Buying, Storing, and Cooking

Kristine Napier, M.P.H., R.D.

The prime rule of fresh fish buying is choose what's freshest in the case that day. If you have a choice of several types of fresh fish, select what you enjoy most or what you have a recipe for. If you can't find fresh, catch what you need in the freezer case.

Perhaps you want fish highest in omega-3s, those special fats found in fish that help reduce heart disease risk. We've listed good omega-3 picks in two groups, according to omega-3 content. That said, though, rest assured that any fish meal is a great way to diversify protein intake. Let's take a look:

- *Best omega-3 catch (supplies about 1.4 grams omega-3s per 3-ounce serving):*

  All varieties of salmon (except lox)

  Pacific and jack mackerel

  Whitefish (except smoked)

  Pickled Atlantic herring

  European anchovies

WHY DOESN'T FISH TASTE GOOD WHEN I COOK IT?

You're not alone if you say you can't cook fish—but it's easier than you think! Two common reasons that fish doesn't turn out tasting good at home are:

- Starting with less than fresh fish. When fish is past its prime, the taste is "off." No matter how much you try, it will never taste great. Solution: start with only fresh fish. See the next section for buying guidelines.
- Cooking it too long. While fish is extremely easy to cook, the time between done just right and overdone is literally minutes. Overdone fish is chewy, rubbery, dry, and tasteless. Solution: Time fish carefully. See the next section for easy guidelines.

- *Second omega-3 choice (supplies 0.8 to 1.1 grams omega-3s per 3-ounce serving):*

  Atlantic mackerel

  Rainbow trout

  Atlantic sardines *(choose a brand packed in sardine oil to get even more omega-3s)*

  Atlantic and Pacific oysters

  Canned white tuna (albacore) *(Note: for many people, this may be the easiest and most inexpensive way to get omega-3s)*

  Swordfish

  Bluefin tuna

  Rainbow smelt

How to Buy Fish: If It Smells Fishy, Walk Away!

Aroma is a key indicator of the quality of fish you buy. Fresh fish has an ocean-breeze aroma, or perhaps no smell at all. When you walk into a fish store or approach the fish counter in a supermarket, are you greeted with the crisp clean scent of salt and ice? These are the only scents—if any—you should smell. If the air is at all rank, vaguely foul, or there is any type of fishy (ammonialike) smell, the fish might not be fresh. Try another store.

The look of the fish is also important. Fresh whole fish has:

- Moist and even slippery skin
- A shiny skin with firmly attached scales (if unscaled) and bright coloring
- Bright red, moist gills
- Firm flesh, which bounces back when touched

- Crystal-clear eyes—not sunken into the surrounding skin

If you prefer the convenience of buying fillets or steaks, look for:

- Firm flesh. Run your hand across the top; if the flesh flakes off, the fish has been in the case too long
- Clear white or red color, depending on the variety of fish
- Even coloring
- Moist appearance

Fresh shellfish guidelines include:

- Clams and oysters in the shell should be alive, and the shells should close tightly when tapped. Gaping shells indicate that the shellfish is dead and not safe to eat.
- Shucked oysters should be plump with a mild odor; they should be creamy in color with a clear liquor or nectar.
- Fresh shrimp have a mild odor and meat that is firm in texture.
- Scallops have a sweetish odor with no excess liquid when bought in packages.

If you are buying cooked shellfish, note the following signs of freshness:

- Cooked crab and lobsters are bright red with no disagreeable odor.
- Cooked shrimp have red color in shells and meat that has a reddish tint.

YES, ENJOY SHELLFISH!

For many years, consumers shied away from shellfish—such as lobster, scallops, and shrimp—hearing they were high in cholesterol. But pass by these succulent gems no longer, as more advanced ways of analyzing food have determined that what was once thought to be cholesterol in many of them—the mollusk variety—is really just a cholesterol-like compound. More good news: this noncholesterol, called sterol, might even stop the body from absorbing cholesterol from other foods. Mollusks include clams, oysters, mussels, scallops, and squid.

Although crustacean shellfish—crab, shrimp, lobster, and crayfish—do have some cholesterol, the amounts aren't high enough to cross them off your grocery list. A 1½ pound Maine lobster has about 140 milligrams of cholesterol, and Alaska king crab has just 42 milligrams per 3½ ounce serving. Another great reason to enjoy these foods: they are very low in calories and fat, and almost all of the fat it does have is the healthier, unsaturated variety. The 3½ ounces of Alaska king crab has only 96 calories and 1.5 grams fat of which just 1/10 of 1 gram is saturated.

How Do I Store Fish?

While it's always best to cook fresh fish the day you buy it, that's not always possible. To store fish for a day or two without freezing:

- Rinse when you arrive home, place in an air- and water-tight container, and cover with ice cubes. If the ice melts, drain and cover with new ice.
- Store fish in the coldest part of the refrigerator.
- Shellfish stores a bit longer than fresh fish. Store clams and mussels up to two days in the refrigerator:

  Place live shellfish in an open container in a single layer covered with a moist cloth.

  Shucked clams and mussels store up to three days in the refrigerator when you place them in a container in their liquor, which is the liquid surrounding them.
- Store frozen fish no more than six months, as after that it tends to lose flavor; double-wrap to retain moisture and flavor.
- Store cooked fish no more than three to four days in the refrigerator (at a maximum of 40°F) in a tightly sealed container. See the food safety section on how to reheat safely.

HOW DO I TELL WHEN FISH IS DONE?

Use these two easy rules:

- Fish flakes easily but shouldn't completely fall apart when you pick it up with a spatula.
- Fish is opaque almost all the way through, with just the faintest amount of translucency in the middle.
- If you use an instant-read or meat thermometer, fish should reach an internal temperature of 145°F.

Don't forget the age-old "carryover cooking" principle: fish will continue to cook even after you remove it from the heat source, so pull it out slightly before it's done to prevent overcooking.

Cooking Fish: It's Easier Than You Think

Cooking fish is much simpler than most people realize. Fish cooked for just the right amount of time is moist and flavorful.

Rule for Cooking Fin Fish

To cook fresh fish just right—deliciously moist—follow the Canadian Cooking Theory, developed by the Canadian Department of Fisheries: ten minutes per inch (2.5 cm) of thickness, measuring fish at the thickest point.

When cooking fish from frozen, cook twenty minutes per inch. This guideline works for all methods of cooking—baking (in a 450°F oven), steaming, sautéing, grilling, and broiling. Thick or thin, you'll know just how long to cook your fish to a gourmet finish.

How to Bake Fin Fish

Here are two simple ways of baking fin fish:

- Baking in a foil packet is a most "unfussy" way to cook fish, and a great way to get started down the path of eating more fish; this method also conserves omega-3s. Figure ten minutes per inch. Measure fish at thickest point to calculate cooking time. For example, fish that is 1½ inches thick requires a cooking time of ten minutes × 1.5 inches, or fifteen minutes.
  1. Place the fish flesh side up (if it has skin).
  2. Season with your favorite herbs and spices.
  3. Top each serving with up to two cups chopped vegetables, such as spinach, bell peppers, onions, zucchini, mushrooms, and tomatoes.
  4. Seal tightly, leaving one small vent.
- Baking in a pan:
  1. Measure the fish at its thickest point; calculate cooking time. For example, fish that is ¾ inch thick requires a cooking time of ten minutes × 0.75 inches, or seven to eight minutes.
  2. Spray an oven-safe pan with nonstick cooking spray, or line the pan with foil.
  3. Place the fish flesh side up (if it has skin).
  4. Season with your favorite herbs and spices.
  5. Top with slices of lime, lemon, and/or orange to add flavor and ensure moisture.

How to Sauté Fin Fish

Sautéing is a way to get dinner on the table quickly. To sauté:

1. Measure the fish at its thickest point to calculate cooking time (see Canadian Cooking Theory, page 594).
2. Spray a nonstick pan with nonstick cooking spray.
3. Add a measured, small amount (1 teaspoon to 1 tablespoon, depending on the amount of fish) of canola, sesame, walnut, or peanut oil (depending on the recipe and flavor desired).
4. Season the oil with chopped garlic, minced fresh garlic, and/or other favorite herbs and spices.
5. Heat the oil and the herbs over low heat for five minutes, allowing the flavors to fully release into the oil.

6. Increase the heat to medium-high; add the fish and sauté each side for half of the total cooking time as calculated. Another guideline: fish is done when it is just about to lose that transparent look in the middle.
7. For the best flavor and texture, serve immediately.

How to Poach Fin Fish

This gentle cooking method is perfect for seafood, because it imparts lots of moisture and does not mask the delicate flavor of the fish. Traditionally, fish is poached in a court bouillon, a broth made by simmering aromatic vegetables and herbs in water together with peppercorns and something acidic, such as lemon juice, vinegar, or white wine.

An easier way to poach is to use vegetable or chicken stock, with or without a bit of wine. Here's how:

1. Use a pan big enough to lay the fish flat.
2. Pour in enough liquid to just barely cover the fish.
3. Place a pan on one or over two burners, depending on the size of the pan.
4. Bring liquid to a gentle simmer, and adjust heat to maintain the simmer.
5. Fish that's 1 inch thick will take fifteen to twenty minutes; there's no need to turn fillets during cooking.

How to Steam Fin Fish

Steaming is another very gentle cooking method that's especially popular in Asian cuisines for cooking seafood. Like baking and poaching, steaming is a great way to save omega-3s. Here are some tips from the steaming pros:

1. Rub the fish with spices, chopped fresh herbs, ginger, garlic, or chili peppers to infuse flavor into the flesh while it cooks.
2. Use a folding steamer basket (or a bamboo steamer—it might be fun to buy one) with enough room for each piece of fish to lie flat.
    a. Pour about 1½ inches of water into a pan that fits the steamer; you can throw some more spices or herbs into the water to infuse a little extra subtle flavor.
    b. Place the steamer over the water, cover the pot, and bring the water to a boil.
    c. Begin checking the fish for doneness after ten minutes.
3. Follow the previous guidelines for sautéing, but add a tablespoon or

two of broth, juice, or water, cover, and steam over medium-low to medium heat.

4. Follow the previous guidelines for baking in foil, but add a tablespoon or two of broth, juice, or water, and wrap tightly (do not vent). Try our recipe for Steamed Fish, Chinese Style on page 464.

How to Grill Fin Fish

Grilling fish is challenging because it requires more baby-sitting than other cooking methods. Make a note that grilling can destroy more omega-3s than other cooking methods due to the high temperatures required by this method.

1. Measure the fish at its thickest point to calculate cooking time (see Canadian Cooking Theory, page 594).
2. Spray the fish with nonstick cooking spray, or brush it very lightly with canola or extra-virgin olive oil (about ½ teaspoon per side is adequate).
3. Leave the skin on to help retain moisture. Even if the skin sticks to the grill, you can remove the flesh easily.
4. When the grill is hot and ready, place the fish around the edges of the grill, away from the hottest part of the fire.
5. Don't try to lift up the fish right away; it will be stuck to the grate for the first couple of minutes, and prying it up to peek at the underside will tear apart the flesh.
6. Once the fish has been on the grill for a couple of minutes it will start to release some of its juices and should no longer be stuck to the grate. Start checking it for color and doneness at this point, and flip it over when it has light grill marks.

Broiling Fish

While broiling is great when you want a fast, simple, hassle-free preparation with delicious results, note that this cooking method can destroy more omega-3s than other methods. Consider baking on a rack farther from the heat source—it takes just a few more moments.

Best Cooking Methods for Specific Types of Fish

Some types of fish are naturally dry, others are moist. Texture also varies from soft to quite meaty. Choose the cooking method which best enhances the fish to further increase enjoyment; some fish is more versatile than others and can be prepared in a variety of ways. Here's a little guidance:

To steam or poach:

- Bass
- Flounder
- Mackerel
- Mahimahi
- Monkfish
- Orange roughy
- Pike
- Pollack
- Salmon
- Grouper
- Skate
- Snapper
- Swordfish
- Tuna
- Whitefish

To grill or broil:

- Bass
- Bluefish
- Butterfish
- Catfish
- Cod
- Flounder
- Halibut
- Mackerel
- Mahimahi
- Mullet
- Orange roughy
- Pollack
- Pompano
- Sablefish
- Salmon
- Shark
- Skate
- Snapper
- Swordfish
- Trout
- Tuna
- Whitefish

To bake:

- Bass
- Bluefish
- Butterfish
- Catfish
- Cod
- Flounder
- Halibut
- Mackerel
- Mahimahi
- Mullet
- Orange roughy
- Pollack
- Salmon
- Skate
- Snapper
- Swordfish
- Trout
- Tuna
- Whitefish

For making chowder and stews:

- Catfish
- Cod
- Haddock
- Halibut
- Monkfish
- Orange roughy
- Pollack

To sauté:

- Bass
- Catfish
- Flounder
- Halibut
- Monkfish
- Mullet
- Orange roughy
- Perch
- Pollack
- Salmon
- Tuna

Mercury in Fish Put into Perspective

Yes, some fish are high in mercury, which means we should all limit how much we eat of them. Pregnant women should be particularly attentive to limiting such fish, because it tends to settle in the brain and nervous system of their developing babies and can cause learning disabilities.

That said, the U.S. Centers for Disease Control and Prevention (CDC) says we should not shy away from all fish because of the fear of mercury. The problem of excessive mercury in fish as opposed to (note the key word *excessive*) the health benefits of fish is "a very difficult message to convey," says epidemiologist Tom Sinks of the National Center for Environmental Health, part of the CDC. "Fish is a vehicle by which people are exposed to mercury. But at the same time, fish is a good source of protein and nutrients, an important part of the diet, and one we want people to eat in a healthy way."

The best advice is to be aware of fish that tend to be high in mercury, and limit how much you eat of these particular varieties. According to the Washington Department of Public Health, these fish tend to be high in mercury:

- Swordfish
- Shark
- Tilefish
- King mackerel

The United States Environmental Protection Agency recommends checking with local and state health departments about freshwater fish caught there.

Canned tuna is another often misunderstood topic. Yes, there is concern about eating too much of it, because some tuna (depending on the waters from which it is fished) can be high in mercury. Just to be on the cautious side, the Washington Department of Public Health recently issued the

CAVIAR CAUTION

If you take medication classified as monoamine oxidase (MAO) inhibitor (used to treat depression and high blood pressure), don't indulge in caviar. These inhibitors stop certain enzymes, or the body's chemical knives, from working properly to break down tyramine. While tyramine is made naturally as the body breaks down protein, the body does not tolerate large amounts of it in the system at any one time. That's because tyramine constricts blood vessels, which causes blood pressure to increase abnormally. Eating foods that contain tyramine, such as caviar, can be very dangerous, as the tyramine will build up in the bloodstream.

following guidelines for how much canned fish is safe to eat each week, based on body weight:

- Body weight 25 to 40 pounds: 1 tablespoon/week
- Body weight 50 to 75 pounds: 2 ounces/week (1/3 can)
- Body weight 75 to 100 pounds: 3 ounces/week (1/2 can)
- Body weight 100 to 125 pounds: 5 ounces/week
- Body weight 125 to 150 pounds: 6 ounces/week (1 can)
- Body weight 150 to 175 pounds: 8 ounces/week
- Body weight 175 to 200 pounds: 9 ounces/week (1 1/2 cans)
- Body weight 200 pounds or more: 10 ounces/week

Pregnant women, no matter what their weight, should limit canned tuna to one 6-ounce can per week.

Note again a *critical perspective:* Even within the world of canned tuna, there are tremendous differences. *Fortunately*, the type of canned fish highest in omega-3s—albacore—is also lowest in mercury. Chunk and chunk-light varieties are also lower in mercury than solid-white or chunk-white types, which tend to be higher.

For the most up-to-date information on mercury advisories and fish:

- Call the U. S. Food and Drug Administration Center for Food Safety and Applied Nutrition Food Information Line (24 hours a day); 1-888-SAFEFOOD
- Visit the FDA's Food Safety Web site, http://www.cfsan.fda.gov
- Environmental Protection Agency http://www.epa.gov/ost/fish

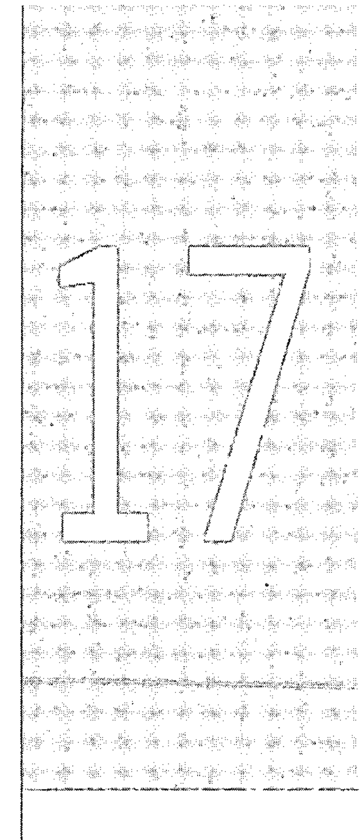

THE ULTIMATE MEAT AND POULTRY BUYING AND USAGE GUIDE

Laura L. Molseed, M.S., R.D., L.D.N.; Lisa C. Peterson, M.S., R.D., C.D.N.;
Jeannie Houchins, R.D.; Barbara Alvarez, M.P.H., R.D., L.D.N.

Which cuts of meat are leanest but still flavorful and tender? What's more versatile: a stewing chicken or a fryer? What's the difference between braising and stewing? We've unraveled all the confusion and compiled the buying, cooking, and storage guides that follow.

Poultry

Chicken and turkey are the most common poultry selections in the United States, but certainly not the only choices. Goose, duck, Cornish hen, and pheasant are now available in many supermarkets.

How do you tell if poultry is fresh? Take a moment to inspect the skin and flesh; poultry should be:

- Unblemished
- Well-plucked, without residual feathers or down
- Free from signs of bleeding
- "Bouncy"—the flesh should give way to slight pressure from your thumb

What weight whole bird should you buy per serving? Purchase one pound (raw weight) per person, but a little more for duck and goose.

Understanding Poultry Label Terms

Poultry labels give you a lot of information. Use our guide to help you understand it.

POULTRY LABEL TERMS

Label Term	Characteristics
Fresh	The bird or its parts have never been below 26°F; this temperature halts microbial activity but allows the surface to remain pliable, yielding to pressure.
Frozen	The bird or parts are held at temperatures below 26°F.
Previously frozen	At some point the bird or its parts have been held at temperatures below 26°F.
Free-range	The bird was raised in a barnyard and given freedom to roam within it and forage for its food instead of being raised in a coop.
Organic	May be coop-raised, but should not have been induced with antibiotics, hormones, or chemicals. They must be raised on certified organic feed for at least 1 year.

Source: USDA and National Agriculture Research Services Web site, National Data Laboratory, Nutrient Database. http://www.nal.usda.gov/fnic/foodcomp.

Matching Cooking Methods with the Bird

Cooking poultry in a variety of ways helps make meals more interesting. Most poultry is extremely versatile and can be prepared using several different methods. With the exception of roasting, refer to the sections later in this chapter for a step-by-step guide to meat and poultry cooking methods.

OPTIMAL COOKING METHODS FOR SPECIFIC TYPES OF POULTRY

Name	Description	Optimal Cooking Method(s)
Cornish game hens	Very small birds, tender meat; usually ¾ to 2 pounds	All cooking methods, but usually roasted
Broiler (chicken or duckling)	Small, tender birds; chicken is usually 1 to 2 pounds, duckling is 2 to 4 pounds	All cooking methods, but usually prepared with dry heat
Fryer (chicken or duckling)	Small birds, very tender; usually 2 to 4 pounds	All cooking methods are appropriate

Name	Description	Optimal Cooking Method(s)
Roaster (chicken or duckling)	Small to medium birds; 3 to 6 pounds	Usually roasted but suitable for all cooking methods
Stewing hen, turkey, goose, or duck	Medium, old female birds, tough meat; 3 to 6 pounds	Slow, moist heat is best
Capon (castrated male)	Young male bird, tender meat; 5 to 8 pounds	All cooking methods
Young hen or Tom turkey	Very tender young bird; 8 to 22 pounds	All cooking methods
Yearling turkey	Mature bird, but still tender; 10 to 30 pounds	Usually roasted
Young goose or gosling	Young, tender bird; 6 to 10 pounds	Usually roasted
Guinea hen or fowl (pheasant)	Tender bird; 1.6 to 3.3 pounds	Usually roasted

How to Roast Poultry

When roasting a whole bird, additional fat is not needed, as the poultry naturally bastes itself. Roasting with the skin is best, as the fat layer is directly under the skin and the skin helps seal the moisture in the bird, minimizing the risk of its drying out. Remove and discard the skin just prior to serving. Basting the bird with its own juice drippings periodically throughout the cooking process will bump up moisture. Follow these easy instructions to enjoy roasted poultry:

1. Preheat the oven to 450°F.
2. Remove the giblets and neck from the cavity of the bird; rinse the cavity well inside and out.
3. Place the bird in a roasting pan; season the bird inside and out.
4. Place in the oven. For larger birds, reduce the temperature to 325°F to 350°F immediately; for smaller birds reduce the temperature after thirty minutes. The initial higher temperature browns the outside quickly, sealing in the juices.

TO STUFF OR NOT TO STUFF?

Most food safety professionals recommend not stuffing poultry because of the chance that the stuffing will not reach a temperature high enough to destroy bacteria that could lead to food-borne illness. If you do choose to stuff, do so just before placing poultry in the oven. Fill the cavity loosely, allowing room for expansion. Check the temperature of the stuffing in the middle, making sure it reaches 165°F.

ARE POP-UP THERMOMETERS AN ACCURATE WAY TO CHECK THE TEMPERATURE OF A ROASTED BIRD?

The pop-up thermometer is simply a guide indicating when the bird is *close* to being cooked through. Rely on only a meat or instant-read thermometer to tell when poultry is cooked through.

5. Brown Cornish game hens and other small birds on the stove top prior to placing in the oven (they will not brown adequately by the time they finish cooking).

The following table provides approximate times for cooking poultry. The only sure way, however, to know when poultry is cooked through is to check the temperature with a meat or instant-read thermometer. For whole birds, check the temperature in the innermost part of the thigh (between the thigh and the breast); it should reach 180°F. If cooking individual pieces, the temperature should reach 170°F.

APPROXIMATE ROASTING TIMES FOR POULTRY
(Rely on only a meat or instant-read thermometer)

Type of Poultry	Roasting Time (350°F)
Chicken, whole stuffed	
3 to 4 pounds	1½ to 2 hours
5 to 7 pounds	2¼ to 2¾ hours
Chicken, whole unstuffed	
3 to 4 pounds	1¼ to 1½ hours
5 to 7 pounds	2 to 2¼ hours
Chicken parts	
Breast halves, bone in	30 to 40 minutes
Boneless breasts	20 to 30 minutes
Legs, thighs, or wings	40 to 50 minutes
Cornish game hens	50 to 60 minutes (prebrowned)
Turkey, whole unstuffed	
8 to 12 pounds	2¾ to 3 hours
12 to 14 pounds	3 to 3¾ hours
14 to 18 pounds	3¾ to 4¼ hours
18 to 20 pounds	4¼ to 4½ hours
20 to 24 pounds	4½ to 5 hours
Turkey, whole stuffed	
8 to 12 pounds	3 to 3½ hours
12 to 14 pounds	3½ to 4 hours
14 to 18 pounds	4 to 4¼ hours
18 to 20 pounds	4¼ to 4¾ hours
20 to 24 pounds	4¾ to 5¼ hours
Turkey breast	
4 to 6 pounds	1½ to 2¼ hours
6 to 8 pounds	2¼ to 3¼ hours
Duckling, whole	30 to 35 minutes per pound
Duckling, breast or parts	2 hours
Goose, whole 8 to 12 pounds	2½ to 3 hours or more

Beef and Pork

Purchase the leanest cut of meat that matches your budget and recipe. Refer to the lists that follow for the leanest cuts of beef and pork, each listed with their recommended cooking techniques.

The ten leanest cuts of beef and the best cooking methods:

- Eye round steak: pan-broil, grill, moist-cook
- Eye round roast: roast, moist-cook
- Top round steak: stir-fry, pan-broil, broil, or grill
- Top round roast: roast
- Round tip steak, thin cut: stir-fry, pan-broil
- Top sirloin steak: stir-fry, pan-broil, broil, grill
- Top loin steak: stir-fry, pan-broil, broil, grill
- Tenderloin steak: stir-fry, pan-broil, broil, grill
- Tenderloin roast: roast, grill
- Flank steak: stir-fry, broil, grill, moist-cook

The eight leanest cuts of pork and the best cooking methods:

- Tenderloin: roast, grill, sauté
- Boneless sirloin chop: sauté, grill, braise
- Boneless loin roast: roast
- Boneless top loin chop: roast, grill, sauté, braise
- Loin chop: roast, grill, sauté, braise
- Boneless sirloin roast: roast
- Rib chop: roast, grill, sauté, braise
- Boneless rib roast: roast

BEEF AND PORK: TEMPERATURES AND VISUAL CUES OF DONENESS

Type of Meat	Visual	Temperature
Ground meat including patties, sausages, meat loaf, meatballs	• Centers are no longer pink and juices are clear	160°F
Whole cuts like roasts, chops and steaks (bone-in or boneless). Includes beef, veal, pork, and lamb.	• Medium-rare: red, warm, and juicy center • Medium: dark-pink to pink, hot and juicy center • Well done: tan, hot, and slightly moist center	145°F 160°F 170°F
Leftovers	Piping hot with steam	165°F
Fresh ham	Hot, moist, and light tan center with a hint of blush	160°F
Fully cooked ham (smoked, spiral-sliced, etc.)	Heated through	140°F

Meat and Poultry Cooking Know-How

Two excellent poultry-cooking techniques are dry and moist. Let's take a look at the many variations within each of these categories.

Sautéing

This stove-top method is typically used for small thin pieces of meat or poultry. Often the cuts are pounded to make them thinner and shorten the cooking time. Thicker cuts are best sautéed on the stove top just long enough to brown them, and then cooked until done in the oven.

- To sauté, place the poultry or meat on the stove in a preheated pan coated with vegetable oil cooking spray. Do not turn until it releases easily from the pan. Peeking to see if it is done or turning it too quickly can interrupt the browning process and decrease taste.
- Try seasoning blends, rubs (or just salt and pepper).

  Rub on the meat up to 12 hours before cooking (refrigerate covered tightly until cooking).

  If salting poultry, salt right before cooking so that it does not pull the moisture out of the meat.

  When the product is finished cooking, deglaze the pan by adding stock or wine and make a sauce to serve with it.

Grilling or Broiling

This method works well with individual pieces of poultry and tender cuts of meat. Marinades work well to retain moisture, tenderize, and add flavor. Marinate at least thirty minutes and not more than twenty-four hours. *Discard marinating liquid—do not use to pour over meat or as a dipping sauce—as it contains bacteria that can cause food-borne illness.*

For best grilling results:

- Start with a clean grill.
- Before turning on heat, lightly oil the grill grate.
- Preheat the grill and place the item on the grill once it is well heated. Use the palm test to monitor the temperature of the grill if you don't have a built-in thermometer. If you can hold your palm over the grill comfortably for four to five seconds, the grill is probably at an optimal temperature for most grilling purposes.
- Turn the meat only once or twice for best results, flipping when lines have formed on the meat and it releases easily from the grill.

- Cooking times vary according to the cut and thickness as well as the grill's heat.
- To ensure safety, check for doneness with an instant-read thermometer.

Pan-Frying

It *is* possible to fry without adding a lot of extra fat. Use an oil that can be heated to higher temperatures, such as canola or peanut oils, because heating the hot oil decreases the amount of fat absorbed into the meat and also ensures the shortest possible cooking time, which helps retain moisture.

- Heat the oil to 365°F; test with a frying thermometer.
- Fry in small batches. Cold meat lowers the oil temperature, and large batches lower it even more.

Stir-Frying

This Asian-inspired, popular method of cooking strips or chunks of poultry and meat, vegetables, and other ingredients over very high heat can be a healthful alternative. For best results:

- Cut food into small pieces, which ensures quicker cooking and therefore less oil absorption.
- Use a very small amount of oil (1 teaspoon to 2 tablespoons, depending on the amount of food); stretch it by adding broth or wine.
- Stir food constantly over a high heat.

Moist-Cooking

Moist-cooking techniques, such as braising and stewing, work well with tougher cuts of meat and older birds (such as stewing hens). Casseroles, too, are great ways to make tough meat or poultry more moist, flavorful, and tender. Cook meat or poultry first, and then assemble the casserole. For either method:

- Sear in a small amount of oil or fat along with some highly flavored vegetables, such as onions, garlic, and/or shallots. A high enough temperature is extremely important for optimal browning.
- Add liquid (broth, juice, water, and/or wine) and other ingredients (such as vegetables), cover, and simmer.
- Cooking time is shorter for stewing than for braising, but longer simmering further tenderizes the meat and adds flavor.

Safe Food Handling in the Store, in the Car, at Home

Get the most from the money you've spent on meat and poultry by practicing a few simple food-safety strategies. In the store:

- Look for freshness in packaging:

  Reach only for packages free of tears.

  Pass over leaking packages and choose one that is dry.

  Check the "sell by" or "use by" date.
- Place meat and poultry in plastic bags provided near the meat case. Seal as tightly as possible. Bagging meat and poultry helps prevent cross-contamination of other foods in your cart.
- Position meat and poultry on the bottom of your cart, away from ready-to-eat foods.

To transport food from the store to your home safely:

- Load meat and poultry into the coolest part of your car, such as a spot away from sun and the heater.
- In hot weather, load meat into an ice-filled cooler if the supermarket is more than thirty minutes away.

In your home:

- Refrigerate or freeze meat and poultry immediately upon arriving home.
- Store meat and poultry in the original packaging bolstered with another layer—plastic wrap, aluminum foil, or storage bags—to prevent both leaks and freezer burn.
- Check the refrigerator temperature. It should be 40°F or below (refer to chart later in this chapter for information on how long poultry can be held in the refrigerator).
- Check the freezer temperature, which should be 0°F or below (refer to the table that follows for recommended storage times).

To thaw frozen meat and poultry:

- Place in a container that can catch thawing juices.
- Allow twenty-four hours per four pounds of whole poultry.

  Allow three to nine hours for poultry pieces.

  Allow three to five hours per pound for roasts.

  Allow twenty-four hours for a 1½-inch-thick package of ground or cubed meat.

  Allow twelve hours to thaw 1-inch-thick chops and steaks.

- For quicker thawing:

  Place frozen poultry in a leak-proof bag and submerge in cold tap water; change the water every thirty minutes.
- Cook immediately after thawing and before refreezing.
- For microwave thawing, refer to the manufacturer's directions for time and power settings.

While preparing food:

- Wash hands before and after handling raw meat. During food preparation, wash hands after handling meat and before touching other food (such as produce).
- Marinate meat and poultry covered and in the refrigerator.
- Wash knives, bowls, and counter tops with hot, soapy water (or place in the dishwasher).
- Sanitize cutting boards with a solution of 1 teaspoon chlorine bleach mixed in 1 quart of water.

Store leftovers safely by:

- Refrigerating or freezing leftover meat and poultry within two hours (one hour during hot weather)
- Discarding leftovers that have been sitting at room temperature for more than two hours
- Removing and storing stuffing in a separate container

When in doubt, throw it out. If food looks or smells unsafe, discard it safely.

HOW LONG DOES POULTRY KEEP IN THE REFRIGERATOR AND THE FREEZER?

Product	Refrigerator	Freezer
Poultry cold cuts/hot dogs	3 to 5 days	1 to 2 months
Poultry salads (home made or purchased)	3 to 5 days	Not recommended
Sausage (fresh, raw)	1 to 2 days	1 to 2 months
Ground poultry	1 to 2 days	3 to 4 months
Fresh, whole poultry	1 to 2 days	1 year (6 months for duck and geese)
Fresh pieces	1 to 2 days	9 months
Cooked products (leftovers)	3 to 4 days	2 to 4 months
Giblets (fresh, uncooked)	1 to 2 days	3 to 4 months
Poultry soups/stews	3 to 4 days	2 to 3 months
Chicken nuggets and patties	1 to 2 days	1 to 3 months

For more information, contact:

National Chicken Council
1015 15th Street NW, Suite 930
Washington, DC 20005-2605
202-296-2622
fax: 202-293-4005
http://www.eatchicken.com

USDA Meat and Poultry Hotline
1-888-mphotline (674-6854)
1-800-256-7072 (TTY)
http://www.mphotline.fsis.usda.gov

National Turkey Federation
1225 New York Ave., Suite 400
Washington, DC 20005
202-898-0100
fax: 202-898-0203
http://www.eatturkey.com

The National Pork Producers Council
7733 Douglas Avenue
Urbandale, IA 50322
515-278-8012
fax: 515-278-8011
http://www.nppc.org

The National Cattlemen's Beef Association
9110 East Nichols Ave. #300
Centennial, CO 80112
303-694-0305
fax: 303-694-2851
http://www.beef.org
http://www.veal.org

American Lamb Board
877-747-4566
http://www.americanlambboard.org
http://www.lambinfo.com

18

MILK AND OTHER DAIRY

Building Strong Bones and More

Deanna Rose, R.D., L.D.N., and Catherine Hoffmann, M.S., R.D.

Milk, yogurt, and other dairy products boast a powerful nutrient package that includes calcium, the most important predictor of bone strength. Including at least three servings daily into your eating plan is an important step toward making and keeping bones strong today *and* tomorrow. In addition to calcium, dairy products are also rich in:

- Potassium (for regulating blood pressure and heart contractions)
- Phosphorus (works with calcium to strengthen bones and teeth, for energy metabolism and healthy cell membranes)
- Protein (for growth, wound healing, thinking, and repairing and replacing cells)
- Vitamin D (another key nutrient for bone strength)
- Vitamin A (for healthy eyes and tissues inside the body)
- Vitamin B_{12} (for healthy red blood cells, making new cells)
- Riboflavin (for healthy red blood cells, skin, and eyes)
- Niacin (for healthy skin, nerves, and digestive system)

How Much Calcium?

The National Academy of Sciences recommends a specific amount by milligram of calcium according to age and gender. We provide that information and go one step further: we converted the milligram amount into the number of dairy servings you need each day.

CALCIUM REQUIREMENTS BY AGE

Age	Calcium Recommended Daily (mg)	Number of Daily Servings
1 to 3	500	2
4 to 8	800	3
9 to 18	1,300	4
19 to 50	1,000	3
Over 50	1,200	4

America's Calcium Intake Is Too Low

America's low calcium intake is recognized as a major public health problem. According to the USDA 1996 study, "Continuing Survey of Food Intakes by Individuals," all age groups fall short of calcium need. For example:

- One out of three kids ages one to five do not get the recommended amount of calcium.
- Approximately two out of three preteens fall short of the calcium they need.
- An astonishing nine out of ten teenage girls and seven out of ten teenage boys don't meet daily calcium recommendations. On average, teen girls drink twice as much soda as milk.

While low calcium intake is troublesome at every age, it is especially disconcerting among young people. By about age twenty, people have acquired about 98 percent of their skeletal mass. Building strong bones during childhood and adolescence is the best defense against developing osteoporosis later in life, according to USDA nutrition experts.

Adult women and people over age fifty have even greater trouble getting the calcium they need. According to the USDA report:

- Among people age fifty and older, less than 15 percent—or less than one in six—take in enough calcium.
- Half of all adult women in this country do not drink even one glass of milk daily.

Although bones have stopped growing in length, they continue to grow in density until about age thirty. After that, adequate calcium helps maintain bone strength. As you can see, we need calcium at every age to keep standing strong. Take action today to reduce risk of future osteoporosis and fractures.

Do I Get Enough Calcium in Lower-Fat Dairy?

Absolutely—and your heart will thank you, too. Reap all the calcium of whole milk—and all the other nutrients—for much fewer calories and fat grams. In addition, most reduced-fat dairy has more calcium than the regular fat varieties. The following chart compares the fat content of dairy products.

COMPARISON OF FAT IN MILK

Type of Milk	Other Names	Total Fat Grams per 8 Ounces (1 Cup)
Fat free	Nonfat, skim	<0.5
Low fat	1%	3
Reduced fat	2% fat	5
Whole milk	3.25% fat	8

Use More Yogurt, Get More Calcium

- Spoon flavored yogurt on the top of pancakes or waffles.
- Substitute plain yogurt for half of the mayonnaise called for in chicken, potato, or tuna salads.
- Use yogurt as a base for dips; stir in favorite herbs and spices.
- Top baked potatoes with yogurt instead of sour cream.
- Add a dollop to garnish a cream soup (instead of sour cream).
- Blend yogurt with ice and fresh fruit for a healthy smoothie drink.

Can I Enjoy Dairy If I Am Lactose Intolerant?

There are many solutions for enjoying dairy foods if you are lactose intolerant, a condition in which the body cannot easily break down lactose, the sugar in milk. When this happens, a person can experience gastrointestinal discomfort and/or diarrhea. There are varying degrees of lactose intolerance, but most people can still enjoy some dairy.

Try these strategies for including dairy products if you have a problem digesting lactose:

- Look for lactose-reduced or lactose-free milk.
- Ask your physician about taking a supplement that can help you digest lactose.

- Try yogurt instead of milk, as the cultures help break down lactose.
- Choose hard cheeses, such as cheddar and Swiss, which are naturally lower in lactose.
- Go for smaller portions, such as one-half cup of milk at a time.
- Team up dairy foods with other foods, as dairy is often easier to digest when there is other food in the stomach.

Tips for Using More Dairy

Try some of these great ideas for pouring more milk into your diet:

- Use low-fat milk instead of water when making:

  Instant hot cocoa

  Hot cereals

  Canned soups

  Boxed rice dishes

  Muffin and pancake mixes

  Risotto or couscous (substitute up to half the water with low-fat milk)
- Instead of plain ice, freeze fat-free milk or yogurt in ice-cube trays for thickening smoothies and milkshakes.
- Make fluffier scrambled eggs and omelets by whisking in 2 tablespoons of milk for each egg used.
- Cook fresh or frozen corn ears in lightly salted milk instead of water for a sweeter and more flavorful taste.

More Help in the Kitchen Using Dairy Products

Here we've gathered some of the most common questions regarding storing, using, and freezing dairy products.

How long can I keep milk once I've opened it? Check the date on the container. This refers to the latest date by which the product was meant to be sold. It is used by the dairy industry to indicate the age of individual packages and does not reflect the shelf life of the product.

To preserve the quality of milk and other dairy foods:

- Refrigerate milk at 40°F or less as soon as possible after purchase. Temperatures above 40°F reduce the shelf life of dairy products.
- Rotate dairy products in your refrigerator.
- Return the milk container to the refrigerator immediately.
- Never return unused milk to the original container.

- Use proper containers to protect milk from exposure to sunlight, bright daylight, and strong fluorescent light. This helps prevent milk from picking up other flavors in the refrigerator; it also reduces the chance that light-sensitive nutrients (such as riboflavin, ascorbic acid, and vitamin B_6) will break down.

Can I cut away the mold on cheese and then use the rest? If mold develops on cheese, discard ½ inch of cheese on all sides of the visible mold. The exception is mold-ripened cheeses such as Roquefort and blue. In general, most molds are harmless, although some produce toxins that can diffuse into the cheese. Undesirable mold occurs when cheeses are improperly wrapped and consequently exposed to air.

Can I freeze milk and cheese? What is the best way to thaw them? With the exception of butter, ice cream, frozen yogurt, and other frozen dairy desserts, freezing of most dairy foods (e.g., milk, cream, yogurt, milk puddings, soft cheeses) is not recommended. Although naturally hard, semihard, and processed cheeses can be frozen, this affects their texture, causing them to become crumbly and mealy after thawing. However, they are suitable for cooking or use in salads or salad dressing.

If frozen, cheeses should be thawed slowly in the refrigerator for twenty-four hours and then used as soon as possible after thawing.

The following are other cheese cooking and storage tips:

- Store cheeses in waxed paper or parchment paper in the refrigerator to allow them to breathe and therefore last longer.
- Keep cheese in the refrigerator before grating or shredding for the best consistency.
- Four ounces of hard cheese equals 1 cup of shredded cheese.
- Shred or cut cheese into small pieces before melting, or use shredded cheese blends.
- If using cheese in a sauce, add it to the sauce after it comes off the heat, to keep it from separating. Shredding or grating the cheese helps it melt into the sauce more quickly.

Handling Eggs Safely at Home

Like raw meat, poultry, and fish, eggs are perishable. Even unbroken, clean, fresh shell eggs may contain *Salmonella* Enteritidis (SE) bacteria that can cause food-borne illness. While the number of eggs affected is quite small, the risk is always there. To be safe, eggs must be properly handled, refrigerated, and cooked.

Bacteria can be on the outside of a shell egg because the egg exits the hen's body through the same passageway as feces are excreted. That's why eggs are washed and sanitized at the processing plant. Nevertheless, bacteria can be inside an uncracked, whole egg. Contamination may be due to bacteria within the hen's ovary or oviduct before the shell forms around the yolk and the white. Salmonella doesn't make the hen sick. It is also possible for eggs to become infected by SE fecal contamination through the pores of the shells after they're laid.

Enjoy eggs safely by following the advice of the Food Safety and Inspection Service of the USDA:

- Don't eat raw eggs. This includes "health food" milk shakes with raw eggs, Caesar salad, Hollandaise sauce, and any other foods like homemade mayonnaise, ice cream, or eggnog made from recipes in which the raw egg ingredients are not cooked.
- Buy clean eggs. At the store, choose Grades A or AA eggs with clean uncracked shells. Make sure they've been refrigerated in the store.
- Refrigerate eggs. Take eggs straight home and store them immediately in the refrigerator set at 40°F or slightly below. Store them in the grocery carton in the coldest part of the refrigerator and not in the door.
- Use eggs within recommended times.

  Use raw shell eggs within three to five weeks. Hard-cooked eggs will keep refrigerated for one week.

  Use leftover yolks and whites within four days.
- If eggs crack on the way home from the store, break them into a clean container, cover it tightly, refrigerate, and use within two days.
- Freeze eggs for longer storage (up to one year).

  Eggs should not be frozen in their shells.

  To freeze whole eggs, beat the yolks and the whites together.

  Egg whites can be frozen by themselves.
- If eggs freeze accidentally in their shells, keep them frozen until needed (but discard those with cracked shells).

  Defrost them in the refrigerator.

  Discard any with cracked shells.
- Handle eggs safely. Wash hands, utensils, equipment, and work areas with warm soapy water before and after contact with eggs and dishes containing eggs.
- Don't keep eggs—including Easter eggs—out of the refrigerator more than two hours.
- Serve cooked eggs and dishes containing eggs immediately after cooking, or place in shallow containers for quick cooling and refrigerate at once for later use. Use within three to four days.

- Cook eggs.

  Many cooking methods can be used to cook eggs safely, including poaching, hard boiling, scrambling, frying, and baking.

  Eggs must be cooked thoroughly until the yolks are firm. Scrambled eggs should not be runny.

  Casseroles and other dishes containing eggs should be cooked to 160°F as measured with a food thermometer.

- Use safe egg recipes.

  Egg mixtures are safe if they reach 160°F, so homemade ice cream and eggnog can be made safely from a cooked base.

  Dry meringue shells are safe, as are divinity candy and seven-minute frosting.

  Meringue-topped pies should be safe if baked at 350°F for about fifteen minutes.

  Chiffon pies and fruit whips made with raw, beaten egg whites may not be safe. Substitute whipped cream or whipped topping.

  To make key lime pie safely, heat the lime (or lemon) juice with the raw egg yolks in a pan on the stove, stirring constantly, until the mixture reaches 160°F. Then combine it with the sweetened condensed milk and pour it into a baked piecrust.

  Cook egg dishes such as quiche and casseroles to 160°F as measured with a food thermometer.

A Guide to Egg Products

The term "egg products" refers to eggs that have been removed from their shells for processing. Basic egg products include whole eggs, whites, yolks, and various blends, with or without nonegg ingredients that are processed and pasteurized. They are available in liquid, frozen, and dried forms. No-cholesterol refrigerated or frozen egg substitutes consist of egg whites, artificial color, and other nonegg additives.

Are Egg Products Pasteurized?

Yes. The 1970 Egg Products Inspection Act requires that all egg products distributed for consumption be pasteurized. They are rapidly heated and held at a minimum-required temperature for a specified time. This destroys Salmonella but it does not cook the eggs or affect their color, flavor, nutritional value, or use. Dried whites are pasteurized by heating in the dried form.

Can Egg Products Be Used in Uncooked Foods?

Although they have been pasteurized, egg products are best used in a cooked product (which reaches an internal temperature of 160°F). Egg products can be substituted in recipes typically made with raw eggs that aren't cooked to 160°F, such as Caesar salad and homemade mayonnaise. Even though egg products are pasteurized, for optimal safety it is best to start with a cooked base, especially if serving high-risk people—those with health problems, the very young, the elderly, and pregnant women.

Buying Tips for Egg Products

- Containers should be tightly sealed.
- Frozen products should show no sign of thawing.
- Purchase refrigerated products kept at 40°F or below.
- Avoid hardened dried-egg products.

Maximum Storage Times for Egg Products

- Use frozen egg products within one year.
- If the container for liquid products bears a "use by" date, observe it.
- For liquid products without an expiration date, store unopened cartons at 40°F or below for up to seven days (not over three days after opening).
- Don't freeze opened cartons or refreeze frozen cartons that have been thawed.
- Unopened dried-egg products can be stored at room temperature as long as they are kept cool and dry. After opening, keep refrigerated.
- Use reconstituted products immediately or refrigerate and use that day.

NUTRITIONAL VALUES OF EGGS AND EGG PRODUCTS

Product	Calories	Total Fat (grams)	Protein (grams)
Whole egg, extra-large	90	6	7
Whole egg, large	70	5	6
Egg white	15	0	4
Liquid egg substitute (¼ cup)	50	2	8
Liquid egg white (¼ cup)	30	0	6

For further information about eggs and safe egg handling contact:

USDA Meat and Poultry Hotline
1-800-535-4555 (toll-free nationwide)
1-800-256-7072 (TTY)
FDA Food Information Line:
1-888-SAFEFOOD (toll-free nationwide)
http://www.fsis.usda.gov

19

HELP IN THE KITCHEN

Substitutions and Equivalents

Dorothy Chen-Maynard, Ph.D., R.D.; Barbara LaVella M.B.A., R.D., L.D.; Linda McDonald, M.S., R.D.;
Barbara Clonninger, M.S., R.D.,L.D.; Sandy Kapoor, Ph.D., R.D., F.A.D.A

Have you ever been in the middle of baking cookies and realized you didn't have just one ingredient? What about wondering if the box of rice you have is large enough to feed a crowd? We've all tried to recall how many cups are in a gallon (why is that so hard to remember?). Use the three information-packed tables in this chapter for everyday solutions to kitchen encounters:

- Ingredient substitutions
- Food equivalents
- Equivalent measures

You will also find more specific information in the fruit, grain, legume, and vegetable chapters.

[illegible]TITUTIONS

	Amount	Substitutes
[illegible]e	1 teaspoon	• ½ teaspoon cinnamon and ½ teaspoon ground cloves
Apple pie spice	1 teaspoon	• ½ teaspoon cinnamon, ¼ teaspoon nutmeg, and ⅛ teaspoon cardamom
Arrowroot starch	1 teaspoon	• 1 tablespoon flour • 1½ teaspoons cornstarch
Baking powder	1 teaspoon	• ¼ teaspoon baking soda plus ⅝ teaspoon cream of tartar • ¼ teaspoon baking soda plus ½ tablespoon vinegar • ⅓ teaspoon baking soda plus ½ teaspoon cream of tartar
Bay leaf	1 whole	• ¼ teaspoon cracked bay leaves
Beef stock base, instant	2 teaspoons	• 1 beef bouillon cube
Beef stock base, instant	4 teaspoons dissolved in 1¼ cups water	• 1 10½-ounce can condensed, beef bouillon or consommé
Bread crumbs, dry	⅓ cup	• 1 slice of bread
Bread crumbs, soft	¾ cup	• 1 slice of bread
Broth, beef or chicken	1 cup	• 1 bouillon cube dissolved in 1 cup boiling water • 1 teaspoon powdered broth base in 1 cup boiling water
Catsup	1 cup	• 1 cup tomato sauce, ½ cup sugar, and 2 tablespoons vinegar (for use in cooking)
Chicken stock base, instant	1½ teaspoons	• 1 chicken bouillon cube
Chicken stock base, instant	1 tablespoon dissolved in 1 cup water	• 1 cup canned or homemade chicken broth or stock
Chili sauce	1 cup	• 1 cup tomato sauce, ¼ cup brown sugar, 2 tablespoons vinegar, ¼ teaspoon cinnamon, dash each of ground cloves and allspice
Chives, finely chopped	2 teaspoons	• 2 teaspoons finely chopped green onion tops
Chocolate chips, semisweet	1 ounce	• 1 ounce sweet cooking chocolate
Chocolate, semisweet	1 ounce	• 1 ounce unsweetened chocolate plus 4 teaspoons sugar
Chocolate, semisweet pieces, melted	6-ounce package	• 2 squares unsweetened chocolate plus 2 tablespoons shortening and ½ cup sugar
Chocolate, unsweetened	1 ounce or square	• 3 tablespoons cocoa plus 1 tablespoon butter or margarine • 3 tablespoons carob powder plus 2 tablespoons water
Cocoa	¼ cup or 4 tablespoons	• 1 ounce (square) chocolate (decrease fat by ½ tablespoon
Cornmeal, self-rising	1 cup	• ⅞ cup plain cornmeal, 1½ tablespoons baking powder and ½ teaspoon salt • Equivalent: 1 pound = 3 cups

Ingredient	Amount	Substitutes
Corn syrup	1 cup	• 1 cup sugar plus ¼ cup liquid (use whatever liquid is called for in the recipe) • 1 cup honey
Corn syrup, dark	1 cup	• ¾ cup light corn syrup and ¼ cup light molasses
Cornstarch (for thickening)*	1 tablespoon	• 2 teaspoons arrowroot • 2 tablespoons all-purpose flour • 4 to 6 teaspoons quick-cooking tapioca
Cream cheese		• The same amount of part-skim milk ricotta cheese or low-fat cottage cheese blended or processed until smooth
Cream of tartar	½ teaspoon	• 1½ teaspoons lemon juice or vinegar
Flour, all-purpose white flour	1 cup	• ½ cup whole wheat flour plus ½ cup all-purpose flour Tip: It is generally recommended that you replace no more than half the all-purpose white flour with whole-wheat flour.
Flour, self-rising	1 cup sifted	• 1 cup sifted all-purpose flour plus 1½ teaspoons baking powder and ½ teaspoon salt
Garlic	1 clove, small	• ⅛ teaspoon garlic powder or ¼ teaspoon instant minced garlic
Gelatin, flavored	3 ounces	• 1 tablespoon plain gelatin and 2 cups fruit juice
Herbs, dried	1 teaspoon	• 1 tablespoon fresh, finely cut
Herbs, fresh	1 tablespoon, finely cut	• 1 teaspoon dried herbs • ½ teaspoon ground herbs
Honey	1 cup	• 1¼ cups sugar plus ¼ cup liquid (use liquid called for in recipe)
Lemon	1 teaspoon juice	• ½ teaspoon vinegar
Milk, buttermilk	1 cup	• 1 cup plain yogurt
Milk, fat-free	1 cup	• 6 tablespoons nonfat dry milk powder and enough water to make one cup, or follow manufacturer's directions
Onion	1 small	• ¼ cup chopped fresh onion • 1 to 2 teaspoons minced onion • 1 teaspoon onion powder
Rum	¼ cup	• 1 tablespoon rum extract plus 3 tablespoons liquid (use liquid called for in recipe or water)
Sugar, confectioners' or powdered	1 cup	• ¾ cup granulated sugar
Tomato juice	1 cup	• ½ cup tomato sauce plus ½ cup water
Tomatoes, fresh	2 cups, chopped	• 16-ounce canned
Tomatoes, chopped	16-ounce can	• 3 fresh medium • 16-ounce can stewed

(continued)

INGREDIENT SUBSTITUTIONS *(continued)*

Ingredient	Amount	Substitutes
Yeast, active dry	1 tablespoon	• 1 cake (3/5 ounce), compressed (2/3 ounce) • 1 package active dry yeast

*Liquids thickened with cornstarch will be somewhat translucent, while flour gives a more opaque appearance. Cornstarch will thicken a liquid almost immediately. A flour-based sauce or gravy must be cooked longer to thicken and will have a flourlike taste if undercooked. According to *The Joy of Cooking* (Scribner, 1997), when using flour as a substitution for cornstarch in sauces and gravies, simmer the sauce for about 3 minutes *after* it has thickened to help avoid a raw taste of flour.

- Cornstarch-thickened liquids are more likely to thin if overheated, cooked too long, or reheated.
- Whether you use cornstarch or flour, mix it with a little cold water or other cold liquid, about two parts liquid to one part thickener, before adding it to the rest of the liquid.
- (Note: when you mix flour with fat to make a roux for use as a thickener, do not dissolve it in liquid first.)

Sources: North Dakota State University Extension Service; University of Nebraska Cooperative Extension in Lancaster County; Utah State University Extension; Oleane Carden Zenoble, "Ingredient Substitution and Equivalent Chart," Circular HEto585, Alabama Cooperative Extension Service, Auburn University.

How Many Cups in a Pound of . . .? Helpful Food Equivalents

Ever wonder how many cups of flour there are in a five-pound bag? How many eggs it takes to yield a cup cooked and chopped? The following tables will help you solve these everyday dilemmas.

DAIRY PRODUCT EQUIVALENTS

(All amounts are approximate and may vary depending on food item size, peel, manufacturers' packing, etc.)

Food	This Amount	Equals
Butter or margarine	1 pound	2 cups
	1 stick	½ cup; ⅓ cup clarified
	1 ounce	2 tablespoons
Cheese		
Cottage	1 pound	2 cups
Cream	3-ounce package	⅓ cup
Parmesan	8 ounces	1½ cups grated
Eggs, hard cooked	8 medium eggs	3¼ cups chopped
Milk, evaporated or sweetened condensed	13- or 14-ounce can	1¼ cups to 1¼ cups + 1 tablespoon
Whipped topping, frozen	8-ounce carton	3½ cups
Whipping cream	1 cup liquid	2 cups whipped
Yogurt	3 cups	1 cup yogurt "cheese"

ABOUT YOGURT CHEESE

Enjoy this creamy spread on toast, bagels, and more without the fat of cream cheese—and with lots more protein. You need one quart of yogurt (low-fat plain or vanilla, depending on intended use), a paper coffee filter, a sieve, and a 2- to-3-cup bowl. Make yogurt cheese by following these easy steps:

1. Line a sieve with a paper coffee filter; balance the sieve securely atop the bowl.
2. Transfer the yogurt to the lined sieve.
3. Cover and place in the refrigerator overnight, or at least eight hours.

Liquid from the yogurt drains into the bowl, and the thickened cheese in the sieve is ready for use. Add herbs, spices, chopped vegetables, or dried fruit to flavor the cheese.

MEAT, SEAFOOD, POULTRY, AND MEAT-SUBSTITUTE EQUIVALENTS

Food	This Amount	Equals
Bacon, raw	1 pound	Average: 16 to 24 slices
Bacon, sliced, cooked	1 pound	1 to 1½ cups crumbled
	1 slice	1 tablespoon crumbled
Beef, cooked, diced	1 pound	3 cups
Beef, ground	1 pound	2 cups; 12 ounces (cooked)
Chicken breast half	1 each	½ cup cooked, chopped
Chicken broth	13¾ ounce can	1¾ cups
Chicken, bone in	3 pounds	2½ to 3 cups cooked, diced
Chicken, boned	1 pound	3 cups cooked, diced
Chicken, canned	5-ounce can	½ cup drained
Clams, in shell	8 quarts	1 quart shucked
Clams, shucked	1 quart	2 to 3 cups chopped
Crabmeat, canned	6½-ounce can	1 cup flaked
Crab, whole, in shell	1 pound	⅔ cup flaked; 6 to 7 ounces edible crab
Ham, cooked	1 pound	2 cups ground; 3 cups diced
Lobster	2½ pound whole	2 cups cooked meat
Mussels, unshucked	1 quart	1 cup meat or 25 mussels
Oysters, shucked	1 pound	1 pint or 12 medium
Peanut butter	18-ounce jar	2 cups
Scallops, bay	1 pound	100 scallops; 2 cups
Scallops, sea	1 pound	30 scallops; 2 cups
Shrimp, canned	4½-ounce can	½ cup
Shrimp, frozen, large size	7 ounces	1 cup cooked
Shrimp, raw, in shell	1 pound	1 cup cleaned, shelled, cooked; 51 to 60 small; 43 to 50 medium; 31 to 35 large; 26 to 30 extra large; 21 to 24 jumbo
Tofu	1 pound	2 cups crumbled; 1¾ cups puréed
Tofu, firm	1 pound	2½ cups cubed

DRY GOODS AND SPICE EQUIVALENTS

Food	This Amount	Equals
Allspice, ground	1 ounce	¼ cup plus 1½ teaspoon
Baking mix (Bisquick®)	60-ounce box	14 cups
Basil, dried	1 ounce	¾ cup
Basil, fresh	½ ounce	1 cup chopped leaves
Bay leaf	1 whole	¼ to ½ teaspoon broken; ⅛ to ¼ teaspoon crushed
Bread crumbs	8-ounce package	2 cups
Bread, dried	1 slice	⅓ cup crumbs
Bread, fresh	1 slice	¾ cup soft cubes
Bread, loaf	1 pound	12 cups croutons; 16 to 18 regular slices
Bread, toasted	1 slice	¼ cup dry crumbs
Bulgur wheat	1 pound	8 cups cooked; 2¾ cups
Cardamom	1 pod	18 to 20 seeds; 1 teaspoon ground
Chocolate, baking	1 ounce	1 square
Chocolate chips	6 ounces	1 cup
Chocolate wafers	20 each	1 cup finely crushed
Cinnamon, ground	1 ounce	4 tablespoons
Cinnamon, stick	1 stick	1 teaspoon ground
Cloves, whole	1 teaspoon	¾ teaspoon ground
Cocoa powder	4 ounces	1 cup
Corn bread	8-inch square pan	4 cups crumbled for stuffing
Corn syrup	11½-ounce bottle	1 cup
Cornflakes	1 pound	16 cups
	3 cups	1 cup crushed
Cornmeal	1 pound	16 cups cooked; 3 cups
Cornstarch	4½ ounce box	1 cup
Couscous	7 ounces	2½ to 3 cups cooked; 1 cup raw
Cracker meal	14-ounce box	2¾ cup
Crackers, graham	14 to 15	1 cup finely crushed
Crackers (round, oval, or square, about the size of a saltine)	1 roll	35 whole crackers; 1½ cups finely crushed
	28 each	1 cup finely crushed
	1 pound	4½ cups finely crushed; 130 to 140 crackers
Dill plant, fresh or dried	3 heads	1 tablespoon dill seed
Flour, whole wheat	1 pound	3½ cups sifted
Flour, all-purpose, unsifted	1 pound	4 cups sifted; 3⅓ cups unsifted
	¼ ounce	1 tablespoon
	5 ounces	1 cup unsifted
	2 ounces	½ cup unsifted
Flour, cake	1 pound	4½ cups sifted
	3 ounces	1 cup
Flour, pastry, unsifted	1 pound	4 cups; 4½ cups sifted
Flour, rice, unsifted	1 pound	3 cups; 3½ cups sifted
Flour, rye	1 pound	4½ to 5 cups sifted
Garlic salt	1 teaspoon	⅛ teaspoon garlic powder plus ⅞ teaspoon salt
Garlic, fresh	1 head	8 to 15 cloves
	1 large clove	½ teaspoon garlic powder; 1½ teaspoon minced

Food	This Amount	Equals
Garlic, fresh *(continued)*	1 small clove	⅛ teaspoon garlic powder; ½ teaspoon minced
Gelatin	¼ ounce package	1 scant tablespoon
Gingersnaps	15 each	1 cup finely crushed
Ginger, crystallized	1 tablespoon	1 teaspoon ground
Ginger, fresh	1-inch piece	1 tablespoon grated or chopped
Ginger, fresh, chopped	1 tablespoon	1 teaspoon ground
Grits, quick cooking	1 pound	3 cups; 10 cups cooked
	1 cup raw	3⅓ cups cooked
Herbs, fresh, chopped	1 tablespoon	½ teaspoon crushed, dried
Honey	12 ounces	1 jar
Horseradish, fresh	1 tablespoon	2 tablespoons bottled
	1½ pounds	2¾ cups peeled, grated
Lemongrass	2 stalks	1 tablespoon finely chopped
Marshmallows, miniature	10 each	1 large
	1 cup	110 each
	10½-ounce package	5½ cups
Marshmallows, regular	1-pound package	65 regular
	10½-ounce package	45 regular
	1 cup	11 regular
Mayonnaise	32-ounce jar	4 cups
Mint, fresh leaves	1 cup	¼ cup dried leaves
Mustard, dry	1-ounce jar	5 tablespoons
	1 teaspoon	1 tablespoon prepared mustard
Mustard, prepared	8-ounce container	1 cup
	1 ounce	2 tablespoons
Nutmeats	4½ ounces nuts,	1 cup chopped
Nutmeg, whole	1 whole	2 teaspoons grated
Nuts		
Almonds, chopped	3 ounces	1 cup
Almonds, ground	3¾ ounces	1 cup
Almonds, in shell	1 pound	1 to 1¾ cups shelled
Almonds, paste	8 ounces	1¾ cups
Almonds, sliced or slivered	3 ounces	1 cup
Almonds, without shell	1 pound	3½ cups
Almonds, whole	5 ounces	1 cup
Filberts, in shell	1 pound	1½ cups shelled
Filberts, whole	5 ounces	1 cup
Macadamia	5-ounce container	1 cup
Peanuts in shell	5-ounce container	1 cup shelled
	1 pound	2¼ cups shelled
Peanuts, without shell	1 pound	3 cups
Pecans, halves	3¾ ounces	1 cup
Pecans, in shell	1 pound	2¼ cups shelled
Pecans, pieces	2 ounces	½ cup
Pecans, without shell	1 pound	4 cups
Pistachios, in shell	1 pound	3½ to 4 cups; 2 cups shelled
Pistachios, without shell	1 pound	3½ to 4 cups

(continued)

DRY GOODS AND SPICE EQUIVALENTS *(continued)*

Food	This Amount	Equals
Nuts *(continued)*		
Walnuts, chopped	1 pound	3½ cups
	4½ ounces	1 cup
Walnuts, halves	1 pound	4 cups
Walnuts, in shell	1 pound	1½ cups shelled
Oats, rolled	1 pound	5 cups uncooked
	1 cup	1¾ cups cooked
Parsley, dried	1 teaspoon	2 sprigs fresh; 1 tablespoon fresh, chopped
Parsley, fresh	1 bunch	1½ cups chopped; 2 ounces
Pasta		
Lasagna	1 pound	16 to 24 noodles
Macaroni, dry	1 cup	2½ cups cooked
	1 pound	4 cups; 8 cups cooked
Manicotti	1 pound	10 to 12 pieces
Noodles	1 cup	1¼ cups cooked
	1 pound	10 cups; 12 cups cooked
Spaghetti, dry	4 ounces	4 cups cooked
	1 pound	8 to 9 cups cooked
Peppermint, dried	1 tablespoon	¼ cup chopped fresh mint
Pine nuts (pignoli)	5 ounces	1 cup
Popcorn, unpopped	¼ cup kernels	8 cups popped
Poppy seeds	1 ounce	3 tablespoons
Rice, brown, uncooked	1 cup	4 cups cooked
Rice, instant	1 pound	4 cups; 8 cups cooked
Rice, long-grain, dry	2 pounds	14 cups cooked
	1 cup	3 cups cooked
	7 ounces	1 cup cooked
	2 pounds	4¾ cups
Rice, wild	1 pound	3 cups; 9 to 10 cups cooked
Rosemary, fresh	4-inch stem	¼ teaspoon dried leaves
Sage, fresh	12 leaves	1 teaspoon dried
Sage, fresh, chopped	1 tablespoon	1 teaspoon dried
Spearmint, dried	1 tablespoon	¼ cup chopped fresh mint
Stuffing mix	8 ounces	4 cups
Sugar, cube	1 cube	½ teaspoon
Sugar, brown	7 ounces	1 cup packed
	1 pound	2¼ cups packed
Sugar, confectioners', unsifted	4 ounces	1 cup
	1 pound	4 to 4½ cups sifted; 3 to 3¾ cups unsifted
Sugar, granulated	1 pound	2 cups
Sunflower seeds, in shell	7 ounces	¾ cup shelled nuts
Taco seasoning, dry	1¼-ounce package	4 tablespoons
Tapioca, quick	8 ounces	3¾ cups cooked; 1½ cups uncooked
Thyme, fresh	1 sprig	½ teaspoon dried
Vanilla bean, scraped	1-inch bean	1 teaspoon extract
Vanilla extract	1 ounce	2 tablespoons plus 1½ teaspoons

Food	This Amount	Equals
Vanilla wafers	22 each	1 cup finely crushed
	12-ounce box	88 wafers
Vegetable shortening	1 pound	2½ cups
	6¾ ounces	1 cup
Wheat berries, uncooked	1 cup	3 cups cooked
Wheat, cracked, uncooked	1 cup	3 to 3½ cups cooked
Wonton wrappers	1 pound	60 wrappers
Yeast, active dry	¼-ounce package	2¼ teaspoons
Yeast, compressed	2-ounce cake	3 ¼-ounce packages dry
Egg and Egg Product Equivalents		
Egg product	1 pound	8 eggs; 2 cups
	¼ cup	1 egg
Egg whites	1 large	2 tablespoons
Egg whites (large)	7 to 8 whites	1 cup
Egg whole (large)	1 each	3 tablespoons
	4 to 5 each	1 cup
Egg yolks	1 large	1 tablespoon plus 1½ teaspoons
Egg yolks (large)	12 yolks	1 cup
Eggs, cooked	1 large	6 hard-cooked slices
	4 large	1 cup hard-cooked, chopped

EQUIVALENT MEASURES

This Much	Is the Same As	This Much	Is the Same As
1 gallon	4 quarts	⅜ cup	6 tablespoons
1 quart	2 pints	⅓ cup	5⅓ tablespoons
1 pint	2 cups	¼ cup	4 tablespoons
1 bushel	4 pecks	⅛ cup	2 tablespoons
1 peck	8 quarts	1⁄16 cup	1 tablespoon
1 cup	16 tablespoons	1 tablespoon	3 teaspoons
⅞ cup	14 tablespoons or 1 cup minus 2 tablespoons	¾ tablespoon	2⅓ teaspoons
		⅔ tablespoon	2 teaspoons
¾ cup	12 tablespoons	½ tablespoon	1½ teaspoons
⅔ cup	10⅔ tablespoons	⅓ tablespoon	1 teaspoon
⅝ cup	10 tablespoons	¼ tablespoon	¾ teaspoon
½ cup	8 tablespoons	Pinch or dash	1⁄16 teaspoon

Sources: Utah State University Extension; Oleane Carden Zenoble, "Ingredient Substitution and Equivalent Chart," Circular HE-585, Alabama Cooperative Extension Service, Auburn University.

Recipe Index

Index